Spine Injuries in Athletes

Editor

Andrew C. Hecht, MD

Chief, Spine Surgery
Mount Sinai Hospital and Mount Sinai Health System
Director, Mount Sinai Spine Center
Associate Professor Orthopaedic and Neurosurgery
Mt. Sinai Medical Center and Icahn School of Medicine
New York, New York

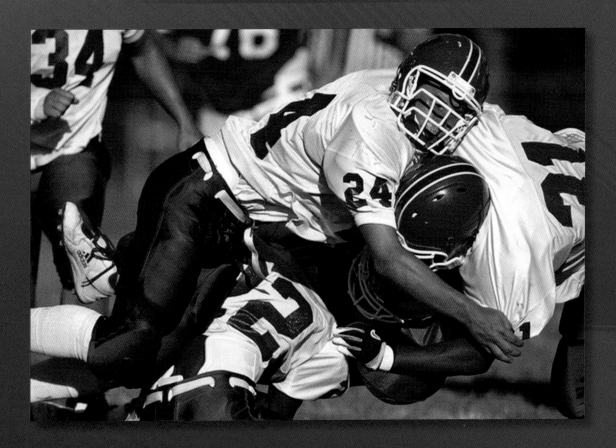

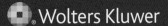 Wolters Kluwer

Philadelphia · Baltimore · New York · London
Buenos Aires · Hong Kong · Sydney · Tokyo

AAOS
AMERICAN ACADEMY OF
ORTHOPAEDIC SURGEONS

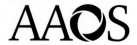

AMERICAN ACADEMY OF ORTHOPAEDIC SURGEONS

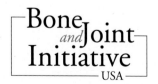

Acquisitions Editor: Brian Brown
Product Development Editor: Kate Heaney
Production Project Manager: David Orzechowski
Design Coordinator: Elaine Kasmer
Manufacturing Coordinator: Beth Welsh
Marketing Manager: Dan Dressler
Prepress Vendor: Aptara, Inc.

Library of Congress Cataloging-in-Publication Data

Names: Hecht, Andrew C., editor.
Title: Spine injuries in athletes / editor, Andrew C. Hecht.
Description: Philadelphia : Wolters Kluwer, [2017] | Includes
   bibliographical references.
Identifiers: LCCN 2016051267 | ISBN 9781496360267
Subjects: | MESH: Athletic Injuries | Spinal Injuries
Classification: LCC RA645.S66 | NLM WE 737 | DDC
   617.4/82044–dc23
LC record available at https://lccn.loc.gov/2016051267

I dedicate this book to my children Oliver and Layla, your growth and kindness is a constant source of joy and pride. Both of you will make our world a better place.

To my wife Elana, it is my greatest honor to share my life and love with you.

—Andrew C. Hecht

"I've missed more than 9000 shots in my career. I've lost almost 300 games. 26 times, I've been trusted to take the game winning shot and missed. I've failed over and over and over again in my life. And that is why I succeed."

—Michael Jordan

Contributors

Laith Al-Shihabi, MD
Fellow, Hand Surgery
Mary S. Stern Fellowship
Cincinnati, Ohio

Howard S. An, MD
Professor and Director of Spine Surgery
Orthopaedic Surgery
Rush University Medical Center
Chicago, Illinois

Lindsay M. Andras, MD
Assistant Professor
Children's Orthopaedic Center
Children's Hospital Los Angeles
Los Angeles, California

Nomaan Ashraf, MD, MBA
Assistant Clinical Professor
Orthopaedic Surgery
Mount Sinai Medical Center
New York, New York

Julian E. Bailes, Jr, MD
Chairman
Department of Neurosurgery
NorthShore University Health System
Evanston, Illinois

Evan Baird, MD
Assistant Professor
Orthopaedic Surgery
Icahn School of Medicine at Mount Sinai
New York, New York

Vin Shen Ban, MA, MB, BChir, MRCS, MSc, AFHEA
Research Fellow
Department of Neurological Surgery
University of Texas Southwestern Medical Center
Dallas, Texas

Kelley E. Banagan, MD
Associate Professor of Orthopaedics
Department of Orthopaedics
University of Maryland, Baltimore
Baltimore, Maryland

Ronnie Barnes, ATC
Senior Vice President of Medical Services
Head Athletic Trainer
New York Giants
New York, New York

Rahul Basho, MD
Director of Spine Surgery
Orthopaedic Surgery
Hannibal Regional Hospital
Hannibal, Maryland

H. Hunt Batjer, MD, FACS
Chair
Department of Neurological Surgery
University of Texas Southwestern Medical Center
Dallas, Texas

Gordon R. Bell, MD
Emeritus Staff
Cleveland Clinic
Former Director
Center for Spine Health
Cleveland, Ohio

Mitchel Berger, MD
Chairman
Department of Neurological Surgery
University of California, San Francisco
San Francisco, California

Micah Blais, MD
Resident
Orthopaedic Surgery
Massachusetts General Hospital
Boston, Massachusetts

Christopher M. Bono, MD
Chief, Orthopaedic Spine Service
Brigham and Women's Hospital
Associate Professor
Orthopaedic Surgery
Harvard Medical School
Boston, Massachusetts

Barrett Boody, MD
Resident Physician
Department of Orthopaedic Surgery
Northwestern Memorial Hospital
Chicago, Illinois

Javier Cárdenas, MD
Director
Barrow Concussion and Brain Injury Center
Department of Neurology
Barrow Neurological Institute
St. Joseph's Hospital and Medical Center
Phoenix, Arizona

Michael J. Cendoma, MS, ATC
Program Director
Sports Medicine Concepts, Inc.
Livonia, New York

Haroon Fiaz Choudhri, MD
Professor
Department of Neurosurgery
Augusta University
Augusta, Georgia

Tanvir Choudhri, MD
Co-Director
Neurosurgery Spine Program
Department of Neurosurgery
Icahn School of Medicine at Mount Sinai
New York, New York

Alexis Chiang Colvin, MD
Associate Professor
Department of Orthopaedic Surgery
Mount Sinai Hospital
New York, New York

Leah G. Concannon, MD
Clinical Assistant Professor
Department of Rehabilitation Medicine
Division of Sports and Spine
University of Washington
Seattle, Washington

Aristides I. Cruz, Jr., MD
Assistant Professor
Department of Orthopaedic Surgery
The Warren Alpert Medical School
Brown University
Providence, Rhode Island

Peter DeLuca, MD
Associate Professor
The Rothman Institute
Thomas Jefferson University
Philadelphia, Pennsylvania

Shah-Nawaz M. Dodwad, MD
Orthopaedic Surgery Spine Fellow
Department of Orthopaedic Spine Surgery
Northwestern University Memorial Hospital
Chicago, Illinois

Andrew B. Dossett, MD
Orthopaedic Spine Surgeon
Carrell Clinic
Dallas, Texas

Siatta B. Dunbar, DO, CAQSM
Sports Medicine Physician
Sports and Orthopedic Care
Fairview Health Services
Burnsville, Minnesota

Richard G. Ellenbogen, MD
Chairman
Neurological Surgery
University of Washington School of Medicine
Seattle, Washington

Michael G. Fehlings, MD, PhD
Professor of Neurosurgery
Department of Surgery
University of Toronto
Toronto, Ontario

John M. Flynn, MD
Richard M. Armstrong Jr Professor of Orthopedic Surgery
Department of Pediatric Orthopedic Surgery
The Children's Hospital of Philadelphia
Philadelphia, Pennsylvania

Tristan Fried, BS
Research Assistant
The Rothman Institute
Thomas Jefferson University
Philadelphia, Pennsylvania

Heath P. Gould, BS
Medical Student
Case Western Reserve University School of Medicine
Cleveland, Ohio

Colin M. Haines, MD
Physician
Department of Spine Surgery
Cleveland Clinic
Cleveland, Ohio

Mitchel B. Harris, MD, FACS
Chief, Orthopedic Trauma
Department of Orthopedic Surgery
Brigham and Women's Hospital
Boston, Massachusetts

Andrew C. Hecht, MD
Chief, Spine Surgery
Mount Sinai Hospital and Mount Sinai Health System
Director, Mount Sinai Spine Center
Associate Professor Orthopaedic and Neurosurgery
Mt. Sinai Medical Center and Icahn School of Medicine
New York, New York

John G. Heller, MD
Baur Professor of Orthopaedic Surgery
Department of Orthopaedic Surgery
Emory University School of Medicine
Atlanta, Georgia

Stanley A. Herring, MD
Clinical Professor
Departments of Rehabilitation, Orthopaedics and
*   Sports Medicine and Neurological Surgery*
University of Washington
Seattle, Washington

Wellington Hsu, MD
Clifford C. Raisbeck Distinguished
  Professor of Orthopaedic Surgery
Department of Orthopaedic Surgery
Northwestern University Feinberg School of Medicine
Chicago, Illinois

Andre M. Jakoi, MD
Fellow
Department of Orthopedic Surgery
University of Southern California
Los Angeles, California

Ehsan Jazini, MD
Chief Orthopaedic Resident
Department of Orthopaedics
University of Maryland, Baltimore
Baltimore, Maryland

Tyler J. Jenkins, MD
Physician
Department of Orthopaedic Surgery
Northwestern University Feinberg School of Medicine
Chicago, Illinois

Kevin L. Ju, MD
Spine Surgery Fellow
Department of Orthopaedic Surgery
Emory University
Atlanta, Georgia

William J. Kemp, MD
Resident—Neurosurgery PGY-2
Department of Neurosurgery
Cleveland Clinic
Cleveland, Ohio

Jun Sup Kim, MD
Orthopaedic Surgery Resident
Department of Orthopaedic Surgery
Mount Sinai
New York, New York

Michael Kordecki, DPT, SCS, ATC
Physical Therapist and Athletic Trainer
Praxis Physical Therapy
Vernon Hills, Illinois

Melissa A. Lancaster, PhD
Postdoctoral Fellow
Department of Neurosurgery
Medical College of Wisconsin
Milwaukee, Wisconsin

Brian C. Liem, MD
Clinical Assistant Professor
Department of Rehabilitation Medicine,
  Division of Sports and Spine
University of Washington
Seattle, Washington

Steven C. Ludwig, MD
Chief of Spine Surgery
Department of Orthopaedics, Spine Division
University of Maryland, Baltimore
Baltimore, Maryland

Allan R. Martin, MD
Neurosurgery Resident, PGY-5
Division of Neurosurgery
Department of Surgery
University of Toronto
Toronto, Ontario
Canada

Steven McAnany, MD
Spine Surgery Fellow
Department of Orthopaedics
Emory University Hospital
Atlanta, Georgia

Michael A. McCrea, PhD
Professor
Department of Neurosurgery
Medical College of Wisconsin
Milwaukee, Wisconsin

Thomas Mroz, MD
Director
Center for Spine Health
Cleveland Clinic
Cleveland, Ohio

Lindsay D. Nelson, PhD
Assistant Professor
Department of Neurosurgery
Medical College of Wisconsin
Milwaukee, Wisconsin

Brian Neri, MD
Chief
Division of Orthopaedic Sports
ProHealthcare Associates, LLP
Lake Success, New York

Kenneth Nwosu, MD
Orthopaedic Surgery Resident
Department of Orthopaedic Surgery
Harbor—UCLA Medical Center
Torrance, California

Alpesh A. Patel, MD
Associate Professor
Department of Orthopaedic Surgery
Northwestern University
Chicago, Illinois

Diana Patterson, MD
Physician
Department of Orthopaedic Surgery
Mount Sinai Hospital
New York, New York

Margot Putukian, MD, MSPH
Director of Athletic Medicine
Head Team Physician
Assistant Medical Director
Princeton University Health Services
Princeton University
Princeton, New Jersey

Sheeraz Qureshi, MD, MBA
Associate Professor
Orthopaedic Surgery
Icahn School of Medicine at Mount Sinai
New York, New York

K. Daniel Riew, MD
Professor
Department of Orthopedic Surgery
Columbia University Medical Center
New York, New York

Timothy T. Roberts, MD
Surgical Spine Fellow
Center for Spine Health
Cleveland Clinic
Cleveland, Ohio

Brett D. Rosenthal, MD
Resident Physician
Department of Orthopaedic Surgery
Northwestern University
Chicago, Illinois

Rajiv Saigal, MD, PhD
Affiliate
Department of Neurological Surgery
University of California, San Francisco
San Francisco, California

Gregory D. Schroeder, MD
Spine Research and Clinical Fellow
The Rothman Institute
Thomas Jefferson University
Philadelphia, Pennsylvania

Mark Seeley, MD
Clinical Instructor
Department of Orthopaedic Surgery
Geisinger Medical Center
Danville, Pennsylvania

Christie Stawicki, BA
Research Fellow—Spine Division
The Rothman Institute
Thomas Jefferson University
Philadelphia, Pennsylvania

Erik E. Swartz, PhD, ATC, FNATA
Professor and Chair
Department of Kinesiology
University of New Hampshire
Durham, New Hampshire

Eeric Truumees, MD
Director of Spine Trauma
Seton Brain and Spine Institute
Brackenridge University Hospital
Austin, Texas

Alexander R. Vaccaro, MD, PhD, MBA
President, Spine
The Rothman Institute
Philadelphia, Pennsylvania

Frank H. Valone III, MD
Postdoctoral Fellow
Department of Orthopaedic Spine Surgery
Washington University
St. Louis, Missouri

Jeffrey C. Wang, MD
Professor
Department of Orthopaedic Surgery
University of Southern California
Keck School of Medicine of the
*   University of Southern California*
Los Angeles, California

Robert G. Watkins, MD
Co-Medical Director
Marina Spine Center
Marina Del Rey Hospital
Marina Del Rey, California

Robert G. Watkins IV, MD
Co-Medical Director
Marina Spine Center
Marina Del Rey Hospital
Marina Del Rey, California

Tristan B. Weir, BS
Spine Research Fellow
Department of Orthopaedics
University of Maryland, Baltimore
Baltimore, Maryland

Leigh J. Weiss, ATC, PT/DPT, SCS
Assistant Athletic Trainer
Physical Therapist
New York Giants
New York, New York

Foreword

Robert G. Watkins, Sr., MD

What is a spine-in-sports surgeon or spine-in-sports specialist? The spine surgery community was initially skeptical. Demand for subspecialization in this area came from orthopaedic surgeons, team doctors, trainers, agents, and most of all, from the players.

Orthopaedic surgeons who specialize in sports medicine have a unique understanding of the complexities of specialized injuries and surgeries. Trainers and physical therapists who are often the primary health care providers understand the value of a spinal surgeon concentrating on sports injuries of the spine. Agents want the best team of subspecialists for their clients. Players who have a spinal injury want an expert in this critical area. Players who can play with broken bones and injured joints may find that being temporarily paralyzed or having a weakness and sciatica is a whole different ball game.

The spine-in-sports specialist must enjoy and understand his patient's sport and the demands of his patient's job. The spine-in-sports surgeon must have a complete understanding of comprehensive non-operative and postoperative spine rehabilitation programs. If your patient desires to return to a high-performance level, the surgeon must have a complete sports-specific rehabilitation program for him. You have to enjoy and appreciate talking to athletes, trainers, and everyone involved with the care of the athlete. You must assume responsibility of the best care and advice to your patient. The basic premise is to put the athlete first and foremost as your patient; give him the best advice and always obtain his opinion concerning his injury and his return to his sport; come up with a clearly executable plan; and then establish a line of communication to transmit the exact plan to everyone concerned with your patient.

This monograph is the experience of some of the best specialists in this important subspecialty area, the spine in sports, and the care of the athlete with spinal problems and injuries.

Robert G. Watkins, Sr., MD
Co-Medical Director
Marina Spine Center
Marina Del Rey Hospital
Marina Del Rey, California

Introduction and Overview of Cases

Andrew C. Hecht, MD

The athlete with a spine injury represents one of the most challenging clinical problems for sports medicine physicians, physical therapists, athletic trainers, orthopaedic surgeons, and spine surgeons. These injuries affect athletes of all ages and ability levels. The evaluation of the injured athlete starts even before kickoff. Understanding the epidemiology of the most devastating injuries and high-risk behaviors that affect athletes is critical because it reinforces the need to prevent these injuries through proper technique and strict avoidance of high-risk behaviors such as spear tackling or cross-checking from behind. The understanding of the unique high-risk behaviors in certain sports can often prevent the most devastating outcomes. Proper on-field management and evaluation will be discussed extensively, as this is a source of great consternation for team physicians and athletic trainers. The text will emphasize a "how to" and practical approach to the management of these injuries. The best evidence and suggestions will be made for not only the on-field management but for transport and pharmacologic management. All teams in the National Football League (NFL) and National Hockey League (NHL) have defined protocols for the acute management of the injured player (on field and in transport). The National Collegiate Athletic Association has also implemented many important on-field protocols.

The text will also discuss the most common clinical problems that confront all practitioners taking care of athletes. Many chapters will emphasize differential diagnosis and others how to treat specific clinical entities. This book will provide not only didactic content and outline of controversy but will also emphasize the practical reality of taking care of elite athletes and weekend warriors. Each chapter, when applicable, will emphasize return to play criteria and decision making. The most common injury patterns affecting the cervical and lumbar spine will be discussed. The most common injury patterns will be discussed such as stingers/burners, cervical cord neurapraxias, cervical disk herniation, cervical stenosis, congenital cervical anomalies, cervical trauma, lumbar disk herniation, spondylolysis/spondylolisthesis, lumbar degenerative disk disease, pelvic and hip disorders that mimic spine problems, thoracic disk herniation, as well as issues that confront the aging athlete. Lastly, the final section will discuss the important topics of concussion. The key leaders from the NFL Brain and Spine committee have organized a cohesive practical approach to outlining the condition, giving practical on-field management strategies and how to determine return to play even in the days and weeks that follow.

The final chapter of this text is a round table discussion of experts in the field of spine injuries in athletes discussing several clinical scenarios affecting the cervical and lumbar spine. Each case involves a clinical scenario that will discuss in detail down its winding path to emphasize decision making and return to play. The answers to these clinical scenarios can also be found in the ensuing chapters.

1. A professional football player with a C4-5 disk herniation with arm weakness that has failed conservative care. What are the surgical options? When can the player return to play? Do you need to establish definitive evidence of fusion before returning to

play? Is there a role for disc replacement? What if he gets a nonunion? What if the original clinical problem affected two disks rather than one?

2. A collegiate football player with multiple stingers who has congenital cervical stenosis. Can he return to play? How soon?

3. A football player with a cervical cord neurapraxia. What if he has a cervical disk herniation or congenital cervical stenosis in that setting? When can he return to play? If he has congenital cervical stenosis can he return after a laminoplasty? What if the CCN is in the absence of any cervical stenosis or lesion of any kind?

4. An elite 17-year-old tennis player with acute fracture of the pars interarticularis (spondylolysis) that has edema on magnetic resonance imaging consistent with acute injury. How should this be further worked up? What is the role of bracing? How long? Should these ever be repaired?

5. College hockey player with NHL prospects with a grade 1-2/4 lytic L5-S1 spondylolisthesis with back pain and leg pain secondary to foraminal stenosis at L5-S1. What is the role of conservative care? If he has a fusion, when can he return to play? Will there be a performance issue secondary to the fusion?

6. A football player with a healed cervical facet fracture with incongruity and mild neck pain? What about contiguous cervical spinous fracture non-unions where there is wide splaying of the spinous processes on flexion and extension but no pain?

7. What is the role of steroids or thermal cooling with an incomplete spinal cord injury in an elite athlete?

I am extremely fortunate to have had the chance work with exceptional contributors who have vast experience in taking care of spine problems in elite athletes. This text is not only based on published clinical evidence but also on the practical hands on experience of the various contributors from their respective fields. I also want to thank Drs. Watkins, Vaccarro, Hsu, Ludwig, and Dossett as well as Erik Schwartz for their collective wisdom and contributions. I want to thank both Drs. Bajer and Ellenbogen for organizing this important concussion section of this text as well as the various experts. This text is unique in that it reflects the true interdisciplinary collaboration between orthopaedic spine surgeons, neurosurgeons, sports medicine physicians, athletic trainers, physiatry, and neuropsychology. I wanted to thank the American Academy of Orthopaedic Surgeons, the National Athletic Trainers' Association, and the NFL Brain and Spine Committee for supporting this endeavor.

Finally, I want to thank those individuals who have shared the journey with me thus far including mentors at Emory Spine Center, Harvard, and Mount Sinai; my residents and fellows; and most importantly my children, Oliver and Layla, and my wife, Elana.

Contents

Contributors   iv

Foreword   viii

Introduction and Overview of Cases   ix

SECTION 1 General   1
Section Editor: Steven C. Ludwig, MD

1 **The Epidemiology of Spine Injuries in Athletes**   2
Barrett Boody, MD
Brett D. Rosenthal, MD
Shah-Nawaz M. Dodwad, MD
Alpesh A. Patel, MD

2 **Biomechanics of the Spine in Sports and Prevention Considerations**   11
Eeric Truumees, MD
Erik E. Swartz, PhD, ATC, FNATA

3 **Rehabilitation of Athletes After Spine Injury and Spine Surgery**   22
Robert G. Watkins IV, MD
Michael Kordecki, DPT, SCS, ATC

4 **On-Field Evaluation and Transport of the Injured Athlete**   32
Tristan B. Weir, BS
Michael J. Cendoma, MS, ATC
Ehsan Jazini, MD
Kelley E. Banagan, MD
Steven C. Ludwig, MD

5 **Spinal Cord Injury: Pharmacologic Agents, Thermal Cooling, and Timing of Interventions**   40
Allan R. Martin, MD
Michael G. Fehlings, MD, PhD

6 **Diagnostic Imaging of Sports-Related Spinal Disorders**   51
Mitchel B. Harris, MD, FACS
Micah Blais, MD

7 **Spine Injuries in Pediatric Athletes**   59
John M. Flynn, MD
Mark A. Seeley, MD
Aristides I. Cruz, Jr., MD

8 **Role of the Spine Surgeon with Professional Sports Teams, Agents, and Coaches**   69
Robert G. Watkins, MD

SECTION 2 Cervical Spine Injuries in Athletes   **73**
Section Editors: Andrew C. Hecht, MD
Alexander R. Vaccaro, MD, PhD, MBA

9   **Differential Diagnosis of Upper Extremity Disorders (Neck and Arm Pain)**   **74**
Laith Al-Shihabi, MD
Howard S. An, MD

10 **Stingers and Burners**   **86**
Andrew B. Dossett, MD

11 **Cervical Cord Neurapraxia**   **92**
Frank H. Valone III, MD
K. Daniel Riew, MD

12 **Cervical Disk Herniation in Athletes**   **100**
Andrew C. Hecht, MD
Steven McAnany, MD
Sheeraz Qureshi, MD, MBA

13 **Congenital Cervical Anomalies and Special Needs Athletes**   **112**
Jun Sup Kim, MD
Evan Baird, MD
Lindsay Andras, MD
Nomaan Ashraf, MD, MBA

14 **Degenerative Disorders of the Cervical Spine and Cervical Stenosis**   **123**
Kevin L. Ju, MD
John G. Heller, MD

15 **Fractures of the Cervical Spine and Spinal Cord Injuries**   **134**
Gregory D. Schroeder, MD
Tristan Fried, BS
Christie Stawicki, BA
Peter Deluca, MD
Alexander R. Vaccaro, MD, PhD, MBA

SECTION 3 Lumbar Spine   **145**
Section Editor: Wellington Hsu, MD

16 **Incidence of Low Back Pain in Athletes and Differential Diagnosis
and Evaluation of Athletes with Back or Leg Pain**   **146**
Kenneth Nwosu, MD
Christopher M. Bono, MD

17 **Spondylolysis and Spondylolisthesis in Immature and Adult Athletes**   **154**
Rahul Basho, MD
Andre M. Jakoi, MD
Jeffrey C. Wang, MD

18 **Lumbar Disk Herniation in Immature and Adult Athletes**   **163**
Tyler J. Jenkins, MD
Wellington Hsu, MD

19 **Lumbar Degenerative Disk Disease and Spinal Stenosis in Athletes**   **172**
Heath P. Gould, BS
Colin M. Haines, MD
William J. Kemp, MD
Timothy T. Roberts, MD
Thomas Mroz, MD

20 Piriformis Syndrome, Sacral Stress Fractures, and
Hip Labral Disorders   **181**
Diana Patterson, MD
Brian Neri, MD
Alexis Chiang Colvin, MD

21 Lumbar Spine Disorders in Aging Athletes   **194**
Gordon R. Bell, MD

22 Thoracic Injuries and Pain Syndromes in Athletes   **203**
Tanvir Choudhri, MD
Haroon Fiaz Choudhri, MD
Julian E. Bailes, Jr., MD

SECTION 4 Concussion   **217**
Section Editors: Richard G. Ellenbogen, MD
H. Hunt Batjer, MD, FACS

23 Concussion: Introduction—The Controversy   **218**
Vin Shen Ban, MA, MB, BChir, MRCS, MSc AFHEA
Richard G. Ellenbogen, MD
H. Hunt Batjer, MD, FACS

24 Definitions of Sports Concussion, Initial Diagnosis, and On-Field Evaluation   **227**
Leah G. Concannon, MD
Brian C. Liem, MD
Stanley A. Herring, MD

25 Determining Short-Term Prognosis and Return to Play   **244**
Margot Putukian, MD, MSPH
Siatta B. Dunbar, DO, CAQSM

26 Neuropsychological Testing in the Treatment and Management of
Sport-Related Concussion   **254**
Melissa A. Lancaster, PhD
Lindsay D. Nelson, PhD
Michael A. McCrea, PhD

27 Postconcussion Syndrome   **262**
Javier Cárdenas, MD

28 Concussion: Long Term Sequelae—The Controversy   **270**
Rajiv Saigal, MD, PhD
Mitchel Berger, MD

SECTION 5 Roundtable Discussion of the Experts   **277**

29 Spine and Sports: A Roundtable Discussion   **278**
Andrew C. Hecht, MD
Alexander R. Vaccaro, MD, PhD, MBA
Wellington Hsu, MD
Robert G. Watkins, MD
Andrew Dossett, MD

Index   **285**

SECTION 1

General

1 The Epidemiology of Spine Injuries in Athletes

Barrett Boody, MD • Brett D. Rosenthal, MD • Shah-Nawaz M. Dodwad, MD • Alpesh A. Patel, MD

INTRODUCTION

As the number of competitive athletes continues to rise, training in the diagnosis and management of sport specific spine injuries is essential. During 2013 and 2014, more than 7.7 million high school and 460,000 college students participated in athletics, of whom 1.1 million high school and 70,000 college students participated in football.[1,2] Athletes have a significant number of potential injury exposures during practice and games. For example, in the National Football League (NFL), the estimated yearly average for potential injury exposure events to occur is 177,000 during practice and 35,000 during actual games.[3] Previously, the lack of centralized systems to report and track spine injuries in athletes hindered our ability to document the frequency and circumstances surrounding these events. Over the past 40 years, widespread reporting of spine injuries in athletes has enabled sport organizations to protect athletes by penalizing high-risk player contact, such as spear tackling in football and checking from behind in hockey. As a result, we have seen a decrease in the rate of catastrophic spine injuries.[4–6] Despite improvement in sport regulation and protective equipment, physicians continue to encounter a wide variety of spine pathologies, ranging from back pain to catastrophic neurologic injury.

SPINAL CORD INJURY

The National Spinal Cord Injury Statistics Center (NSCISC) compiles the largest spinal cord injury (SCI) database in the United States, producing yearly reports that review the epidemiology of new cases, as well as trends extending over several decades. In the 2013 report, sporting injuries are listed as the fourth most common etiology of SCI, responsible for 3054 or 9.2% of all reported cases of SCI with only motor vehicle collision (36.5%), falls (28.5%), and violence (14.3%) occurring more frequently. Within the sports-related SCI subgroup, participants between the ages of 16 and 30 years account for the majority of cases (68.5%), with boys and men involved in 89% of SCIs. The sporting activity identified with the highest SCI incidence was snow skiing, ranking 11th in overall etiology and 1st within the sports subgroup with a total of 154 cases. Football ranked 12th overall and 2nd within the sports-related SCI subgroup with a total 145 cases.[7] Schmitt et al investigated causes of SCI in Germany from 1985 to 1997, identifying 1016 cases. They attribute 6.8% of SCIs to being sports related, with the majority of sporting accidents involving downhill skiing ($n = 16$) and horseback riding ($n = 9$). They reported an incidence of serious spine injuries among skiers as 0.01 injuries per 1000 skier-days.

Dr. Patel or an immediate family member has received royalties from Amedica, Biomet, and Ulrich Medical USA; serves as a paid consultant to Amedica, DePuy, a Johnson & Johnson Company, Pacira, Relievant, and Zimmer; has stock or stock options held in Amedica, Cytonics, Nocimed, and Vital5; has received nonincome support (such as equipment or services), commercially derived honoraria, or other non-research–related funding (such as paid travel) from Springer; and serves as a board member, owner, officer, or committee member of AAOS, the American Orthopaedic Association, the AO Spine North America, Cervical Spine Research Society, Journal of the American Academy of Orthopaedic Surgeons, North American Spine Society, Surgical Neurology International, and Wolters Kluwer Health. None of the following authors or any immediate family member has received anything of value from or has stock or stock options held in a commercial company or institution related directly or indirectly to the subject of this article: Dr. Boody, Dr. Dodwad, and Dr. Rosenthal.

Tator et al reviewed hockey injuries in Canada between 1966 and 1996, identifying 243 spine injuries with 90% occurring from C1 to T1. The most common reported injury morphologies were burst fractures and fracture-dislocations. Approximately 40% of injuries involved checking from behind, and 77% involved checking into the boards.[8] Although football is associated with a higher occurrence of SCI, the rate of SCI in ice hockey is nearly three times higher. Of the 207 players with neurologic injuries, 108 (52%) were permanent injuries, and 52 (25%) were complete injuries, with 8 deaths related to SCI. Only 31 of the 243 SCIs were reported before 1982; however, this is likely attributable to the lack of a centralized reporting system. The Canadian Ice Hockey Spinal Injuries Registry was established in 1981 and shortly thereafter in 1984 began reporting the significant hazard of checking from behind into the boards that prompted the subsequent rule changes in 1985 banning this action.[6] Tator et al demonstrated a continued decline in the annual incidence of spine injuries in his Think First Canadian Ice Hockey Spinal Injuries registry with 40 spine injuries and 5 severe SCIs with permanent neurologic deficits occurring between 2000 and 2005. In 2005, Tator et al reported a 69% decrease in the incidence of SCIs in participants ages 18 years and older compared with before 2001.[6]

● FOOTBALL-SPECIFIC CERVICAL SPINE INJURIES

Spine-related complaints are common among football players, with nearly 11,500 football related neck injuries presenting yearly to emergency departments in the United States.[9] Mall et al reviewed 2208 NFL spine and axial skeleton injuries over 11 seasons, 44.7% of which involved the cervical spine (**Table 1-1**).[3] They found the injury with the greatest average time missed from play was thoracic disk herniation (189 days) followed by cervical fracture (120 days) and cervical disk herniation (85 days). They estimated NFL players totaled 386,688 potential game injury exposures and 1,947,750 potential practice injury exposures over the 11-season time period. Muscular injuries were the most common reported injury (41.2%) followed by nerve injury (21.4%), disk injury (11.4%), and fractures (3.7%).[3]

Cervical spine pathology has been shown to have a significant negative impact on NFL players' careers. Schroeder and colleagues reported on 143 NFL athletes from 2003 to 2011 with prior cervical spine pathology, the most common diagnoses being spondylosis (87 players), stenosis (30 players), and cervical sprain or strain

(24 players). They noted that these athletes were less likely to be drafted and had less total games played, with no difference in total games started or performance scores compared with other football players without prior cervical spine diagnoses.[10] Of athletes who had sagittal cervical spine canals smaller than 10 mm, no differences were shown in the number of games or years played or in performance scores. Also, these players with cervical stenosis had no reported neurologic injuries. Furthermore, 7 athletes with prior cervical spine surgery displayed no difference in career longevity compared with the average NFL player.[10] Meredith and colleagues reviewed outcomes in 16 NFL players with cervical disk herniations undergoing operative versus nonoperative treatment. They noted that 1 of 3 (33%) surgically managed and 8 of 13 (61%) conservatively treated players eventually returned to play.[11] They concluded that nonoperative management of NFL players can be successful in the management of cervical disk herniations, with return to play (RTP) predicated on complete relief of symptoms and no cord compression on follow up MRI.[11]

Catastrophic Cervical Spine Injuries

The safety of American football has been substantially improved by efforts to identify and report player injuries. From 1971 to 1975, Torg and colleagues reported on 259 cervical fracture-dislocations with an incidence of 4.14 per 100,000 exposures, 99 cases of quadriplegia with an incidence of 1.58 per 100,000 exposures, and 77 deaths related to severe neck injuries.[12] As a result of the reported significant morbidity and mortality of cervical spine injuries, headfirst contact or spear tackling was banned by the National Collegiate Athletic Association's football rules committee and high school football governing bodies. After these rule changes, reported cervical spine fractures decreased 70%, and traumatic quadriplegia decreased 82% from 1976 to 1987.[4,13]

Boden et al reviewed 196 catastrophic cervical spine injuries occurring in high school and college football players between 1989 and 2002 and found that 76 athletes during their study had an injury that resulted in quadriplegia. Quadriplegic injuries had an incidence of 0.50 per 100,000 high school and 0.82 per 100,000 college participants with a 1.65 times higher risk in the collegiate football players. The position played at the time of injury was identified in 70 players with the defensive back position having the highest quadriplegic injury occurrence of 44.3% followed by special teams players at 18.3% and then linebackers with 17.1%. They identified spear tackling as the cause in 88% of

● TABLE 1-1 Cervical spine injuries in athletes

Author	Sport	Type of Study	Demographics	Pathology	Outcomes of Interest
Tator[7]	Hockey	Retrospective	Amateur and professional, 1966–1996	243 spine injuries (fracture and/or dislocation and neurologic deficits) identified in Canadian Ice Hockey Spinal Injuries Registry	Push or check from behind in 40%, impact with boards in 77%; ~50% of injuries occurred in 16- to 20-year old athletes
Tator et al[6]	Hockey	Retrospective	Amateur and professional, 2000–2005	40 spine injuries (fracture and/or dislocation and neurologic deficits) identified in Canadian Ice Hockey Spinal Injuries Registry	82.8% spine injuries within cervical spine; push or check from behind in 35%, impact with boards in 64.8%; five (12.5%) severe injuries identified (complete and incomplete SCIs)
Mall et al[3]	Football	Retrospective	NFL players (professional), 2000–2010	2208 spine or axial skeleton injuries identified (7% of overall injuries) from NFL registry	Most common spine injury was muscular (41.2%); nerve injury and fractures accounted for 21.4% and 3.7%, respectively; on average, 25.7 days missed because of spine injuries; 987 (44.7%) of injuries occurred in cervical spine with 14 SCIs reported
Schroeder et al[9]	Football	Retrospective cohort	American football athletes attending NFL combine, 2003–2011	143 players with cervical spine diagnoses (2965 evaluated athletes)	Athletes with cervical spine diagnoses less likely to be drafted and lower total NFL games played than athletes without cervical spine diagnoses; players with history of cervical spine surgery or congenital stenosis with no difference in career longevity or performance
Torg et al[11]	Football	Retrospective	Amateur and professional, 1971–1975	1,275,000 estimated player exposures; retrospective data collection	259 cervical fracture-dislocations, 99 cervical fracture-dislocations resulting in permanent quadriplegia; 77 deaths from severe neck injuries
Boden et al[5]	Football	Retrospective	High school and collegiate (amateur), 1989–2002	196 catastrophic cervical spine injuries; incidences, 1.10 and 4.72 per 100,000 high school and collegiate players, respectively, using National Center for Catastrophic Sports Injury Research registry	76 cases of quadriplegia; 43 cases of cervical CN, with 16 players returning to sport (no additional CCN reported)
Torg et al[15]	Football	Retrospective cohort	Amateur and professional	45 athletes with CCN	Ratio of spinal canal to vertebral body diameter on lateral radiographs <0.8 with 93% sensitivity, 59% specificity for CCN; because of the low incidence of CCN (7.3 per 10,000), PPV reported as 0.2%
Charbonneau et al[17]	Football	Retrospective	Collegiate athletes (amateur), 2010 season	244 players; 64 (26%) episodes of brachial neurapraxia (stingers)	59% of stingers reported to medical staff; 14% of players reported >1 stinger during 2010 season; 62% lifetime prevalence of stingers; no statistically significant effect of protective equipment

CCN = cord neurapraxia, NFL = National Football League, PPV = positive predictive value, SCI = spinal cord injury.

these catastrophic events.[5] Boden et al further reviewed fatalities related to high school and college football between 1990 and 2010, noting 164 noncontact and 79 traumatic causes of fatalities, estimating approximately 4 deaths annually. Cervical fractures were the cause in 4 mortality cases, and the most common causes of death were related to cardiac (100 players), brain injury (62 players), and heat illness (38 players).[14] They found that the fatality rates related to cervical spine fracture were greatly reduced from previously reported rates, an improvement they believed reflected the rule changes regarding spear tackling.[14]

Cervical Cord Neurapraxia

Cervical cord neurapraxia (CCN), also referred to as transient quadriplegia, is commonly caused by a hyperextension and/or axial compression mechanism with transient bilateral upper and/or lower symptoms of pain, weakness, and/or paresthesias and occur in approximately 0.2 per 100,000 high school and 2 per 100,000 college football players.[15] Boden et al retrospectively identified 196 significant cervical injuries between 1989 and 2002 in high school and college football players as reported to the National Center for Catastrophic Sports Injury Research. They identified 42 athletes with CCN (23 high school and 20 college players). The concluded that the mean incidences were 0.17 per 100,000 high school players and 2.05 per 100,000 college players, concluding a risk ratio of 12.2 for college compared with high school football players. Of the 43 patients identified with CCN, only 12 patients had duration of symptoms recorded. Neurologic symptoms of less than 15 minutes were present in 5 patients, between 15 minutes and 24 hours in 5, and longer than 24 hours in 2 patients with eventual full recovery in all 12 patients.[5]

Torg et al evaluated the relationship of congenital cervical stenosis to CCN in football players, noting a relationship in the subaxial spine lateral radiograph that a canal-to-vertebral body diameter ratio of less than 0.8 correlated with CCN.[16] Ninety-three percent of players reporting CCN had a Torg ratio of less than 0.8. The authors concluded that the Torg ratio had a high sensitivity of 93% but a low specificity of 59%. The overall low incidence of CCN (~7.3 per 10,000 college football athletes) gives the Torg ratio a low positive predictive value (PPV) of 0.2%, limits the utility of the measure in identifying at-risk athletes in contact sports, and should not be used as a screening tool to deem a player ineligible to participate in contact sports.[16]

Cervical Nerve Root or Brachial Plexus Neurapraxia

Neurapraxia of the cervical nerve roots or brachial plexus are also known as "stingers" and can clinically manifest as transient unilateral upper extremity pain, weakness, or paresthesias. Three mechanisms for stingers are commonly described as potential causes: (1) compression of cervical nerve roots with hyperextension and lateral flexion, (2) a "pincer"-type mechanism from hyperextension with infolding of the ligamentum flavum, and (3) traction and stretching of the brachial plexus with direct contact to the supraclavicular region.[15] Between 26% and 65% of college football players report stingers over the course of their college careers, most often in lineman, defensive ends, and linebackers.[17,18] Significant associations for stingers were a personal history of prior stingers and total years played, yet there was no identifiable association with type of equipment used, age, body mass index, or strength training regimen. Charbonneau and colleagues reviewed the occurrence of stingers in 244 football players over the course of the 2010 season at four Canadian universities, noting that only 38 of 64 (59%) of stingers were reported to medical staff, with only 2 injuries evaluated by physicians.[18]

Forty-seven percent of college football players with stinger injuries display cervical stenosis less than 13 mm.[19] The duration of stingers is commonly reported as brief, with fewer than 10% describing symptoms lasting more than 24 hours.[18] Page and Guy examined the utility of screening contact athletes with the Torg ratio, evaluating 125 football players at the University of South Carolina, ultimately identifying 14 players reporting stingers. They found that those with Torg ratios less than 0.8 was four times more likely to experience stingers, with a sensitivity and specificity of 71% and 68%, respectively. However, the low occurrence of stingers lead to a 22% PPV for the screening tool, which is significantly low and not clinically meaningful as a screening tool for asymptomatic players.[20]

Recurrence of stingers is reported as high as 87%, with 14% of football players reporting more than one stinger within a single season.[18,21] Reviewing recurrent stingers in 55 contact athletes, Levitz et al describe the most common mechanism as cervical extension with ipsilateral lateral deviation in 83% of recurrent injuries. Radiographic evaluation of those with recurrent stingers showed 53% with congenital stenosis (**Figure 1-1**) and 93% with disk disease or foraminal narrowing.[19,21]

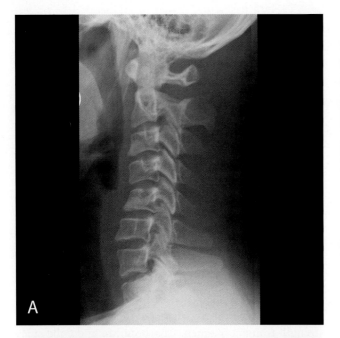

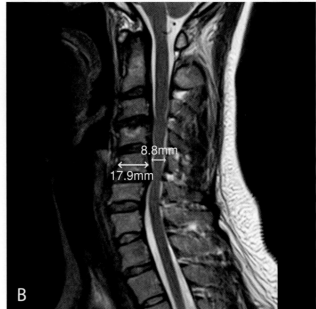

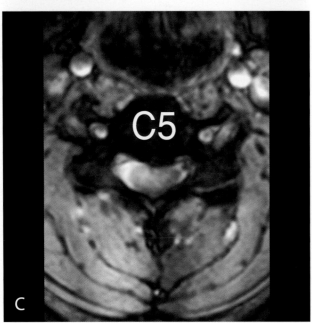

FIGURE 1-1 A 26-year-old noncontact female athlete presents with complaints of neck pain. (**A**) A lateral cervical radiograph with congenital stenosis, C5 to C6 DDD, and focal kyphosis. Sagittal (**B**) and axial T2 MRI images (**C**) of the same patient's cervical spine. Congenital stenosis is measured at C5 (8.8 mm) with cord compression. The patient's neck pain was managed conservatively, and she was allowed to return to play.

● THORACOLUMBAR SPINE INJURIES

Athletes can experience significant morbidity associated with thoracolumbar spine injuries. In the general population, 65% of adults report having experienced low back pain compared with the athletic population, in which the incidence of low back pain is much lower at 30%.[22,23] Kolt and Kirkby reviewed injuries in elite and sub-elite gymnasts, identifying a total of 349 injuries in 64 gymnasts over an 18-month period (**Table 1-2**). Spine and trunk injuries accounted for 17.2% of total injuries, with the low back injury subgroup accounting for 86.6% of spine and trunk injuries.[24] Sward and coworkers reported an incidence of low back pain in 65.4% and 84.6% of elite female and male gymnasts, respectively, over a 2-year period.[25] Hutchinson similarly reported an incidence of low back pain in 86% of elite rhythmic gymnasts over a 7-week period.[26] Goldstein et al reviewed screening MRI findings in female gymnasts, finding a substantial increase in disk and bony pathology for pre-elite (1 of 11 or 9%) compared with

TABLE 1-2	Thoracolumbar spine injuries in athletes				
Author	**Sport**	**Type of Study**	**Demographics**	**Pathology**	**Outcomes of Interest**
Kolt and Kirkby[23]	Gymnastics	Prospective	64 Australian elite and sub-elite gymnasts over 18 months	Of 349 reported injuries, 14.9% occurred in the lumbar spine	Sub-elite gymnasts more commonly reported injuries to the lower back (19.4% vs. 9.2%); elite gymnasts spent 21% of the year training at less than full capacity because of injury
Stracciolini et al[27]	Any	Retrospective	2133 children (5–17 years old) seen at a sports medicine clinic	210 spine injuries, $n = 80$ and $n = 130$ for male and female athletes, respectively	Majority of injuries classified as overuse in nature (female athletes, 93.9%; male athletes, 81.3%); traumatic etiology noted in 18.8% of male athletes and 6.2% of female athletes
Soler and Calderon[28]	Any	Retrospective	3152 elite Spanish athletes	253 athletes found to have spondylolysis (8.02% prevalence)	Athletes with spondylolysis reported higher incidence of low back pain (46.2% vs. 23.5%; $P < 0.01$); 84.3% of lesions at L5 level; 30% of spondylolysis lesions had associated spondylolisthesis, with female athletes displaying higher rates of spondylolisthesis (41% vs. 25%; $P < 0.05$).
Muschik et al[33]	Any	Retrospective	86 young athletes with spondylolysis with or without spondylolisthesis, between 6 and 20 years old	36 athletes had progression of spondylolisthesis (average progression, 10.5%) over an average of 4.8 years	Despite progression in 36 of 86 athletes, no symptoms were reported
Earhart et al[39]	Baseball	Retrospective	MLB (professional) players, 1980–2009	69 reported symptomatic lumbar disk herniations in 64 players	RTP averaged 97.5% and 96.6% for operative and nonoperative management, respectively; operative treatment experienced a longer recovery time (8.7 months vs. 3.6 months; $P < 0.001$)
Hsu et al[40]	Any	Retrospective	Professional American football, baseball, hockey, and basketball athletes, 1972–2008	342 athletes with identified lumbar disk herniation	82% of athletes returned to sport after treatment, with average career length of 3.4 years; athletes undergoing operative treatment returned to play 81% of the time; 62.3% of athletes remained active at 2 years; baseball players experienced the highest RTP (96%)

MLB = Major League Baseball, RTP = return to play.

Olympic level (5 of 8 or 63%) gymnasts, suggesting an association between increased intensity and length of training and average hours of training per week with increased abnormalities seen on spine MRI.[27]

Spondylolysis and Spondylolisthesis

Although the cause of low back pain in the general population can be attributable to various causes, the cause of back pain in younger athletes often involves posterior element injuries. Up to 40% of young athletes with low back pain lasting more than 3 months display pars abnormalities, with an overall incidence of 15% in college football players and 11% in gymnasts.[22] Stracciolini et al reviewed 2133 pediatric athletic injuries, aged 5 to 17 years, seen between 2000 and 2009 and found higher rates of spine injuries in female athletes (11.3%) compared with male athletes (8.2%) as well as in athletes 13 to 17 years old.[28] Of the pediatric athletes who reported spine injuries, Stracciolini et al found that 81.3% of injuries in male athletes and 93.9% of injuries in female athletes were classified as overuse injuries with spondylolysis present in half of male athletes and one third of female athletes presenting for spine-related complaints.[28] They also reported that the most common sports for spine injuries were gymnastics, dancing, and figure skating in female athletes and football, ice hockey, and soccer in male athletes.[28]

Reviewing 3152 Spanish elite athletes, Soler and Calderon found an overall incidence of spondylolysis of 8.02% compared with a 6% prevalence in the general population.[29,30] The authors further noted an increased incidence of spondylolysis in athletes participating in throwing sports (12 of 45 participants; 26.7%), artistic gymnastics (19 of 112 participants; 17.0%), and rowing (13 of 77 participants; 16.9%).[29] They also identified that 30.3% of the 253 athletes with spondylolysis had evidence of spondylolisthesis with subgroup analysis showing an increased incidence in female compared with male athletes.[29]

There is no clear evidence that athletic activity leads to spondylolisthesis progression; however, Lonstein suggests that athletes who have anterolisthesis of 25% to 50% (Meyerding grade 2) should consider avoiding gymnastics or other high-risk or high-impact sports.[31] Spondylolisthesis progression occurs in 4% to 5% of athletes, with further slip unlikely after reaching skeletal maturity.[32,33] Muschik et al followed 86 child and adolescent competitive athletes, 6 to 20 years old, participating in intensive training of more than 20 hours per week with radiographically confirmed spondylolysis or spondylolisthesis over an average of 4.8 years. In their study, the initial average anterior translation was $10.1 \pm 11.6\%$ with final measurements of 13.8 +/− 11.0%, concluding that 80% of the spondylolisthesis progression occurred before entry into the study.[34] Only one athlete with spondylolisthesis during the study period demonstrated an increase in anterior translation greater than 20% of the caudad vertebral body anterior to posterior diameter, beginning at 7% translation before the study and progressing to 31% at the conclusion of study. Therefore, their recommendation was that patients with mild spondylolisthesis do not need to avoid competitive sports.

Sacral and Pedicle Stress Fractures

Stress fractures are another source of low back pain with a reported incidence of 14% in the lumbar and pelvic region and approximately 1% in the chest and ribs.[35] Shah and Stewart reviewed sacral stress fractures as a potential cause of athletic low back pain and found 25 of 27 cases (92%) had negative findings on initial radiographs, with bone scan being the most common method of diagnosis.[36] They reported that the underlying cause of these sacral stress fractures is abnormal bone loading

and bone quality as well as leg length discrepancy.[36] Pedicle stress fractures are a rare cause of low back pain in adolescents, described mostly in case reports.[37–39] Parvataneni et al presented a case report of bilateral pedicle stress fractures in a female athlete.[39]

Disk Herniation

Earhart et al reviewed outcomes for surgical versus nonoperative management of lumbar disk herniation in Major League Baseball (MLB) players, identifying 69 athletes (40 operative and 29 nonoperative).[40] They noted an overall 97% rate of RTP by 6.6 months with significantly delayed RTP in the operative group of 8.7 months compared with the nonoperative group of 3.6 months. Furthermore, there was no significant difference between operative and nonoperative treatment for time to RTP for pitchers (8.0 months vs. 5.7 months, respectively; $P = 0.25$). However, there was a significant delay in RTP with operatively managed hitters returning in 9.4 months compared with nonoperative treatment with players returning to play in 2.6 months. Significant conclusions are difficult to draw from this data because baseline severity and duration of symptoms leading up to treatment were not reported and may have had a significant impact on surgical outcome. Similarly, Hsu and colleagues reported on outcomes after management of 342 athletes with lumbar disk herniation who participated in one of four professional sports in North America from 1972 to 2008, including football, baseball, hockey, and basketball. Their findings demonstrated similar RTP for surgical and nonoperative management (81% vs. 84%) at 3-year follow-up.[41] The 68 MLB players with lumbar disk herniations displayed the highest RTP rate among the four sports regardless of treatment (42 players treated operatively with 96% RTP and 26 players treated nonoperatively with 97% RTP). However, players receiving nonoperative treatment played more games after the injury (471 vs. 256; $P = 0.05$). It is difficult to draw significant conclusions from this given the inherent limitations within the study. The 138 NFL players displayed the greatest improvement from surgery, with operative treatment in 101 players resulting in 78% RTP with an average of 36 subsequent games versus nonoperative treatment in 37 players, resulting in 59% RTP and 20 subsequent games.[41]

Although less common than lumbar disk herniations, thoracic disk herniations can be a significant source of disability. Gray and colleagues reported 4 thoracic level disk herniations of 275 reported disk herniations (2%) in

NFL players between 2000 and 2012, with greater days and games lost (mean, 189 days, 72 practices, and 17 games missed) for thoracic level herniations compared with cervical and lumbar disk herniation (cervical disk herniations with a mean of 93 days, 113 practices, and 15 games missed and lumbar disk herniations with a mean of 51 days, 39 practices, and 11 games missed).[42] Other less frequently reported thoracic spine injuries include spinous process avulsion fractures of the cervicothoracic region.[43]

CONCLUSION

Clinicians caring for athletes encounter a wide array of spine pathology, ranging from low back pain to catastrophic SCIs. Advanced imaging has increased our ability to identify the underlying etiology of athletic spine morbidity but has unclear prognostic significance with degenerative disk disease. An understanding of the epidemiology of spine injuries in athletes is crucial for physicians to better diagnose and manage this patient population.

REFERENCES

1. National Collegiate Athletic Association: *Estimated Probability of Competing in College Football*. Available at: http://www.ncaa.org/about/resources/research/football. Accessed September 9, 2016.

2. National Collegiate Athletic Association: *Probability of Competing in Sports Beyond High School*. Available at: http://www.ncaa.org/about/resources/research/probability-competing-beyond-high-school. Accessed September 9, 2016.

3. Mall NA, Buchowski J, Zebala L, Brophy RH, Wright RW, Matava MJ: Spine and axial skeleton injuries in the National Football League. *Am J Sports Med* 2012;40(8): 1755–1761.

4. Banerjee R, Palumbo MA, Fadale PD: Catastrophic cervical spine injuries in the collision sport athlete, part 1: Epidemiology, functional anatomy, and diagnosis. *Am J Sports Med* 2004;32(4):1077–1087.

5. Boden BP, Tacchetti RL, Cantu RC, Knowles SB, Mueller FO: Catastrophic cervical spine injuries in high school and college football players. *Am J Sports Med* 2006;34(8):1223–1232.

6. Tator CH, Provvidenza C, Cassidy JD: Spinal injuries in Canadian ice hockey: An update to 2005. *Clin J Sports Med* 2009;19(6):451–456.

7. Schmitt H, Gerner HJ: Paralysis from sport and diving accidents. Clinical journal of sport medicine: official journal of the Canadian Academy of Sport Medicine. 2001;11(1):17–22.

8. Tator CH, Carson JD, Cushman R: Hockey injuries of the spine in Canada, 1966–1996. *CMAJ* 2000;162(6): 787–788.

9. Delaney JS, Al-Kashmiri A: Neck injuries presenting to emergency departments in the United States from 1990 to 1999 for ice hockey, soccer, and American football. *Br J Sports Med* 2005;39(4):e21.

10. Schroeder GD, Lynch TS, Gibbs DB, et al: The impact of a cervical spine diagnosis on the careers of National Football League athletes. *Spine* 2014;39(12):947–952.

11. Meredith DS, Jones KJ, Barnes R, Rodeo SA, Cammisa FP, Warren RF: Operative and nonoperative treatment of cervical disc herniation in National Football League athletes. *Am J Sports Med* 2013;41(9):2054–2058.

12. Torg JS, Quedenfeld TC, Burstein A, Spealman A, Nichols C 3rd: National football head and neck injury registry: Report on cervical quadriplegia, 1971 to 1975. *Am J Sports Med* 1979;7(2):127–132.

13. Torg JS, Vegso JJ, O'Neill MJ, Sennett B: The epidemiologic, pathologic, biomechanical, and cinematographic analysis of football-induced cervical spine trauma. *Am J Sports Med* 1990;18(1):50–57.

14. Boden BP, Breit I, Beachler JA, Williams A, Mueller FO: Fatalities in high school and college football players. *Am J Sports Med* May 2013;41(5):1108–1116.

15. Rihn JA, Anderson DT, Lamb K, et al: Cervical spine injuries in American football. *Sports Med* 2009;39(9):697–708.

16. Torg JS, Naranja RJ Jr, Pavlov H, Galinat BJ, Warren R, Stine RA: The relationship of developmental narrowing of the cervical spinal canal to reversible and irreversible injury of the cervical spinal cord in football players. *J Bone Joint Surg Am* 1996;78(9):1308–1314.

17. Shannon B, Klimkiewicz JJ: Cervical burners in the athlete. *Clin Sports Med* 2002;21(1):29–35, vi.

18. Charbonneau RM, McVeigh SA, Thompson K: Brachial neuropraxia in Canadian Atlantic University sport football players: What is the incidence of "stingers"? *Can J Med* 2012;22(6):472–477.

19. Meyer SA, Schulte KR, Callaghan JJ, et al: Cervical spinal stenosis and stingers in collegiate football players. *Am J Sports Med* 1994;22(2):158–166.

20. Page S, Guy JA: Neurapraxia, "stingers," and spinal stenosis in athletes. *South Med J* 2004;97(8):766–769.

21. Levitz CL, Reilly PJ, Torg JS: The pathomechanics of chronic, recurrent cervical nerve root neurapraxia. The chronic burner syndrome. *Am J Sports Med* 1997;25(1):73–76.

22. Dunn IF, Proctor MR, Day AL: Lumbar spine injuries in athletes. *Neurosurg Focus* 2006;21(4):E4.

23. Borg-Stein J, Elson L, Brand E: The aging spine in sports. *Clin Sports Med* 2012;31(3):473–486.

24. Kolt GS, Kirkby RJ: Epidemiology of injury in elite and sub-elite female gymnasts: A comparison of retrospective and prospective findings. *Br J Sports Med* 1999;33(5):312–318.

25. Sward L, Hellstrom M, Jacobsson B, Peterson L: Back pain and radiologic changes in the thoraco-lumbar spine of athletes. *Spine* 1990;15(2):124–129.

26. Hutchinson MR: Low back pain in elite rhythmic gymnasts. *Med Sci Sports Exerc* 1999;31(11):1686–1688.

27. Goldstein JD, Berger PE, Windler GE, Jackson DW: Spine injuries in gymnasts and swimmers. An epidemiologic investigation. *Am J Sports Med* 1991;19(5):463–468.

28. Stracciolini A, Casciano R, Levey Friedman H, Stein CJ, Meehan WP 3rd, Micheli LJ: Pediatric sports injuries: A comparison of males versus females. *Am J Sports Med* 2014;42(4):965–972.

29. Soler T, Calderon C: The prevalence of spondylolysis in the Spanish elite athlete. *Am J Sports Med* 2000;28(1):57–62.

30. Fredrickson BE, Baker D, McHolick WJ, Yuan HA, Lubicky JP: The natural history of spondylolysis and spondylolisthesis. *J Bone Joint Surg Am* 1984;66(5):699–707.

31. Lonstein JE: Spondylolisthesis in children. Cause, natural history, and management. *Spine* 1999;24(24):2640–2648.

32. Frennered AK, Danielson BI, Nachemson AL: Natural history of symptomatic isthmic low-grade spondylolisthesis in children and adolescents: A seven-year follow-up study. *J Pediatr Orthop* 1991;11(2):209–213.

33. Saraste H: Long-term clinical and radiological follow-up of spondylolysis and spondylolisthesis. *J Pediatr Orthop* 1987;7(6):631–638.

34. Muschik M, Hahnel H, Robinson PN, Perka C, Muschik C: Competitive sports and the progression of spondylolisthesis. *J Pediatr Orthop* 1996;16(3):364–369.

35. Changstrom BG, Brou L, Khodaee M, Braund C, Comstock RD: Epidemiology of stress fracture injuries among US high school athletes, 2005–2006 through 2012–2013. *Am J Sports Med* 2015;43(1):26–33.

36. Shah MK, Stewart GW: Sacral stress fractures: an unusual cause of low back pain in an athlete. *Spine* 2002;27(4): E104–E108.

37. Amari R, Sakai T, Katoh S, et al: Fresh stress fractures of lumbar pedicles in an adolescent male ballet dancer: Case report and literature review. *Arch Orthop Trauma Surg* 2009;129(3):397–401.

38. Sirvanci M, Ulusoy L, Duran C: Pedicular stress fracture in lumbar spine. *Clin Imaging* 2002;26(3):187–193.

39. Parvataneni HK, Nicholas SJ, McCance SE: Bilateral pedicle stress fractures in a female athlete: case report and review of the literature. *Spine* 2004;29(2):E19–E21.

40. Earhart JS, Roberts D, Roc G, Gryzlo S, Hsu W: Effects of lumbar disk herniation on the careers of professional baseball players. *Orthopedics* 2012;35(1):43–49.

41. Hsu WK, McCarthy KJ, Savage JW, et al: The Professional Athlete Spine Initiative: Outcomes after lumbar disc herniation in 342 elite professional athletes. *Spin J* 2011;11(3):180–186.

42. Gray BL, Buchowski JM, Bumpass DB, Lehman RA Jr, Mall NA, Matava MJ: Disc herniations in the National Football League. *Spine* 2013;38(22):1934–1938.

43. Menzer H, Gill GK, Paterson A: Thoracic spine sports-related injuries. *Curr Sports Med Rep* 2015;14(1): 34–40.

2 Biomechanics of the Spine in Sports and Prevention Considerations

Eeric Truumees, MD • Erik E. Swartz, PhD, ATC, FNATA

• INTRODUCTION

In sports, spine injuries occur across a wide spectrum from acute high-energy trauma to a chronic, repetitive overuse lesion. Appropriate diagnosis, management, and return to play for an athlete who has sustained a spine injury requires a reasonable understanding of the biomechanical mechanism of the injury. Whether the problem is low back pain that limits the athlete's ability to train and compete or a devastating, destabilizing cervical spine dislocation with **spinal cord injury** (SCI), four aspects of the biomechanical milieu are important.

The first aspect to consider is *what is the mechanism of injury*? Each sport is associated with unique loading and injury patterns.[1] Participation in any single sport may have acute or chronic effects on the spine, and in some cases, both. Examples of this include cycling, which can lead to high-energy impacts from crashes compared with the lumbar strain phenomena associated with the sustained posture common with endurance riding. Even acute injuries lie along a continuum of levels of imparted energy from repetitive micro-loading to devastating point loading. These issues may be interrelated because back and neck pain may impact subsequent training and readiness for competition. A second aspect to consider is

which part of the spine is affected? Each region offers a very different biomechanical milieu. Understanding spinal biomechanics regionally and globally will assist the clinician in diagnosis, treatment, prevention, and rehabilitation strategies. Third, *which tissue was predominantly affected*? Although ligamentous sprain may be benign in some parts of the body, spinal ligament disruption may be devastating. Recognizing the variable impacts of sports-related injury on the muscles, joints, and bones of the spine offers the best first guide to treatment. Fourth, consider that *each individual athlete's personal characteristics affect his or her vulnerability to different injuries*. A number of studies have shown differences in risk rates for male and female athletes. Similar differences exist for children, adolescents, adults, and older athletes. Understanding your player's predisposing factors is another key step in proper diagnosis, rehabilitation, and the prevention of further injury.

The scope of this chapter and the available evidence prevent us from going into detail in every sport or every clinical circumstance. However, it is reasonable to use "best available evidence" and extrapolate from the data available to the unique combination of factors involved in the management of a given athlete's injury.

Dr. Swartz or an immediate family member serves as a board member, owner, officer, or committee member of the Athletic Training and Sports Health Care, the Journal of Athletic Training, and the New Hampshire Musculoskeletal Institute. Dr. Truumees or an immediate family member has received royalties from Stryker; has stock or stock options held in Doctor's Research Group; has received research or institutional support from Globus Medical and Relievant; has received nonincome support (such as equipment or services), commercially derived honoraria, or other non-research–related funding (such as paid travel) from the North American Spine Society; and serves as a board member, owner, officer, or committee member of AAOS, AAOS Now, the Journal of Bone and Joint Surgery—American, the Journal of the American Academy of Orthopaedic Surgeons, the North American Spine Society, the Spine, and The Spine Journal.

BIOMECHANICAL VULNERABILITY BY TISSUE TYPE

The spine's functions are both biomechanical and protective in nature. The biomechanical functions include transmitting body weight during ambulation and allowing for flexibility and motion of the extremities during activities of daily living. The spine also serves to protect the spinal cord; cauda equina; and along with the rib cage, major organs of the thoracic cavity. To understand the vulnerability of the spine and its contents to injury from sports, one must understand the material characteristics of the individual tissues involved and the ways in which the anatomic elements of the spine move together. Depending on the sport and the mechanism of injury, the spine may be subjected to compression, tension, shear, and rotational forces, often at the same time. Although the stability and weight-bearing ability of the thigh can be disrupted by a simple fracture of the femur, the spine requires several structures to be disrupted before stability is lost. This is not to suggest that incomplete disruption of tissues associated with a spinal level are not of clinical significance. In fact, the concept of a **functional spinal unit (FSU)** may be helpful in identifying spinal structures at risk.[2] The FSU is a useful model for how these elements come together. The FSU consists of wo adjacent vertebral bodies, the interconnecting intervertebral disk, the articulating facet joints, and the segmental components of ligaments and muscles.

Injury will occur when those extrinsic forces exceed the intrinsic strength of the spine and its encasing soft tissues. Because these tissues work together as a unit, the strength and function of the muscles impact the likelihood of disk or bone injury. For example, coactivation of adjacent trunk muscle units may help direct forces along an efficient pathway. In this way, forces are not focused on a vulnerable area, and tissue failure may be avoided.

Soft Tissue Injuries

As with sports injuries to the bone and joints of the spine, most musculoligamentous injuries occur through indirect loading. Direct blows rarely lead to bony injuries in the spine but occasionally affect the soft tissues.[3] Indirect loading injuries can occur either with acute, high-energy mechanisms or with chronic overuse, high-repetition mechanisms. Typically, acute musculoligamentous injuries to the spine are caused by violent rotational or bending forces.[4] Chronic musculoligamentous injury is more common and often results from sustained high-repetition activities. Although nondestabilizing, these injuries can result in debilitating symptoms.[4] Rowing, for instance,

has a 22% incidence of back injury and a 9% incidence of rib cage injury from continuous, repetitive motion, particularly through the pull of the serratus anterior.[5]

Although musculoligamentous injuries certainly can and do occur in the cervical and thoracic spine, lumbar strain is the most common cause of low back pain in athletes. Here, too, a spectrum of injury from simple muscle bundle irritation without disruption to intrasubstance tearing of the muscle fibers or fascia is possible. Injury to the various spinal ligaments, or sprains, may also occur. In the cervical spine, ligament disruption to the transverse atlantal ligament, for example, resulting from focal hyperflexion of the upper cervical spine, can lead to a devastating neurologic injury.[6] More common, and more benign, are spinal ligamentous injuries involving the supra- and interspinous ligaments of the thoracolumbar region. These ligaments typically function as elastic stabilizers for the spinal segment and assist in extension. They are typically injured with abrupt segmental flexion.

When a significant rotational moment is added to a flexion injury, additional damage to the lumbar facet joint capsules or thoracic costovertebral joints may be seen. Higher energy trauma may lead to additional injury to the spinal ligaments, such as the anterior and posterior longitudinal ligaments (ALL and PLL), but these are almost always in combination with disk or bone injuries and discussed elsewhere.

Joint Injuries

Critical components in the biomechanics of the FSU come from the articulations, which include the intervertebral disk and the facet joints. As with musculotendinous injury, disk injuries in sports span a wide spectrum from traumatic, massive annulus disruption to repetitive traumas leading to degeneration. The zygapophyseal joints (facets) may be injured at any level of the spine. The relative risk, causative mechanisms, and implications on spinal stability vary by region and are discussed later.[7]

Mechanically, the intervertebral disk has two main functions: axial load transmission (a burden carried mainly by the nucleus pulposus) and ROM, particularly rotation (carried out by the annulus fibrosis). Hence, compromise of one structure, the nucleus or annulus, through a distinct biomechanical pattern can lead to injurious effects in the other structure. For example, most disk herniations are thought to occur after a series of repetitive traumas has created small rents and tears between annular fibers. Later, asymmetric axial loads on the disk may force a portion of the nucleus pulposus to migrate through the zone of annular weakness and into the spinal canal. Because the posterior longitudinal ligament is rarely injured in this context, the herniation is more typically posterolateral.[8] Symptomatic disk herniation are more common in the lower lumbar spine than in the upper lumbar and thoracic spine.[9] When they do occur in the thoracic spine, they are typically below T8.[9,10] Risk for these injuries increases for patients in their fourth and fifth decades. With higher energy trauma in younger patients, the PLL and the annulus are acutely and massively disrupted, allowing a larger portion of disk material to enter the canal centrally. In professional sports, upper lumbar and thoracic disk injuries are not particularly common and are typically attributed to contact injuries such as blocking and tackling.[11]

In the cervical spine, the articular pillars, which include the lateral masses and facet joints, carry a far greater percentage of the axial load passing through the segment than in the thoracolumbar spine.[12] The inherent stability conferred by the rib cage offers relative protection to the thoracic facets, but injuries still may be seen. With slight medial angulation, the thoracic facets are oriented vertically in the coronal plane. This orientation limits the thoracic spine's flexion and extension but allows for lateral bending and rotation. Excessive or rapid flexion or extension may lead to facet joint fracture. Lumbar facet joint injury is more common.[13] These lesions are thought to occur when a rotational injury overwhelms the stabilizing effect of facet capsule.

Another spinal articulation that has recently gotten more attention recently is the sacroiliac (SI) joint. SI joint dysfunction may result from repetitive lumbopelvic rotational loading mechanisms.[14,15] Sweep rowers and cross-country skiers are thought to be at higher risk.[16]

Bony Injuries

Sport activities can cause a variety of fractures in the cervical, thoracic, and lumbar spine. Some of these injuries are more aptly included with musculotendinous injuries such as isolated transverse or spinous process fractures. Sadly, however, destabilizing fractures and fracture-dislocations are also seen after athletic pursuits. As with the soft tissue and joint injuries already discussed, most of these injuries occur through indirect loading. Direct injury to a spinous process or the coccyx leading to fracture can also occur, but these are typically more benign injuries in terms of their mechanical impact on spinal stability.[17,18] Sports-related bony injury from indirect loading is divided into acute fractures and repetitive microtrauma or stress fractures.

In the thoracolumbar spine, stress fractures occurring in spinous processes, transverse processes, pars interarticularis, or ribs can result from overuse activities. Although a number of factors interact to cause these injuries, three are most important biomechanically: degree of loading, frequency of loading, and bone quality.[19] Understandably, as the degree (rate or force) or frequency increases, even in the presence of healthy bone, risk of stress fracture increases. Prevention strategies therefore require that one or more of these factors be addressed.

Spinous process avulsion fracture can occur either through acute injury or through repetitive muscular shear injury. These injuries are most common in the lower cervical or upper thoracic spine, where they are termed *clay-shoveler fractures*. This region may be affected more frequently in sports emphasizing the overlying shoulder girdle musculature. Single and multiple spinous process avulsions have been reported in a number of sports, including golf, rock climbing, baseball, and wrestling.[20–22]

More common are defects in the pars interarticularis. Such spondylolysis is most common at L5 and is a common cause of low back pain in younger athletes. In one study, low back pain in young athletes was thought to be related to a stress fracture 48% of the time.[23] Spondylolysis can occur more cranially in the spine. These injuries are rare in thoracic spine because the limited arc of flexion and extension is less likely to stress the pars interarticularis. A finite element investigation concluded that multilevel spondylolysis was more likely due to genetic than mechanical factors.[24] A biomechanical analysis has suggested that athletes with cervical spondylolysis not return to contact sports.[25]

Stress fractures of the sacrum are uncommon, mostly typically seen in runners and volleyball players.[26] Repetitive impact loading is thought to be the most significant risk factor. The role of decreased bone density in the incidence of these injuries continues to be debated.[27]

Acute fractures are more severe injuries, particularly in the cervical spine, and are typically caused by higher energy spinal loading activities, such as skiing, rugby, and football. These often involve a common mechanism, an axial load, and are discussed in the next section.

In the thoracic spine, axial loading and flexion forces may cause compression fractures, in which the anterior column fails while the posterior bone and ligamentous structures remain intact. Because of the inherent stability from the ribs and sternum, thoracic compression fractures rarely require operative treatment.[7,28] In an athletic population, adequate bone healing and muscle rehabilitation have typically occurred to allow return to sport by 3 months.[29]

With higher levels of energy imparted and the addition of flexion and rotational moments, more severe fracture patterns such as burst, translation rotation, and flexion-distraction fracture can be seen.[30–32] These injuries are more likely to lead to true spinal destabilization and confer a higher risk of SCI.

Spinal Cord Injury

The most feared aspect of any athletic injury to the spine is the possibility of damage to the neurologic tissues (the cauda equina, the nerve roots, and the spinal cord, in particular). The overall incidence of SCI varies drastically by anatomic region and sport type. However, sports are reported to be the second most common cause of SCI in patients younger than 30 years of age.[33] The most common mechanism of injury in sport leading to a cervical SCI is an axial load, such as with head-initiated strikes in diving, football, skiing, and horseback riding.[34,35]

● REGIONAL BIOMECHANICS OF THE SPINE

Just as each tissue type carries a different risk of injury and different types of injury, the regional differences in pathomechanics of the spine offer different opportunities for prevention.

Cervical

In terms of potentially devastating, sports-related spine trauma, head and neck injuries typically get the most attention. Because the mechanisms for acute and chronic head or neck injury often share the common mechanism of head-initiated contact, a variety of prevention efforts are underway. Many of these efforts seek to address the pathomechanics of the most common injury patterns. In the 1970s, better helmets led to an increased use of head during tackling. This "spear tackling" led to an epidemic in which as many as 70% of nonfatal cervical spine injuries in football resulted from head impacts.[36,37]

From a biomechanical perspective, the relatively small size of the cervical spine relative to the size of the head means that only 20% of its overall stability comes from the osteoligamentous structures.[38] The other 80% arises from the strong anterior and posterior neck muscles. As such, there is significant overlap between cervical ROM and neck strength on the one hand and the types and severity of head and neck injuries on the other. Theoretically, for example, athletes may reduce their head acceleration in an impact by contracting their cervical musculature, which serves to increase the effective mass of their head.[39,40] Unlike a whiplash scenario in motor vehicle accidents, athletic collisions in which the neck stops the head rarely impart enough energy to cause injury relative to those in which the neck must stop the torso.[41] As mentioned, most cervical spine injuries occur in conjunction with a head strike. So, appropriate prevention and return to play recommendation require an understanding of the dynamics of cervical spine injury.[42]

Initially, the common hypothesis was that head movement caused the spine to exceed its ROM. This, in turn, lead to a cervical spine injury.[43] However, in 1972, Roaf first suggested a mechanistic model based on forces and bending moments acting on the cervical spine.[44] Later, seminal studies by Bauze and Ardran and Nightingale et al demonstrated that severe cervical spine injuries, including bilateral facet dislocations and compression-flexion injuries, could occur within the normal arc of motion.[45,46]

More recently, these models have been updated with the concept of buckling, which arose to explain how multiple, noncontiguous and disparate injuries can occur.[42,46,47] In experimental studies, cervical spine buckling has been shown to precede injury. This buckling forces the spine into a complex shape with some regions of pure compression, compression-flexion, and compression-extension.[42,46,48–50] This model explains why high-energy collisions are not needed to create devastating injury patterns (**Figure 2-1**) . To stop the moving torso, depending on the position of the head and the alignment of the cervical spine, only a small percentage of body weight is needed to disrupt the cervical spine. In one study, only 16 kg of mass at a velocity of 3.1 m/s was required.[46,51]

There are three important time points after these head-first impacts: the initial head-strike and the force vectors on the cervical spine that follow moments later followed by the continuing movement of the body. In an unhelmeted impact to the top of the skull, a large, 8-kN force is generated but dissipates within milliseconds. Although there is initially no force on the cervical spine, a few milliseconds later, the still moving torso will exert profound compression between the head and body across the cervical spine. Helmets markedly reduce head impact forces to under 4 kN but do not protect the neck because cervical spine injury occurs shortly after head strike. In fact, certain helmets may increase the chance of cervical spine injury by holding the head to the impact surface longer.[42] Referred to as "pocketing," upon impact, the head sinks into the helmet's interior padded surface rather than being allowed to deflect off and away from the impact surface.[51] Then, as the torso keeps moving, the "held" head forces the cervical spine into positions of hyperflexion or extension, depending on the point of impact of the skull. With or without a helmet, the position of the neck at the moment of impact has a critical effect on the chance, severity, and type of cervical spine injuries seen. Typically, a position of slight flexion is thought to be more dangerous than facial or back of the head impacts.[46,51,52]

The fact that cervical spine injuries are not more common is probably explained by the high normal cervical ROM. For example, the cervical spine can flex to more than 96° without injury.[53] Thus, with most head impacts, the athlete is able to bend the head and neck out of the path of the moving torso. Decreased cervical flexibility decreases the ability of the head and neck to flex or extend away from the torso's path of loading and thereby prevent injury.[43,54]

A head strike in which the head is already moving in an escape direction allows the cervical musculature to push the head in this same direction. This limits the force passing through the cervical spine and significantly lowers the risk for injury. Directly perpendicular strikes confer a greater risk for injury.[42,51] A change in impact surface orientation as little as 15° may mark the difference between catastrophic and no neck injury.[42]

Both head and neck injuries are best prevented by limiting the common mechanism, head impacts. In 1976, a rules change in football requiring "heads-up" tackling reduced these injuries by nearly 50%. A heads-up block and tackling approach mitigates neck injury by reducing the chance of impact to the top of the head.[49,50] A "heads-up" block allows the neck to "escape" into extension after the initial collision and has been clinically shown to reduce the frequency of cervical spine injury.[50]

Although preflexion of the neck may increase injury risk, a number of studies have demonstrated fractures in unconstrained, naturally curved cervical spines.[36,42,46,49,51,55]

In other contact sports, such as hockey, improved protective gear for the head, face, and body has not decreased the incidence of catastrophic spine injuries.[56] Other sports offer different prevention pathways. For example, in very high-speed sports such as automobile racing, newer constraint systems limiting cervical spine flexion and extension have been used. In diving sports, efforts to prevent shallow water dives are most effective,[57] and in sliding sports such as baseball, discouraging the behavior of head-first sliding reduces the risk of spine injury. Ultimately, the goal is to design head protection

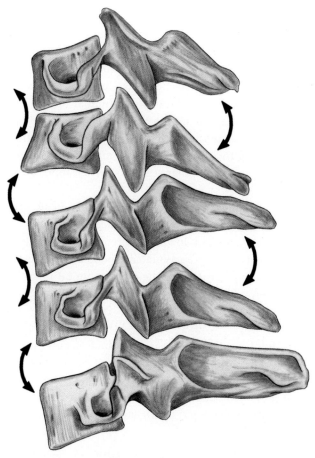

FIGURE 2-1 Buckling effect in the cervical column under axial load. (Reprinted from Swartz EE, Floyd RT, Cendoma M: Cervical spine functional anatomy and the biomechanics of injury due to compressive loading. *J Athl Train* 2005;40(3):155–161.)

systems or techniques that match the injury pattern associated with that sport; in some, it may be to minimize constraints to head motion, but in others, it may be to maximize the constraint.

Thoracic Spine

Sports-related injuries to thoracic spine are far less common than cervical and lumbar injuries because of the relatively more stable biomechanical support afforded by the thoracic cage.[58] This forms a veritable fourth column that restricts flexion-extension while allowing rotation because of the costovertebral joint and linkage to the sternum.[59] A complete rib cage with an intact sternum increases thoracic spine stability in flexion-extension, lateral bending, and axial rotation by up to 40%.[7,28] The combined structures of the thoracic region provide powerful axial rotation, which adds power to the torsional force generation from the shoulder region in sports such as in tennis and pitching in baseball.

Thoracolumbar Junction

In the lower thoracic spine, the ribs are attached to a single vertebral body and do not attach to the sternum anteriorly. Additionally, the facet joints transition from a coronal orientation in the lower thoracic spine to an oblique sagittal orientation in the lumbar spine. This increased sagittal orientation permits increased mobility in flexion and extension and more limitation of rotation. Furthermore, the transition from a more rigid thoracic region to a mobile lumbar region renders it more prone to injury.

When standing, the T10 to L2 sagittal alignment is relatively straight. In this position, the center of mass lies anterior to T10. With loading, therefore, there is a flexion moment at the thoracolumbar junction.[58] As a result, compression fractures are the most common injury at 52% followed by transverse process fractures at 37%.[60]

Lumbar and Lumbo-Sacro-Pelvic Spine

In the lumbar spine, load bearing is increasingly carried through the disks anteriorly. Chronic overloading can lead to spondylotic change. Acute loading may lead to compression or burst fractures. With sports injuries, destabilizing spine fractures are less common.

● SPORT-SPECIFIC BIOMECHANICS

Although aggressive, full-contact sports, such as American football and rugby, receive the most attention in many medical circles, other sports with repetitive spinal loading patterns can also cause debilitating injuries, including rowing, gymnastics, and golf.[2,58] In contrast, newer adventure sports (e.g., X-games) such as snowboarding, skateboarding, and BMX involve high speeds and vertical heights with associated high-energy collisions fueling the incidence of catastrophic spinal injuries. Therefore, when seeking to treat or prevent spinal injury in athletes, understanding the mechanisms of injury most typically associated with the specific sport and its associated training programs is critical. It is important to understand regional differences in training and play surfaces as well.[61,62]

Running and Weight Lifting

Up to 70% of recreational and competitive runners sustain some type of spinal overuse injury. Not all of these are musculotendinous injuries. A number of studies have identified early degenerative changes in the disks and facets of runners over the long term.[63]

Other epidemiologic studies have found little increased risk of lumbar degeneration in competitive and elite runners.[64-66] Running has been identified as a risk factor for sacral stress fracture.[67,68]

In 2004, Schmitt and others reported a retrospective cohort study to clarify occurrence of vertebral osteophytes and other degenerative changes in the lumbar spine in former elite track and field athletes.[69] Although no long-term differences in functional limitations were seen in these athletes, the highest degree of radiographic change was seen in high jumpers and throwing athletes. The authors concluded that these disciplines load the spine more than running sports. In an assessment of CT scan data from the Framingham Heart Study, heavy physical activity was associated with severe lumbar facet osteoarthritis, but this association was not seen in runners.[70]

Other studies support heavy physical activity, outside of running, but including jumping, as a risk factor for lumbar degeneration.[58] Although the authors could not attribute clinical significance to the finding, one study found that throwing athletes and high jumpers had more lumbar vertebral osteophytes than other types of athletes.[69]

Weight lifting, whether for competition or training purposes, has been shown to cause both acute overload injuries, such as compression fractures, and an increased rate of lumbar degenerative disease. In one study, 80% of male weight lifters showed signs of degenerative disk disease at the age of 40 years.[71] Weight lifters may also present with of strains and sprains of the spinal musculature and ligaments, spondylolysis, spondylolisthesis, and herniated nucleus pulposus. Although rare, catastrophic injuries can occur when the athlete uses poor technique and tries to lift too much weight.[72] Prevention requires that weight be keep close to the body to shorten the moment arm. With dead lifts, for example, the "sumo style" with the feet spread apart significantly lowers that compressive force through the L4 to L5 facets.[73] Weight belts have been shown to increase intraabdominal pressure during squat lifting, thereby decreasing spinal compression and shear forces.[74]

Training or competition that requires asymmetric spinal loading may be associated with specific injury patterns. In one study, scoliosis was detected in up to 80% of athletes with an asymmetric load on the trunk and shoulders, such as javelin throwers and tennis players. The curvature was small, however, and not associated with back pain.[60]

Contact Sports and Gymnastics

Contact sports, such as football or hockey, involve the instantaneous transmission of high-force loads to the spine. When overloaded, the tissues of the spine might be disrupted. This loading can accelerate lumbar disk and facet degeneration. For these athletes, the risk of chronic low back pain rates is proportional to their years of involvement in the sport.[75]

Football interior linemen are at increased risk for acute and chronic spinal injury.[36,50] Blocking entails repeated axial loads, hyperextension, and torsional strain on the spine, which can lead to spondylolysis.[76] As with football linemen, gymnasts often undergo axial loading and hyperextension of the lumbar spine, resulting in spondylolysis. The incidence of pars interarticularis injury is 11% in young gymnasts compared with less than 3% in the age-matched general population.[77] Gymnasts also often perform on apparatuses on which a miss may lead to a fall from a significant height, leading to axial force overload.

Golf and Swimming

Back pain from repetitive loading is fairly well studied in golf.[78,79] This pain has been shown to correlate with decreased lumbar spine extension, lead hip internal rotation, and decreased distance of the knee to the examination table when the ipsilateral hip is flexed, abducted, and externally rotated.[80] As a result, some have suggested that increasing hip ROM using physical therapy modalities can help to prevent low back pain in golfers.

In water sports, the buoyancy of water decreases axial loading of the spine. Lumbar torsion and extension forces can be significant with swimming, however. This is particularly true when performing laps with repetitive movements, such as freestyle, breast stroke, or back stroke. For example, during the rolling motion of a freestyle stroke, if the whole body is not rolling as a unit, torsional strain to the thoracolumbar spine can occur.[81] Some strokes, such as the breast and butterfly strokes, exaggerate lumbar extension through the lumbar spine.[82,83] Despite limited axially loading, one study found that athletes who participated in sports requiring significant rotation, including swimming and baseball, exhibited significantly greater disk degeneration on MRI compared with nonathletes.[62] In water sports, cervical spine injuries have been identified primarily with diving caused by head impacts.[84] However, repetitive stress injuries may also occur during turns with poor head and body position.

Cycling

As with winter sports, a variety of high-impact collision injuries can occur with cycling. Repetitive loading injuries are a bit more sport specific in that, depending on the type cycling, various mechanically unfavorable postures may be maintained for long periods. With endurance road racing, the cervical spine may be maintained in hyperextension. With most cycling, the lumbar spine assumes a posture of at least mild kyphosis.[85,86] Loading the lumbar spine in flexion increases intradiscal pressure.[87] The degree to which the lumbar paraspinals encounter strain is a function of amount the cyclist loads the pedals and his or her position on the bicycle. Increasing load or torque to pedals or crank has been shown to increase lumbar paraspinal activation.[86,88] Lumbar strain injuries have been commonly reported with endurance bicycling in road racers,[89] triathletes,[90] and recreational riders,[91-93] These loads may be partly mitigated through proper gear selection and bicycle fitting. At this point, however, the evidence that "best fit" interventions improve in spine complaints remain limited.[91-93] Changing saddle geometry through cut-outs may affect pelvic angle and, secondarily, lumbar lordosis.[94]

● BIOMECHANICALLY RELEVANT PATIENT CHARACTERISTICS

We know certain athletes are at greater risk for spine injury than others. For example, the greatest predictor of low back pain in athletes is prior low back pain.[71,77] Many of these risk factors are mechanical, others not.

For example, the different biomechanical aspects offered by the spines of athletes of different ages leads to varied injury patterns. For our purposes, a child's spine exhibits a fairly adult pattern of loading after age 8 years. For athletes younger than 8 years, there is a significant head–weight mismatch that renders the upper cervical spine more vulnerable. Given that much sport-related spine trauma arises from collision, enforcement of proper age and weight classes is important for younger athletes to avoid critical player size mismatches and resulting collision injury.[2]

With repetitive loading injuries, the permanent mechanical changes caused by overtraining of the adolescent skeleton are not as clear for the spine.[95,96] The most common example of this type of injury is isthmic spondylolisthesis.[60] During periods of rapid growth, athletes may lack balance of bone, ligament, and muscle strength. The spine, as with the rest of the skeleton, is at greater risk of injury during growth, especially during the adolescent growth spurt.[2,60] Protective proprioception is negatively affected after significant height change.[2] Certainly, the biochemistry and biomechanics of the disk are age related, and thus, adolescent and older athletes may have different concerns with regards to the diagnosis, treatment, and prognosis after injury to the spine.[71]

The impact of lumbar flexibility on back pain is controversial. In a 3-year longitudinal study in Finnish hockey and soccer players, skaters, and gymnasts, ROM was related to back pain. The authors concluded that loss of lumbar extension mobility causes overloading of the low back and, ultimately, low back pain.[97] Sward and colleagues measured hip and spine ROM in 116 elite Swedish athletes representing wrestling, gymnastics, soccer, and tennis. Significant differences were seen, although the authors were not sure if these differences represented a long-term training effect or merely natural selection of individuals better physically suited to their sports.[98] Independent of the cause, the spine definitely works differently in athletes of different types. Other studies have not correlated flexibility and back pain, although these studies were limited to collegiate athletes only.[99,100] Certainly, younger patients exhibit a different range of injuries than young adults. Older athletes may be more prone to low-energy, repetitive loading injuries.

Gender-based anatomic differences have been shown to affect female athletes' vulnerability to certain injuries, such as anterior cruciate ligament tears.[101] Similar biomechanical factors may also impact injury risk and prevention strategies for spinal injuries. For example, lower neck circumference and lower cervical muscle strength are thought to increase vulnerability to head and neck injuries.[102] Bone loss rapidly increases an athlete's risk for both acute bone injury, such as compression fracture, but also more chronic bone disruption such as sacral stress fracture. The female athlete triad—disordered eating, amenorrhea, and osteoporosis—has long been identified as one source of bone loss. This triad is more common in endurance sports or activities in which appearance is judged such as figure skating, gymnastics, and ballet.[103,104]

Even male elite athletes, especially in low-impact sports, may exhibit bone loss. Several studies have shown that high-volume bicyclists experience bone demineralization.[105-107] Most affected were lean male athletes who only rode bicycles for exercise and had done so at high levels for prolonged periods of time. As a result, endurance bicycling not recommended for those known to have low bone density.

● SUMMARY

In this chapter, we sought to describe the biomechanics of the spine relevant to its vulnerability to athletic injury. Although the available data remain too limited to cover every sport and permutation of injury pattern with patient vulnerability, working from a basic framework such as this will hopefully assist caregivers as they seek to:

- Prevent injury in vulnerable or at-risk patients.
- Work with coaches and training staff to address wide-ranging risk factors across a team.
- Offer guidance to a sport's governing body to improve protective gear, rules, and training to reduce the risk of injury across the sport more globally.

For a patient presenting with symptoms, an understanding of the biomechanics of a sport and that athlete's individual vulnerabilities may improve the diagnostic process while improving decision making for treatment and return to sport. To achieve these aims, we recommend a systematic approach to understand the clinical presentation. It may be useful to think of this environment in terms of the three-dimensional matrix presented at the beginning of this chapter. The likelihood and severity of injury is based on the convergence of each dimension of that matrix. Understanding this matrix will allow the practitioner to appropriately characterize the continuum of athletic spinal afflictions from lower energy, repetitive loading injuries to devastating, high-energy impacts.

REFERENCES

1. Maxwell C, Spiegel A: The rehabilitation of athletes after spinal injurie, in Watkins R, ed. *The Spine in Sports*. Philadelphia, PA, Hanley & Belfus, 1990, pp 281–292.

2. Khan N, Husain S, Haak M: Thoracolumbar injuries in the athlete. *Sports Med Arthrosc* 2008;16(1):16–25.

3. Benson ER, Schutzer SF: Posttraumatic piriformis syndrome: Diagnosis and results of operative treatment. *J Bone Joint Surg Am* 1999;81(7):941–949.

4. Watkins R: *The Spine in Sports*. St. Louis, MO, Mosby, 1996.

5. Hosea TM, Hannafin JA: Rowing injuries. *Sports Health* 2012;4(3):236–245.

6. Banerjee R, Palumbo MA, Fadale PD: Catastrophic cervical spine injuries in the collision sport athlete, part 2: Principles of emergency care. *Am J Sports Med* 2004;32(7):1760–1764.

7. Horton WC, Kraiwattanapong C, Akamaru T, et al: The role of the sternum, costosternal articulations, intervertebral disc, and facets in thoracic sagittal plane biomechanics: A comparison of three different sequences of surgical release. *Spine (Phila Pa 1976)* 2005;30(18):2014–2023.

8. Hochschuler S: *The Spine in Sports.* Philadelphia, PA, Hanley & Belfus, 1990.

9. Yoshihara H: Surgical treatment for thoracic disc herniation: An update. *Spine (Phila Pa 1976)* 2014;39(6):E406–412.

10. Stillerman CB, Chen TC, Couldwell WT, et al: Experience in the surgical management of 82 symptomatic herniated thoracic discs and review of the literature. *J NeuroSurg* 1998;88(4):623–633.

11. Gray BL, Buchowski JM, Bumpass DB, et al: Disc herniations in the National Football League. *Spine (Phila Pa 1976)* 2013;38(22):1934–1938.

12. Truumees E, Demetropoulos CK, Yang KH, Herkowitz HN: Effects of disc height and distractive forces on graft compression in an anterior cervical discectomy model. *Spine (Phila Pa 1976)* 2002;27(22):2441–2445.

13. Beresford ZM, Kendall RW, Willick SE: Lumbar facet syndromes. *Curr Sports Med Rep* 2010;9(1):50–56.

14. Timm KE: Sacroiliac joint dysfunction in elite rowers. *J Orthop Sports Phys Ther* 1999;29(5):288–293.

15. Lindsay DM, Meeuwisse WH, Vyse A, et al: Lumbosacral dysfunctions in elite cross-country skiers. *J Orthop Sports Phys Ther* 1993;18(5):580–585.

16. Schwarzer AC, Aprill CN, Bogduk N: The sacroiliac joint in chronic low back pain. *Spine (Phila Pa 1976)* 1995;20(1):31–37.

17. Kazemi M, Pieter W: Injuries at the Canadian National Tae Kwon Do Championships: A prospective study. *BMC Musculoskelet Disord* 2004;5:22.

18. Hodges SD, Eck JC, Humphreys SC: A treatment and outcomes analysis of patients with coccydynia. *Spine J* 2004;4(2):138–140.

19. Hall SJ: Mechanical contribution to lumbar stress injuries in female gymnasts. *Med Sci Sports Exerc* 1986;18(6):599–602.

20. Yamaguchi KT Jr, Myung KS, Alonso MA, Skaggs DL: Clay-shoveler's fracture equivalent in children. *Spine (Phila Pa 1976)* 2012;37(26):E1672–1675.

21. Kang DH, Lee SH: Multiple spinous process fractures of the thoracic vertebrae (Clay-Shoveler's Fracture) in a beginning Golfer: A case report. *Spine (Phila Pa 1976)* 2009;34(15):E534–537.

22. Cantu RC, Mueller FO: Catastrophic football injuries: 1977-1998. *Neurosurgery* 2000;47(3):673–675; discussion 675–677.

23. Micheli LJ: Sports following spinal surgery in the young athlete. *Clin Orthop Relat Res* 1985(198):152–157.

24. Sairyo K, Sakai T, Yasui N, et al: Newly occurred L4 spondylolysis in the lumbar spine with pre-existence L5 spondylolysis among sports players: Case reports and biomechanical analysis. *Arch Orthop Trauma Surg* 2009;129(10):1433–1439.

25. Sasa T, Yoshizumi Y, Imada K, et al: Cervical spondylolysis in a judo player: A case report and biomechanical analysis. *Arch Orthop Trauma Surg* 2009;129(4):559–567.

26. Johnson AW, Weiss CB Jr, Stento K, Wheeler DL: Stress fractures of the sacrum. An atypical cause of low back pain in the female athlete. *Am J Sports Med* 2001;29(4):498–508.

27. Shah MK, Stewart GW: Sacral stress fractures: An unusual cause of low back pain in an athlete. *Spine (Phila Pa 1976)* 2002;27(4):E104–108.

28. Watkins RT, Watkins R 3rd, Williams L, et al: Stability provided by the sternum and rib cage in the thoracic spine. *Spine (Phila Pa 1976)* 2005;30(11):1283–1286.

29. Elattrache N, Fadale PD, Fu FH: Thoracic spine fracture in a football player. A case report. *Am J Sports Med* 1993;21(1):157–160.

30. Myers B, Woolley C, Slotter T, et al: The influence of strain rate on the passive and stimulated engineering stress-large strain behavior of the rabbit tibialis anterior muscle. *J Biomech Eng* 1998(120):126–132.

31. Nightingale R, Camacho D, Armstrong A, et al: Inertial properties and loading rates affect buckling modes and injury mechanisms in the cervical spine. *J Biomech* 2000;33:191–197.

32. Penning L: Acceleration injury of the cervical spine by hypertranslation of the head. Part II. Effect of hypertranslation of the head on cervical spine motion: Discussion of literature data. *Eur Spine J* 1992;1:13–19.

33. Gill SS, Boden BP: The epidemiology of catastrophic spine injuries in high school and college football. *Sports Med Arthrosc* 2008;16(1):2–6.

34. Boden B: Direct catastrophic injury in sports. *J Am Acad Orthop Surg* 2005;13:445–454.

35. Cantu R: Cervical spine injuries in the athlete. *Semin Neurol* 2000;20:173–178.

36. Torg JS, Quedenfeld TC, Burstein A, Set al: National football head and neck injury registry: Report on cervical quadriplegia, 1971 to 1975. *Am J Sports Med* 1979;7(2):127–132.

37. Albright JP, Moses JM, Feldick HG, et al: Nonfatal cervical spine injuries in interscholastic football. *JAMA* 1976;236(11):1243–1245.

38. Schmidt JD, Guskiewicz KM, Blackburn JT, et al: The influence of cervical muscle characteristics on head impact biomechanics in football. *Am J Sports Med* 2014;42(9):2056–2066.

39. Mihalik JP, Guskiewicz KM, Marshall SW, et al: Head impact biomechanics in youth hockey: comparisons across playing position, event types, and impact locations. *Ann Biomed Eng* 2012;40(1):141–149.

40. Mihalik JP, Guskiewicz KM, Marshall SW, et al: Does cervical muscle strength in youth ice hockey players affect head impact biomechanics? *Clin J Sport Med* 2011;21(5):416–421.

41. Huelke DF, Mackay GM, Morris A, Bradford M: A review of cervical fractures and fracture-dislocations without head impacts sustained by restrained occupants. *Accid Anal Prev* 1993;25(6):731–743.

42. Nightingale RW, Richardson WJ, Myers BS: The effects of padded surfaces on the risk for cervical spine injury. *Spine (Phila Pa 1976)* 1997;22(20):2380–2387.

43. Kazarian L: Injuries to the human spinal column: Biomechanics and injury classification. *Exerc Sport Sci Rev* 1981;9:297–352.

44. Roaf R: International classification of spinal injuries. *Paraplegia* 1972;10(1):78–84.

45. Bauze RJ, Ardran GM: Experimental production of forward dislocation in the human cervical spine. *J Bone Joint Surg Br* 1978;60-B(2):239–245.

46. Nightingale RW, McElhaney JH, Richardson WJ, et al: Experimental impact injury to the cervical spine: Relating motion of the head and the mechanism of injury. *J Bone Joint Surg Am* 1996;78(3):412–421.

47. Shear P, Hugenholtz H, Richard MT, et al: Multiple noncontiguous fractures of the cervical spine. *J Trauma* 1988;28(5):655–659.

48. Myers BS, Winkelstein BA: Epidemiology, classification, mechanism, and tolerance of human cervical spine injuries. *Crit Rev Biomed Eng* 1995;23(5-6):307–409.

49. Torg JS, Sennett B, Pavlov H, et al: Spear tackler's spine. An entity precluding participation in tackle football and collision activities that expose the cervical spine to axial energy inputs. *Am J Sports Med* 1993;21(5):640–649.

50. Torg JS, Vegso JJ, O'Neill MJ, Sennett B: The epidemiologic, pathologic, biomechanical, and cinematographic analysis of football-induced cervical spine trauma. *Am J Sports Med* 1990;18(1):50–57.

51. Nightingale RW, McElhaney JH, Richardson WJ, Myers BS: Dynamic responses of the head and cervical spine to axial impact loading. *J Biomech* 1996;29(3):307–318.

52. Panjabi MM, Oda T, Crisco JJ 3rd, et al: Experimental study of atlas injuries. I. Biomechanical analysis of their mechanisms and fracture patterns. *Spine (Phila Pa 1976)* 1991;16(10 suppl):S460-S465.

53. Roaf R: A study of the mechanics of spinal injuries. *J Bone Joint Surg Br* 1960;42(4):810–823.

54. Winkelstein BA, Myers BS: The biomechanics of cervical spine injury and implications for injury prevention. *Med Sci Sports Exerc* 1997;29(7 suppl):S246–S255.

55. Yoganandan N, Stemper BD, Pintar FA, et al: Cervical spine injury biomechanics: Applications for under body blast loadings in military environments. *Clin Biomech (Bristol, Avon)* 2013;28(6):602–609.

56. Stuart MJ, Smith AM, Malo-Ortiguera SA, et al: A comparison of facial protection and the incidence of head, neck, and facial injuries in Junior A hockey players. A function of individual playing time. *Am J Sports Med* 2002;30(1):39–44.

57. Gabrielsen M: *Diving Injuries: The Etiology of 486 Case Studies with Recommendations for Needed Action.* Ft. Lauderdale, FL, NOVA University Press, 1990.

58. Menzer H, Gill GK, Paterson A: Thoracic spine sports-related injuries. *Curr Sports Med Rep* 2015;14(1):34–40.

59. Berg EE: The sternal-rib complex. A possible fourth column in thoracic spine fractures. *Spine (Phila Pa 1976)* 1993;18(13):1916–1919.

60. Sward L: The thoracolumbar spine in young elite athletes. Current concepts on the effects of physical training. *Sports Med* 1992;13(5):357–364.

61. Reid DC, Saboe L: Spine fractures in winter sports. *Sports Med* 1989;7(6):393–399.

62. Hangai M, Kaneoka K, Hinotsu S, et al: Lumbar intervertebral disk degeneration in athletes. *Am J Sports Med* 2009;37(1):149–155.

63. Jacobs SJ, Berson BL: Injuries to runners: a study of entrants to a 10,000 meter race. *Am J Sports Med* 1986;14(2):151–155.

64. Woolf SK, Glaser JA: Low back pain in running-based sports. *South Med J* 2004;97(9):847–851.

65. Ribaud A, Tavares I, Viollet E, et al: Which physical activities and sports can be recommended to chronic low back pain patients after rehabilitation? *Ann Phys Rehabil Med* 2013;56(7-8):576–594.

66. Raty HP, Kujala UM, Videman T, et al: Lifetime musculoskeletal symptoms and injuries among former elite male athletes. *Int J Sports Med* 1997;18(8):625–632.

67. Mundt DJ, Kelsey JL, Golden AL, et al: An epidemiologic study of sports and weight lifting as possible risk factors for herniated lumbar and cervical discs. The Northeast Collaborative Group on Low Back Pain. *Am J Sports Med* 1993;21(6):854–860.

68. Eller DJ, Katz DS, Bergman AG, et al: Sacral stress fractures in long-distance runners. *Clin J Sport Med* 1997;7(3):222–225.

69. Schmitt H, Dubljanin E, Schneider S, Schiltenwolf M: Radiographic changes in the lumbar spine in former elite athletes. *Spine (Phila Pa 1976)* 2004 29(22):2554–2559.

70. Suri P, Hunter DJ, Boyko EJ, et al: Physical activity and associations with computed tomography-detected lumbar zygapophyseal joint osteoarthritis. *Spine J* 2015;15(1):42–49.

71. Tall RL, DeVault W: Spinal injury in sport: Epidemiologic considerations. *Clin Sports Med* 1993;12(3):441–448.

72. Gallo RA, Reitman RD, Altman DT, et al: Flexion-distraction injury of the thoracolumbar spine during squat exercise with the smith machine. *Am J Sports Med* 2004;32(8):1962–1967.

73. Cholewicki J, McGill SM, Norman RW: Lumbar spine loads during the lifting of extremely heavy weights. *Med Sci Sports Exerc* 1991;23(10):1179–1186.

74. Lander JE, Hundley JR, Simonton RL: The effectiveness of weight-belts during multiple repetitions of the squat exercise. *Med Sci Sports Exerc* 1992;24(5):603–609.

75. Gerbino PG, d'Hemecourt PA: Does football cause an increase in degenerative disease of the lumbar spine? *Curr Sports Med Rep* 2002;1(1):47–51.

76. Gatt CJ Jr, Hosea TM, Palumbo RC, Zawadsky JP: Impact loading of the lumbar spine during football blocking. *Am J Sports Med* 1997;25(3):317–321.

77. Spencer CW 3rd, Jackson DW: Back injuries in the athlete. *Clin Sports Med* 1983;2(1):191–215.

78. Gluck GS, Bendo JA, Spivak JM: The lumbar spine and low back pain in golf: A literature review of swing biomechanics and injury prevention. *Spine J* 2008;8(5):778–788.

79. Lindsay DM, Vandervoort AA: Golf-related low back pain: A review of causative factors and prevention strategies. *Asian J Sports Med* 2014;5(4):e24289.

80. Vad VB, Bhat AL, Basrai D, et al: Low back pain in professional golfers: the role of associated hip and low back range-of-motion deficits. *Am J Sports Med* 2004;32(2):494–497.

81. Kenal KA, Knapp LD: Rehabilitation of injuries in competitive swimmers. *Sports Med* 1996;22(5):337–347.

82. Wanivenhaus F, Fox AJ, Chaudhury S, Rodeo SA: Epidemiology of injuries and prevention strategies in competitive swimmers. *Sports Health* 2012;4(3):246–251.

83. Thomas PL: Thoracic back pain in rowers and butterfly swimmers—costo vertebral subluxation. *Br J Sports Med* 1988;22(2):81.

84. Albrand OW, Walter J: Underwater deceleration curves in relation to injuries from diving. *Surg Neurol* 1975;4(5):461–464.

85. Griskevicius J, Linkel A, Pauk J: Research of cyclist's spine dynamical model. *Acta Bioeng Biomech* 2014;16(1): 37–44.

86. Usabiaga J, Crespo R, Iza I, et al: Adaptation of the lumbar spine to different positions in bicycle racing. *Spine (Phila Pa 1976)* 1997;22(17):1965–1969.

87. Nachemson A: The load on lumbar disks in different positions of the body. *Clin Orthop Relat Res* 1966;45:107–122.

88. Rohlmann A, Zander T, Graichen F, et al: Spinal loads during cycling on an ergometer. *PLoS One* 2014;9(4):e95497.

89. Clarsen B, Krosshaug T, Bahr R: Overuse injuries in professional road cyclists. *Am J Sports Med* 2010;38(12):2494–2501.

90. Andersen CA, Clarsen B, Johansen TV, Engebretsen L: High prevalence of overuse injury among iron-distance triathletes. *Br J Sports Med* 2013;47(13):857–861.

91. Asplund C, Webb C, Barkdull T: Neck and back pain in bicycling. *Curr Sports Med Rep* 2005;4(5):271–274.

92. Dettori NJ, Norvell DC: Non-traumatic bicycle injuries: A review of the literature. *Sports Med* 2006;36(1):7–18.

93. Thompson MJ, Rivara FP: Bicycle-related injuries. *Am Fam Physician* 2001;63(10):2007–2014.

94. Bressel E, Larson BJ: Bicycle seat designs and their effect on pelvic angle, trunk angle, and comfort. *Med Sci Sports Exerc* 2003;35(2):327–332.

95. Gannon LM, Bird HA: The quantification of joint laxity in dancers and gymnasts. *J Sports Sci* 1999;17(9):743–750.

96. Tsai L, Wredmark T: Spinal posture, sagittal mobility, and subjective rating of back problems in former female elite gymnasts. *Spine (Phila Pa 1976)* 1993;18(7):872–875.

97. Kujala UM, Taimela S, Oksanen A, Salminen JJ: Lumbar mobility and low back pain during adolescence. A longitudinal three-year follow-up study in athletes and controls. *Am J Sports Med* 1997;25(3):363–368.

98. Sward L, Eriksson B, Peterson L: Anthropometric characteristics, passive hip flexion, and spinal mobility in relation to back pain in athletes. *Spine (Phila Pa 1976)* 1990;15(5):376–382.

99. Twellaar M, Verstappen FT, Huson A, van Mechelen W: Physical characteristics as risk factors for sports injuries: A four year prospective study. *Int J Sports Med* 1997;18(1):66–71.

100. Nadler SF, Wu KD, Galski T, Feinberg JH: Low back pain in college athletes. A prospective study correlating lower extremity overuse or acquired ligamentous laxity with low back pain. *Spine (Phila Pa 1976)* 1998;23(7):828–833.

101. Cheung EC, Boguszewski DV, Joshi NB, et al: Anatomic Factors that may predispose female athletes to anterior cruciate ligament injury. *Curr Sports Med Rep* 2015;14(5):368–372.

102. Silver JR, Silver DD, Godfrey JJ: Injuries of the spine sustained during gymnastic activities. *Br Med J (Clin Res Ed)* 1986;293(6551):861–863.

103. Nattiv A, Agostini R, Drinkwater B, Yeager KK: The female athlete triad. The inter-relatedness of disordered eating, amenorrhea, and osteoporosis. *Clin Sports Med* 1994;13(2):405–418.

104. Yeager KK, Agostini R, Nattiv A, Drinkwater B: The female athlete triad: disordered eating, amenorrhea, osteoporosis. *Med Sci Sports Exerc* 1993;25(7):775–777.

105. Campion F, Nevill AM, Karlsson MK, et al: Bone status in professional cyclists. *Int J Sports Med* 2010;31(7): 511–515.

106. Nichols JF, Palmer JE, Levy SS: Low bone mineral density in highly trained male master cyclists. *Osteoporos Int* 2003;14(8):644–649.

107. Nichols JF, Rauh MJ: Longitudinal changes in bone mineral density in male master cyclists and nonathletes. *J Strength Cond Res* 2011;25(3):727–734.

3 Rehabilitation of Athletes After Spine Injury and Spine Surgery

Robert G. Watkins IV, MD • Michael Kordecki, DPT, SCS, ATC

INTRODUCTION

Return to activity after spinal injury, with or without surgery, mainly depends on a proper rehabilitation program. Whether the patient is a professional athlete, recreational athlete, or injured worker, the goal is the same: restore normal movement patterns and strength to the hips, legs, and spine, which will allow restoration of the highest level of function with the least amount of pain. To accomplish this goal, the physician, patient, physical therapist, and employer all have to work in coordination. A structured and graduated rehabilitation program allows all concerned parties to monitor and guide recovery.

LUMBAR SPINE

Evaluation

The first step in recovery after a spinal injury or surgery is to determine the "root cause" of the problem. Often spinal injuries are the result of years of poor movement patterns. Many patients present with similar patterns of movements and postures that, left uncorrected, will not only lead to acute injuries but will also cause chronic pain and deterioration of the lumbar spine.[1,2]

A history and comprehensive physical examination are the first steps in addressing the "root cause." The history is used to help determine whether the problem is acute or long term. If the patient complains of back pain

---

Dr. Kordecki or an immediate family member is an employee of Abbvie; and has stock or stock options held in Abbvie. Dr. Watkins IV or an immediate family member has received royalties from Aesculap/B. Braun, Amedica, Medtronic Sofamor Danek, and Pioneer; is a member of a speakers' bureau or has made paid presentations on behalf of Aesculap/B. Braun and Medtronic Sofamor Danek; and serves as a paid consultant to Aesculap/B. Braun, Amedica, and Medtronic Sofamor Danek.

that is more local to a specific area, a facet joint could be the problem. If a patient complains of pain that is more "beltlike," the problem could be more muscular in nature. If the patient complains of leg, buttock, or thigh pain that "shoots or radiates," the problem is more likely to involve the neurologic structures of the spine. If the patient wakes up in the morning feeling stiff and sore and the pain is alleviated with movement, it is more likely to be muscular or arthritic in origin. Conversely, if a patient wakes up feeling better and experiences more pain as the day goes by, especially in the buttocks and legs, the pain is usually neurogenic in nature.

The physical examination is used to evaluate the patient's movement patterns. Basic biomechanics dictate human beings are designed to ambulate and move primarily from the hips, knees, and ankles rather than the lumbar spine. The spine is meant for cushioning, shock absorption, and stability. In many cases, because of rapid growth in the younger population or lack of general exercise in older patients, the hip flexors and hamstrings become tight. The gluteal muscles and abdominal muscles become weak, and the individual loses the ability to move normally. When this happens, hip, knee, and ankle motion are limited, and the spine is forced into a resting position of hyperextension (**Figure 3-1**). As this occurs, hip motion is substituted by excessive motion at the lumbar spine, which puts significant pressure on the facet joints and disks, leading to facet and disk pathology. A simple gait analysis will reveal typical patterns seen in patients with low back pathology. They often demonstrate loss of true heel strike caused by a tight gastroc and soleus. The legs are externally rotated because of tight hip flexors and rotators and weakness in the gluteal muscles. The patients pull themselves along using the hamstrings rather than pushing themselves forward by using the gluteal muscles and extending the hips. The pelvis is maintained in an anterior tilt because of a lack of abdominal strength, tight hip flexors, and weak gluteal muscles. In turn, the lumbar spine is

---

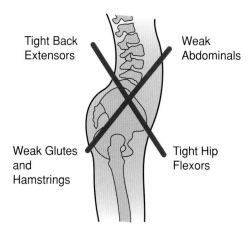

FIGURE 3-1 Improper pelvic position.

in a position of extreme hyperextension, locking the facet joints and overloading the posterior aspect of the disk.

Range of motion (ROM) measurements are taken to determine the patient's basic flexibility. When assessing flexibility, care must be taken to maintain a neutral spine throughout the examination. A modified straight-leg raise is used to test the hamstrings. Results greater than 15° of short of neutral indicates a positive test result. The quadriceps are compared from a supine position (heel to buttock) to a prone position. Any discrepancies between the two positions indicates tightness in the quadriceps. The patient's hip flexors should be assessed using the Thomas test. Motion less than 5° below neutral is indicative of a positive test result. The hip rotators and piriformis are tested in supine with the hip flexed to 50° to determine their length. Normally, the hip should rotate at least 30° and adduct 40° for a normal test result. The Obers test is performed in the sidelying position to test the length of the iliotibial band and tensor fascia latae. Normally, the hip should adduct to 45° with the knee straight without rotating the spine.

The next step in the physical examination is the manual muscle test. Close attention should be paid to the strength of the hip flexors, gluteal muscles, hamstrings, and abdominals. The gluteal muscles should be tested as both hip external rotators and hip extensors.

Rehabilitation

The rehabilitation program is a system of exercises that produces functional movement patterns and coordinated core strength for the hips, abdominal muscles, and low back muscles. Athletic functions such as throwing, swinging, and lifting, as well as activities of daily living require normal movement patterns and coordinated muscle strength to achieve maximum performance while protecting the spine. Lumbar spine rehabilitation begins

with establishment of pain-free neutral position. Balance and coordination are added into the program with endurance exercises. By building endurance strength centered on a neutral pain-free position, postinjury and postsurgical rehabilitation can begin relatively early because it avoids extreme and painful ROMs.

The rehabilitation program is a five-level program that gradually increases in strength, endurance, and proprioceptive demands (**Table 3-1**, on page 24). Level 1 starts in a neutral pain-free position with specific stretching exercises for the legs and hips and isometric exercises that train the core muscles to protect the spine (**Figure 3-2**). In the acute postoperative period, motion through the spine can cause mechanical trauma and exacerbate symptoms. Patients are taught to strictly maintain a neutral pain-free position while performing the basic stretching and core stabilization exercises (**Figure 3-3**).[1] The program accelerates to increasing intensity and compromised positions with balance and coordination

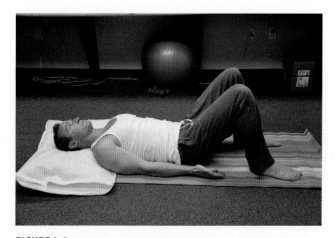

FIGURE 3-2 Neutral pain-free spine position.

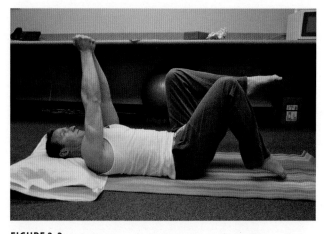

FIGURE 3-3 Maintain neutral pain-free spine position while moving the arms, legs, or both.

Dead Bug	Partial Sit-Ups	Bridging	Prone	Quadriped	Wall Slide	Ball	Aerobic	Sports
A	B	C	D	E	F	G	H	
1. Supported arms, marching legs, 2 min or supported legs, extended arms, 2 min	Forward, hands on chest, 10 reps	Double-leg supported, 2 sets × 10 reps	Alternating arm or leg lifts, 1 set × 10 reps, hold 2 sec	Alternate arm or leg, 1 set × 10 reps, hold 2 sec. Each side	45°, 10 reps, hold 5 sec	Double supported leg press, arms at side, 10 reps, hold 2 sec	Walk: land or water	None
2. Unsupported, alternate opposite arms and legs, 3 min	Forward, hands on chest, 3 sets × 10 reps	Double-leg supported, 2 sets × 20 reps. May add weights to hips	Alternating opposite arm and leg lifts, 2 sets × 10 reps, hold 5 sec. Each side	Alternating opposite arm and leg, 2 sets × 10 reps, hold 5 sec. Each side	90°, 10 reps × 20 sec	Double supported leg press, arms overhead, 10 reps, hold 2 sec	10–20 min: walk, bike, elliptical, swim	Rotator cuff exercises, scapular stabilization, light throw, flat foot shoot, skate
3. Unsupported, alternate opposite arms and legs 7 min	Forward, right, left, 3 sets × 10 reps	Single-leg supported, alternate opposite leg extended, 3 sets × 20 reps, each side. May add weight	On ball, flys, swim, supermans, 2 sets × 20 reps, hold 5 sec	Alternating opposite arm and leg, 2 sets × 20 reps, hold 5 sec, each side. May add weights	90°, 10 reps × 30 sec. Lunges 1 min	Arms on chest, ball sit-ups, 20 reps, hold 2 sec: forward, right, left	20–30 min: run, bike, Elliptical, swim	Rotational exercises, swinging, shooting, throwing, striding on field. Weight room (protected)
4. Unsupported, alternate opposite arms and legs, 10 min. May add weights	Weight on chest: forward, right, left, 3 sets × 20 reps	On ball, single-leg extended, 4 sets × 20 reps, each side. May add weight	On ball, flys, swim, supermans with weights, 2 sets × 20 reps, hold 5 sec. Walkout/pushups 3 sets × 5 reps	Alternating opposite arm and leg, 3 sets × 20 reps, hold 5 sec, with weights	90°, weights at side, 10 reps × 30 sec. Lunges with weights at side 3 min	Weight on chest, ball sit-ups, 30 reps, hold 5 sec: forward, right, left	45 min: run, bike, elliptical, swim	Sport-specific exercises, short sprints, cutting, practice with team
5. Unsupported, alternate opposite arms and legs, 15 min. May add weights	Weights overhead: forward, right, left, 3 sets × 30 reps	On ball, single-leg extended, 5 sets × 20 reps, each side. May add weight	On ball, flys, swim, supermans with weights, 4 sets × 20 reps, hold 5 sec. Walkout/pushups 4 sets × 10 reps	Alternating opposite arm and leg, 3 sets × 20 reps, hold 15 sec, with weights	90°, weights with arms extended, 10 reps × 30 sec. Lunges with weights in front 5 min	Weight in extended arms, 30 reps, hold 5 sec: forward, right, left. May add pulleys, weighted stick	60 min: run, bike, elliptical, swim	Gradual return to sport

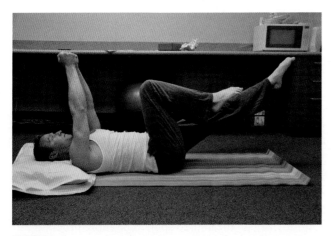

FIGURE 3-4 Increasing difficulty while maintaining a neutral spine.

exercises as long as the patient is able to maintain a pain-free state (**Figure 3-4**). If a particular exercise exacerbates symptoms, then exercise is modified, decreased, or discontinued.

Almost every postoperative patient is encouraged to ambulate immediately after surgery. The goal is to walk several times a day for a comfortable distance. Postsurgical rehabilitation is initiated when soft tissues have adequately healed, symptoms have sufficiently stabilized, and the stability of the anatomic structures is acceptable. Typically, a physical therapy program that focuses on a stretching program with a neutral spine can be started 2 to 4 weeks after a single level lumbar laminotomy or discectomy, 6 to 8 weeks after a multilevel laminotomy or laminectomy, 6 to 8 weeks after an artificial disk replacement, and 6 to 12 weeks after a fusion. Restoring normal mobility in the ankles, knees and hips while maintaining a neutral spine will help reduce mechanical stress from the bony and muscular structures of the lumbar spine. This in turn will help reduce pain and improve function in a timely manner.[3]

The stretching portion of the program can begin as soon as the surgical incisions are healed, typically 14 to 21 days after surgery. The stretching exercises are all performed in a neutral spine position slowly and deliberately without pain to protect the healing tissue. Each stretch is held for 10 full seconds and repeated 7 to 10 times twice day. The stretching portion of the program will be maintained throughout the entire rehabilitation process and continue after discharge.

To properly stretch the muscles of calf, the stretch is performed in the standing position without shoes. Care is taken so the lumbar spine is not allowed to fall into a position of hyperextension. The patient stands with his or her hands on the wall and slowly bends at the elbows and ankles while the heels stay firmly planted on the ground.

This ensures that the motion takes place at the ankle and not the arch of foot. The spine stays neutral throughout.

Stretching the hamstrings is done in supine. Performing the stretch in supine keeping the contralateral leg flat on the ground ensures the proper position of the pelvis in a neutral position. The stretch can be performed through a doorway or on a post (**Figure 3-5**). The leg being stretched is gently extended until a slight tension is felt in the hamstring and the knee is in full extension. If the knee cannot extend fully or the contralateral leg comes off the ground, the patient is too close and must back away to proper position. Attempting to stretch the hamstrings in standing or long sitting will only cause excessive flexion in the lumbar spine, placing stress on the disks and spinal extensors (**Figure 3-6**).

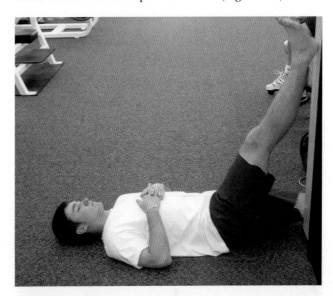

FIGURE 3-5 Proper hamstrings stretch.

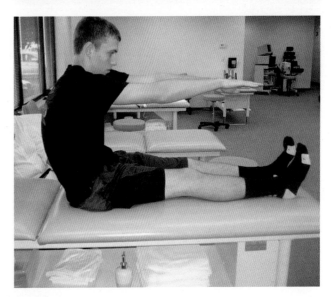

FIGURE 3-6 Improper hamstrings stretch.

Stretching the quadriceps should initially be done in the prone position with a firm pillow under the pelvis to help maintain a neutral spine (**Figure 3-7**). The heel is gently pulled toward the buttock until a gentle stretch is felt in the front of thigh.

The hip flexor stretch is performed in the high-kneeling position (**Figure 3-8**). The patient shifts his or her weight forward and tightens the buttock muscle of the leg being stretched. The shoulders and the pelvis move together as the stretch is performed, moving the hip toward extension. Care must be taken to maintain the lumbar spine in a neutral position throughout the exercise. Using the high-kneeling position and hyperextending the spine by throwing the shoulders back will only lock the facet joints and place unwanted stress on the healing tissues (**Figure 3-9**).

In testing of professional golfers, Major League baseball players, and other athletes, it has been well demonstrated that the coordination of trunk muscles produces maximum control of the spine.[4] Coordinated strength is more effective than uncoordinated strength. Each of the trunk muscles fires in an exact sequence in relation to each other for particular actions. This coordinated strength protects the spine from injury and produces the desired athletic result. The trunk stabilization program is a five-level strength and conditioning program. The patient or athlete progresses through eight different exercises rated 1 through 5 in difficulty. The entire program starts with finding a neutral pain-free position for the spine and strictly holding it in that position while performing the exercises. This makes it possible to begin postoperative conditioning earlier because it avoids the extremes of motion through the injured spine. The entire program can be performed with relatively simple exercise equipment: exercise balls, hand weights, and pulleys (**Figure 3-10**).

The rehabilitation of an injured athlete begins with level 1 core stabilization training. The key is to learn the proper technique. Proper technique is simply maintaining

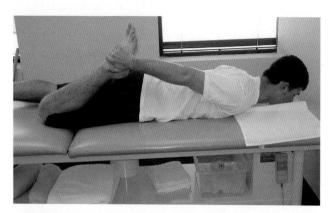

FIGURE 3-7 Prone quadriceps stretch.

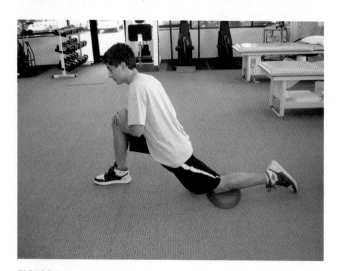

FIGURE 3-8 Proper hip flexor stretch.

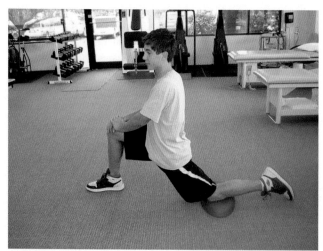

FIGURE 3-9 Improper hip flexor stretch.

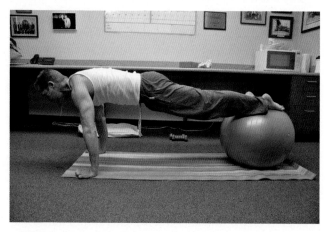

FIGURE 3-10 Neutral spine while doing a plank on an exercise ball.

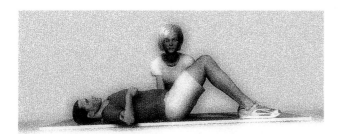

FIGURE 3-11 Pelvic tilt to maintain a neutral spine.

the neutral spine position. This is accomplished using the pelvic tilt maneuver (**Figure 3-11**). By properly tilting the pelvis using the abdominal and gluteal muscles, the patient places the lumbar spine in a neutral position. After the patient learns the neutral position, he or she is taught to maintain this position while performing all levels of the rehabilitation program.

A proper pelvic tilt has three components. First and foremost, the abdominal muscles must fire correctly. Most patients have a tendency to attempt to fire the abdominals using the "draw-in" maneuver (DIM). It has been shown that the DIM is a very poor technique used to establish abdominal control. With the DIM, the patient is actually elevating the rib cage away from the pelvis and stretching the rectus abdominis rather than causing a contraction. The transverse abdominis and oblique muscles do very little. A correct technique to engage the entire abdominal muscle group is called the abdominal bracing technique (ABT). Using the ABT creates a pushing-out maneuver that draws the pelvis up toward the rib cage using the rectus abdominis and transverse abdominis as well as the internal and external oblique groups.[5] The second component and the third component occur together. The gluteal muscles fire, and the pelvis tips in a posterior direction. By performing the pelvis tilt correctly, the lumbar spine is held in a neutral position.

After the patient demonstrates the ability to perform and hold a proper tilt, the exercises can begin. No movement of the spine is allowed. By doing this, the patient will not only avoid exacerbations in the early postoperative period but will also develop proper timing through proprioceptive feedback of the core muscles. The goals during both the stretching and strengthening phases include stability through the spine, going slow, and deliberate execution with all levels of exercise. Feedback ensuring no motion of the spine is critical. At first feedback is tactile and eventually becomes internal as the patient advances to higher levels. It is not a matter of brute strength; instead, it is a matter of doing the technique properly.

When the athlete has established proper technique at level 1 of the program, he or she is advanced through the five levels of increasing difficulty. The trunk stabilization program is categorized into levels, which helps the patient, therapist, trainer, doctor, and so on stay on the same page in regards to return to activity. Level 1 consists of establishing neutral pain-free position. Upon completing level 2, most patients can return to low-impact exercises such as bicycle, elliptical, and swimming. After level 3, most patients can return to running, skating, soft-toss throwing, and shooting. Competitive athletes should complete level 4 before returning to sport-specific exercises that involve significant force and extremes of motion. Professional athletes should maintain level 5 before and during return to play (RTP). RTP depends on:

1. Achieving the proper level of the stabilization program; for recreational golfers and tennis players, it is level 3; for professional athletes, it is level 5
2. Obtaining good aerobic conditioning; the key to aerobic conditioning is to diversify the aerobic exercise
3. Performing sports-specific exercises
4. Returning slowly to the sport
5. Continuing the stabilization exercise after the athlete returns to sport

The trunk stabilization program has been divided into five levels of eight categories (see Table 3-1). The graduated nature of this exercise program allows a patient to go from a neutral, pain-free position for the spine in a very safe, controlled position to very advanced strengthening exercises conducted in a somewhat precarious position, requiring balance and coordination. The therapist's objective is to teach the patient how to do the exercises correctly. Regardless of how advanced the exercise, strict spine stability must be maintained. Often a patient with advance faster in one category than another category. Patients may be doing the level 3 in dead bug exercises yet only level 2 in prone exercises. The therapist will advance the patient quicker in some exercises as long as the patient is able to perform the specific exercise correctly without pain.

For example, in category A, the sit-ups are done with the feet on the floor; the back in the neutral, pain-free position and the arms clasped across the chest. Then with an elevation of the head and back, the patient performs a slight hold and then returns to neutral position (**Figure 3-12**). The exercise is then progressively increased, adding weights to the chest and then finally with arms extended forward. There is no need to fully sit up; the patient should just lift until the shoulder blades are off the mat.

The bridging exercises are done by lifting the pelvis off the floor while strictly maintaining the neutral,

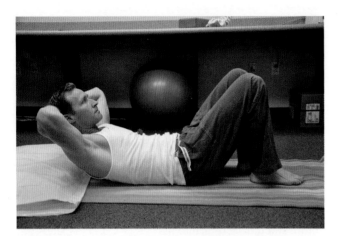

FIGURE 3-12 Partial sit-up returning to a neutral lumbar spine.

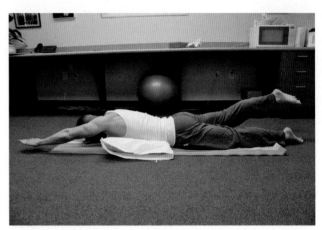

FIGURE 3-14 Prone exercise while not hyperextending the spine.

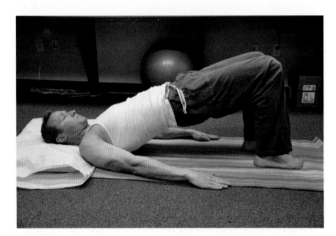

FIGURE 3-13 Bridging while maintaining a neutral lumbar spine.

movements into lumbar extension (**Figure 3-14**). Alternate arm and leg extensions require good trunk control to prevent hyperextension.

Ball exercises provide a platform that requires higher levels of coordination and proprioceptive control to maintain strict stability. Initially, the therapist may need to provide tactile feedback to achieve this. The leg press begins with just a simple balancing exercise, rolling on the ball, and maintaining control of the ball throughout the motions. Prone exercises of supermans, swimming and shoulder abduction challenge the abdominals and gluteals to prevent hyperextension (**Figure 3-15**). Prayer exercises and push-ups demand upper abdominal control to maintain stability. Applying resistive forces with batons increases the challenges in all planes of motion. Always start slow to ensure a stable spine position.

The wall slide exercises can begin with a gentle flexion of the knees and with no real lower extremity or back strain. This is an easy exercise, initially, that can be begun in the immediate postoperative period. Quadriceps

pain-free position (**Figure 3-13**). The lifting is done primarily with the legs and muscles of the core. The core muscles stabilize the low back and abdominal region. The pelvis remains in a neutral position.[6,7] The back is not arched into a hyperextended position. Hyperextending the lumbar spine locks the facet joints while putting the spine extensors and abdominal muscles in a mechanically insufficient position. Pain with this maneuver is often produced by loss of control of pelvis, allowing it to tilt in an anterior position, causing hyperextension in the lumbar spine. If the maneuver is done properly, the patient will use the gluteal hamstrings and muscles of the core to stabilize the pelvis and back.[8] Holding this bridged position helps isolate trunk musculature in a different fashion than the dead bug exercises. This is progressed through a one leg bridge on the ball and weights may be added to the trunk and extended legs.

Exercises done in the prone position challenge the ability to strictly maintain the neutral position. Initially, a cushion under the stomach can assist avoiding

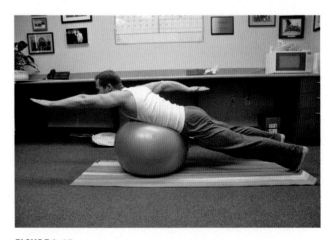

FIGURE 3-15 Supermans while not hyperextending the spine.

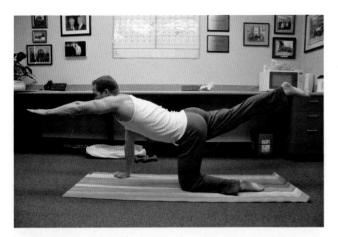

FIGURE 3-16 Quadruped exercises while maintaining a neutral spine.

strength is directly proportional to the ability to work in a bent forward position in a lifting job, and most important, the quadriceps exercises are a reflection of the ability of a patient to use the legs for bending and lifting rather than the back. Patients with weak quads and tightness of the hamstrings and calf muscles lock their knees and bend at the waist, which is exactly the opposite of what we want for a patient with back pain. The wall slide progresses through a full 90°, with longer periods of holding. The addition of weights and extended arms increase the difficulty of the maneuver. The transition from the initial stage of identifying neutral position and maintaining that proceeds through a series of unsupported arm and leg motion exercises. Actively having the patient activate the abdominals and gluteals to maintain neutral spine position enhances quadriceps function and provides desired closed chain proprioceptive feedback.

Quadruped positions offer unique challenges in that there is less tactile feedback (**Figure 3-16**). The patient needs to develop better internal proprioceptive feedback mechanisms to strictly maintain the neutral spine position. The patient must learn to hold this position while progressing from more simple leg or arm lifts to alternate arm and leg lifts without and then with weights. Use of a stick lying across the pelvis will give feedback if lost position occurs on the frontal or transverse plane; however, feedback in the sagittal plane must be monitored internally by the patient or assisted by therapist hand feedback.

Aerobic exercise is important for general conditioning. Choosing the right type of exercise is important. An effective strategy is diversification. Those who rely only on running or jogging may be predisposed to strains and sprains. Pool walking is an excellent solution for many patients and can commence as soon as 3 weeks postoperatively. More complex and sophisticated types of aerobic

conditioning must be approached carefully. Nordic Track and swimming for untrained patients can result in an exacerbation of their condition. A diversified approach to aerobic conditioning is less likely to produce overuse syndromes. Be aware of proper technique and make sure equipment is fitted appropriately. With the VersaClimber and stepmasters, the key is to have the appropriate height step. We use the VersaClimber with a very narrow step. The aerobic conditioning is there without getting the pelvic tilting that you get with too high of a step. The same is true with the Exercycle. The seat should be low enough that the feet are not reaching down for the pedals, producing rocking of the pelvis on the seat. Running is a stiffening exercise, prone to development of contractures and weaknesses in isolated areas that are not used. If running technique is poor, the likelihood of compensatory dysfunction is high. Taking time to review running technique is worthwhile. Skipping rope is an excellent technique for trunk strength. The slight bent forward flexion posture, locking the back in a neutral position, and maintaining trunk control while producing the aerobic exercise can produce very tight trunk control while getting aerobic conditioning.

Key to the program is strictly maintaining the neutral position with all exercises. Not allowing spine motion will not only limit pain and injury; more importantly, it will develop the coordinated firing patterns of core muscles. The exercises challenge the patient in different planes of motion, including the anterior and posterior sagittal plane, right and left frontal plane, and right and left transverse plane. If a patient has difficulty in with a certain exercise, category determine what plane of motion is the suspect. This will help direct the stabilization progression. Core strengthening is neurologic retraining as much as it is physiological strengthening. Precise application will enhance results.

● CERVICAL SPINE

Rehabilitation is initiated after the pain has improved. Trunk stabilization and chest-out posture exercises can be performed without increasing intradiscal pressure. These exercises reinforce ideal posture, thereby increasing intervertebral foraminal height and decreasing the weight of the head.

Return to play after cervical spine surgery depends on healing of the surgical structures, neurologic recovery, and rehabilitation. A foraminotomy for posterior foraminal stenosis has the least significant anatomic structures to heal. The cervical muscles and facet capsule may heal in 6 weeks. A posterior discectomy probably will take longer for the annular defect to heal, approximately 8 to 12 weeks. A fusion typically takes 3 to 6 months to heal. The time for the surgical structures to heal does not equal RTP. The athlete must complete a well-organized rehabilitation and sport-specific program before RTP.

When the postoperative pain has subsided (typically 4–6 weeks), physical therapy and rehabilitation begin. To eliminate a rounded shoulder, forward head posture. One of the goals of rehabilitation is to create a neutral cervical spine. To accomplish this goal, the lumbar spine and thoracic spine should be rehabilitated back to a neutral position in an effort to allow as much normal function as possible in the neck. A lumbar spine that is stuck in hyperextension will force more kyphosis in the thoracic spine, which in turn creates excessive hyperextension (lordosis) in the cervical spine. Excessive kyphosis is brought about by excessive tightness across the chest and weakness in the parascapular muscles.[9] Exercises that stretch the chest can be done in the standing position. While the patient uses a doorway, the shoulders are held at 90° of abduction and 90° of external rotation (**Figure 3-17**). The patient then performs a pelvic tilt and while keeping the spine neutral slowly walks forward to stretch the chest and

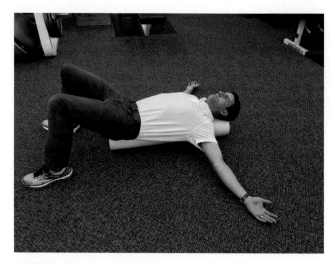

FIGURE 3-18 Foam roller stretch.

pectoralis minor. A more advanced exercise can be done in the supine position over a foam roller (**Figure 3-18**). Specific strength exercises that target the rhomboids, middle trapezius, and latissimus are critical elements in restoring scapular position.[10] Proper scapular position in turn improves the inclination of the thoracic spine.[9] A neutral thoracic spine allows the cervical spine to realign itself with the help of some isometrics. Rehabilitation at this stage focuses on proper performance of the strength exercises. Patients who demonstrate scapular weakness often have a difficult time moving the scapula to the retracted position properly. Often a patient will create retraction in the scapula by extending the shoulder. Extending the shoulder causes the humerus to push the scapula back toward the spine. If this occurs, the muscles of scapular retraction do not engage and therefore will remain weak. When done properly, the scapular moves *first* followed by movement of the arm. The most basic scapular exercise is the "scapula set." The scapular set can be done in standing and then progressed to the sidelying position and finally prone. The patient is taught to properly retract the shoulder blades without moving the humerus in the glenoid. A more advanced exercise can be done in standing using exercise bands to provide resistance to the motion of scapular retraction and shoulder extension. If this exercise is done properly the scapula will move first to the fully retracted position, and then the shoulder will move secondarily.

After proper scapular control is established, common exercises such as "Y's" and "T's" can also be used to strengthen the parascapular muscles (**Figures 3-19** and **3-20**).[11] When done correctly, these exercises also help strengthen the extensor muscles of the cervical and thoracic spine. "Y's" and "T's" can be done first in the prone

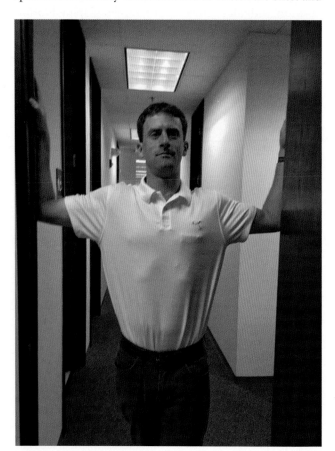

FIGURE 3-17 Doorway stretch.

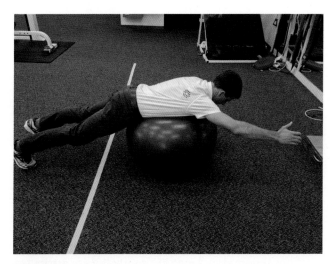

FIGURE 3-19 Prone scapular exercise "y."

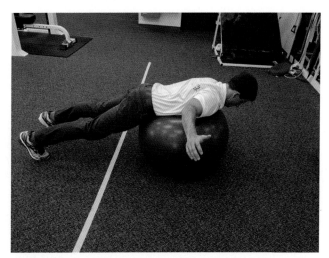

FIGURE 3-20 Prone scapular exercise "t."

position with a pillow under the thorax while the patient performs a pelvic tilt. Using this position keeps the cervical spine from being forced into hyperextension while at the same time allowing the scapula to move against gravity carrying the weight of the arm as resistance. "Y's" and "T's" can be progressed to the prone position over an exercise ball as long as the patient is pain free and can perform the exercises correctly.

The athlete must establish neutral spine stabilization before progressing to balance and coordination exercises. Sport-specific exercises are gradually introduced as long as the athlete remains asymptomatic.

● KEY POINTS

- A systematic and comprehensive rehabilitation program is essential to return athletes to a high level of function.
- The lumbar rehabilitation program is a system of exercises that produces functional movement patterns and coordinated core strength for the hips, abdominal muscles, and low back muscles.
- Cervical spine rehabilitation consists of chest-out posture exercises that decrease the effective weight of the head, open intervertebral foramen, and open thoracic outlet.

REFERENCES

1. Granata KP, Marras WS: Cost–benefit of muscle co-contraction in protecting against spinal instability. *Spine* 2000;25:1398–1404.

2. Hodges PW, Richardson CA: Inefficient muscular stabilization of the lumbar spine associated with low back pain. A motor control evaluation of transversus abdominis. *Spine (Phila Pa 1976)* 1996 Nov 15;21(22):2640–50.

3. Vezina MJ, Hubley-Kozey CL: Muscle activation in therapeutic exercises to improve trunk stability. *Arch Phys Med Rehabil* 2000;81:1370–1379.

4. Watkins RG, Uppal GS Perry J, et al: Dynamic electromyographic analysis of trunk musculature in professional golfers. *Am J Sports Med* 1996;24(4):535–538.

5. Gardner-Morse MG, Stokes IA: The effects of abdominal muscle coactivation on lumbar spine stability. *Spine* 1998;23:86–91.

6. Cholewicki J, VanVliet JJ: Relative contribution of trunk muscles to the stability of the lumbar spine during isometric exertions. *Clin Biomech* 2002;17(2):99–105.

7. Vera-Garcia FJ, Elvira JL, Brown SH, McGill SM: Effects of abdominal stabilization maneuvers on the control of spine motion and stability against sudden trunk perturbations. *J Electromyogr Kinesiol* 2007;17: 556–567.

8. McGill SM, Grenier S, Kavcic N, Cholewicki J: Coordination of muscle activity to assure stability of the lumbar spine. *J Electromyogr Kinesiol* 2003;13(4):353–359.

9. Wang CH, McClure P, Pratt NE, Nobilini R: Stretching and strengthening exercises: Their effect on the three-dimensional scapular kinematics. *Arch Phys Med Rehabil* 1999;80(8):923–929.

10. Kibler W, Sciascia A, Wilkes T: Scapular dyskinesis and its relation to shoulder injury. *J Am Acad Orthop Surg* 2012; 20:364–372.

11. Cools AM, Dewitte V, Lanszweert F, et al: Rehabilitation of scapular muscle balance. *Am J Sports Med* 2007;35: 1744–1751.

4 On-Field Evaluation and Transport of the Injured Athlete

Tristan B. Weir, BS • Michael J. Cendoma, MS, ATC • Ehsan Jazini, MD • Kelley E. Banagan, MD • Steven C. Ludwig, MD

INTRODUCTION

According to the National Spinal Cord Injury Statistical Center, sports-related injuries ranked fourth behind vehicular accidents, falls, and violence as the most common causes of spinal cord injury (SCI). Sporting activities accounted for 7.93% of the 4628 cases admitted to sites contributing to the database from September 2005 to May 2012.[1] Although the thoracolumbar spine is susceptible to injury during sports, the focus remains on the cervical spine because of the higher injury incidence and more profound morbidity. All of the 223 SCIs reported in American football between 1977 and 2001 involved the cervical spine.[2]

American football is associated with the greatest number of catastrophic cervical spine injuries for all sports in the United States.[3] Generally, catastrophic cervical spine injuries in American football have declined since the early 1970s. The NATA reports that an average of 7.8 catastrophic cervical spine injuries resulting in incomplete recovery and 6 resulting in quadriplegia were reported in American football between 1997 and 2006.[4] Alarmingly, double-digit catastrophic cervical spine injuries were reported during three of the four years between 2003 and 2006; only 1999 showed double-digit numbers between 1991 and 2002. As recent as 2015, 14.3% of the direct fatalities reported in American football were attributed to cervical spine fracture.[5]

The risk of catastrophic cervical spine injury in other sports has also been reported. Although American football is associated with the greatest number of catastrophic cervical spine injuries, the incidence of nonfatal, direct catastrophic injuries in ice hockey, lacrosse, men's hockey, and gymnastics is higher than in American football.[3,4]

Although severe catastrophic spine injuries are rare in sports, their profound morbidity demands a systematic protocol for injury prevention. On-field stabilization and transport of the injured athlete is essential to minimize or prevent further injury and requires a well-practiced and team-based approach. Sport-specific regulations and proper coaching aid in the primary prevention of SCI, but the initial management of such events begins with preseason planning by the team physician, athletic trainer, and emergency medical services (EMS).[6] This chapter provides an overview of prevention measures, pregame planning, on-field assessment, stabilization and transfer

Dr. Banagan or an immediate family member is an employee of Johnson & Johnson; and has received nonincome support (such as equipment or services), commercially derived honoraria, or other non-research–related funding (such as paid travel) from Orthofix. Dr. Ludwig or an immediate family member has received royalties from DePuy, a Johnson & Johnson Company; is a member of a speakers' bureau or has made paid presentations on behalf of DePuy, a Johnson & Johnson Company, and Synthes; serves as a paid consultant to DePuy, a Johnson & Johnson Company, Globus Medical, K2Medical, and Synthes; has stock or stock options held in ASIP, ISD; has received research or institutional support from AO Spine North America Spine Fellowship Support,

Globus Medical, K2M Spine, OMEGA, and Pacira; has received nonincome support (such as equipment or services), commercially derived honoraria, or other non-research– related funding (such as paid travel) from Thieme, QMP; and serves as a board member, owner, officer, or committee member of the American Board of Orthopaedic Surgery, the American Orthopaedic Association, the Cervical Spine Research Society, the Journal of Spinal Disorders and Techniques, *and Smiss. Neither of the following authors nor any immediate family member has received anything of value from or has stock or stock options held in a commercial company or institution related directly or indirectly to the subject of this article: Dr. Jazini and Dr. Weir.*

techniques, and equipment management concepts that medical personnel should consider when developing an emergency action plan and on-field response protocols for the potentially spine-injured athlete (Video 4-1).

● PREVENTION: RULES, TECHNIQUES, AND EDUCATION

The on-field management of SCI begins by preventing the injury from occurring. Primary prevention of SCI in athletes consists of implementing and enforcing rules, teaching proper technique, and educating athletes and coaches in concepts that promote safety. This is especially important for football and ice hockey because they are the team sports associated with a greater risk of SCI.[2]

In 1976, an upward trend of fatalities from head and neck trauma in American football led the National Operating Committee on Standards for Athletic Equipment to ban spearing, or using the head as the initial point of contact during blocks and tackles.[1,6] Spearing can result in cervical injury through axial loading and cervical flexion.[7] In the seasons following the implementation of rules regarding spearing, there was a dramatic decrease in permanent cervical spine injuries, from 20 cases per year before 1976 to only 7.2 cases per year in the 1990s.[2] However, recent studies show that the incidence of spearing remains high despite implementation of rules banning spearing. Some have argued that rule changes regarding spearing would be more effective at reducing the incidence of spearing if properly enforced.

Educating players, coaches, and officials regarding the rationale for rules regarding spearing and the consequences of such technique is a vital component of any effective prevention program. Educating players and coaches in proper tackling techniques that do not place the head and neck in danger of injury is also a vital component of an effective injury prevention program. The combination of enacting and enforcing appropriate rules and educating players, coaches, and officials is attributed to a reduction in the number of permanent cervical injuries.[7]

Ice hockey has implemented similar guidelines to help reduce the incidence of cervical spine injuries, including penalties for checking players from behind. Checking does not allow players to adequately protect themselves and may lead to head-on collisions against the rink wall.[8] Education of young players helps to prevent such dangerous occurrences. Studies from the 1980s clearly illustrate a gap in education of youth hockey players because players were unaware of the consequences of checking from behind or leading a check with their head.[8] The Safety Towards Other Players (STOP) Patch Program requires youth hockey players to wear a STOP symbol on the back of their jerseys as a reminder to avoid checking from behind. Educational programs, along with regulation changes, have a proven track record of promoting player safety and should be continued.[9]

● PREGAME PLANNING

Preparation for cervical trauma in the athlete begins in the offseason by creating and practicing a cervical trauma protocol, obtaining the equipment needed for the protocol, and identifying a hospital that can continue the athlete's care after an injury has occurred. The protocol must be tailored to the specific sport by accounting for variables related to that activity, including the surface of play and the equipment worn by the athletes. It is very important for athletic programs to have an Emergency Action Plan (EAP) developed in conjunction with local EMS.[10]

The team medical personnel should become familiar with the type of equipment worn by the players each season because new models of gear may require different tools and techniques to remove padding in the event of an accident. The tools typically required for running a cervical trauma protocol include instruments for neurologic testing, a back board, a cervical collar, tools for removing the athlete's protective gear, and advanced airway supplies.[11]

If an athlete sustains an on-field injury, the team physician or athletic trainer typically leads the cervical spine protocol while the other members of the rescue team follow the leader's commands. The leader should encourage rehearsals with the rescue team at least annually, and each member of the medical team should be versed in her or his role in the protocol.[12] Before each sporting event, the medical team should take inventory of their equipment and review the spine trauma protocol.[7] This is essential when working with new members from the medical staff because there are variations in protocol from team to team. Communication between the EMS and the rescue team promotes a smooth transition from on-field management to the athlete's transport to a preplanned hospital that can definitively manage the athlete's injuries.[7] Controversy still exists surrounding the timing of definitive treatment for cervical trauma, but the receiving hospital should be able to perform the needed treatment with an available neurosurgeon or orthopaedic spine surgeon.[13,14] Additionally, the athlete's emergency contact information should be updated yearly and be easily accessible on the field in the event that a player sustains an injury during a game or practice.[11] Sports medicine teams should conduct a "time out" before each athletic event to review of items mentioned earlier to ensure familiarity with medical staff, athletic trainers, EMS, and each team.

● INITIAL ASSESSMENT: ON THE FIELD

The initial assessment of the athlete begins with on field attentiveness, and the medical staff observing the mechanism of injury (i.e., "spear tackling" or "checking"). Extremity movement and vocalization can be assessed from a distance as the medical team approaches the injured athlete. Athletes with loss of consciousness or altered mental status are assumed to have a cervical spine injury until proven otherwise. For this reason, only the medical staff should be permitted to manipulate the athlete because excessive movement and jostling of the player can lead to primary or secondary injury of the cervical spine.[15] Considerable movement of the athlete

may result when equipment needs to be removed from the athlete. During management of an equipment-laden athlete, the medical team will need to consider the appropriateness and timing of equipment removal. This is a decision that each medical team will make while determining a course of action that promotes the safest handling of the injured athlete.

A standard emergency assessment of the athlete's airway, breathing, circulation, and neurologic function (disability) should be performed to identify any potentially life-threatening injuries, for which EMS must be contacted (Video 4-2).[16] Signs and symptoms that should prompt the rescue team to initiate the cervical spine injury protocol are loss of consciousness, altered mental status, bilateral neurologic symptoms, and focal spine pain or tenderness.[12] A low Glasgow Coma Scale score, especially at or below 8, is associated with cervical spine injury.[12,16] See **Figure 4-1** for an algorithm for the on-field assessment of the cervical spine in athletes.[17] After a cervical injury has been ruled out in a conscious athlete, specific symptoms should be elicited, and a physical examination is required, including a neurologic assessment.[16]

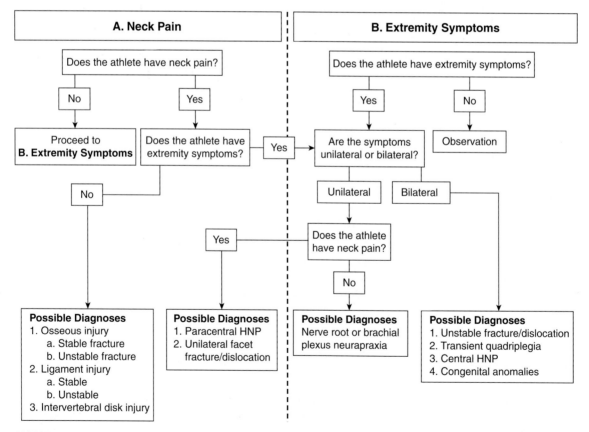

FIGURE 4-1 Algorithm for the on-field assessment of an athlete's cervical spine based on neck pain (**A**) or extremity symptoms (**B**). HNP = herniated nucleus pulposus. (Reprinted from Banerjee R, Palumbo MA, Fadale PD: Catastrophic cervical spine injuries in the collision sport athlete, part 1: Epidemiology, functional anatomy, and diagnosis. *Am J Sports Med* 2004;32(4):1077–1087.)

● STABILIZATION AND TRANSPORT OF THE ATHLETE

Neutral cervical stabilization should occur as soon as the rescue team recognizes a potential SCI (Video 4-3). In a supine athlete, the medical staff leader assumes a cephalad position and stabilizes the cervical spine by grasping the mastoid processes and cupping the palms over the occiput (**Figure 4-2**).[18] If the patient is wearing a helmet, the leader should stabilize the cervical spine in a similar fashion without removing the helmet. Applying traction to the head is not recommended because it may increase distraction and lead to secondary damage.[18] Sometimes the head must be moved to assume a neutral position. This is contraindicated only if moving the player's head causes increased pain, loss of neurologic function, or muscle spasm or if restricted motion is present.[12]

Assessing a prone player requires a "prone log roll technique" to return the athlete to the supine position. A minimum of four trained personnel familiar with the technique is recommended to roll the athlete—one each at the head, shoulders, hips, and legs. Larger bodies may require more rescuers to smoothly roll the player. If the head is turned to one side, the leader instructs the other three rescuers to line up on the side opposite to the face. The leader maintains a neutral position of the athlete's cervical spine and directs the rescuers to synchronously pull the athlete toward them. The leader uses a crossed-arm technique to maintain a neutral position of the cervical spine, resulting in uncrossed arms at the end of the log roll. The log roll should be delayed until a back board is available in the stable, conscious athlete. A fifth rescuer can slide a back board between the athlete and medical personnel at the midpoint of the roll, which accomplishes rolling and transferring in one movement of the athlete. This is important because each movement of the athlete can cause further neurologic injury. An unconscious, unstable athlete must be immediately rolled from prone to supine to assess the player's condition, regardless of the presence of a back board.[11]

Several potentially vital considerations must be assessed when examining the spine-injured athlete, such as impaired perfusion, ventilation, neurogenic shock, and cardiac shock. Impaired ventilation can arise from an upper airway obstruction caused by a foreign body, injury to the airway, or impaired consciousness. Alternatively, injury to the C3 to C5 region of the spinal cord can cause a loss of diaphragmatic motion and ventilation because the nerve roots that make up the phrenic nerve arise from this region of the spinal cord. When the player is in a supine position, assessing the athlete's cardiovascular

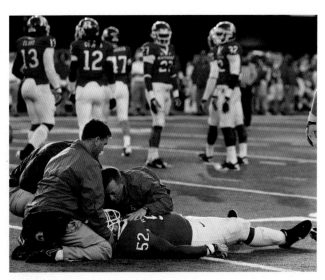

FIGURE 4-2 Eric LeGrand paralyzed from a spear tackle. (AP Photo.)

status is the first step in the protocol. If a loss of sympathetic tone is present, resulting in neurogenic shock, fluids and, occasionally, vasopressors will help stabilize the player. In the event of cardiac shock, the shoulder pads must be removed to expose the chest for cardiopulmonary resuscitation and defibrillation.[7] Commotio cordis is another life-threatening condition that requires prompt access to the athlete's chest for defibrillation and may occur in the setting of a cervical spine injury. This results from blunt trauma to the chest during ventricular repolarization, resulting in an R-on-T phenomenon and subsequent ventricular fibrillation.[19]

Gaining access to the airway without causing secondary damage is a top priority before respiratory compromise ensues.[7] While keeping the cervical spine in a neutral position, a jaw thrust helps prevent the tongue from obstructing the airway and should be initiated before the facemask is removed.[7,20,21] The jaw thrust is effective for most unconscious athletes, and a head tilt, chin lift is not typically recommended because this maneuver increases cervical spine movement and can cause further injury.[4,11,16,20] If the jaw thrust does not adequately open the airway, the helmet should be removed using the pack and fill method followed by a reattempt at a jaw thrust.[22] If this is still unsuccessful, check for obstruction and insert an airway adjunct. Foreign bodies, secretions, and vomitus can all obstruct the airway and should be removed to keep the airway patent.[7] Because of the risk of concomitant head trauma, nasopharyngeal airways should not be used for a suspected cervical spine injury.[21] When the airway is open, ventilator support with a portable barrier device or a bag valve mask may still be

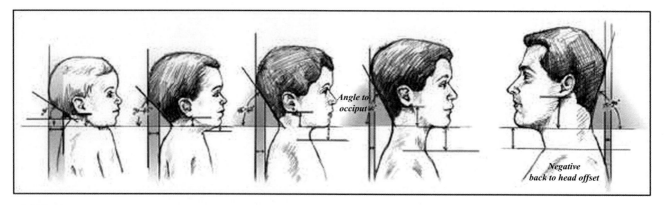

Angle to occiput

Negative back to head offset

FIGURE 4-3 Relationship between the occiput and shoulders. (Reprinted from Nemeth J: Case study: A new approach to stabilization of the cervical spine in infants. *The Academy Today* 2005;1:1.)

needed. If conservative airway measures fail, the most experienced member of the team may have to establish an advanced airway (laryngeal mask airway or endotracheal intubation). Some evidence suggests that advanced airways produce less cervical motion than a jaw thrust and are recommended when properly trained personnel are present.[4,20] If a cervical collar is in place before intubation, the anterior collar should be removed to allow for an enhanced ability to open the patient's mouth to allow for intubation.[23]

Transferring the stable patient to a back board can be performed with either the log roll or the lift and slide technique. The log roll was discussed earlier as the first step to manage a prone athlete. The player can be rolled directly onto the back board if one is immediately present. In a supine player, however, the log roll transfer to a back board may cause more axial rotation and lateral flexion of the cervical spine compared with the lift and slide technique.[24,25] Despite the increased risk of cervical motion, reasons to log roll a player onto a back board include very heavy or broad athletes, having fewer than eight people present to perform a lift and slide, and having rescuers present who are more familiar with the log roll technique.[11] The lift and slide technique is performed with the rescue leader at the player's head and two rescuers on either side of the chest, pelvis, and legs. The leader instructs the other rescuers to lift the athlete 4 to 6 inches off the ground, and the eighth rescuer slides the back board under the athlete. The player can then be set down synchronously at the leader's command.[26] This technique likely results in less cervical motion because of the linear movement of the athlete in the vertical direction compared with the arc motion of the log roll that requires more precise coordination between the rescuers.[26] Therefore, the lift and slide is less susceptible to

cause iatrogenic injury to the athlete and is usually the preferred option. Supportive straps and blocks are used to immobilize the player's head neutrally on the back board.

Although cervical spine injuries are relatively rare in youth athletes, it is necessary to recognize important considerations in the on-field management of youths and adults. The head of a child grows at a relatively faster rate than the body, and a child's head has a more dorsally displaced occiput in relation to the shoulders (**Figure 4-3**).[27] The larger head-to-body ratio and the anatomy of the pediatric cervical spine result in cervical flexion when the child is lying supine on a back board.[28] This has led to the use of spine boards with either thoracic elevation via padding or an occipital depression with a board cutout to establish a neutral cervical spine position in children younger than 8 years old.[29] Children older than 8 years old are managed according to adult recommendations, using a standard back board and leaving the helmet and shoulder pads in place.[30] Although general recommendations have been made, studies have not identified a single reliable method to stabilize the cervical spine in pediatric patients.[31] To decrease the excessive movement of a child, cervical collars and tape are additional considerations to assist with stability when preparing for the transfer of a pediatric athlete on a spine board.[32]

The spine-injured athlete must be transferred quickly and safely from the accident site to a hospital. Considerations for choosing the mode of transportation include the distance of travel, peak traffic hours, and the severity of the injury.[33] Ground (ambulance) and air (helicopter or fixed wing aircraft) transport are both viable options for spine-injured athletes. When proper precautions are exercised, there is no difference in negative outcomes when comparing land and air transport.[33] Therefore, one must consider clinical, geographic, and logistical factors when choosing a safe and expedited mode of transportation for a spine-injured athlete.

The use of corticosteroids in the setting of acute cervical SCIs is controversial. The National Acute Spinal Cord Injury Studies no longer recommends corticosteroids to treat cervical spine injuries because steroids are associated with severe pneumonia, sepsis, and death.[34] The American Association of Neurological Surgeons and Congress of Neurological Surgeons concluded that "treatment with methylprednisolone for either 24 or 48 hours is recommended as an option in the treatment of patients with acute spinal cord injuries that should be undertaken only with the knowledge that the evidence suggesting harmful side effects is more consistent than any suggestion of clinical benefit."[35] Nevertheless, clinicians should be aware of using corticosteroids as an option to manage SCIs in athletes. However, the spine-injured athlete represents a unique consideration, and current evidence suggests that steroids may be useful in this setting because care is usually initiated within minutes of injury, and these are typically isolated injuries. This is covered more extensively in Chapter 5.

● MANAGEMENT OF THE ATHLETE'S PROTECTIVE PADDING

Protective padding worn by American football players serves to prevent injury but also acts as a variable that affects the on-field management in a suspected cervical spine injury (Video 4-4). The on-field management of padding most often involves the safe, rapid removal of the facemask to gain access to the airway. The techniques to remove facemasks from American football helmets have evolved as new helmet models have been introduced to the game. Prior recommendations suggested cutting the loop straps holding the facemask in place as a fast and efficient option, but this also results in head movement that could result in secondary injury.[36] Cutting the loop straps bypasses screw removal failure because of rust, spinning of the screw without loosening, and obliterating the screw face.[36] Cordless screwdrivers, however, remove facemasks more rapidly, with less torque, and cause less head motion than cutting the loop straps.[4] Failure to remove screws with a cordless screwdriver may be much rarer than one would expect. Studies have shown a 94% screw removal rate with a cordless screwdriver,[37] and a 100% facemask removal rate when combined with backup cutting tools.[38] Helmet manufacturers have now also created partial and full quick-release mechanisms to assist with facemask removal. These helmets allow for rapid facemask removal with little head movement and eliminate the variables associated with the screws, cordless screwdriver, and cutting tools.[39] The facemask should almost always be removed before transport regardless of airway status. The decision to remove equipment before transport should be based on several logistical factors, including the medical status of the injured.

The shoulder pads and helmet of American football players are typically left in place to help support in-line stabilization until they become a liability to the medical team's ability to complete critical care tasks (Video 4-5).[4,11,39] The medical team will also consider equipment removal before transport of the athlete from the prehospital care setting. The appropriateness and timeliness of equipment removal will be decided based on the team's decision regarding how to provide the safest handling and transport of the injured athlete (Video 4-6). Certain situations require the helmet, shoulder pads, or both to be removed. For instance, (1) the facemask cannot be removed in an acceptable timeframe when respiratory compromise is a concern, (2) the helmet does not allow for proper ventilation even after the facemask is removed, (3) the helmet does not fit properly and allows movement of the head even with the chin strap in place, and (4) the shoulder pads are too loose and prevent proper immobilization of the athlete on the back board.[11,15,40]

New shoulder pad designs also allow for more rapid shoulder pad removal with less movement of the cervical spine.[39,40] Two techniques currently in use for shoulder pad removal have been described before this technology. The first is the torso-lift technique, which involves one rescuer straddling the athlete's torso, pulling the player to a 45° angle while keeping the buttocks and lower extremities flat on the spine board, and sliding the pads laterally as a unit. The second is the flat-torso or levitation technique. At least six trained personnel raise the athlete, split the front of the pads, and remove them from the back before placing the athlete back on the spine board. Newer systems allow the pads to separate down the midline to allow for the lateral removal of each half over the extremities without the need for this added motion.[40] Although on-field shoulder pad removal has yet to become standard practice, it does provide full access to the airway and chest, allow for the use of a cervical collar, obviate the need for pad removal in the ambulance, and allow for immediate radiologic tests in the emergency department.[40] More research is still necessary to determine how shoulder pad accessories, such as rib protectors, will affect the removal of these new shoulder pad designs. Information about unique circumstances in other sports such as hockey and lacrosse can be found in Video 4-7.

● SUMMARY

The on-field management of SCI in athletes requires preparedness and organization of the team's medical personnel. Prevention of cervical injuries in athletes begins with proper coaching and rule implementation in the preseason, and the development and rehearsal of a cervical spine protocol helps prevent primary or secondary neurologic dysfunction after an injury occurs. Medical personnel must have a high index of suspicion for cervical injuries and a low threshold for implementing the necessary precautions. Stabilization of the athlete's spine in a neutral position is the first step in management of a potential SCI. This is followed by managing the airway, breathing, circulation, and other vital functions of the athlete. Several methods of back board transfer exist, but the medical personnel should use the technique they are most familiar with. Finally, the proper management of an athlete's protective gear begins in the offseason by becoming familiar with the different types of equipment and practicing their removal.

REFERENCES

1. National Spinal Cord Injury Statistical Center: *Fact Sheet: Recent Trends in Causes of SCI*. Birmingham, AL, University of Alabama at Birmingham, 2012.

2. Cantu RC, Mueller FO: Catastrophic spine injuries in American football, 1977–2001. *Neurosurgery* 2003; 53(2):358–362; discussion 362–353.

3. Kucera KL, Yau R, Cox Thomas L, Wolff C: *Catastrophic Sports Injury Research. Thirty-Second Annual Report*. Chapel Hill, NC, The University of North Carolina, 2015.

4. Swartz EE, Boden BP, Courson RW, et al: National athletic trainers' association position statement: acute management of the cervical spine-injured athlete. *J Athl Train* 2009;44(3):306–331.

5. Kucera KL, Klossner D, Colgate B, Cantu RC: *Catastrophic Sport Injury Research. Annual Survey of Football Injury Research 1931–2015*. National Center for Catastrophic Sport Injury Research, 2016.

6. Mueller F, Kucera K, Cox L: Catastrophic sports injury research, in National Center for Catastrophic Sport Injury Research, ed: *Thirty-First Annual Report, Fall 1982-Spring 2013*. Chapel Hill, NC, University of North Carolina, 2013.

7. Banerjee R, Palumbo MA, Fadale PD: Catastrophic cervical spine injuries in the collision sport athlete, part 2: Principles of emergency care. *Am J Sports Med* 2004;32(7):1760–1764.

8. Tator CH, Edmonds VE: National survey of spinal injuries in hockey players. *Can Med Assoc J* 1984;130(7):875–880.

9. Houghton KM, Emery CA: *Position Statement on Bodychecking in Youth Ice Hockey*. Canadian Paediatric Society, 2012. Ottawa, ON Canada.

10. Andersen J, Courson RW, Kleiner DM, McLoda TA: National Athletic Trainers' Association position statement: Emergency planning in athletics. *J Athl Train* 2002; 37(1):99–104.

11. Sanchez AR, Sugalski MT, LaPrade RF. Field-side and prehospital management of the spine-injured athlete. *Curr Sports Med Rep* 2005;4(1):50–55.

12. Swartz EE, Del Rossi G: Cervical spine alignment during on-field management of potential catastrophic spine injuries. *Sports Health* 2009;1(3):247–252.

13. Fehlings MG, Vaccaro A, Wilson JR, et al: Early versus delayed decompression for traumatic cervical spinal cord injury: Results of the Surgical Timing in Acute Spinal Cord Injury Study (STASCIS). *PLoS One* 2012;7(2):e32037.

14. Liu Y, Shi CG, Wang XW, et al: Timing of surgical decompression for traumatic cervical spinal cord injury. *Int Orthop* 2015;39(12):2457–2463.

15. Bailes JE, Petschauer M, Guskiewicz KM, Marano G: Management of cervical spine injuries in athletes. *J Athl Train* 2007;42(1):126–134.

16. Zahir U, Ludwig SC: Sports-related cervical spine injuries: on-field assessment and management. *Semin Spine Surg* 2010;22:173–180. Published by Elsevier Inc. Presented at the Seminars in Spine Surgery, 2010.

17. Banerjee R, Palumbo MA, Fadale PD: Catastrophic cervical spine injuries in the collision sport athlete, part 1: Epidemiology, functional anatomy, and diagnosis. *Am J Sports Med* 2004;32(4):1077–1087.

18. Lennarson PJ, Smith DW, Sawin PD, Todd MM, Sato Y, Traynelis VC: Cervical spinal motion during intubation: Efficacy of stabilization maneuvers in the setting of complete segmental instability. *J Neurosurg* 2001; 94(2 suppl):265–270.

19. Marcolini EG, Keegan J: Blunt cardiac injury. *Emerg Med Clin North Am* 2015;33(3):519–527.

20. Waninger KN, Swartz EE: Cervical spine injury management in the helmeted athlete. *Curr Sports Med Rep* 2011;10(1):45–49.

21. Jaworski CA: Advances in emergent airway management. *Curr Sports Med Rep* 2002;1(3):133–140.

22. Jacobson B, Cendoma M, Gdovin J, Cooney K, Bruening D: Cervical spine motion during football equipment-removal protocols: A challenge to the all-or-nothing endeavor. *J Athl Train* 2014;49(1):42–48.

23. Goutcher CM, Lochhead V: Reduction in mouth opening with semi-rigid cervical collars. *Br J Anaesth* 2005;95(3):344–348.

24. Del Rossi G, Heffernan TP, Horodyski M, Rechtine GR: The effectiveness of extrication collars tested during the execution of spine-board transfer techniques. *Spine J* 2004;4(6):619–623.

25. Del Rossi G, Horodyski M, Powers ME: A Comparison of spine-board transfer techniques and the effect of training on performance. *J Athl Train* 2003;38(3):204–208.

26. Del Rossi G, Horodyski MH, Conrad BP, Di Paola CP, Di Paola MJ, Rechtine GR: The 6-plus-person lift transfer technique compared with other methods of spine boarding. *J Athl Train* 2008;43(1):6–13.

27. Nemeth J: Case study: A new approach to stabilization of the cervical spine in infants. *The Academy Today* 2005;1:1.

28. Herzenberg JE, Hensinger RN, Dedrick DK, Phillips WA: Emergency transport and positioning of young children who have an injury of the cervical spine. The standard backboard may be hazardous. *J Bone Joint Surg Am* 1989;71(1):15–22.

29. Nypaver M, Treloar D: Neutral cervical spine positioning in children. *Ann Emerg Med* 1994;23(2):208–211.

30. Treme G, Diduch DR, Hart J, Romness MJ, Kwon MS, Hart JM: Cervical spine alignment in the youth football athlete: recommendations for emergency transportation. *Am J Sports Med* 2008;36(8):1582–1586.

31. Curran C, Dietrich AM, Bowman MJ, Ginn-Pease ME, King DR, Kosnik E: Pediatric cervical-spine immobilization: Achieving neutral position? *J Trauma* 1995;39(4):729–732.

32. Huerta C, Griffith R, Joyce SM: Cervical spine stabilization in pediatric patients: evaluation of current techniques. *Ann Emerg Med* 1987;16(10):1121–1126.

33. Theodore N, Aarabi B, Dhall SS, et al: Transportation of patients with acute traumatic cervical spine injuries. *Neurosurgery* 2013;72(suppl 2):35–39.

34. Hurlbert RJ, Hadley MN, Walters BC, et al: Pharmacological therapy for acute spinal cord injury. *Neurosurgery* 2015;76(suppl 1):S71–S83.

35. Pharmacological therapy after acute cervical spinal cord injury. *Neurosurgery* 2002;50(3 suppl):S63–S72.

36. Swartz EE, Norkus SA, Armstrong CW, Kleiner DM: Face-mask removal: Movement and time associated with cutting of the loop straps. *J Athl Train* 2003;38(2):120–125.

37. Decoster LC, Shirley CP, Swartz EE: Football face-mask removal with a cordless screwdriver on helmets used for at least one season of play. *J Athl Train* 2005;40(3):169–173.

38. Copeland AJ, Decoster LC, Swartz EE, Gattie ER, Gale SD: Combined tool approach is 100% successful for emergency football face mask removal. *Clin J Sport Med* 2007;17(6):452–457.

39. Swartz EE, Mihalik JP, Decoster LC, Al-Darraji S, Bric J: Emergent access to the airway and chest in american football players. *J Athl Train* 2015;50(7):681–687.

40. Kordecki M, Smith D, Hoogenboom B: The Riddell Ripkord system for shoulder pad removal in a cervical spine injured athlete: A paradigm shift. *Int J Sports Phys Ther* 2011;6(2):142–149.

5 Spinal Cord Injury: Pharmacologic Agents, Thermal Cooling, and Timing of Interventions

Allan R. Martin, MD • Michael G. Fehlings, MD, PhD

INTRODUCTION

Sport-related injuries are the fourth leading cause of traumatic spinal cord injury (SCI) in the United States, and are particularly prevalent in the 16- to 30-year-old age group.[1] Previously considered an untreatable condition, the chance for meaningful recovery after SCI has improved dramatically because of the discovery of numerous treatments and management strategies. This chapter summarizes the current best practices in management of acute SCI and highlights several emerging therapies that are candidates for clinical translation.

PATHOPHYSIOLOGY OF SPINAL CORD INJURY

Before discussing potential therapeutic agents for SCI, it is important to first elaborate on the pathophysiology of specific injury mechanisms. The biologic processes in traumatic SCI can be divided into primary and secondary injury followed by regeneration and functional recovery. Primary injury describes the immediate cellular and extracellular damage incurred by destructive forces and energy transfer. Secondary injury involves a cascade of mechanisms beginning immediately and lasting for weeks, including ischemia, vasospasm, thrombosis, inflammatory cytokines, breakdown of the blood–brain barrier, ion-mediated cellular damage, glutamate-related excitotoxicity, oxidative cellular damage, peroxidation of membrane lipids, sodium- and calcium-mediated cell

Neither of the following authors nor any immediate family member has received anything of value from or has stock or stock options held in a commercial company or institution related directly or indirectly to the subject of this article: Dr. Fehlings and Dr. Martin.

injury, and apoptosis (**Figure 5-1**).[2] The remaining spinal cord tissue bridges are precarious, and therefore secondary injury can be exacerbated by extrinsic factors such as mechanical instability that allows for repetitive trauma and systemic factors such as hypoxia, hypotension, and metabolic derangements that further injure the compromised tissue. After the acute phase, the spinal cord subsequently undergoes a period of limited repair, which is stimulated by cellular signaling and includes resolution of edema, remodeling of the disrupted blood–spinal cord barrier, axonal sprouting, remyelination, and reconnection of synapses (synaptic plasticity). However, this period of repair can also be negatively affected by the formation of a glial scar at the injury site, which hinders neural regeneration. Each of the individual mechanisms occurring at each stage after injury presents a potential target for intervention, and many such therapeutic agents are currently in various stages of research.

NEUROPROTECTION

The primary goal of current SCI management is avoidance of additional injury, which involves a number of different strategies that fall under the category of neuroprotection. Preservation of viable spinal cord tissue is enhanced by careful avoidance of repeat trauma, support of hemodynamic function, timely spinal cord decompression, and focused regulation of the inflammatory response.

Supportive Measures

The optimal management of SCI relies on supportive measures provided by all types of health professionals, beginning in the field with first responders who identify a

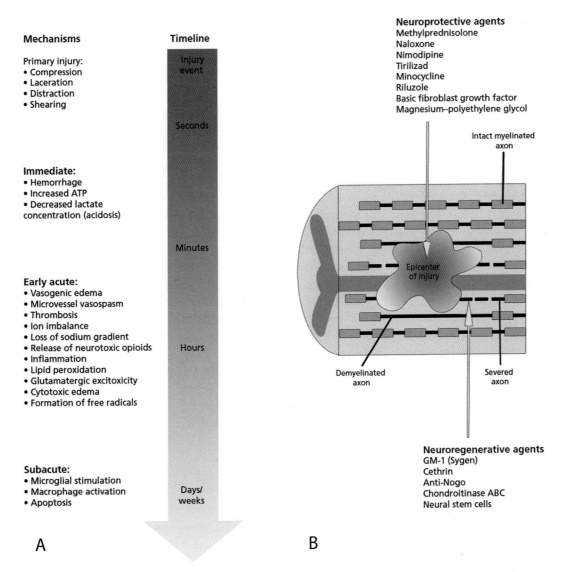

FIGURE 5-1 **A,** Primary and secondary mechanisms of injury determining the final extent of spinal cord damage. The primary injury event starts a pathobiological cascade of secondary injury mechanisms that unfold in different phases within seconds of the primary trauma and continuing for several weeks thereafter. **B,** Longitudinal section of the spinal cord after injury. The epicenter of the injury progressively expands after the primary trauma as a consequence of secondary injury events. This expansion causes an increased region of tissue cavitation and, ultimately, worsened long-term outcomes. Within and adjacent to the injury epicenter are severed and demyelinated axons. The neuroprotective agents listed act to subvert specific secondary injuries and prevent neural damage, and the neuroregenerative agents act to promote axonal regrowth after damage has occurred. ATP = adenosine triphosphate. (Reprinted from Wilson JR, Forgione N, Fehlings MG: Emerging therapies for acute traumatic spinal cord injury. *Canadian Medical Association Journal* 2013;185(6):485–492. © Canadian Medical Association (2013). This work is protected by copyright and the making of this copy was with the permission of the Canadian Medical Association Journal (www.cmaj.ca) and Access Copyright. Any alteration of its content or further copying in any form whatsoever is strictly prohibited unless otherwise permitted by law.)

potential injury, correctly immobilize the spine, and carefully transport the patient to a specialized trauma center. It is the responsibility of the trauma team to quickly assess and prioritize all injuries while maintaining spinal alignment and hemodynamic stability. The spinal surgeon should be involved in this process as early as possible to perform a complete physical examination, help guide imaging investigations, and lead clinical decision making. Expedient transfer to an intensive care unit (ICU) with

respiratory, cardiac, and hemodynamic monitoring is critical because it has been shown to improve morbidity, mortality, and neurologic outcomes.[3] Levi et al[4] established in 1993 that hypotension caused by neurogenic shock is common in patients with SCI (primarily in cervical, motor-complete injuries), and prompt and aggressive treatment appeared to improve mortality and neurologic outcomes. A subsequent observational study of 77 SCI patients by Vale et al[5] suggested that maintaining a mean arterial pressure (MAP) above 85 mm Hg with crystalloids, or vasopressors, or both for 7 after following injury showed markedly improved neurologic outcomes compared with historical control participants, leading to the American Association of Neurological Surgeons (AANS) and the Congress of Neurological Surgeons (CNS) guideline of maintaining MAP at 85 to 90 mm Hg for 7 days.[2]

Early Decompression of the Spinal Cord

After SCI, the spinal cord frequently faces ongoing mechanical compression, causing focal ischemia. Decompression may involve anterior or posterior surgery (or a combined approach) to remove tissues such as bone, disk, and blood that are compressing the spinal cord, often followed by an instrumented reconstruction with metallic implants such as screws, hooks, rods, or plates. Alternatively, in cases of dislocations of the spine, decompression may involve a closed-reduction maneuver under cervical traction. Closed reduction has been established as a safe intervention in awake patients who do not have additional rostral injuries, and this treatment is effective in approximately 80% of cases to relieve spinal cord compression and restore alignment.[6]

The issue of the optimal timing of spinal cord decompression has been debated within the surgical community because of concerns of the risk of surgery and an antiquated notion of the futility of surgery. However, recent evidence has provided clear justification that spinal cord decompression should be performed as quickly as possible,[7,8] which is consistent with previous evidence from animal studies.[9] A prospective study titled Surgical Timing in Acute Spinal Cord Injury Study (STASCIS) showed that patients undergoing surgery within 24 hours of injury have improved outcomes compared with those undergoing decompression after 24 hours.[10] More specifically, the early group (mean time to decompression, 14.2 hours) was 2.8 times more likely to achieve a 2-grade American Spinal Injury Association Impairment Scale (AIS) improvement compared with the late group (mean, 48.3 hours). STASCIS also confirmed the safety of early surgery, with equivalent complication rates between early versus late decompression (24% vs. 30%; $P = 0.21$). Two other observational studies have also been conducted in large cohorts, confirming the benefits of early surgery, although one study found no benefit in the subgroup of AIS A patients.[7,8] A European multicenter study, spinal cord injury-prospective, observational European multicenter study (SCI-POEM), is now underway, with similar methodology to STASCIS.[11] Considering the compelling evidence in favor of early surgical decompression, early SCI should be performed as quickly as medically and logistically feasible.

Induced Hypothermia

The use of induced hypothermia dates back to ancient Greece, where physicians treated traumatic brain injuries (TBIs) by cooling with ice baths.[12] The use of induced hypothermia was cast into the media spotlight in 2007 when a professional football player was treated with systemic hypothermia after sustaining a cervical SCI, recovering the ability to walk several months later.[13] Reports are unclear if the initial injury was truly motor complete or incomplete (AIS B or C), but his final neurologic status appears to be a highly functional AIS D. Moreover, it is unclear how much of the recovery was related to the treatment with induced hypothermia, early surgical decompression, intensive rehabilitation, or spontaneous recovery. However, related research in animal models of SCI has demonstrated a substantial benefit with intravascular cooling to a level of moderate hypothermia (32°–34°C), attenuating some of the mechanisms of secondary injury.[14] Cooling of the spinal cord has also been used in humans, with intraoperative application of cold saline directly over the spinal cord, but no benefits were established, and the practice has been largely abandoned.[15] Levi et al[16] recently reported on a pilot study of systemic hypothermia in the acute management of 14 AIS A patients, which demonstrated the safety of this treatment with equivalent complication rates and a trend toward neurologic improvement (43% vs. 21%). However, further research is needed before this treatment is widely adopted, prompting the initiation of a phase II study to provide further evidence.[17]

Neuroprotective Pharmaceutical Agents

A large number of potential neuroprotective drugs have been investigated for numerous neurologic disorders, including stroke, Alzheimer disease, amyotrophic lateral sclerosis (ALS), TBI, and SCI. Unfortunately, only a small number of these have demonstrated therapeutic benefits, and further development is needed to identify agents with greater efficacy. The mechanisms of action of neuroprotective agents are often nonspecific, offering the possibility of using one compound to treat multiple diseases. In conditions with an acute onset, such as SCI, TBI, and stroke, the efficacy of neuroprotective treatments tends to strongly depend on the timing of administration, posing a substantial barrier to implement successful clinical trials. Furthermore, enrolment in a clinical trial requires that a diagnosis can be confidently made and consent obtained before administration of the treatment, which can be time consuming and render the treatment ineffective. The design of SCI clinical trials has evolved to overcome these barriers, with many trials including a strict time window (treatment within 12 or 24 hours) and having dedicated research personnel quickly obtain consent and perform treatment administration immediately on arrival to the hospital. The field of SCI research is vast, and a large number of neuroprotective medications have been the subject of human or animal studies. The following sections focus on only the most promising neuroprotective pharmaceutical agents.

Methylprednisolone

Methylprednisolone (MP) is available as an intravenous (IV) infusion and is among the most potent corticosteroids, inhibiting inflammation and membrane lipid peroxidation. MP is the most studied neuroprotective agent for SCI and was previously used widely because animal studies have shown strong benefits and the National Acute Spinal Cord Injury Study (NASCIS) 2 clinical trial demonstrated modest benefits in humans. However, MP has been the subject of substantial debate and controversy, including the fact that the 2002 AANS/CNS guidelines suggested MP as a "treatment option," but the more recent 2013 version of the guidelines reversed this to "treatment not recommended" without substantial new evidence. In fact, a recently published Cochrane review synthesized the literature on MP, including six randomized controlled trials (RCTs) and several observational studies, and suggested that MP had evidence of efficacy and should remain a treatment option.[2,18] This review included a meta-analysis that demonstrated no neurologic benefit in the overall data but a 4-point improvement on American Spinal Injury Association (ASIA) motor score when initiated within 8 hours. The analysis also identified a trend toward decreased mortality rates with MP but increased rates of wound infection and gastrointestinal bleeding. Critics of MP have argued that there is clear evidence of increased complications, but the improved efficacy is only seen in subgroup analysis, as was performed in the Cochrane review and in the original publication of NASCIS 2 results.[2] However, it is important to note that the decision to perform subgroup analysis with the 8-hour time window in NASCIS 2 was made a priori rather than post hoc. It is also notable that the STASCIS data showed a 44% reduction in overall complications among patients who received MP, likely because the population was confined to cervical injuries, and wound infections are more common at lower

levels.[10] Furthermore, it is increasingly being recognized that cervical SCI has a greater potential for recovery than thoracolumbar injuries, indicating that future studies will be better powered by including only the cervical injury population.[19] In light of the evidence from the Cochrane review, which comprises the highest level of the evidentiary pyramid, MP should remain a treatment option because it most likely offers a small neurologic benefit with modest additional risks. The optimal candidates for MP are young, healthy patients with cervical injuries treated within 8 hours who will undergo early surgical decompression and stabilization within 24 hours, based on work from the STASCIS trial.[19] However, it must be stressed that this is an ongoing controversy within the SCI community, and SCI groups other than the AANS/CNS are likely to make differing recommendations regarding the use of MP.

Riluzole

Riluzole is a voltage-gated sodium channel blocker that reduces aspects of secondary injury, such as glutamatergic excitotoxicity and astrocytosis.[20] This drug was initially developed for treatment of ALS, receiving regulatory approval in the 1990s. Riluzole slows the degeneration of motor neurons and prolongs survival in ALS patients, albeit with a mean improvement of only 2 to 3 months in this typically aggressive disease.[21] In animal models of SCI, riluzole attenuates the secondary injury cascade and improves behavioral outcomes such as locomotion.[20] Recently, a phase I/II clinical study in SCI that treated 36 patients (AIS A, B, or C, 28 cervical and 8 thoracic) with riluzole showed an improvement of 15.5 points on the ASIA motor score compared with matched registry control participants ($P = 0.02$).[22] The multicenter phase II/III RCT Riluzole in SCI Study (RISCIS) is now underway in several countries around the world, only enrolling patients with cervical SCI.[23]

Minocycline

Minocycline is a derivative of the acne medication tetracycline, possessing antibiotic and anti-inflammatory properties and having an established safety profile. It appears to have multiple mechanisms of action in SCI, including the inhibition of microglial activation, tumor necrosis factor α (TNF-α), nitric oxide synthase (NOS), and metalloproteinases.[24,25] Preclinical research has demonstrated benefits of minocycline in SCI, with improved motor function, reduced lesion size, and a greater preservation of axons.[24,25] A small single-center RCT of minocycline versus placebo in 44 patients with cervical or thoracic SCI showed a weak trend toward improvement on ASIA motor scores (6 points; $P = 0.20$).[26] However, it was noted that the cervical subgroup of 25 patients demonstrated substantially greater improvement (14 points; $P = 0.05$).[26] These results have prompted a multicenter phase III RCT titled Minocycline in Acute Spinal Cord Injury (MASC), which is now underway and is also focused solely on the cervical injury population.[27]

Granulocyte Colony-Stimulating Factor

Granulocyte colony-stimulating factor (G-CSF) is an endogenous hormone and cytokine best known for its role in inducing the mobilization of stem cells from bone marrow into the blood. Preclinical studies have also identified several nonhematopoietic functions of G-CSF, offering a neuroprotective effect in both SCI and stroke that appears to preserve myelin, promote angiogenesis, and attract stem cells to the injury site while also inhibiting TNF-α and interleukin-1 (IL-1).[28] A pilot study using IV injection of G-CSF in 16 human participants demonstrated safety and tremendous efficacy, with all 16 patients showing improvement in AIS grade.[29] A subsequent multicenter nonrandomized controlled study also showed intriguing results, with 15 of 17 participants receiving G-CSF improving at least one AIS grade.[30] Further research of this promising therapeutic agent is anticipated, but a larger scale trial has yet to be announced.

Inhibitors of Glutamate-Related Excitotoxicity

Similar to riluzole and fibroblast growth factor (FGF), a number of other potential therapies involve the targeted reduction of glutamate-related excitotoxicity. GM-1 ganglioside (Sygen) is a membrane protein that reduces glutamatergic excitotoxicity and apoptosis and enhances neuritic sprouting.[31] Unfortunately, a multicenter RCT with 797 patients treated within 72 hours of injury showed no neurologic improvement at 1-year,[31] leading to the AANS/CNS guideline of "treatment not recommended."[3]

Magnesium (Mg) is a well-known neuroprotective agent that has been used previously in several neurologic disorders, working through several possible mechanisms, including noncompetitive antagonism of glutamate N-methyl-D-aspartate receptor (NMDA) receptors, reduction of free radicals, and inhibition of inflammatory cytokines.[32] One animal study used a formulation of Mg chloride in polyethylene glycol (PEG) to allow greater penetration of the blood-brain barrier, which facilitated better locomotor recovery than MP.[33] PEG has also been investigated for potential neuroprotective properties, such as preserving or resealing axonal membranes and reducing oxidative stress.[34] A multicenter phase II trial is currently investigating a formulation of Mg and PEG called AC105.[35]

● REGENERATIVE THERAPIES

The concept of regenerative medicine revolves around the growth of new tissues and cells, primarily based on the induction and amplification of endogenous repair mechanisms. The notion of spinal cord regeneration comes directly from nature because certain reptiles and the zebrafish have shown remarkable capacity to regrow lost tissues, including the spinal cord. However, the application of regenerative approaches to humans is far from straightforward because our natural ability of neural regeneration is extremely limited. The optimal timing of regenerative strategies also remains to be determined because there is an inherent trade-off between intervening early, when some treatments might have higher efficacy, and intervening late, which can avoid subjecting patients who would have made a good recovery without intervention to unnecessary risk. There is an array of emerging pharmaceuticals, cell-based therapies, and structural implants that could all have a substantial impact as potential treatments.

Rho Inhibitors

The Rho family of GTPases are key to a signaling pathway that regulates the cytoskeleton and motility, ultimately inhibiting neuronal growth.[36] Inhibition of Rho or other parts of the pathway tends to stimulate neurite growth, profoundly improving motor function in animal models of SCI.[36] Cethrin is a Rho inhibitor that has been investigated in a phase I/IIa study in which it was applied directly to the dura mater intraoperatively.[37] The results in 48 SCI patients demonstrated virtually no motor improvement in thoracic cases, but patients with cervical injuries recovered 18.6 (±19.3) ASIA motor score points, trending toward significance compared with historic control participants.[37] Patients with thoracic injuries also showed a trend toward sensory improvement.[38] A phase III clinical trial is currently being planned.[39] Several other pharmaceutical agents have also shown Rho inhibition, including the commonly used NSAIDs. Preclinical work has demonstrated that ibuprofen induces increased axonal sprouting.[40] A current phase I clinical trial is now investigating ibuprofen in human patients with SCIs at a dosage of 2400 mg/d over 4 weeks.[41]

Nogo-A Inhibitors

The myelin protein Nogo-A, in a similar fashion as the Rho pathway, strongly inhibits neurite growth. The intrathecal injection of monoclonal antibodies that are specific for Nogo-A, blocking its activity, improves regeneration in rats and primates.[42,43] A phase I clinical trial with intrathecal pump delivery of such an antibody, developed by Novartis and called ATI355, involving 51 patients has been completed, but results have not been published.[44]

Fibroblast Growth Factors

Zebrafish possess the unique ability to completely regenerate a functional spinal cord after transection. This has inspired tremendous research into the cellular signaling mechanisms behind this trait, and it appears that the family of FGF molecules provide the key signals to form a glial bridge, allowing axons to grow over as a scaffold.[45] The specific mechanisms of FGF appear to vary between acidic (aFGF) and basic (bFGF) forms but include the reduction of glutamatergic excitotoxicity and the induction of axonal sprouting and growth. IV or intrathecal administration of bFGF has been shown to dramatically improve hindlimb function in rats with SCI.[46] A current phase II RCT is now evaluating a recombinant analog of bFGF developed by Asubio, called SUN13837, which has been specifically engineered to avoid the undesirable effect of fibroblast proliferation.[47]

Chondroitinase ABC

An important barrier to regenerative therapies, particularly in the chronic phase of SCI, is the glial scar that forms at the injury site.[48] This is composed of a dense area of extracellular matrix produced by reactive astrocytes and microglia over the initial months after injury. The scar not only blocks the absorption and penetration of potential regenerative therapeutics, but it also inhibits neurite outgrowth. Chondroitinase ABC is an enzyme that degrades sugar chains and chondroitin sulphate proteoglycans within the scar, with demonstrated benefits in rodents.[48] Several research groups are now adopting a combinatorial treatment approach, combining chondroitinase ABC with other regenerative therapies such as anti–Nogo-A.[49] A human formulation of chondroitinase ABC is not yet available, but its development is currently in progress.

Cell-Based Therapies

Stem cells and other cell-based therapies are perhaps the most exciting and intriguing potential therapy in SCI to repopulate injured neurons and regenerate the injured tissue. Unfortunately, a number of studies using a variety of cell types (stem cells, activated macrophages, bone marrow stromal cells, Schwann cells) in humans have shown poor cell survival or a lack of neurologic benefit (**Table 5-1**).[50-58] These studies typically injected the cells into the spinal cord (percutaneously or during surgery), most often in the acute period after SCI. Few adverse events were encountered, but these pilot studies had smaller cohorts and were not powered to detect neurologic or functional improvements. Some researchers have argued that these treatments may provide more benefit through indirect mechanisms such as cell signalling and structural support.[58] Many cell types, including Schwann cells and neural precursors, secrete trophic factors and inhibitory signals that can enhance neurite sprouting and neuronal survival and improve functional outcomes in animal studies.[59] Several larger phase II clinical trials are now underway, which should offer better insight into the efficacy of these treatments.[60-62] In addition, newer techniques have recently allowed the production induced pluripotent stem cells, which can then be further induced to specific cell types such as neurons.[63] It remains to be determined if further refinements to these cell-based treatments can fulfill the dream of substantial spinal cord regeneration.

Implanted Scaffolds

A potentially complementary strategy to regenerative pharmaceuticals and cell treatments is the surgical implantation of a structural material that bridges the lesion site and encourages axonal regrowth. Several types of synthetic and biologic tissues have been developed and investigated in animal studies. It is important that these materials are biocompatible, biodegradable, and have appropriate mechanical properties such as porosity (for axons), elasticity, and adhesion with surrounding tissues.[64] Synthetic designs, such as multichannel hydrogel polymer grafts, have been tested in animals, but axons tend to stop growing if the gap is greater than 1 cm. Current research is exploring the incorporation of bioactive molecules and living cells into these implants.[64] An alternative approach is the implantation of peripheral nerve tissue, which has the desirable properties of having existing conduits for axonal regrowth and Schwann cells that secrete neurotrophic factors.[65] Unfortunately, this technique has had low success in animals because of difficulty with axons exiting the graft, which is also affected by glial scarring. Recent work using chondroitinase ABC appears to have overcome this issue, restoring function in rodent models.[66] An entirely different approach

TABLE 5-1 Potential therapeutic agents: Pharmacologic, cell based, and implanted materials

Class	Type	Agent	Description	Completed or Ongoing Studies
Neuroprotective	Temperature	Hypothermia	The induction of moderate hypothermia (33C) through intravascular or extrinsic cooling	Case-control study of 14 AIS A patients; trend toward neurologic improvement (43% vs. 21%)[16]
	Pharmaceutical	Methyl-prednisolone	Potent corticosteroid that inhibits inflammation, administered IV	Subgroup analysis shows modest (4-point) motor improvement with 24-hour MP initiated within 8 hours[18]
		Riluzole	Voltage-gated sodium channel blocker; mitigates glutamatergic toxicity; administered orally	Riluzole-treated cervical injury subgroup ($n = 28$) improved 15.5 points* more than matched control participants ($P = 0.02$); no benefit in thoracic ($n = 8$)[22]; phase II/III RISCIS trial underway[23]
		Minocycline	Tetracycline anti-inflammatory; reduces microglial activation, TNF-α; inhibits NOS and metalloproteinases; administered IV	Minocycline-treated cervical injury subgroup ($n = 25$) improved 14 points* compared with placebo ($P = 0.05$)[26]; phase III MASC trial underway[27]
		G-CSF	Endogenous glycoprotein attracts stem cells, preserves myelin, suppresses TNF-α and IL-1, and promotes angiogenesis; administered IV	Two early phase studies with IV injection showed safety and AIS grade improvements in 16 of 16 (100%) and 15 of 17 (88%) of patients, respectively[28,29]
		FGFs	Signals glia to forms "glial bridge" over which regenerating axons can traverse; reduces glutamate-related excitotoxicity; administered IV	Recombinant basic FGF (SUN13837) engineered to avoid stimulating fibroblast proliferation is subject of phase II RCT[44]
		Mg; PEG	Magnesium: glutamate NMDA receptor antagonist; anti-inflammatory; PEG helps Mg cross BBB; preserves axonal membranes; administered IV	Proprietary formation of Mg–PEG (AC105) now under investigation in multicenter phase II trial[35]
Regenerative	Pharmaceutical	Cethrin	Inactivates Rho or its downstream target ROK to stimulate neurite growth; administered intraoperatively (extradural)	Cethrin-treated cervical patients improved 18.6 (±19.3) points* (trend over historic control participants)[37]; phase III trial is planned[39]
		NSAIDs	Inhibitory properties on the Rho pathway, prompting increased axonal sprouting; administered orally	Phase I trial of ibuprofen currently underway[41]
		Anti–Nogo-A antibodies	The myelin protein Nogo-A is a potent inhibitor of neurite growth; administered intrathecally (via pump)	Phase I trial of anti–Nogo-A antibody (ATI355) completed; results pending publication[44]
		Chondroitinase ABC	Degrades sugar chains and chondroitin sulphate proteoglycans within glial scar; promotes axonal regrowth; administered intraspinally	Design of human formulation underway; phase I trial anticipated
		Hepatocyte growth factor	Neurotrophic factor and promotes angiogenesis; administered intraspinally	Phase I/II study of recombinant human HGF (KP-100IT) currently underway
	Cell based	BMSCs	Marrow cells include stem cells and other cells at varying maturation, spun to yield only mononuclear cells; mechanism is both cell signalling and repopulation of injured cells; administered intraspinally	Phase II trial of intraspinal cells and GM-CSF intravenously in 35 AIS A patients; nonsignificant improvement over control participants[57]; a separate study of BMSCs injected intraspinally in thoracic AIS A patients is ongoing[62]
		Adult neural stem cells	Allogeneic cells extracted from CNS of healthy donors (possibly from the subventricular zone)	A proprietary product is the subject of an ongoing phase II study[61]

Class	Type	Agent	Description	Completed or Ongoing Studies
		Adipose-derived stem cells	Cells extracted and incubated; unclear if reprogrammed to pluripotency; administered intraspinally	A phase II study inserting cells intraoperatively is underway[60]
		Schwann cells	Autologous cells obtained from sural nerve; administered intraspinally	Phase I trial of 33 chronic thoracic SCI patients showed safety but no improvement[55]
		Human embryonic stem cells	Cells derived from human embryos, cultured and injected intraspinally	Study by Geron Corp (Menlo Park, CA) stopped before completion after four patients received intraspinal injections
	Tissue based	Bioengineered scaffolds and tissue grafts	Synthetic and/or biologic tissues providing structural construct are implanted or injected to bridge the injury and permit axonal regrowth; administered intraspinally	No human studies to date

TABLE 5-1 Potential therapeutic agents: Pharmacologic, cell based, and implanted materials (*Continued*)

*Points refer to American Spinal Injury Association (ASIA) motor score points.

AIS = ASIA Impairment Scale, BBB = blood–brain barrier, BMSC = bone marrow stromal cell, CNS = central nervous system, FGF = fibroblast growth factor, GM-CSF = granulocyte macrophage-colony stimulating factor, HGF = human growth factor, IV = intravenous, MASC = Minocycline in Acute Spinal Cord Injury, Mg = magnesium, MP = methylprednisolone, NMDA = N-methyl-D-aspartate receptor, NOS = nitric oxide synthase, PEG = polyethylene glycol, RCT = randomized controlled trial, RISCIS = Riluzole in SCI Study, ROK = Rho-associated Kinase, SCI = spinal cord injury, TNF-α = tumor necrosis factor α.

Reproduced from Martin AR, Aleksanderek I, Fehlings MG: Diagnosis and acute management of spinal cord injury: Current best practices and emerging therapies. *Curr Trauma Rep* 2015;1:169–181, with permission from Springer Business + Science.

utilizes self-assembling peptides that form cylindrical nanotubes.[67,68] These molecules are injectable and can be modified to incorporate neurotrophic factors, but further research is needed to assess their value in SC.

FUTURE DIRECTIONS

At present, it is unclear which of the various approaches will provide SCI patients with substantially improved recovery. Looking forward, it is highly likely that SCI management will consist of combinatorial treatments that address different aspects of secondary injury and regeneration. These treatments will almost certainly involve elements of neuroprotection administered as quickly as possible after injury as well as regenerative approaches, most likely delivered using a combination of drugs, cell-based therapies, and implanted materials at multiple time points of intervention. The path ahead is not straightforward because the complexity of implementing these treatments is high, but the potential dramatic impact these approaches can have on individuals with SCI clearly justifies taking on this challenge.

SUMMARY

Great progress has been made in the treatment of patients with traumatic SCI over the past several decades, offering the possibility of meaningful recovery to a much greater

number of patients. A vast number of additional therapeutic agents are emerging that have the potential to offer substantial improvements in neurologic and functional outcomes, focused in the areas of neuroprotection or regeneration. However, most of these agents have yet to successfully show benefits in humans and be translated to clinical use, severely limiting the array of available treatment options. Despite this fact, the field of SCI research has great momentum and there is good reason to expect that additional treatments that improve neurological outcomes will soon be available (**Table 5-2**).

TABLE 5-2 Strategies to optimize outcomes in athletes with acute spinal cord injury

- Immediately immobilize the spine (cervical collar, spine board with head immobilization, careful transfers) and transport the patient to a trauma center.
- Maintain oxygenation and hemodynamic parameters, including mean arterial pressure above 85 mm Hg.
- Consider administering intravenous methylprednisolone within 8 hours of injury (particularly in cervical injuries), using the dosing regimen of initial bolus dose of 30 mg/kg followed by an infusion of 5.4 mg/kg/h for 23 hours.
- Perform surgical decompression and stabilization as early as possible to mitigate ischemia and additional tissue injury caused by ongoing spinal cord compression.
- Consider the use of emerging neuroprotective and regenerative therapies after sufficient evidence of their safety and efficacy has been accumulated.

REFERENCES

1. Sci-Info-Pages: *Spinal Cord Injury Facts & Statistics.* Available at: http://www.sci-info-pages.com/facts.html. Accessed September 10, 2015.

2. Rowland JW, Hawryluk GW, Kwon B, Fehlings MG: Current status of acute spinal cord injury pathophysiology and emerging therapies: Promise on the horizon. *Neurosurg Focus* 2008;25:E2.

3. American Association of Neurological Surgeons (AANS) and the Congress of Neurological Surgeons (CNS), Section on Disorders of the Spine and Peripheral Nerves. Guidelines for the Management of Acute Cervical Spine and Spinal Cord Injuries. 2013.

4. Levi L, Wolf A, Belzberg H: Hemodynamic parameters in patients with acute cervical cord trauma: Description, intervention, and prediction of outcome. *Neurosurgery* 1993;33(6):1007–1016; discussion 1016–1017.

5. Vale FL, Burns J, Jackson AB, Hadley MN: Combined medical and surgical treatment after acute spinal cord injury: Results of a prospective pilot study to assess the merits of aggressive medical resuscitation and blood pressure management. *J Neurosurg* 1997;87(2):239–246.

6. Gelb DE, Aarabi B, Dhall SS: Treatment of subaxial cervical spinal injuries. *Neurosurgery* 2013;72:187–194.

7. Dvorak MF, Noonan VK, Fallah N, et al: The influence of time from injury to surgery on motor recovery and length of hospital stay in acute traumatic spinal cord injury: An observational Canadian cohort study. *J Neurotrauma* 2014;32(9):645–654.

8. Wilson JR, Singh A, Craven C, et al: Early versus late surgery for traumatic spinal cord injury: The results of a prospective Canadian cohort study. *Spinal Cord* 2012;50:840–843.

9. Furlan JC, Noonan V, Cadotte DW, Fehlings MG: Timing of decompressive surgery of spinal cord after traumatic spinal cord injury: An evidence-based examination of pre-clinical and clinical studies. *J Neurotrauma* 2011;28: 1371–1399.

10. Fehlings MG, Vaccaro A, Wilson JR, et al. Early versus delayed decompression for traumatic cervical spinal cord injury: results of the Surgical Timing in Acute Spinal Cord Injury Study (STASCIS). *PloS One.* 2012;7:e32037.

11. ClinicalTrials.gov: *Surgical Treatment for Spinal Cord Injury (SCI-POEM).* Available at: http://www.clinicaltrial.gov/ct2/show/NCT01674764. Accessed November 20, 2014.

12. Jones WHS: *Hippocrates,* 472 ed. Heinemann, London, 1923.

13. Kwon BK, Mann C, Sohn HM, et al: Hypothermia for spinal cord injury. *Spine J* 2008;8:859–74.

14. Lo TP, Cho K-S, Garg MS, et al: Systemic hypothermia improves histological and functional outcome after cervical spinal cord contusion in rats. *J Comp Neurol* 2009; 514:433–448.

15. Dietrich WD, Levi AD, Wang M, Green BA: Hypothermic treatment for acute spinal cord injury. *Neurotherapeutics* 2011;8:229–239.

16. Levi AD, Casella G, Green BA, et al: Clinical outcomes using modest intravascular hypothermia after acute cervical spinal cord injury. *Neurosurgery* 2010;66:670–677.

17. ClinicalTrials.gov: *Efficacy of Intravenously Instituted Hypothermia Treatment in Improving Functional Outcomes in Patients Following Acute Spinal Cord Injury.* Available at: http://www.clinicaltrial.gov/ct2/show/NCT01739010. Accessed November 20, 2014.

18. Bracken MB: Steroids for acute spinal cord injury. *Cochrane Database Syst Rev* 2012;1:CD001046.

19. Fehlings MG, Wilson JR, Cho N: Methylprednisolone for the treatment of acute spinal cord injury: counterpoint. *Neurosurgery* 2014;61:36–42.

20. Schwartz G, Fehlings MG: Evaluation of the neuroprotective effects of sodium channel blockers after spinal cord injury: Improved behavioral and neuroanatomical recovery with riluzole. *J Neurosurg* 2001;94:245–256.

21. Bensimon G, Lacomblez L, Meininger V; the ALS/Riluzole Study Group: A controlled trial of Riluzole in Amyotrophic Lateral Sclerosis. *N Engl J Med* 1994; 330:585–591.

22. Grossman RG, Fehlings MG, Frankowski RF, et al: A prospective, multicenter, phase I matched-comparison group trial of safety, pharmacokinetics, and preliminary efficacy of riluzole in patients with traumatic spinal cord injury. *J Neurotrauma* 2014;31:239–55.

23. ClinicalTrials.gov: *Riluzole in Spinal Cord Injury (RISCIS) trial.* Available at http://www.clinicaltrials.gov/show/NCT01597518. Accessed November 20, 2014.

24. Festoff BW, Ameenuddin S, Arnold PM, et al: Minocycline neuroprotects, reduces microgliosis, and inhibits caspase protease expression early after spinal cord injury. *J Neurochem* 2006;97:1314–1326.

25. Wells JEA, Hurlbert RJ, Fehlings MG, Yong VW: Neuroprotection by minocycline facilitates significant recovery from spinal cord injury in mice. *Brain* 2003;126:1628–1637.

26. Casha S, Zygun D, McGowan MD, et al: Results of a phase II placebo-controlled randomized trial of minocycline in acute spinal cord injury. *Brain* 2012;135:1224–1236.

27. ClinicalTrials.gov: *Minocycline in Acute Spinal Cord Injury (MASC).* Available at: http://www.clinicaltrial.gov/ct2/show/NCT01828203. Accessed November 21, 2014.

28. Kawabe J, Koda M, Hashimoto M, et al: Granulocyte colony-stimulating factor (G-CSF) exerts neuroprotective effects via promoting angiogenesis after spinal cord injury in rats. *J Neurosurg Spine* 2011;15:414–21.

29. Takahashi H, Yamazaki M, Okawa A, et al: Neuroprotective therapy using granulocyte colony-stimulating factor for acute spinal cord injury: A phase I/IIa clinical trial. *Eur Spine J* 2012;21:2580–2587.

30. ClinicalTrials.gov: *Study to Evaluate the Efficacy, Safety, and Pharmacokinetics of SUN13837 Injection in Adult Subjects with Acute Spinal Cord Injury (ASCI)*. Available at: http://www.clinicaltrial.gov/ct2/show/NCT02260713. Accessed November 21, 2014.

31. Geisler FH, Coleman WP, Grieco G, Poonian D; the Sygen Study Group: The Sygen multicenter acute spinal cord injury study. *Spine* 2001;26(24 suppl):S87–S98.

32. Kwon BK, Tetzlaff W, Grauer JN, Beiner J, Vaccaro AR: Pathophysiology and pharmacologic treatment of acute spinal cord injury. *Spine J* 2004;4:451–464.

33. Kwon BK, Roy J, Lee JH, et al: Magnesium chloride in a polyethylene glycol formulation as a neuroprotective therapy for acute spinal cord injury: Preclinical refinement and optimization. *J Neurotrauma* 2009;26:1379–1393.

34. Luo J, Borgens R, Shi R: Polyethylene glycol immediately repairs neuronal membranes and inhibits free radical production after acute spinal cord injury. *J Neurochem* 2002;83:471–480.

35. ClinicalTrials.gov Website. A Phase 2 Double-blind, Randomized, Placebo-controlled Study to Determine the Safety, Tolerability and Potential Activity of AC105 Following a Regimen of 6 Doses Over 30 Hours in Patients With Acute Traumatic Spinal Cord Injury (SCI) as Compared to Patients Treated With Placebo. http://clinicaltrials.gov/ct2/show/NCT01750684 Accessed November 20, 2014.

36. Dergham P, Ellezam B, Essagian C, et al: Rho signaling pathway targeted to promote spinal cord repair. *J Neurosci* 2002;22:6570–6577.

37. Fehlings MG, Theodore N, Harrop J, et al: A phase I/IIa clinical trial of a recombinant Rho protein antagonist in acute spinal cord injury. *J Neurotrauma* 2011;28:787–796.

38. McKerracher L, Anderson KD: Analysis of recruitment and outcomes in the phase I/IIa Cethrin clinical trial for acute spinal cord injury. *J Neurotrauma* 2013;30:1795–1804.

39. ClinicalTrials.gov: *Cethrin in Acute Cervical Spinal Cord Injury (CACSCI) Trial*. Available at: http://www.clinicaltrials.gov/ct2/show/NCT02053883. Accessed November 20, 2014.

40. Wang X, Buddel S, Baughman K, et al: Ibuprofen enhances recovery from spinal cord injury by limiting tissue loss and stimulating axonal growth. *J Neurotrauma* 2009;26:81–95.

41. ClinicalTrials.gov: *The Rho-Inhibitor Ibuprofen for the Treatment of Acute Spinal Cord Injury: Investigation of Safety, Feasibility and Pharmacokinetics*. Available at: http://www.clinicaltrial.gov/ct2/show/NCT02096913. Accessed November 20, 2014.

42. Liebscher T, Schnell L, Schnell D, et al: Nogo-A antibody improves regeneration and locomotion of spinal cord-injured rats. *Ann Neurol* 2005;58:706–719.

43. Freund P, Schmidlin E, Wannier T, et al: Nogo-A-specific antibody treatment enhances sprouting and functional recovery after cervical lesion in adult primates. *Nat Med* 2006;12:790–792.

44. ClinicalTrials.gov Website. *Study to Evaluate the Efficacy, Safety, and Pharmacokinetics of SUN13837 Injection in Adult Subjects With Acute Spinal Cord Injury (ASCI)*. http://www.clinicaltrial.gov/ct2/show/NCT02260713. Accessed November 21, 2014.

45. Goldschmidt Y, Sztal TE, Jusuf PR, Hall TE, Nguyen-Chi M, Currie PD: Fgf-dependent glial cell bridges facilitate spinal cord regeneration in zebrafish. *J Neurosci* 2012; 32(22):7477–7492.

46. Rabchevsky AG, Fugaccia I, Turner AF, et al: Basic fibroblast growth factor (bFGF) enhances functional recovery following severe spinal cord injury to the rat. *Exp Neurol* 2000;164:280–291.

47. ClinicalTrials.gov: *Acute Safety, Tolerability, Feasibility and Pharmacokinetics of Intrath. Administered ATI355 in Patients with Acute SCI*. Available at: http://www.clinicaltrials.gov/show/NCT00406016. Accessed November 21, 2014.

48. Bradbury EJ, Moon LD, Popat RJ, et al: Chondroitinase ABC promotes functional recovery after spinal cord injury. *Nature* 2002;416:636–640.

49. Zhao RR, Andrews MR, Wang D, et al. Combination treatment with anti-Nogo-A and chondroitinase ABC is more effective than single treatments at enhancing functional recovery after spinal cord injury. *Eur J Neurosci.* 2013;38:2946–61.

50. Geffner LF, Santacruz P, Izurieta M, et al: Administration of autologous bone marrow stem cells into spinal cord injury patients via multiple routes is safe and improves their quality of life: Comprehensive case studies. *Cell Transplant* 2008;17:1277–1293.

51. Syková E, Homola A, Mazanec R, et al: Autologous bone marrow transplantation in patients with sub-acute and chronic spinal cord injury. *Cell Transplant* 2006;15:675–687.

52. Deda H, Inci MC, Kurekci AE, et al: Treatment of chronic spinal cord injured patients with autologous bone marrow-derived hematopoietic stem cell transplantation: 1-year follow-up. *Cytotherapy* 2008;10:565–574.

53. Mackay-Sim A, Feron F, Cochrane J, et al: Autologous olfactory ensheathing cell transplantation in human paraplegia: a 3-year clinical trial. *Brain* 2008;131:2376–2386.

54. Lima C, Escada P, Pratas-Vital J, et al: Olfactory mucosal autografts and rehabilitation for chronic traumatic spinal cord injury. *Neurorehabil Neural Repair* 2010;24:10–22.

55. Saberi H, Moshayedi P, Aghayan HR, et al: Treatment of chronic thoracic spinal cord injury patients with autologous Schwann cell transplantation: an interim report on safety considerations and possible outcomes. *Neurosci Lett* 2008;443:46–50.

56. Knoller N, Auerbach G, Fulga V, et al: Clinical experience using incubated autologous macrophages as a treatment for complete spinal cord injury: Phase I study results. *J Neurosurg Spine* 2005;3:173–181.

57. Yoon SH, Shim YS, Park YH, et al: Complete spinal cord injury treatment using autologous bone marrow cell transplantation and bone marrow stimulation with granulocyte macrophage-colony stimulating factor: phase I/II clinical trial. *Stem Cells* 2007;25:2066–2073.

58. Lammertse DP, Jones LA, Charlifue SB, et al: Autologous incubated macrophage therapy in acute, complete spinal cord injury: Results of the phase 2 randomized controlled multicenter trial. *Spinal Cord* 2012;50:661–671.

59. Ruff CA, Wilcox JT, Fehlings MG. Cell-based transplantation strategies to promote plasticity following spinal cord injury. *Exp Neurol* 2012;235:78–90.

60. ClinicalTrials.gov: *Transplantation of Autologous Adipose Derived Stem Cells (ADSCs) in Spinal Cord Injury Treatment*. Available at: http://www.clinicaltrial.gov/ct2/show/NCT02034669. Accessed November 20, 2014.

61. ClinicalTrials.gov: *Study of Human Central Nervous System (CNS) Stem Cell Transplantation in Cervical Spinal Cord Injury*. Available at: http://www.clinicaltrials.gov/ct2/show/NCT02163876. Accessed November 21, 2014.

62. ClinicalTrials.gov: Autologous Bone Marrow Cell Transplantation in Persons with Acute Spinal Cord Injury: An Indian Pilot Study. Available at: http://www.clinicaltrial.gov/ct2/show/NCT02260713. Accessed November 21, 2014.

63. Warren L, Manos PD, Ahfeldt T, et al: Highly efficient reprogramming to pluripotency and directed differentiation of human cells with synthetic modified mRNA. *Cell Stem Cell* 2010;7(5):618–630.

64. Wang M, Zhai P, Chen X, et al: Bioengineered scaffolds for spinal cord repair. *Tissue Eng Part B Rev* 2011;17:177–194.

65. Cote MP, Amin AA, Tom VJ, Houle JD: Peripheral nerve grafts support regeneration after spinal cord injury. *Neurotherapeutics* 2011;8:294–303.

66. Lee YS, Lin CY, Jiang HH, et al: Nerve regeneration restores supraspinal control of bladder function after complete spinal cord injury. *J Neurosci* 2013;33:10591–10606.

67. Tysseling-Mattiace VM, Sahni V, Niece KL, et al: Self-assembling nanofibers inhibit glial scar formation and promote axon elongation after spinal cord injury. *J Neurosci* 2008;28:3814–3823.

68. Liu Y, Ye H, Satkunendrarajah K, et al: A self-assembling peptide reduces glial scarring, attenuates post-traumatic inflammation and promotes neurological recovery following spinal cord injury. *Acta Biomater* 2013;9:8075–8088.

6 Diagnostic Imaging of Sports-Related Spinal Disorders

Mitchel B. Harris, MD, FACS • Micah Blais, MD

● INTRODUCTION

Spinal injuries in athletes range widely in terms of severity, etiology, and the acuity with which diagnostic imaging should be obtained. Sports-related activities are the second most common cause of subaxial cervical spine injuries, behind only motor vehicle collisions.[1] Although these injuries are relatively uncommon, they can be associated with significant morbidity and mortality and often require urgent imaging.[2] On the other end of the spectrum, lumbar disk herniation is a commonly seen injury pattern in older athletes that rarely requires imaging in the acute setting.[3] The objective of this chapter is to highlight injury patterns that are commonly seen in athletes of all ages and to identify current, evidence-based approaches to management and decision making regarding imaging. We will approach these disorders by grouping the conditions into two major categories: (1) acute and traumatic and (2) chronic and atraumatic (**Table 6-1**).

● ACUTE AND TRAUMATIC CONDITIONS

Cervical Spine Trauma

Cervical spinal cord injury (SCI) is a relatively uncommon yet potentially devastating injury associated with participation in sports. In a review of the National Center for Catastrophic Sports Injury Research database, Boden et al estimated the incidence of catastrophic cervical spine injury in high school and college football players to be 1.10 and 4.72 per 100,000 participants respectively.[4] Although hockey, wrestling, and rugby are also associated

with cervical spine trauma, football is the most commonly implicated sport in the United States. The incidence of sports-related catastrophic SCIs has decreased over the past 30 years because of multitude of factors, including rule changes regarding "spearing" tackling techniques and athlete education.[5] Despite these improvements, these injuries still occur and are associated with significant morbidity and therefore require appropriate management and imaging to ensure optimal patient outcomes.

The initial management of acute cervical spine injury should be managed in the same way as any other trauma patient, with focus on adherence to Advanced Trauma Life Support (ATLS) protocols. Specific concerns regarding on-field management and helmet removal techniques are covered elsewhere in this text. Much research effort has been devoted toward the development of systematic approaches to imaging of adult spine injury in the

TABLE 6-1	Differential diagnosis of lower back pain in athletes
Spinal Diagnoses	**Nonspinal Diagnoses**
Muscle or ligament strain	Intrapelvic or gynecologic (e.g., ovarian cysts)
Degenerative disk disease	Renal disease
Isthmic spondylolysis (no slip)	Sacroiliac joint dysfunction
Isthmic spondylolisthesis	
Fact syndrome	
Ring apophyseal injury (adolescents)	
Sacral stress fracture	
Central disk herniation (without radiculopathy)	
Sacralization of L5 or transverse process impingement	
Facet stress fracture	
Acute traumatic facet fracture	
Discitis or osteomyelitis	
Neoplasm	

(From Bono CM: Low-back pain in athletes. *J Bone Joint Surg Am.* 2004;86-A(2):382–396 with permission.)

emergency department (ED) setting. The two most commonly used approaches are the Canadian C-spine rules and National Emergency X-radiography Utilization Study (NEXUS) criteria.[6] These guidelines are systematic and evidence based and provide a high level of sensitivity in detection of cervical spine injury.[7] Although only a small percentage of ED complaints are sports related, these algorithms should provide a foundation for decision making regarding imaging for adult athletes with concern for cervical spine injury. It is important to note, however, that the applicability of these rules to the athletic population is not absolute and still requires interpretation on the part of the provider. For example, cervical neurapraxia (also known as a "stinger" or "burner") is a common injury sustained while playing football that results in paresthesias involving the upper extremities and is often the result of an axial load to the head. Strict application of the Canadian C-spine rules to such a patient would identify two "high-risk factors" that would mandate radiography. In actuality, these patients are rarely acutely imaged, and the symptoms usually resolve without incident.

Although NEXUS and the Canadian C-spine rules provide a useful approach to management of adult (athletic) cervical spine trauma, their applicability to pediatric athletes (particularly those younger than the age of 8 years old) is questionable.[8] Children younger than the age of 8 years old have a more horizontal orientation of their facet joints, which allows for greater flexion/extension mobility. Additionally, younger children have wedge-shaped vertebral bodies as well as incomplete fusion of vertebral synchondroses.[9] Therefore, the

fulcrum of cervical spine flexion/extension is more cranial in children younger than the age of 8 years (C2–C3) and moves more caudally as the spine matures until reaching a level of C5 to C6 in adolescence.[10] The net effect of this shift is that whereas children younger than 8 years old are more likely to sustain injuries at or above C3, older children are typically injured below this level. Leonard et al retrospectively identified patient factors that are associated with the presence of cervical spine injury in pediatric trauma patients.[11] However, even in the presence of one or more of these factors, an evidence-based approach to imaging pediatric patients has not yet been developed. As a result, many individual pediatric emergency centers have attempted to implement institutional-level protocols for imaging patients with suspected cervical spine trauma (Figure 6-1). Although studies have shown that these measures have decreased the amount of time elapsed between presentation and collar clearance, their applicability in terms of a decision-making tool for imaging remains uncertain, and their deployment is far less universal than the adult protocols.[12]

For providers evaluating pediatric patients with suspected cervical spine injury, the initial evaluation usually includes a thorough physical examination and plain film radiographs of the cervical spine (anteroposterior [AP], lateral, and odontoid views).[13] Flynn et al found that MRI can be useful in evaluation of pediatric patients, particularly in evaluating obtunded patients or patients with equivocal radiographs.[14] Although CT is more sensitive than MRI in detecting bony injury in the cervical spine, it is less commonly used in pediatric patients because of concerns surrounding radiation exposure.

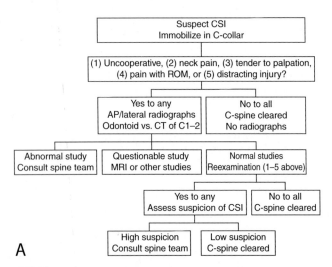

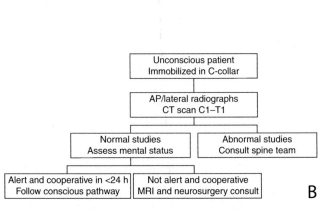

FIGURE 6-1 Pediatric imaging algorithm: conscious (**A**) and unconscious (**B**). AP = anteroposterior, CSI = Cervical Spine Injury, ROM = range of motion. (Adapted from Lee SL, Sena M, Greenholz SK, Fledderman M: A multidisciplinary approach to the development of a cervical spine clearance protocol: Process, rationale, and initial results. *J Pediatr Surg* 2003;38(3):358–362.)

Additionally, Adelgais et al found that the use of helical CT in the ED setting was associated with increased ED lengths of stay and research usage (see Figure 6-1 and **Boxes 6-1** and **6-2**).[15]

Cervical nerve root neurapraxias are the result of acute cervical spine trauma with resulting numbness and tingling involving the upper extremities. They represent the most common peripheral nerve injuries, and up to 50% to 65% of college football players have reported experiencing these injuries at least once in their careers.[16] Even though these injuries are commonly seen among athletes, a fair amount of debate exists within the medical community in regards to deciding between allowing immediate return to play (RTP) versus further workup and imaging. The first step for the provider is to distinguish a routine "burner" or "stinger" from a more dangerous condition. Specifically, involvement of more than one extremity, involvement of the lower extremities, associated headache or altered mental status, significant neck pain, or decreased neck range of motion (ROM) should all raise concern for possible fracture or associated SCI (or both), and the patient should be managed with spinal precautions pending further imaging.[17]

Athletes who experience true "burners" or "stingers" present with sensations of pain or numbness involving a single upper extremity. The exact mechanism of nerve stretch or injury is unclear, but it is believed to be attributable either to traction on the peripheral nerve at the level of the brachial plexus or impingement at the level of the exiting nerve root. The symptoms are typically transient and quite often will have resolved by the time that the patient comes off of the field of play for evaluation.[18] Although little evidence exists regarding the management of these injuries, RTP without imaging can be considered in an athlete who sustains his or her first "burner" and is also found to have the following: normal neurovascular examination results; normal, pain-free cervical spine ROM; normal pain-free shoulder ROM; and a negative Spurling's test result.[19] Imaging should be considered in athletes with recurrent episodes, persistent symptoms, or symptoms involving more than one extremity.[17] In patients with recurrent or persistent pain, paresthesias, or weakness involving a single upper extremity, MRI or electromyographic studies can be obtained to further localize the level and site of compression.[20] Despite this relatively clear distinction, Levitz et al evaluated 55 athletes with recurrent "burners" and found that 53% had cervical stenosis and 87% had evidence of disk disease on MRI.[21]

It is also important for the managing provider to distinguish between cervical nerve root and cervical cord neurapraxia (CCN). CCN is a afar less commonly seen

---

BOX 6-1   NEXUS

1. No midline cervical tenderness
2. No focal neurologic deficit
3. Normal alertness
   a. Glasgow Coma Scale score of 15
   b. No disorientation to person, place, time, or events
   c. Ability to remember three objects in 5 minutes
   d. Appropriate response to external stimuli
4. No intoxication
5. No painful, distracting injury
   a. Examples: long bone fractures, visceral injury requiring surgical consultation, large lacerations, crush injuries, or large burns

---

BOX 6-2   Canadian C-spine rules criteria

A. Is there any high-risk factor that mandates radiography?
   1. Age 65 years or older
   2. Dangerous mechanism
      a. Fall from 1 m (or five stairs)
      b. Axial load to the head (e.g., diving accidents)
      c. Motor vehicle collisions at high speed (>100 km/h)
      d. Motorized recreational vehicle accident
      e. Ejection from a vehicle
      f. Bicycle collision with an immovable object
   3. Paresthesias in extremities
B. Is there any low-risk factor that allows safe assessment of ROM? Patients who do not have any of the following low-risk factors should be radiographed and are not suitable for ROM testing:
   a. Simple rear-end motor vehicle collision
   b. Sitting position in ED
   c. Ambulatory at any time since injury
   d. Delayed onset of neck pain
   e. Absence of midline C-spine tenderness
C. ROM testing
   a. Is the patient able to actively rotate neck 45° to the left and right (regardless of pain)? If so, imaging is not indicated.

ED = emergency department, ROM = range of motion.
(From Leonard JC, Kuppermann N, Olsen C, et al: Factors associated with cervical spine injury in children after blunt trauma. *Ann Emerg Med.* 2011;58(2):145–155. doi: 10.1016/j.annemergmed.2010.08.038. Epub 2010 Oct 29 with permission.)

---

condition compared with root neurapraxia, with one estimate at only 7 per 10,000 football participants in the United States.[22] It is commonly associated with participation in sport and presents as bilateral loss of sensation with or without associated motor deficits that can range from mild to complete. This entity is commonly associated with spinal stenosis; therefore, the provider should obtain advanced imaging (either CT myelogram or MRI) to assess for the degree of functional canal space available.[23,24] Because of this association with canal stenosis, isolated CT or plain film evaluation of patients with bilateral symptoms is insufficient.

Thoracic and Lumbar Spine Trauma

Acute sports-related injuries involving the thoracic spine include fracture and disk herniation. Cadaveric studies have shown that the rib cage provides tremendous stability against rotational and axial forces acting on the thoracic spine.[25] It is somewhat surprising that athletic involvement is a commonly implicated cause of thoracolumbar spine injury. In fact, Wang et al reviewed the causes of traumatic vertebral body fractures over a 10-year period and found that participation in sports resulted in fractures of the thoracic and lumbar spine more commonly than the cervical spine or sacrum.[26] Although these acute injuries are commonly seen in adult trauma and can be associated with sport participation, far less research has been focused on determining how and when to obtain imaging for patients with these injuries.

The first question facing providers in managing these patients is to address the likelihood of a fracture being present. In a 2013 guideline, the Eastern Association for the Surgery of Trauma stated that all patients with a history of blunt abdominal or chest wall trauma "without complaints of [thoracic, lumbar or sacral] pain that have normal mental status, as well as normal neurological and physical examinations may be excluded from [spinal] injury by clinical examination alone, without radiographic imaging,

provided that there is no suspicion of high-energy mechanism or intoxication with alcohol or drugs."[27] However, a recent study performed by Inaba et al found that up to 21.6% of patients with normal physical exam (no tenderness to palpation in thoracic/lumbar midline, deformity/stepoff, positive neurologic findings) still had clinically significant fractures requiring a thoracolumbosacral orthosis or surgery. Instead, the authors found that a combination of physical examination with pertinent history factors (high-risk mechanism, age older than 60 years old) improved the sensitivity of their screening tool to 98.9%.[28] Application of these principles and findings suggests that a patient younger than 60 years of age presenting with a history of blunt thoracic or abdominal trauma sustained while participating in sports without any concerning neurologic or physical examination findings does not require imaging.

For patients who do have a history or findings concerning for further imaging, the next decision for the provider is to determine which modality is appropriate. Plain films have been shown to have inferior sensitivity, specificity, and negative predictive value for fracture compared with CT.[29] Although helical CT has demonstrated 99% sensitivity in the detection of thoracic and lumbar fracture, its utility for the detection of soft tissue injury) is much more limited.[30] In most Western ED settings, initial evaluation in the trauma bay of a patient who has sustained thoracolumbar trauma with concerning physical examination findings includes a multidirectional CT scan evaluation of the thoracolumbar spine.[31]

The next step for practitioners is to determine whether MRI is warranted. The aforementioned Eastern Association for the Surgery of Trauma guidelines recommends that "MRI should be considered in consultation with the spine service for MultiDetector Computed Tomography (MDCT) findings suggestive of neurologic involvement and of gross neurologic deficits."[29]

An additional study by Winklhofer et al reviewed MRIs performed on 100 patients with CT-confirmed fractures and found that CT alone revealed 162 fractures, and CT combined with MRI detected 192 fractures. Using the Thoracolumbar Injury Classification and Severity (TLICS) Scale cutoff score of 5 for a transition from likely nonoperative management to consideration of surgical intervention, this study found that 24% of injuries could be reclassified from non-operative management when MRI was added to the initial evaluation.[32] Therefore, MRI should be considered in a patient with a documented CT finding or fracture concerning for neurologic compromise with associated neurologic findings on physical examination (**Table 6-2**).[33]

TABLE 6-2 Thoracolumbar injury classification and severity (TLICS) score	
Variable	**Points**
Injury morphology	
Compression	1
Burst	+1
Translation or rotation	3
Distraction	4
Neurologic status	
Intact	0
Nerve injury	2
Cord, conus medullaris	
Incomplete	3
Complete	2
Cauda equina	3
Posterior Ligamentous Complex (PLC) integrity	
Intact	0
Indeterminate	2
Injured	2

(From Lee JY, Vaccaro AR, Lim MR, et al: Thoracolumbar injury classification and severity score: a new paradigm for the treatment of thoracolumbar spine trauma. *J Orthop Sci.* 2005;10(6):671–675 with permission.)

Atraumatic and Chronic Back Pain

Low back pain is a commonly seen complaint among athletes, particularly wrestlers, gymnasts, and linemen.[34] For adult athletes at all levels of competition, lumbar disk degeneration or herniation is a common etiology of pain.[35] Ong et al found that Olympic athletes presenting with complaints of lower back pain had both higher prevalence and severity of disk disease than nonathlete control participants.[36] Disk degeneration and herniation have been observed radiographically at a high rate in even asymptomatic athletes.[37] Furthermore, lower back pain is also commonly seen as a chief complaint among adolescents as well.[38] Imaging decisions regarding suspected lumbar disk disease or herniation vary greatly depending on the level of athletic involvement.

For recreational adult athletes, acute imaging is rarely indicated in the absence of a progressive motor or sensory deficit or new-onset bowel or bladder dysfunction.[39] The presence of these "red flag" symptoms raises concerns for cord compression or cauda equina syndrome and necessitates urgent acquisition of advanced imaging (MRI or CT myelography). However, the vast majority of recreational athletes with atraumatic back pain do not have any concerning symptoms, and acute imaging for these patients has not been shown to have any positive impact on short- or long-term outcomes.[40,41] These patients should be counseled that their symptoms will likely resolve without surgical intervention, and they should expect to see significant symptomatic improvement within 6 weeks of conservative management.[42,43]

The approach to imaging of elite or professional athletes with suspected lumbar disk herniation is significantly different. Hsu found that professional football players who were treated operatively for lumbar disk herniation were able to participate in a greater number of games postinjury without any significant difference between pre- and postinjury performance scores.[44] Whereas the natural history of lower back pain managed nonoperatively can take up to 12 months for full recovery, the duration of recovery for elite athletes who have undergone microdiscectomy ranged from 2.8 to 8.7 months in one series.[45] With the goal of earliest possible return to sport in mind, management of elite athletes with suspected disk herniation trends more toward surgical intervention. Therefore, MRI should be obtained at the soonest possible opportunity to evaluate pathology and assess the patient's suitability for surgical intervention.

Spondylolysis is another common cause of atraumatic back pain in athletes, particularly in adolescents who participate in activities requiring repetitive hyperextension.[46] In one study by Micheli et al, 47% of pediatric patients with low back pain had radiographic evidence of pars defect.[47] For young patients with a concerning history and reproduction of pain with hyperextension, imaging is indicated. Particularly in pediatric patients, the need for proper diagnosis is weighed against the goal of limiting radiation exposure. Miller et al found that 75% of spondylolysis was viewable on AP and lateral plain films alone without any further imaging required. In the setting of negative plain films but a concerning history, a decision to pursue advanced imaging such as single-photon emission computed tomography (SPECT) or bone scan should be considered only after failed empiric conservative therapy with bracing, physical therapy, and NSAIDS.[48] Although commonly asymptomatic on its own, spondylolisthesis can also be found on imaging obtained as part of evaluation of lower back pain attributable to spondylolysis.[49,50] The initial diagnosis is typically made with plain films. Particularly in prepubescent athletes as well as with patients of any age with a greater than 50% listhesis, monitoring for progression of the slip with serial lateral plain films is recommended.

● SUMMARY

Athletes are at risk for a variety of SCIs and disorders, particularly those who participate in contact sports. When making decisions regarding imaging of these conditions, the provider must consider patient factors such as age, the mechanism of injury, the nature of the symptoms, and the patient's examination status. In general, an athlete who has sustained cervical spine trauma and remains neurologically intact with no cervical spine tenderness and relatively unimpeded normal neck motion does not require further imaging. A single episode of isolated unilateral upper extremity pain and paresthesia in the setting of cervical spine trauma is consistent with a diagnosis of a "stinger" or "burner." Provided that the patient's symptoms quickly resolve, he or she does not require imaging. Cervical spine tenderness, decreased ROM of the cervical spine, and a new onset of neurologic deficit (particularly those involving more than one extremity) are potentially signs of more significant neurologic injury that necessitate further imaging. With a mechanism concerning for potential cervical spine fracture, multidirectional CT scan is the imaging modality of choice. Similarly, in patients younger than the age of 60 years who have sustained blunt abdominal or pelvic trauma and present with a benign physical examination and no associated neurologic symptoms or signs, further imaging is unnecessary. However, new neurologic deficit, midline tenderness to palpation, or palpable "step-off" should raise concerns for potential injury and necessitate initial evaluation with a CT.

Although the approach to management of patients with acute spine trauma is essentially universal regardless of age and level of athletic performance, the approach to atraumatic back pain differs greatly between recreational and professional athletes. For non-elite athletes with low back pain consistent with lumbar disk herniation, neither imaging nor surgical intervention is indicated in the absence of a neurologic deficit or symptoms concerning for cauda equina syndrome. Conversely, elite athletes' need for early return to sport often drives them toward seeking surgical intervention (i.e., microdiscetomy) because it has been shown to allow these athletes earlier return to sport at levels comparable to their preinjury status.[51,52] Therefore, in elite athletes with suspected lumbar disk herniation, MRI shortly after injury allows for providers to identify potential surgical candidates.

Atraumatic lower back pain is also a commonly seen entity among pediatric and adolescent athletes. Although the majority of these symptoms are nonspinal and involve the adjacent musculature, spondylolysis and spondylolisthesis are commonly seen entities within these age groups. AP and lateral plain films of the lumbar spine are first-line imaging studies to be obtained in patients with history and physical examination concerning for these conditions. Even in the setting of negative plain films (which can happen up to 25% of the time), advanced imaging such as SPECT or MRI should only be obtained after a failed course of empiric non-operative therapy.

● CASE EXAMPLE

HPI: 19M otherwise healthy male on sideline after using poor tackling technique and "spearing" an opposing player with his helmet. Patient states that he initially felt "numb and tingly" in his right arm but it has since resolved. He denies any LUE or BLE symptoms and denies any associated neck pain. He denies any history of similar episodes in the past.

Past Medical History: None

Meds: None

Allergies: None

Social History: Noncontributory

Physical Exam:

GEN: NAD

PSYCH: Appropriate affect. Alert and oriented to person, place, and time. Patient is able to recall 3/3 items and is not amnestic to the event.

MSK: No cervical midline tenderness. No pain with active or passive ROM of the shoulders. Patient is ambulatory with normal gait and able to rotate his head 45° in both directions.

NEURO: 5/5 strength in BLE and BUE in all muscle groups. Sensation is intact to light touch in bilateral upper and lower extremity dermatomes.

Discussion

Using both Canadian and NEXUS criteria, the patient does not meet any criteria for further imaging in the absence of persistent UE symptoms, cervical midline tenderness, or focal neurologic deficit.[17] This patient's symptoms are most consistent with cervical nerve root neurapraxia (aka "burner" or "stinger"). Although there is little evidence regarding RTP criteria for patients sustaining a "burner," there is no indication for immobilization or further imaging in a patient whose symptoms have resolved and without a history of previous cervical root neurapraxia. If the patient was complaining of persistent neck pain; had persistent RUE symptoms, involvement of the LUE or lower extremities, or an abnormal neurologic examination; or had been found to have cervical midline tenderness, immediate immobilization with cervical collar and further imaging would be indicated.

REFERENCES

1. Murphy RF, Davidson AR, Kelly DM, Warner WC Jr, Sawyer JR: Subaxial cervical spine injuries in children and adolescents. *J Pediatr Orthop* 2015;35(2):136–139.

2. Bailes JE, Hadley MN, Quigley MR, Sonntag VK, Cerullo LJ: Management of athletic injuries of the cervical spine and spinal cord. *Neurosurgery* 1991;29(4):491–497.

3. Chou R, Fu R, Carrino JA, Deyo RA: Imaging strategies for low-back pain: Systematic review and meta-analysis. *Lancet* 2009;373(9662):463–472.

4. Boden BP, Tacchetti RL, Cantu RC, Knowles SB, Mueller FO: Catastrophic cervical spine injuries in high school and college football players. *Am J Sports Med* 2006;34(8):1223–1232.

5. Bailes JE, Petschauer M, Guskiewicz KM, Marano G: Management of cervical spine injuries in athletes. *J Athl Train* 2007;42(1):126–134.

6. Kanwar R, Delasobera BE, Hudson K, Frohna W: Emergency department evaluation and treatment of cervical spine injuries. *Emerg Med Clin North Am* 2015;33(2):241–282.

7. Duane TM, Young A, Mayglothling J, Wilson SP, Weber WF, Wolfe LG, Ivatury RR: CT for all or selective approach? Who really needs a cervical spine CT after blunt trauma. *J Trauma Acute Care Surg* 2013;74(4):1098–1101.

8. Viccellio P, Simon H, Pressman BD, Shah MN, Mower WR, Hoffman JR; NEXUS Group: A prospective multicenter study of cervical spine injury in children. *Pediatrics* 2001;108(2):E20.

9. Jones TM, Anderson PA, Noonan KJ: Pediatric cervical spine trauma. *J Am Acad Orthop Surg* 2011;19(10): 600–611.

10. d'Amato C: Pediatric spinal trauma: injuries in very young children. *Clin Orthop Relat Res* 2005;(432):34–40.

11. Leonard JC, Kuppermann N, Olsen C, et al; Pediatric Emergency Care Applied Research Network. Factors associated with cervical spine injury in children after blunt trauma. *Ann Emerg Med* 2011;58(2):145–155.

12. Lee SL, Sena M, Greenholz SK, Fledderman M: A multidisciplinary approach to the development of a cervical spine clearance protocol: Process, rationale, and initial results. *J Pediatr Surg* 2003;38(3):358–362; discussion 358–362.

13. Tat ST, Mejia MJ, Freishtat RJ: Imaging, clearance, and controversies in pediatric cervical spine trauma. *Pediatr Emerg Care* 2014;30(12):911–915; quiz 916–918.

14. Flynn JM, Closkey RF, Mahboubi S, Dormans JP: Role of magnetic resonance imaging in the assessment of pediatric cervical spine injuries. *J Pediatr Orthop* 2002; 22(5):573–577.

15. Adelgais KM, Grossman DC, Langer SG, Mann FA: Use of helical computed tomography for imaging the pediatric cervical spine. *Acad Emerg Med* 2004;11(3): 228–236.

16. Levitz CL, Reilly PJ, Torg JS: The pathomechanics of chronic, recurrent cervical nerve root neuropraxia. *Am J Sports Med* 1997;25:73–76.

17. Standaert CJ, Herring SA: Expert opinion and controversies in musculoskeletal and sports medicine: Stingers. *Arch Phys Med Rehabil* 2009;90(3):402–406.

18. Castro FP: Stingers, cervical cord neurapraxia, and stenosis. *Clin Sports Med* 2003;22:483–492.

19. Safran MR: Nerve injury about the shoulder in athletes, part 2: long thoracic nerve, spinal accessory nerve, burners/stingers, thoracic outlet syndrome. *Am J Sports Med* 2004;32(4):1063–1076.

20. Bettencourt RB, Linder MM: Treatment of neck injuries. *Prim Care* 2013;40(2):259–269.

21. Levitz CL, Reilly PJ, Torg JS: The pathomechanics of chronic, recurrent cervical nerve root neurapraxia. The chronic burner syndrome. *Am J Sports Med* 1997;25(1): 73–76.

22. Maroon JC, El-Kadi H, Abla AA, Wecht DA, Bost J, Norwig J, Bream T: Cervical neurapraxia in elite athletes: evaluation and surgical treatment. Report of five cases. *J Neurosurg Spine* 2007;6(4):356–363.

23. Cantu RC: Stingers, transient quadriplegia, and cervical spinal stenosis: Return to play criteria. *Med Sci Sports Exerc* 1997;29(suppl):S233–S235.

24. Torg JS, Naranja RJ, Pavlov H, Galinat BJ, Warren R, Stine RA: The relationship of developmental narrowing of the cervical spinal canal to reversible and irreversible injury of the cervical spinal cord in football players. *J Bone Joint Surg* 1996;78-A:1308–1314.

25. Watkins R 4th, Watkins R 3rd, Williams L, et al: Stability provided by the sternum and rib cage in the thoracic spine. *Spine (Phila Pa 1976)* 2005;30(11):1283–1286.

26. Wang H, Zhang Y, Xiang Q, Wang X, Li C, Xiong H, Zhou Y: Epidemiology of traumatic spinal fractures: experience from medical university-affiliated hospitals in Chongqing, China, 2001–2010. *J Neurosurg Spine* 2012;17(5): 459–468.

27. Sixta S, Moore FO, Ditillo MF, et al; Eastern Association for the Surgery of Trauma. Screening for thoracolumbar spinal injuries in blunt trauma: An Eastern Association for the Surgery of Trauma practice management guideline. *J Trauma Acute Care Surg* 2012;73(5 suppl 4):S326–S332.

28. Inaba K, Nosanov L, Menaker J, et al; AAST TL-Spine Multicenter Study Group: Prospective derivation of a clinical decision rule for thoracolumbar spine evaluation after blunt trauma: An American Association for the Surgery of Trauma Multi-Institutional Trials Group Study. *J Trauma Acute Care Surg* 2015;78(3):459–465; discussion 465–467.

29. Berry GE, Adams S, Harris MB, et al: Are plain radiographs of the spine necessary during evaluation after blunt trauma? Accuracy of screening torso computed tomography in thoracic/lumbar spine fracture diagnosis. *J Trauma* 2005;59(6):1410–1413; discussion 1413.

30. Wood KB, Li W, Lebl DR, Ploumis A: Management of thoracolumbar spine fractures. *Spine J* 2014;14(1):145–164.

31. Wilmink JT: MR imaging of the spine: Trauma and degenerative disease. *Eur Radiol* 1999;9(7):1259–1266.

32. Winklhofer S, Thekkumthala-Sommer M, Schmidt D, et al: Magnetic resonance imaging frequently changes classification of acute traumatic thoracolumbar spine injuries. *Skeletal Radiol* 2013;42(6):779–786.

33. Lee JY, Vaccaro AR, Lim MR, et al. Thoracolumbar injury classification and severity score: a new paradigm for the treatment of thoracolumbar spine trauma. *J Orthop Sci.* 2005;10(6):671–675.

34. Swärd L, Hellstrom M, Jacobsson B, Pëterson L: Back pain and radiologic changes in the thoraco-lumbar spine of athletes. *Spine (Phila Pa 1976)* 1990;15(2):124–129.

35. Young JL, Press JM, Herring SA: The disc at risk in athletes: perspectives on operative and nonoperative care. *Med Sci Sports Exerc* 1997;29(7 suppl):S222–S232.

36. Ong A, Anderson J, Roche J: A pilot study of the prevalence of lumbar disc degeneration in elite athletes with lower back pain at the Sydney 2000 Olympic Games. *Br J Sports Med* 2003;37(3):263–266.

37. Rajeswaran G, Turner M, Gissane C, Healy JC: MRI findings in the lumbar spines of asymptomatic elite junior tennis players. *Skeletal Radiol* 2014;43(7):925–932.

38. King HA: Evaluating the child with back pain. *Pediatr Clin North Am* 1986;33(6):1489–1493.

39. Casazza BA: Diagnosis and treatment of acute low back pain. *Am Fam Physician* 2012;85(4):343–350.

40. Chou R, Fu R, Carrino JA, Deyo RA: Imaging strategies for low-back pain: systematic review and meta-analysis. *Lancet* 2009;373(9662):463–472.

41. Kendrick D, Fielding K, Bentley E, Kerslake R, Miller P, Pringle M: Radiography of the lumbar spine in primary care patients with low back pain: Randomised controlled trial. *BMJ* 2001;322(7283):400–405.

42. Artus M, van der Windt D, Jordan KP, Croft PR: The clinical course of low back pain: A meta-analysis comparing outcomes in randomised clinical trials (RCTs) and observational studies. *BMC Musculoskelet Disord* 2014;15:68.

43. Lawrence JP, Greene HS, Grauer JN: Back pain in athletes. *J Am Acad Orthop Surg* 2006;14(13):726–735.

44. Hsu WK: Performance-based outcomes following lumbar discectomy in professional athletes in the National Football League. *Spine (Phila Pa 1976)* 2010;35(12):1247–1251.

45. Nair R1, Kahlenberg CA, Hsu WK: Outcomes of lumbar discectomy in elite athletes: The need for high-level evidence. *Clin Orthop Relat Res* 2015;473(6):1971–1977.

46. Stanitski CL: Spondylolysis and spondylolisthesis in athletes. *Oper Tech Sports Med* 2006;14:141–146.

47. Micheli LJ, Wood R: Back pain in young athletes. Significant differences from adults in causes and patterns. *Arch Pediatr Adolesc Med* 1995;149(1):15–18.

48. Miller R, Beck NA, Sampson NR, Zhu X, Flynn JM, Drummond D: Imaging modalities for low back pain in children: A review of spondylolysis and undiagnosed mechanical back pain. *J Pediatr Orthop* 2013;33(3):282–288.

49. Fredrickson BE, Baker D, McHolick WJ, Yuan HA, Lubicky JP: The natural history of spondylolysis and spondylolisthesis. *J Bone Joint Surg Am* 1984;66(5):699–707.

50. Hu SS, Tribus CB, Diab M, Ghanayem AJ: Spondylolisthesis and spondylolysis. *Instr Course Lect* 2008;57:431–445.

51. Lawrence JP, Greene HS, Grauer JN: Back pain in athletes. *J Am Acad Orthop Surg* 2006;14(13):726–735.

52. Hsu WK: Performance based outcomes following lumbar discectomy in professional athletes in the National Football League. *Spine (Phila Pa 1976)* 2010;35(12):1247–1251.

7 Spine Injuries in Pediatric Athletes

John M. Flynn, MD • Mark A. Seeley, MD • Aristides I. Cruz, Jr., MD

INTRODUCTION

Acute and chronic injuries of the spine can pose significant challenges to young athletes as well as their parents, coaches, trainers, and treating physicians. These injuries can affect participation, performance, and enjoyment of youth sports. Recent evidence has shown that the prevalence of back pain in older children and adolescents may be higher than previously recognized with rates as high as 24% to 36%.[1,2] It has been postulated that this increased prevalence is secondary to the rise in participation of organized youth sports. In 2014 to 2015, an estimated 35 million preadolescents and adolescents participated in organized sports in the United States (Minnesota Amateur Sports Commission, Athletic Footwear Association, *USA Today* Survey, Michigan State). Before more organized sports-specific training, overuse injuries in children were rarely encountered. However, these injuries are now major sources of morbidity in children and adolescents.

The manifestation of both acute and chronic spine injuries in children and adolescents is distinct from that in adults and these injuries can be overlooked by the clinician unaware of the common diagnoses in this subgroup of athletes. Within the general adolescent population, pediatric athletes are an at-risk population with a unique set of diagnoses. Whereas the etiology of back pain in inactive adolescents is often nonspecific,[3] back pain in pediatric athletes is usually due to an identifiable cause.[4] Through careful history and physical examination, supplemented with appropriate imaging, clinicians can often correctly identify the diagnosis in the young athlete, prevent further disability, and allow earlier return to sports.

Dr. Cruz Jr. or an immediate family member serves as a board member, owner, officer, or committee member of the Pediatric Orthopaedic Society of North America.

PEDIATRIC SPINE ANATOMY

Throughout development, the spinal column undergoes changes in both its structure and degree of flexibility, making it more or less susceptible to injury at various stages. The cancellous and cortical bone within the vertebral body also changes throughout development. During the adolescent growth spurt, bone mineralization is delayed, making it susceptible to fracture in part because of the changing bone density and its associated elastic modulus.[5,6] Additionally, because changes in muscle length lag behind longitudinal bone growth, the adolescent growth spurt can cause increased muscle–tendon tightness, thereby increasing the potential risk of injury.

The morphology of the growth plate and its surrounding tissue makes it vulnerable to injury because it is less resistant to deforming forces than either ligaments or bone.[7] Within the developing axial skeleton, the vertebral body contains superior and inferior physes, each with a contiguous ring apophysis (i.e., apophyseal ring) that close at approximately 18 years of age.[8] The cartilaginous epiphysis will subsequently develop into the vertebral endplates as the skeleton matures. The attachment of the apophyseal ring to the annulus fibrosis is through Sharpey's fibers, which are stronger than the fibrocartilaginous junction of the vertebral body. Posteriorly, the apophysis is firmly attached to the posterior longitudinal ligament.

The posterior column consists of the neural arch, pars interarticularis, facet joints, and spinous process. There are three primary growth centers within the posterior arch, one in the spinous process and one located in each of the pedicles, with each closing by 8 years of age.[8] Ossification of the vertebral body occurs in a posterior direction, and this moving transition zone of ossification predisposes the posterior elements to injury. Incomplete ossification of the superior aspect of the pars interarticularis predisposes this region to a stress fracture from the abutting inferior articular facet above.[9]

The morphology of the intervertebral disk also changes throughout development. Unlike the adult population in which degenerative changes of the annulus fibrosis are encountered, adolescent intervertebral disk pathology generally involves the ring apophysis. During axial compression, the forces of the immature spine are transmitted outward to the annulus fibrosis and, if large, can cause an apophyseal ring fracture or a limbus vertebra (herniated disk into the vertebral body). In contrast, the same compressive forces in the adult spine would tear the annulus fibrosis and cause herniation of the nucleus pulposus.

CERVICAL SPINE INJURIES

The cervical spine has a normal lordotic curvature, allowing it to dissipate a significant amount of energy in flexion, extension, rotation, and axial loading. In younger children, normal range of motion (ROM) of the cervical spine is increased at all levels, which subsequently decreases with age. Additionally, the point of maximal mobility is found at higher levels. Children younger than 8 years have their maximal mobility centered between the C1 to C3 vertebrae,[10] predisposing this age group to a higher risk of upper cervical spine injuries.[11] This is also secondary to a child's proportionately larger head, leading to a fulcrum of flexion at C2 to C3. With growth and development, the segment of maximum mobility moves caudally, reaching C5 to C6 by adolescence, where it remains throughout adulthood. Other cervical anatomic factors that differ from adults include horizontally aligned

facet joints; underdeveloped uncinate processes of C3 to C7, leading to flatter articular surfaces; a synchondrosis at the junction of the odontoid and C2 vertebral body; and less developed cervical supporting musculature.[12]

Flexion, combined with axial loading, is a common mechanism of injury implicated in cervical spine injuries in contact sports.[13-15] Cervical flexion decreases the normal lordotic alignment, thereby decreasing the cervical spine's ability to dissipate axial compression. When the maximum energy dissipation is exceeded, the patient may sustain compression or burst fractures with the potential for spinal cord injury (**Figure 7-1**). The fracture pattern will depend on the degree of cervical flexion at the time of injury. In adolescents, flexion fractures generally occur at the C5 and C6 levels because it is the site of maximal mobility. Before the mid-1970s, flexion-type cervical spine injuries were frequently encountered in high school and collegiate football players secondary to spearing (helmet-first football tackles). However, rules banning this form of tackling have dramatically reduced the rate of these injures encountered on the football field.[13] Axial cervical spine injuries can also occur in hockey, gymnastics, diving, and cheerleading.[16-18] Predisposing risk factors in these sports include mechanical increases in acceleration, elevation of the athlete above the playing surface, and violent collisions either with an opponent or an object.

Cervical hyperextension injuries are also encountered in pediatric sports and may result from falls, whiplash injuries, and blows to the anterior head.[15] The anterior cervical soft tissues are less robust than the posterior ligamentous

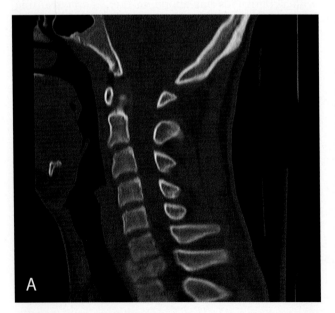
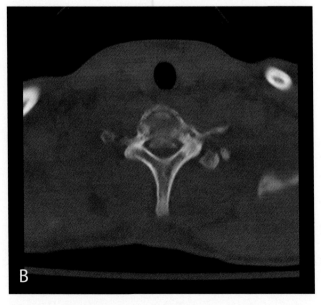

FIGURE 7-1 A 17-year-old male athlete who sustained a C7 burst fracture after a flexion-compression head-on-collision during a rugby match. Axial (**A**) and sagittal (**B**) images show a three-column injury to the spine with a retropulsed fragment into the spinal canal.

structures and confer less resistance to forced hyperextension. Increased cervical instability can be encountered if the hyperextension mechanism of injury is combined with rotation, predisposing the patient to neurologic injury.[19]

● THORACOLUMBAR SPINE INJURIES

Acute injuries to the thoracolumbar spine occur less commonly than cervical spine injuries in the pediatric population and represent fewer than 8% of spine fractures in those younger than 8 years of age.[20] Adolescents are more predisposed to these injures, and sports are the leading cause.[21] When injured, compression fractures are the most common thoracolumbar fracture seen in this age group; however, burst fractures can also occur.[21,22] Axial loading and trunk hyperflexion or hyperextension, as seen in falls landing in a seated position, can predispose to thoracolumbar injury. Gymnastics, diving, snowboarding, and jumping sports have been associated with this mechanism of injury.[18,23]

The majority of thoracolumbar injuries in the pediatric and adolescent population are stable fractures (e.g., spinous process, transverse process, compression fractures) that can be treated nonoperatively. These fractures heal uneventfully and are not associated with growth arrest. Bed rest and activity restriction followed by a thoracolumbosacral orthosis (TLSO) for 4 to 12 weeks is the mainstay

of treatment.[24] Compliance can be difficult in this active patient population, and sports activity is restricted during this period of healing. The athlete can return to sports after undergoing a gradual rehabilitation program in conjunction with radiographic union and resolution of pain.[21]

Burst fractures are a small subset of thoracolumbar fractures in children; however, it is important to recognize these fractures in children because improper management can cause physeal arrest and progressive sagittal or coronal spinal deformity.[22,25] These injuries occur secondary to axial load mechanisms that push the nucleus pulposus, or ring apophysis, or both into the vertebral body, causing it to fracture.[26] Fracture fragments from the vertebral body can retropulse into the spinal canal and compromise neural function; however, in the immature spine, the percentage of canal compromise does not necessarily correlate with the risk of spinal cord injury as is seen with the adult (**Figure 7-2**). Rather, the level of injury in the thoracic spine has been found to be associated with neurologic compromise.[22,27] Absolute indications for surgical treatment of burst fractures are those that are associated with neurologic injury. There is controversy regarding management of neurologically intact patients. Classic surgical indications include those with 40% loss of height, 20 degrees kyphotic deformity, or 40% canal compromise from a retropulsed fragment.[22,28,29] Studies that have assessed operative and nonoperative

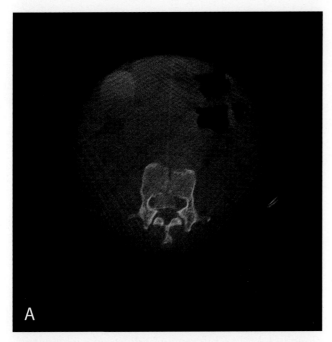
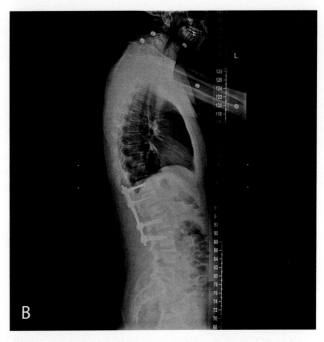

FIGURE 7-2 A 16-year-old female athlete who fell off a horse during show jumping sustaining a L1 burst fracture with a retropulsed fragment into the spinal canal. (**A**) The patient was neurologically intact at presentation, but because there was more than 20° of kyphotic deformity, the patient was taken to the operating room for a posterior spinal fusion from T11 to L3 (**B**).

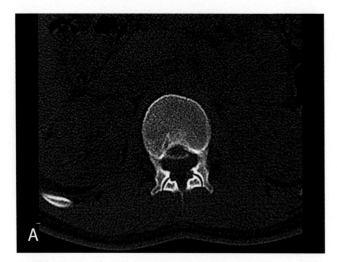
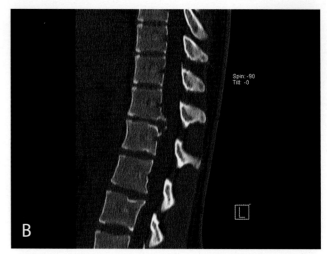

FIGURE 7-3   A 17-year-old cheerleader who presented as an outpatient with a more than 1-month history of low back pain. Axial (**A**) and sagittal (**B**) CT images show a posterior apophyseal ring fracture.

management of burst fractures have shown only minor improvements in the degree of kyphosis with surgical management and no differences in clinical outcomes.[22,25,30]

VERTEBRAL BODY APOPHYSEAL AVULSION FRACTURE

Microtrauma from repetitive flexion and extension of the immature spine can predispose adolescent athletes to an apophyseal ring (i.e., limbus) fracture.[31] Adolescent athletes involved in weight lifting or gymnastics are at particular risk. Ossification of the apophyseal ring occurs at age 4 to 6 years and fuses at age 18 years. Posteriorly, the ring is firmly attached to the annulus fibrosis and posterior longitudinal ligament. With forceful compressive or distraction forces, the osteocartilaginous junction can fail at the attachment of the annulus fibrosis, displacing the fragment posteriorly into the spinal canal (**Figure 7-3**). The most commonly involved levels are at L4 to L5, which occurs in 90% of cases.[32] Certain patient characteristics have been associated with apophyseal ring fracture in adolescents, including lumbarization, sacralization, spinal dysraphism, and irregularities in the end-plate cartilage.[32–34] Obesity has also been implicated, with increased weight placing excessive stress on the lumbar disk, which may predispose to apophyseal fracture.[35]

On examination, the patient will typically guard against flexion and extension secondary to paraspinal muscle spasm. The patient may have a positive straight-leg test or nerve tension signs. Standard radiographs should be obtained; however, it is important to note that the bony avulsion is not always identified on lateral radiographs, making CT or MRI the diagnostic study of choice.[36] Surgical treatment is generally reserved for cases with neural compression or refractory pain. Otherwise, management generally consists of rest, heat, nonsteroidal anti-inflammatory drugs, and progressive rehabilitation program.[31,33]

SPONDYLOLYSIS AND SPONDYLISTHESIS

Lumbar spondylolysis is a common injury in pediatric and adolescent athletes. Whereas the term *spondylolysis* describes a defect in the pars interarticularis, *spondylolisthesis* describes anterior displacement (or "slip") of the superior vertebra relative to the inferior vertebra (**Figure 7-4**). Both conditions may coexist and are often described together in the literature. The condition may affect pediatric and adolescent athletes involved in sports with repetitive loading, twisting, flexion, and extension of the lumbar spine and may account for up to 47% of low back pain in this population.[37]

Etiology and Pathoanatomy

The hallmark of spondylolysis is the defect in the pars interarticularis, which may be unilateral or bilateral and acute or chronic. The lesion is thought to be a chronic stress reaction or stress fracture caused by repetitive flexion and hyperextension or torsional loading of the lumbar spine. It most commonly occurs at L5 and occasionally L4.[38–42] Children and adolescents who participate in sports that require extreme trunk motion (e.g., gymnastics, dancing, golf, racket sports) are at a higher

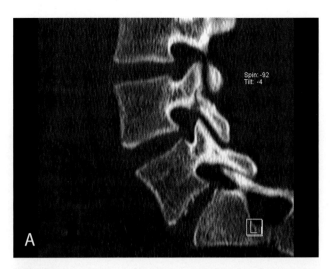
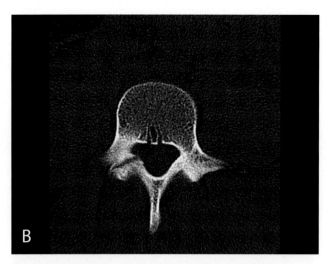

FIGURE 7-4 A 17-year-old football player presented as an outpatient with a 2-week history of lower back pain. Sagittal (**A**) and axial (**B**) images demonstrate a chronic spondylolysis of the right pars intraarticularis. The patient's symptoms resolved with a trial of nonoperative management.

risk for developing low back pain and symptomatic spondylolysis[38–46]; however, spondylolysis can occur in any athletic population.[39]

Anatomic factors have also been shown to be associated with an increased risk of developing spondylolysis. Masharawi et al showed that those with frontally rather than sagittally oriented lumbar facet joints were at greater risk of developing spondylolysis.[47] They also found that at L4, wider interfacet widths, shorter interfacet heights, and shorter or narrower articular facet heights were associated with an increased risk of spondylolysis.[48] Other predisposing factors to spondylolysis include pelvic morphology and spinopelvic balance. Measurements of pelvic incidence, sacral slope, pelvic tilt, and lumbar lordosis have been found to be greater in patients with spondylolisthesis.[49]

Evaluation

History and Physical Examination

Athletes with spondylolysis or spondylolisthesis usually present with axial low back pain as an initial complaint. There is usually no history of acute injury; rather, the pain develops insidiously and is exacerbated by physical activity. Atypical or olisthetic scoliosis caused by muscle spasm may masquerade the spondylolysis or spondylolisthesis. Gait examination may reveal a shortened stride length secondary to hamstring tightness.[41] Examination of the lumbar spine may reveal abnormalities in both the coronal (scoliosis) and sagittal (loss of lumbar lordosis) planes. Lumbar flexion and extension may be limited, and hyperextension often exacerbates symptoms.

Imaging

Anteroposterior (AP) and lateral radiographs of the lumbar spine should be obtained in child or adolescent athletes suspected of having spondylolysis or spondylolisthesis. These images should be taken with the patient standing rather than supine because supine films may not reveal subtle instability. Historically, oblique radiographs of the lumbar spine were recommended to orthogonally visualize the pars interarticularis and any potential defect (i.e., "Scotty dog" sign); however, this is rarely necessary and exposes the young athlete to unnecessary radiation.[50–52] Several authors have assessed the utility of four-view versus two-view radiographs in diagnosing L5 spondylolysis, and many have concluded that two views are adequate.[50,51]

Previously, single-photon emission computed tomography (SPECT) had been the advanced imaging modality of choice for the diagnosis of spondylolysis.[53–57] However, with further improvements in MRI technology, the ability to detect stress reactions is increasing, and some clinicians choose to use this nonionizing radiation modality as a means of assessing injury.[58,59] MRI correctly detects more than 90% of spondylolysis lesions. If the clinical suspicion remains high despite a normal MRI than a SPECT bone can or CT scan can also be used.

Treatment

Nonoperative

The vast majority of pediatric and adolescent athletes diagnosed with symptomatic spondylolysis and low-grade spondylolisthesis improve with nonoperative

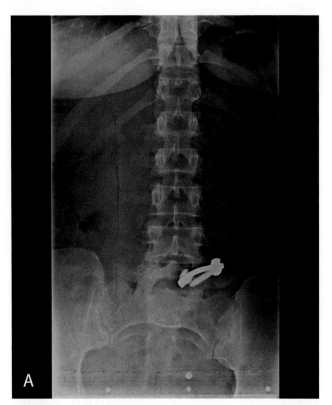
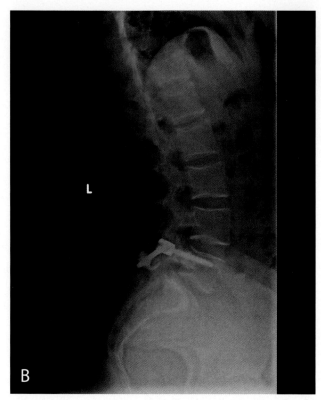

FIGURE 7-5 A, AP radiograph demonstrating left sided L5 pedicle screw with sublaminar hook. **B,** Lateral radiograph demonstrating left sided L5 pedicle screw with sublaminar hook.

treatment. The mainstays of nonoperative management are rest, activity modification, bracing, and gradual return to activity.[60] Rest or activity modification is likely the most important aspect of nonoperative treatment, but compliance is often difficult.[61] If a short period of rest does not quiet symptoms, bracing is used for 8 weeks (and sometimes longer in chronic cases) followed by physical therapy emphasizing hamstring flexibility, core strengthening, and sports hardening. Physical therapy protocols should be initiated when symptoms allow with an emphasis on core strengthening (particularly Williams-type exercises), lumbodorsal fascia stretching, and other "antilordotic" modalities. Bouras and Korovessis performed a comprehensive literature review and determined that conservative treatment in athletes with spondylolysis and low-grade spondylolisthesis results in an 85% success rate.[60]

Operative

Surgical intervention is rarely necessary in pediatric and adolescent athletes with spondylolysis. If, however, symptoms fail to adequately resolve after an appropriate and exhaustive period of comprehensive nonoperative

treatment, surgical intervention can be considered. A new or progressive neurologic deficit is also an indication for surgical treatment.[62] Surgical options for symptomatic spondylolysis without spondylolisthesis are direct repair of the pars defect or single-level instrumented fusion.[63–65] Direct repair of a pars defect can only occur if (1) there is no evidence of translation and (2) the disk space below is normal and without evidence of degeneration. **Figure 7-5** reveals case of a 19-year-old crew rower who had failed more than 1 year of conservative care for a unilateral lysis. She had trials of rest, bracing, and extensive physical therapy but remained symptomatic. She underwent a unilateral pars repair with a pedicle screw and hook with iliac crest bone graft packed into the spondylolytic defect. She returned to full play after 6 months and without any recurring symptoms.

Surgery is indicated for patients with high-grade spondylolisthesis (>50% slip) or if there is radiographic slip progression with or without neurologic symptoms (**Figure 7-6**). Nonoperative treatment for high-grade spondylolisthesis is generally less successful than that for low-grade slips; however, high-grade lesions are rarely encountered in pediatric athletes.

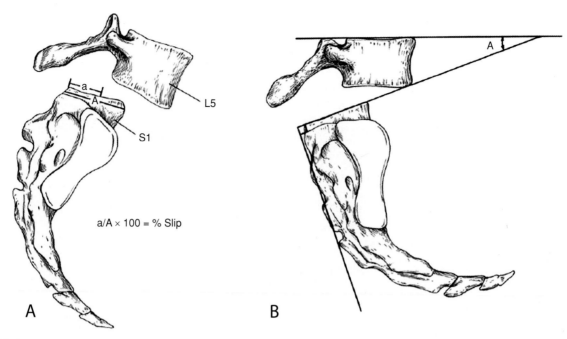

FIGURE 7-6 **A,** The Meyerding classification is used to quantify the degree of spondylolisthesis. Grade 1 is 0% to 25% slip, grade II is 26% to 50% slip, grade III is 51% to 75% slip, and grade IV is 75% to 99% slip. A = width of the superior endplate of S1, a = distance between the posterior edge of the inferior end plate of L5 and the posterior edge of the superior end plate of S1. **B,** Slip angle A quantifies the degree of lumbosacral kyphosis. A value greater than 50% correlates with a significantly increased risk of progression of spondylolisthesis. (Reprinted from Cavalier R, Herman MJ, Cheung EV, et. al. Spondylolysis and spondylolisthesis in children and adolescents: I. Diagnosis, natural history, and nonsurgical management. *J Am Acad Orthop Surg* 2006;14:417-424.)

RETURN-TO-PLAY GUIDELINES

When considering return to sport for adolescent athletes after sustaining a back injury; recommendations should be governed by the diagnosis; the activity level required for the sport; the skeletal maturity of the child; and the willingness of the athlete, parents, and coaches to follow recommendations. In most cases, a period of relative rest will be the initial management of the injured athlete. Activities that cause pain should be strictly avoided until the patient is pain free.[66] Depending on the diagnosis, continued sport participation with activity modification can be individualized, and when the athlete has obtained pain-free ROM as well as normal strength, return to full sports participation can be initiated.

AUTHORS' PREFERRED TREATMENT

Initial evaluation of a child or adolescent athlete with low back pain includes a complete history and physical examination with imaging studies to include AP and lateral radiographs of the lumbar spine. We do not routinely recommend oblique radiographs. In the presence of negative radiograph findings, if the history and physical examination are consistent with symptomatic spondylolysis, treatment is initiated consisting of relative rest, activity modification, cessation of sports activity, and possible TLSO bracing depending on symptoms. If the patient is unable to participate in his or her sport at the time of presentation because of pain, and the patient's symptoms are consistent with spondylolysis, TLSO bracing is initiated. The patient is reevaluated after a period of 8 weeks, and if there is symptomatic improvement, a physical therapy program is initiated concentrating on core muscle strengthening and hamstring stretching. Patients are gradually returned to sport over a period of 3 to 6 months. If the patient is unable to tolerate lumbar hyperextension on examination, bracing is continued for another 4 weeks (**Figure 7-7**).

Persistently symptomatic patients after an appropriate course of nonoperative treatment are infrequent. Operative treatment is only considered in the rare case of high-level athletes in which activity modification or cessation of sport is unacceptable or for patients who have persistent symptoms or pain unresponsive to nonoperative treatment. If, however, the patient and family elect for surgical treatment, return to sport is allowed

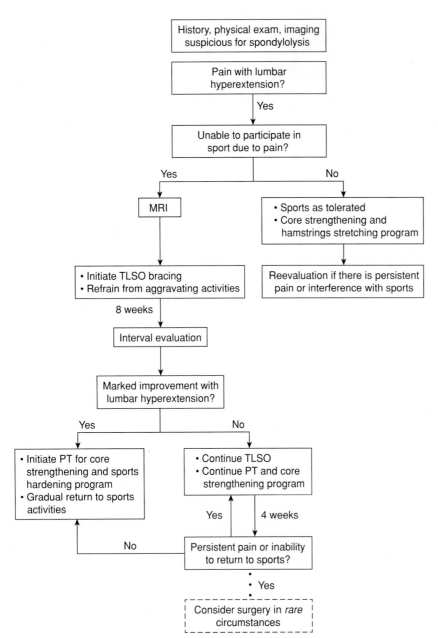

FIGURE 7-7 Proposed treatment algorithm for the treatment of symptomatic lumbar spondylolysis in pediatric and adolescent athletes. PT = physical therapy, TLSO = thoracolumbosacral orthosis.

only after radiographic signs of union and full strength, ROM, and sport-specific exercises can be performed without pain. This is typically after 9 to 12 months postoperatively.

● CONCLUSIONS

Spondylolysis and low-grade spondylolisthesis are common causes of low back pain in pediatric and adolescent athletes. A vast majority of patients respond favorably to nonoperative treatment and are able to return to sport at their same level of activity. It should be stressed to patients and families that relative rest and cessation of the offending activity (i.e., their sport) are the most important aspects of treatment. Surgery is reserved only for recalcitrant cases of spondylolysis or low-grade spondylolisthesis as well as rare cases in athletes with high-grade spondylolisthesis.

REFERENCES

1. Olsen TL, Anderson RL, Dearwater SR, Kriska AM, Cauley JA, Aaron DJ, LaPorte RE: The epidemiology of low back pain in an adolescent population. *Am J Public Health* 1992;82(4):606–608.

2. Watson KD, Papageorgiou AC, Jones GT, Taylor S, Symmons DP, Silman AJ, Macfarlane GJ: Low back pain in schoolchildren: Occurrence and characteristics. *Pain* 2002;97(1–2):87–92.

3. Bhatia NN, Chow G, Timon SJ, Watts HG: Diagnostic modalities for the evaluation of pediatric back pain: A prospective study. *J Pediatr Orthop* 2008;28(2):230–233.

4. Haus BM, Micheli LJ: Back pain in the pediatric and adolescent athlete. *Clin Sports Med* 2012;31(3):423–440.

5. Krabbe S, Christiansen C, Rødbro P, Transbøl I: Effect of puberty on rates of bone growth and mineralisation: With observations in male delayed puberty. *Arch Dis Child* 1979; 54(12):950–953.

6. Carter DR, Hayes WC: Bone compressive strength: the influence of density and strain rate. *Science* 1976; 194(4270):1174–1176.

7. Salter RB: Injuries of the epiphyseal plate. *Instr Course Lect* 1992;41:351–359.

8. Labrom RD: Growth and maturation of the spine from birth to adolescence. *J Bone Joint Surg Am* 2007;89(suppl 1):3–7.

9. Sagi HC, Jarvis JG, Uhthoff HK: Histomorphic analysis of the development of the pars interarticularis and its association with isthmic spondylolysis. *Spine (Phila Pa 1976)* 1998;23(15):1635–1639; discussion 1640.

10. Kewalramani LS, Tori JA: Spinal cord trauma in children. Neurologic patterns, radiologic features, and pathomechanics of injury. *Spine (Phila Pa 1976)* 1980;5(1):11–18.

11. Dietrich AM, Ginn-Pease ME, Bartkowski HM, King DR: Pediatric cervical spine fractures: Predominantly subtle presentation. *J Pediatr Surg* 1991;26(8):995–999; discussion 999–1000.

12. Martin B: Paediatric cervical spine injuries. *Injury* 2005; 36(1):14–20.

13. Torg JS: Epidemiology, pathomechanics, and prevention of football-induced cervical spinal cord trauma. *Exerc Sport Sci Rev* 1992;20:321–338.

14. Waninger KN: Management of the helmeted athlete with suspected cervical spine injury. *Am J Sports Med* 2004; 32(5):1331–1350.

15. Jagannathan J1, Dumont AS, Prevedello DM, Shaffrey CI, Jane JA Jr: Cervical spine injuries in pediatric athletes: Mechanisms and management. *Neurosurg Focus* 2006; 21(4):E6.

16. Torg JS, Gennarelli TA: Catastrophic head and neck injuries. *Adolesc Med* 1991;2(1):155–180.

17. Torg JS, Sennett B, Vegso JJ, Pavlov H: Axial loading injuries to the middle cervical spine segment. An analysis and classification of twenty-five cases. *Am J Sports Med* 1991;19(1):6–20.

18. Caine DJ, Nassar L: Gymnastics injuries. *Med Sport Sci* 2005;48:18–58.

19. Noakes TD Jakoet I, Baalbergen E: An apparent reduction in the incidence and severity of spinal cord injuries in schoolboy rugby players in the western Cape since 1990. *S Afr Med J* 1999;89(5):540–545.

20. Dogan S, Safavi-Abbasi S, Theodore N, et al: Thoracolumbar and sacral spinal injuries in children and adolescents: A review of 89 cases. *J Neurosurg* 2007;106(6 suppl):426–433.

21. Baranto A, Hellström M, Cederlund CG, Nyman R, Swärd L: Back pain and MRI changes in the thoracolumbar spine of top athletes in four different sports: A 15-year follow-up study. *Knee Surg Sports Traumatol Arthrosc* 2009;17(9):1125–1134.

22. Vander Have KL, Caird MS, Gross S, Farley FA, Graziano GA, Stauff M, Segal LS: Burst fractures of the thoracic and lumbar spine in children and adolescents. *J Pediatr Orthop* 2009;29(7):713–719.

23. Michel LJ: Back injuries in gymnastics. *Clin Sports Med* 1985;4(1):85–93.

24. Clark P, Letts M: Trauma to the thoracic and lumbar spine in the adolescent. *Can J Surg* 2001;44(5):337–345.

25. McPhee IB: Spinal fractures and dislocations in children and adolescents. *Spine (Phila Pa 1976)* 1981;6(6):533–537.

26. Junkins EP Jr, Stotts A, Santiago R, Guenther E: The clinical presentation of pediatric thoracolumbar fractures: A prospective study. *J Trauma* 2008;65(5):1066–1071.

27. Lalonde F, Letts M, Yang JP, Thomas K: An analysis of burst fractures of the spine in adolescents. *Am J Orthop (Belle Mead NJ)* 2001;30(2):115–120.

28. Domenicucci M, Preite R, Ramieri A, Ciappetta P, Delfini R, Romanini L: Thoracolumbar fractures without neurosurgical involvement: Surgical or conservative treatment? *J Neurosurg Sci* 1996;40(1):1–10.

29. Schnee CL, Ansell LV: Selection criteria and outcome of operative approaches for thoracolumbar burst fractures with and without neurological deficit. *J Neurosurg* 1997;86(1):48–55.

30. Parisini P, Di Silvestre M, Greggi T: Treatment of spinal fractures in children and adolescents: Long-term results in 44 patients. *Spine (Phila Pa 1976)* 2002;27(18):1989–1994.

31. Watkins RG: Lumbar disc injury in the athlete. *Clin Sports Med* 2002;21(1):147–165, viii.

32. Dietemann JL, Runge M, Badoz A, Dosch JC, Beaujeux R, Bonneville JF, Wackenheim A: Radiology of posterior lumbar apophyseal ring fractures: Report of 13 cases. *Neuroradiology* 1988;30(4):337–344.

33. Epstein NE: Lumbar surgery for 56 limbus fractures emphasizing noncalcified type III lesions. *Spine (Phila Pa 1976)* 1992;17(12):1489–1496.

34. Gennuso R, Humphreys RP, Hoffman HJ, Hendrick EB, Drake JM: Lumbar intervertebral disc disease in the pediatric population. *Pediatr Neurosurg* 1992;18(5–6):282–286.

35. Yen CH, Chan SK, Ho YF, Mak KH: Posterior lumbar apophyseal ring fractures in adolescents: A report of four cases. *J Orthop Surg (Hong Kong)* 2009;17(1):85–89.

36. Peh WC, Griffith JF, Yip DK, Leong JC: Magnetic resonance imaging of lumbar vertebral apophyseal ring fractures. *Australas Radiol* 1998;42(1):34–37.

37. Micheli LJ, Wood R: Back pain in young athletes. Significant differences from adults in causes and patterns. *Arch Pediatr Adolesc Med* 1995;149(1):15–18.

38. Blanda J, Bethem D, Moats W, Lew M: Defects of pars interarticularis in athletes: A protocol for nonoperative treatment. *J Spinal Disord* 1993;6(5):406–411.

39. Congeni J, McCulloch J, Swanson K: Lumbar spondylolysis. A study of natural progression in athletes. *Am J Sports Med* 1997;25(2):248–253.

40. Iwamoto J, Takeda T, Wakano K: Returning athletes with severe low back pain and spondylolysis to original sporting activities with conservative treatment. *Scand J Med Sci Sports* 2004;14(6):346–351.

41. Cavalier R, Herman MJ, Cheung EV, Pizzutillo PD: Spondylolysis and spondylolisthesis in children and adolescents: I. Diagnosis, natural history, and nonsurgical management. *J Am Acad Orthop Surg* 2006;14(7):417–424.

42. d'Hemecourt PA1, Zurakowski D, Kriemler S, Micheli LJ: Spondylolysis: Returning the athlete to sports participation with brace treatment. *Orthopedics* 2002;25(6):653–657.

43. Duggleby T, Kumar S: Epidemiology of juvenile low back pain: a review. *Disabil Rehabil* 1997;19(12):505–512.

44. Jones GT, Macfarlane GJ: Epidemiology of low back pain in children and adolescents. *Arch Dis Child* 2005;90(3):312–316.

45. McMeeken J, Tully E, Stillman B, Nattrass C, Bygott IL, Story I: The experience of back pain in young Australians. *Man Ther* 2001;6(4):213–220.

46. Rebella G: A prospective study of injury patterns in collegiate pole vaulters. *Am J Sports Med* 2015;43(4):808–815.

47. Masharawi YM, Alperovitch-Najenson D, Steinberg N, et al: Lumbar facet orientation in spondylolysis: A skeletal study. *Spine (Phila Pa 1976)* 2007;32(6):E176–E180.

48. Masharawi Y, Dar G, Peleg S, Steinberg N, Alperovitch-Najenson D, Salame K, Hershkovitz I: Lumbar facet anatomy changes in spondylolysis: A comparative skeletal study. *Eur Spine J* 2007;16(7):993–999.

49. Labelle H, Roussouly P, Berthonnaud E, Dimnet J, O'Brien M: The importance of spino-pelvic balance in L5-s1 developmental spondylolisthesis: A review of pertinent radiologic measurements. *Spine (Phila Pa 1976)* 2005;30(6 suppl):S27–S34.

50. Beck NA, Miller R, Baldwin K, et al: Do oblique views add value in the diagnosis of spondylolysis in adolescents? *J Bone Joint Surg Am* 2013;95(10):e65.

51. Miller R, Beck NA, Sampson NR, Zhu X, Flynn JM, Drummond D: Imaging modalities for low back pain in children: a review of spondylolysis and undiagnosed mechanical back pain. *J Pediatr Orthop* 2013;33(3):282–288.

52. Sucato DJ, Micheli LJ, Estes AR, Tolo VT: Spine problems in young athletes. *Instr Course Lect* 2012;61:499–511.

53. Auerbach JD, Ahn J, Zgonis MH, Reddy SC, Ecker ML, Flynn JM: Streamlining the evaluation of low back pain in children. *Clin Orthop Relat Res* 2008;466(8):1971–1977.

54. Bellah RD, Summerville DA, Treves ST, Micheli LJ: Low-back pain in adolescent athletes: Detection of stress injury to the pars interarticularis with SPECT. *Radiology* 1991;180(2):509–512.

55. Collier BD, Johnson RP, Carrera GF, et al: Painful spondylolysis or spondylolisthesis studied by radiography and single-photon emission computed tomography. *Radiology* 1985;154(1):207–211.

56. Spencer HT, Sokol LO, Glotzbecker MP, Grant FD, d'Hemecourt PA, Micheli LJ, Treves ST: Detection of pars injury by SPECT in patients younger than age 10 with low back pain. *J Pediatr Orthop* 2013;33(4):383–388.

57. Takemitsu M, El Rassi G, Woratanarat P, Shah SA: Low back pain in pediatric athletes with unilateral tracer uptake at the pars interarticularis on single photon emission computed tomography. *Spine (Phila Pa 1976)* 2006;31(8):909–914.

58. Saifuddin A, Burnett SJ: The value of lumbar spine MRI in the assessment of the pars interarticularis. *Clin Radiol* 1997;52(9):666–671.

59. Rush JK, Astur N, Scott S, Kelly DM, Sawyer JR, Warner WC Jr: Use of magnetic resonance imaging in the evaluation of spondylolysis. *J Pediatr Orthop* 2015;35(3):271–275.

60. Bouras T, Korovessis P: Management of spondylolysis and low-grade spondylolisthesis in fine athletes. A comprehensive review. *Eur J Orthop Surg Traumatol* 2015;(25 suppl 1):S167–S175.

61. El Rassi G, Takemitsu M, Glutting J, Shah SA: Effect of sports modification on clinical outcome in children and adolescent athletes with symptomatic lumbar spondylolysis. *Am J Phys Med Rehabil* 2013;92(12):1070–1074.

62. Cheung EV, Herman MJ, Cavalier R, Pizzutillo PD: Spondylolysis and spondylolisthesis in children and adolescents: II. Surgical management. *J Am Acad Orthop Surg* 2006;14(8):488–498.

63. Schlenzka D, Remes V, Helenius I, et al: Direct repair for treatment of symptomatic spondylolysis and low-grade isthmic spondylolisthesis in young patients: No benefit in comparison to segmental fusion after a mean follow-up of 14.8 years. *Eur Spine J* 2006;15(10):1437–1447.

64. Westacott DJ, Cooke SJ: Functional outcome following direct repair or intervertebral fusion for adolescent spondylolysis: A systematic review. *J Pediatr Orthop B* 2012;21(6):596–601.

65. Drazin D, Shirzadi A, Jeswani S, et al: Direct surgical repair of spondylolysis in athletes: Indications, techniques, and outcomes. *Neurosurg Focus* 2011;31(5):E9.

66. Li Y, Hresko MT: Lumbar spine surgery in athletes: Outcomes and return-to-play criteria. *Clin Sports Med* 2012;31(3):487–498.

8 Role of the Spine Surgeon with Professional Sports Teams, Agents, and Coaches

Robert G. Watkins, MD

THE SPINE SURGEON

There are a number of complex variations in the role of the spine surgeon as it pertains to the patient's employer and other concerned associates. The base of it all is that the spine surgeon has to establish a proper doctor–patient relationship with every player that he or she treats. It does not matter if the patient is an 18-year-old athlete who will never make it or the top star in the sport. The surgeon must cut through the sports apparatus, the team, and the publicity and be the patient's doctor. Do not be sidetracked by publicity, media, mothers, wives, or the desires of all the other people in your patient's life. Do not try to do anyone a favor; focus on the patient. Base your treatments and prognosis on what is best for your patient. The patient who leads the league in hitting is also a 26-year-old kid who just got married and has a lot of years ahead of him. Talk to your patient and find out the thoughts, and fears concerning his or her career objectives. Analyze the patient's case medically and understand your patient's job.

THE ATHLETE

What does the athlete has to do to succeed in his or her sport? You need to understand the sport and what exactly

Dr. Watkins Sr. or an immediate family member has received royalties from Medtronic Sofamor Danek; is a member of a speakers' bureau or has made paid presentations on behalf of Aesculap/B. Braun, Amedica, and RTI Surgical; serves as a paid consultant to Aesculap/B. Braun, Amedica, and RTI Surgical; serves as a board member, owner, officer, or committee member of the Journal of Neurosurgery *and the* Spine.

your patient's job is. Understand the athlete's position on the field and what he or she physically and mentally has to do to succeed. Understand what training the athlete needs to do, what he or she should. Take the history, examine the patient, review the studies, and add patient's job requirements to your recommended treatment and prognosis. When in doubt, do a complete history and physical on the patient. The surgeon must have an overall objective of accomplishing what his or her patient wants. If it is return to maximum performance, then that should be the objective of the diagnostic and treatment plan. If the patient desires to retire, then adjust the treatment plan accordingly.

THE ATHLETE AND THE SPINE SURGEON

Additionally, the spine surgeon has to make decisions that are in the best long-term interest of the individual patient and must assume the responsibility of the patient's safety while performing his or her job and developing a safe plan of return to high function. The decision to recommend surgery on an athlete's spine must have his or her return to full performance as a major consideration if that is the player's desired outcome. This means that the surgery should be as minimally invasive as necessary to correct the problem so as not to cause secondary symptoms because of the approach, but the surgery must also have the highest chance of success in correcting the problem. A spine surgeon who does only spinal surgeries and has a lot of experience with difficult spine surgeries in patients of all ages adds perspective to the specific problems in athletes. It is important that the surgeon can offer a nonoperative rehabilitation alternative when possible. If the surgeon does not understand and have experience with a good nonoperative rehabilitation program, he or she cannot have a full understanding of the indications and need for surgery. The surgeon must understand the long-term consequences of the surgery; having a lot of experience with patients of all ages helps that understanding.

IF YOU DO NOT KNOW THE REHAB, DO NOT DO THE SURGERY

To have the best opinion as to whether your patient needs surgery, the surgeon must understand and be able to set up a proper nonoperative rehabilitation program that can potentially return the player to play without surgery.

The surgeon and player must discuss the operative and nonoperative options and expectations and agree on a plan of treatment. The surgeon must understand and control the postoperative rehabilitation that safely returns the patient to performance. This is the contraindication to "the microscopic discectomy is a microscopic discectomy no matter who the patient is." If you do not control the postoperative rehabilitation and have an exact plan of action, your surgery will not be successful and your patient will not be able to return to a safe performance level. It is the surgeon's obligation to control the postoperative rehabilitation.

THE ATHLETE'S ENTIRE TEAM

The sports agents that I have dealt with have been open, genuine top professionals who do what is best for their clients and have been very concerned about their clients' health. They have been excellent in supporting my relationship with the players and have supported the recommended medical plans. One of the best agents told me a long time ago: "Doc, you take care of the medicine, and I will take care of the money." The safest area and most appropriate ethical area for the surgeon is to "stick to the medical facts of the case." Contract years and future income are not your concern. Be specific and state the diagnosis and prognosis.

The surgeon must work within the structure of the team and chain of command of the team. The spine specialist chain of command goes through the trainer and the team doctor. The team is your patient's employer. That is the mechanism for your patient to get well and play to her or his maximum capabilities. If your player is to succeed in a team sport, the surgeon must work with the team to enhance the patient's capability and health. The team for the surgeon starts with the trainer. For years, I have ended my spine sports talks with advising "respect the trainers and therapists." If you want good results with your surgeries, you need to treat the trainers on the team with the proper professional respect they deserve. They are such a vital link in this healthcare chain. Often in a difficult spot, they are the player's most immediate personal healthcare provider. Trainers care about their patients and your patient. During the season, they often have 25 patients a day who require treatment. It may take working out a specific program for your patient that is separate from the team to ensure an intense, specific spine treatment with a transition program back into the team environment. Trainers and therapists with the team have both understanding and experience that is helpful for certain sport-specific conditions.

Trainers are part of a team hierarchy whose job centers around the health of the players. They work for the team. A strengthening and conditioning coach knows very well what each player needs to do to perform the job and knows what it takes to get them there. Trainers and coaches must work together to protect your patient and allow maximum performance. Nobody associated with the team wants a broken player who cannot play because of injury or has future problems, and most provide an excellent environment for return to health as well as performance. Again, the patient and surgeon have to work with the team. If your player cannot do the job, the team is obligated to find someone who can, so whether the player can do the job is a decision in which the surgeon, the player, the agent, the trainer, the coach, and management participate. The surgeon doesn't know if the player is good enough to play compared to the other players. Others will decide that. Return to play is obviously an area that requires the surgeon to not only understand the pathology in the individual patient but also the sport and the patient's requirements to perform the sport. The player has a major voice in whether he can perform with the injury. The surgeon, through the rehabilitation program, can allow the player to demonstrate the ability to return.

RETURN TO PLAY

Timing of the return is always a factor of discussion. No one likes to plan a successful return on a certain day and have a reinjury the next day. My usual answer to when players can return is "when they complete their rehab program." It is not an evasion; rather, it is an honest medical answer, and the surgeon must have comprehensively understood postoperative and nonoperative program of rehabilitation for spine injuries in the patients.

These programs are designed for the athlete's return to the sport safely. But that is often not specific enough. A famous older general manager explained that to me by saying, "Dr. Watkins, I'm the general manager of a major league baseball team. My job is to have 25 players ready to play every night. Which 25 is not important, but I have got to have 25, so if you give me an estimated time of return for the player, I will make my plans accordingly." For everyone concerned, the surgeon must give an estimate of time of return to play.

The key to timing of return to play is having a rehabilitation program that can prove to the patient and everyone else that it is safe for her or him to return to a high performance level. A comprehensive rehabilitation program for spine injuries must transition from a progressive endurance, balance-based core program to a sports-specific training program that adds functions of the athlete's exact job while continuing the core program. Our spine rehabilitation program starts with a neutral position balance and coordination endurance core program with five levels of increasing difficulty and transitions. The next transition is back to the team trainers and coaches to further sports-specific training and return to sport. Although nothing can approach the physical and mental intensity of a game day, we want as close to objective proof that the athlete can do the job. The best thing you can do for your patient is take him or her out of the "Do you think you can go today?" situation within a team structure. Set up an objective means and timetable for the athlete's return. Estimating risk in return to a sport is not a very scientific thing. It is often based on the experience of the surgeon. It is not exactly science, but it is a very important aspect of providing care for your patient. The spinal surgeon has to be better than a doctor whose opinion is "never play again if there is any risk to me" because of liability and better than a spine specialist who is a psycho fan of the player's team. You cannot be a surgeon whose decisions are based on the athlete's popularity.

● CONCLUSION

Stick to the facts of the case and make your patient's health, safety, and desire to return to his or her job your sole consideration. Have open, consistent communication with everyone concerned—open, consistent clear communication that tells everyone the same thing. Tailoring the conversation to whom you're talking to is a real trap and is fraught with problems. After an initial consultation, try to tell everyone the same thing in the presence of the patient and then dictate the report in the presence of the patient. Simultaneous communication may not always be possible, but be careful to communicate the same thing to everyone. Others involved often hear what they are expecting to hear. It is also important to put it in writing into the medical records. Understanding potential conflicts in areas of mutual agreement does not take a genius but a concerned surgeon who puts the patient's health first and foremost.

SECTION 2

Cervical Spine Injuries in Athletes

9 Differential Diagnosis of Upper Extremity Disorders (Neck and Arm Pain)

Laith Al-Shihabi, MD • Howard S. An, MD

● INTRODUCTION

By virtue of their frequently overlapping symptoms and examination findings, pathologies of the cervical spine and upper extremity often present a diagnostic challenge to the treating physician. Understanding the differential diagnosis of neck and arm pain can lead to great confusion among many specialists. Making an accurate diagnosis is critical to getting an athlete back on the field of play. Complaints affecting this portion of the body are common in the offices of spine surgeons, sport medicine specialists, and hand surgeons alike. Some patients may find themselves being evaluated by all three, speaking to both the variety of pathologies affecting the upper extremity and the potential difficulty in accurately distinguishing them. Symptoms may result from isolated or combined mechanisms, be acute or chronic in nature, and can be due to causes near to or far from the affected area. This diagnostic challenge is especially true in athletes, who at once may be attuned to subtle extremity dysfunction from one pathology while accepting and tolerating other injuries that do not impair performance. The key to making the correct diagnosis is starting with a broad initial differential diagnosis and then narrow it down with the history and physical examination (H&P). A well-done H&P is the cornerstone of the patient workup and is sufficient to establish the diagnosis in most cases. When it does not, additional tests—including imaging, injections, laboratory studies, and advanced neurologic studies—can be invaluable.

● THE PATIENT HISTORY

Beginning with the presenting complaint, the patient history is used to gather information on the onset, chronicity, and severity of the patient's symptoms. With athletes, the relationship between the symptoms and athletic performance must also be determined. It is important to establish whether the patient is experiencing only one symptom, such as isolated pain, or a constellation of many, such as pain with weakness and numbness. In considering the various etiologies of pain, sensory disturbance, and weakness affecting the upper extremity, an effort should be made to differentiate between potential neurologic versus non-neurologic causes for the patient's symptoms. Although the focus of this chapter is on the differential diagnosis of neurologic upper extremity pathologies, non-neurologic injuries may present similarly or concurrently and should also be considered. A table of commonly encountered injuries to the neck and arm are reviewed in **Table 9-1**.

Neuropathic Pain

- Neuropathic pain can result from a traumatic nerve injury, central or peripheral nerve entrapment, or noncompressive mono- or polyneuropathy.
- Symptoms are classically described as burning or electrical in nature[1,2] and occur in a predictable distribution of affected spinal or peripheral nerves.

Dr. An or an immediate family member has received royalties from U & I and Zimmer; serves as a paid consultant to Bioventis and Stryker; has stock or stock options held in Articular Engineering LLC, Medyssey, Spinal Kinetics, and U & I; has received research or institutional support from Medyssey and Spinalcyte; and serves as a board member, owner, officer, or committee member of the American Journal of Orthopedics and Spine. *Neither Dr. Al-Shihabi nor any immediate family member has received anything of value from or has stock or stock options held in a commercial company or institution related directly or indirectly to the subject of this article.*

TABLE 9-1 Commonly encountered diagnoses in the differential of neck versus arm and shoulder pain in athletes

Diagnosis	Primary Complaint	Associated Symptoms	Pertinent Negatives	Examination Findings and Keys	Clinical Example
Cervical sprain or strain	Paraspinal soreness and tightness Often follows a traumatic event	Pain to anterior cervical muscles or intrinsic and extrinsic cervical muscles	Neurologic symptoms typically absent	Muscular tenderness ROM limited by pain Normal neurologic examination results	"Whiplash" to neck in collision or motor sport athlete
Cervical facet dislocation	New-onset torticollis and loss of motion after high-energy trauma	Neurologic symptoms often present	No extremity tenderness in the absence of extremity injury	Spinal tenderness with asymmetric loss of motion Perform full neurologic exam or MRI before reduction	Rotational injury after "facemask" tackle in American football
Cervical DJD or DDD	Axial neck pain Worst at extremes of motion	Stiffness often present Neurologic symptoms are variably present	Minimal paraspinal tenderness No extremity tenderness	Axial symptoms outweigh radicular symptoms	"Spear tackler's spine" in athlete with a history repetitive axial load to the cervical spine
Cervical radiculopathy	Radiating neurologic pain, numbness, paresthesias, or weakness Pain worsens with distinct movements or positions of the neck	Neck pain may also be present if associated with DDD	Palpation of the symptomatic area does not reproduce pain	Radicular symptoms outweigh axial symptoms Myelopathic signs should be absent in pure radiculopathy Extremity pain improved with shoulder abduction	Radicular symptoms with or without an inciting event May be exacerbated by cervical rotation and upward gaze (e.g., with a tennis serve)
Peripheral nerve injury	Extremity neurologic pain, numbness, paresthesias, or weakness	May be exacerbated by extremity position	No neck pain No exacerbation with neck motion	See Table 9-5	Ulnar neuropathy associated with elbow MCL insufficiency in a pitching athlete
Rotator cuff tear or tendinitis	Shoulder pain and weakness	Pain may radiate to neck	Absence of neurologic symptoms	Symptoms worsen with shoulder abduction Subacromial anesthetic injection improves pain and may improve weakness	Subacromial impingement resulting in rotator cuff tendinitis in an overhead athlete
Glenoid labrum injury	Pain with abduction/external rotation (anterior labrum), adduction or loading (posterior labrum), or overhead activity (superior labrum)	Glenohumeral instability or apprehension with certain arm positions	Absence of neurologic symptoms	Neck pain is infrequent Symptoms maximal when in an "at-risk" position for the shoulder	Shoulder instability after glenohumeral dislocation
Glenohumeral DJD	Shoulder pain or grinding, with or without stiffness	Pain may radiate to neck Pain-limited weakness	Absence of neurologic symptoms	Symptoms are worst at the extremes of shoulder motion Glenohumeral injection improves pain and strength	Accelerated joint wear caused by upper extremity weight bearing in a wheelchair athlete or weight lifter

DDD = degenerative disk disease, DJD = degenerative joint disease, MCL = medial collateral ligament, ROM = range of motion.

- Associated sensory disturbance or weakness within the same spinal or peripheral nerve distribution also indicates a neurologic cause of symptoms.
- Activities that place the nerve in tension or compression may exacerbate symptoms.

Non-Neuropathic Pain

- Fractures and dislocations are associated with the acute onset of sharp pain and deformity (if displaced) relative to a traumatic event. Secondary neurologic injury may also occur, however, as the displacement and energy of the fracture or dislocation increases.
- Inflammatory or degenerative arthritis is characterized by deep-seated aching or painful motion of the affected joint, with the former often improving with activity and the latter worsening. Concomitant swelling and stiffness of the affected joint may also be present.
- Tendinitis, tendinopathy, and tenosynovitis cause a sharp, activity-related pain brought on by resistance against the associated muscle–tendon unit. Palpation the affected tissue should also reproduce the patient's pain complaints. Immobilization of the affected tendon improves symptoms.
- Vascular dysfunction may cause acral pain through either activity-related claudication, chronic ischemia, or reperfusion (as with Raynaud disease). It is frequently associated with cold intolerance and changes or asymmetry in skin temperature.

Neuropathic Weakness

- Traumatic nerve injuries resulting from compression, traction, laceration, or ischemia lead to a disruption in nerve conduction by severing one or more structural components of the nerve.[3,4]
- Acutely, patients experience loss of some or all active motor function of the innervated muscles. Chronic denervation leads to muscle wasting and potential joint contractures due to a loss of balanced motors around the joint.
- Mononeuropathy is most often from nerve compression, either at the spine (following a nerve-root pattern) or peripherally in the extremity. Sensory or motor dysfunction can occur either in isolation or in tandem and should follow the anatomic course of the affected nerve.
- Polyneuropathy is usually secondary to a systemic cause, and etiologies can be genetic, metabolic, infectious, inflammatory, or iatrogenic. Nerve dysfunction

can follow a predictable (e.g., stocking-and-glove) or unpredictable pattern and by definition affects multiple extremities or nerve patterns.

Non-Neuropathic Weakness

- A tendon or intrasubstance muscle rupture is usually associated with a discrete traumatic event, such as with eccentric overload of a muscle, or with atraumatic attritional wear. In both cases, patients report a sudden, isolated inability or weakness with performing a specific joint motion. Numbness and paresthesias are absent, and pain is often minimal in the subacute or chronic presentation.
- Tendinopathy or tenosynovitis often results in pain-limited weakness, in which the onset of pain prevents full force exertion or motion. It can be distinguished from other forms of weakness by restoration of strength with elimination of pain, such as with an anesthetic injection around the tendon.
- Rhabdomyolysis may result from overexertion, causing pain and swelling of the affected muscle belly in association with weakness. Aggressive hydration to prevent renal injury is critical in the acute phase.
- Myopathy or myositis secondary to an infectious, genetic, metabolic, iatrogenic, or other systemic cause may also produce weakness, typically affecting multiple muscles simultaneously.

Sensory Disturbance

- Subjective numbness or paresthesias to the extremity indicate nerve dysfunction at some level. The history should elicit the exact nature and distribution of symptoms and whether they are constant, intermittent, or activity related.
- Whereas bilateral complaints should raise the suspicion of a spinal cord etiology, unilateral symptoms more often indicate a nerve root–level or peripheral cause of nerve dysfunction.

Nerve ischemia secondary to impaired vascular inflow may also produce sensory disturbances.[5,6]

● THE PHYSICAL EXAMINATION

As with the history, the physical examination is performed in a systematic manner that identifies and grades all components of the patient's symptoms. In this way, one or few leading diagnoses are determined, and competing diagnoses can be excluded. Whether the examination is performed by region or by system is unimportant as long as all components of upper extremity function are tested. To facilitate the examination, patients are asked to either change into an examination gown or remove their shirts. The examination begins with a visual inspection of the patient's spine and extremity. With a recent trauma, the examiner should look for signs of injury such as bruising or deformity. The presence and distribution of skin lesions or any asymmetry in the quality of the skin should be noted (**Table 9-2**). If the patient reports either preferential or obligate positioning of the neck or extremity, this should be noted along with the reasons why. Any asymmetry in muscle bulk or tone is also noted. Cervical spine position and motion is tested along with active and passive motion of the upper extremity joints. Any discrepancy in active and passive range of motion (ROM) of a joint must be investigated further. Preserved passive ROM with an absence of active ROM after an acute injury speaks to a disruption in the motors around that joint, either caused by paralysis of or damage to the motor–tendon unit. A chronic injury, on the other hand, may lead to joint contracture and loss of passive motion. Conversely, increased passive motion indicates dysfunction of either the passive stabilizers (bone, ligament) or dynamic stabilizers (muscles, tendons) surrounding a given joint.

Painful areas of the upper extremity are assessed next. In attempting to reproduce the patient's symptoms, it is important to establish whether or not the painful area is directly tender or not. As a general rule, pain originating from neural compression at the cervical nerve root or brachial plexus will not cause tenderness within the extremity even if it causes pain. Similarly, a peripheral nerve may be tender at its site of injury or entrapment but not distally within its territory even if the patient experiences pain there. Spurling's test for cervical nerves or compression, tension, or palpation of a peripheral nerve may cause shooting pain distally; this does not occur with non-neurologic injuries. Instead, with somatic injuries, patients are most often maximally tender at the same location where they experience maximal pain. Specific maneuvers to produce soft tissue impingement or isolate and test specific tendons, ligaments, and other periarticular structures as pain generators are also used to help identify sources of pain in the extremity.

A thorough neurologic examination is critical in the assessment of upper extremity complaints, both to distinguish neurologic from somatic diagnoses and to accurately identify the manifestations of neurologic injury when present. Our preference is to begin centrally and work peripherally in an attempt to identify the location, level, and

TABLE 9-2	Commonly encountered skin lesions and their diagnostic implications
Skin Findings	**Potential Associated Pathology**
Bruising, edema	Fractures, muscle or ligament rupture or contusion, joint dislocation or subluxation
Chronic sores or ulcerations	Loss of protective sensation, vascular insufficiency
Color or temperature changes	Complex regional pain syndrome, cellulitis Raynaud's disease
Hair or nail overgrowth	Complex regional pain syndrome
Vesicles	Herpes zoster, herpes gladiatorum, impetigo
Anhidrosis	Horner syndrome (associated with brachial plexus injury)
Hyperhidrosis	Complex regional pain syndrome

TABLE 9-3	Tests for myelopathy of the cervical spinal cord	
Myelopathic Tests		
Test	**Level**	**Pathologic Findings**
Jaw-jerk reflex	Cranial nerve V (proximal to foramen magnum)	Hyperactive masseter reflex
Scapulohumeral reflex	C3	Scapular elevation or humeral abduction
Biceps reflex	C5	Hyperactive biceps reflex
Brachioradialis reflex	C5–C6	"Inverted" reflex with diminished brachioradialis and hyperactive finger flexor contraction
Hoffman sign	No specific level	Thumb IP or index finger DIP flexion with flicking of the long finger DIP joint
Finger escape sign	No specific level	Inability to maintain extension and adduction of the ulnar digits
Grip-and-release test	No specific level	Early fatigue or slowness with repetitive opening and closing of the hand

DIP = distal interphalangeal, IP = interphalangeal.
Adapted from An HS, Al-Shihabi L, Kurd M: Surgical treatment for ossification of the posterior longitudinal ligament in the cervical spine. *JAAOS* 2014;22:420–429.

symptoms of potential neurologic dysfunction. As such, signs of myelopathy are tested for first and correlated to the level of spinal cord compression (**Table 9-3**). It is important to note that patients may experience dysfunction of

● TABLE 9-4 Testable myotomes, dermatomes, and reflexes for the cranial and cervical nerve root contributions to upper extremity innervation

Cranial and Upper Extremity Nerve Levels

Nerve Level	Myotome	Dermatome	Reflex	Upper Extremity Peripheral Nerve Contributions
CN XI	Trapezius, sternocleidomastoid	None	None	None
C5	Biceps	Lower shoulder and lateral upper arm	Biceps	Dorsal scapular, long thoracic, lateral pectoral, upper and lower subscapular, thoracodorsal, musculocutaneous, axillary, radial, median (variable)
C6	Brachioradialis	Radial forearm and thumb, +/− index finger	Brachioradials	Long thoracic, lateral pectoral, upper and lower subscapular, thoracodorsal, musculocutaneous, axillary, radial, median
C7	Triceps, MCPJ extensors	Posterior forearm and middle finger	Triceps	Long thoracic, lateral pectoral, thoracodorsal, musculocutaneous, radial, median, ulnar (variable)
C8	Finger flexors	Dorso-ulnar forearm, ring and small fingers	None	Medial pectoral, medial antebrachial cutaneous, thoracodorsal, radial, median, ulnar
T1	Finger abduction, PIP and DIP extensors	Volar-ulnar forearm and medial upper arm	None	Medial pectoral, medial antebrachial cutaneous, medial brachial cutaneous, median, ulnar, radial (variable)

CN = cranial nerve, DIP = distal interphalangeal, MCPJ = metacarpophalangeal joint, PIP = proximal interphalangeal.

muscles innervated by nerve roots distal to the level of compression and that the severity of myelopathic findings present on examination may be asymmetric. Neurologic pain is often absent in a "pure" myelopathy but can present if there is concomitant exiting nerve root compression.

The cranial accessory nerve and cervical nerve roots are then tested to assess the function of their myotomes and dermatomes (**Table 9-4**). Dermatomal pain is reproduced using Spurling's test, whereby the head is rotated toward the affected side and the neck is extended while the examiner applies downward pressure to the head (**Figure 9-1**). This compresses the neuroforamina and exacerbates compression of the exiting nerve root; the test has relatively poor sensitivity (30%) but excellent specificity (93%) for nerve root compression.[7] Motor weakness is assessed by comparing a muscle innervated predominantly by a single nerve root on both sides with a 0 to 5 grading scale. A muscle is graded as 5 of 5 if the patient can exert full strength throughout the muscle's ROM that cannot be broken by an examiner. A grade of 4 of 5 is given when full motion is possible against resistance but the patient can either be broken by the examiner or has notable asymmetry in strength. If the patient reports subjective weakness but cannot be broken by the examiner, either weight-based resistance exercises (e.g., a pushup against a wall) or weighted repetitions to failure may be used to quantify the extent of the patient's weakness. A grade of 3 of 5 muscle has full motion against gravity, but not resistance, while a grade of 2 of 5 muscle has full motion only when gravity

resistance is removed. A grade 1 of 5 muscle has discernible voluntary activity, but that is insufficient to overcome the weight of the extremity even in the absence of gravity resistance. Reflexes are tested last, and with compression at the nerve root or distal should produce hyporeflexia when compared with the unaffected side. Hyperreflexia should raise suspicion of myelopathy along with nerve root compression.[8]

The peripheral nerves of the upper extremity are tested last. Although compressive neuropathies are the most commonly encountered pathology of the peripheral nerves in the population at large, posttraumatic nerve palsies and paresthesias (e.g., so-called "burners") are the most commonly encountered peripheral nerve injury in athletes.[9,10] In both cases, nerves are likely to be injured by compression, tension, or laceration at points along their course where space around or excursion of the nerve is constricted (**Table 9-5**). Consequently, the examination is directed toward the assessment of nerve function proximal and distal to the common injury points to localize the level of injury.

● COMMON DIAGNOSTIC DILEMMAS

The overlap in symptoms generated by spinal versus peripheral pathology often leads to misdiagnosis and patient frustration. For this reason, it is valuable to review commonly confused pathologies of the upper extremity and their distinguishing characteristics.

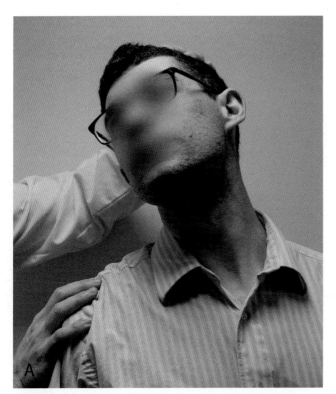
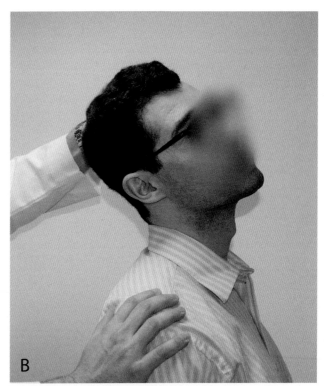

FIGURE 9-1 Front (**A**) and side (**B**) views demonstrating the Spurling maneuver for cervical radiculopathy. The head is rotated toward the affected side, and the cervical spine is extended while the examiner applies downward pressure on the head. Reproduction of radiating extremity pain suggests cervical radiculopathy. Head and cervical spine position can be varied dynamically by the examiner to find the point of maximal radicular symptoms.

C5 Radiculopathy, Suprascapular Nerve Entrapment, and Erb's Palsy Versus Rotator Cuff Tears

C5 radiculopathy, suprascapular nerve entrapment, traumatic Erb's palsy (C5–C6 brachial plexus injury), and rotator cuff tears share symptoms of weakness of shoulder abduction and forward elevation, with pain to the superior and lateral shoulder. Each can result from a trauma incurred in the course of play. Cervical radiculopathy in an athlete presents either acutely after a traumatic disk herniation, facet dislocation, or fracture or chronically in association with degenerative changes to the cervical spine.[11] The suprascapular nerve can be compressed in the suprascapular notch by suprascapular ligament thickening or in the spinoglenoid notch by a cyst associated with wear to the posterior labrum.[12] A traumatic Erb's palsy most frequently results from a fall on to the head and shoulder that places excessive traction on the upper trunks of the brachial plexus, varying in severity from a mild neurapraxia to complete neurotmesis.[13,14] Rotator cuff tears are most often either from attrition against the acromion or occur acutely after eccentric contraction with shoulder dislocation or subluxation.

C5 Radiculopathy

- The patient has a history of acute rotational injury to the cervical spine, chronic axial load (e.g., from a spear tackling technique), or no notable inciting event.
- Pain is unchanged with shoulder motion or improves with abduction.
- Weakness and atrophy involve the deltoid, supra- or infraspinatus, biceps, and other C5-innervated muscles.
- The Spurling's test result is positive.
- Shoulder impingement signs (Neer's, Hawkins, Jobe's) are negative.
- Symptoms are unchanged after injection of the subacromial space with local anesthetic.
- Cervical spine MRI is helpful as a diagnostic test.

Suprascapular Nerve Entrapment

- History of an inciting event is usually lacking, but it may occur more frequently with overhead athletes.
- The patient may have isolated weakness or atrophy of either the supra- and infraspinatus (compression at the suprascapular notch) or the infraspinatus only.
- All other muscles innervated by C5 are unaffected.

TABLE 9-5 The common compression points, symptoms, and examination findings for the upper extremity peripheral nerve compression neuropathies

Peripheral Nerve	Compression Point(s)	Muscles Affected	Symptoms	Exam Findings and Keys
Dorsal scapular	Suprascapular notch, spinoglenoid notch	Suprascapular notch: supraspinatus and infraspinatus Spinoglenoid notch: infraspinatus only	Weak shoulder abduction, external rotation	None
Axillary	Quadrilateral space	Deltoid, teres minor	Weak shoulder abduction, shoulder numbness	"Hornblower" sign: inability to maintain shoulder flexion and external rotation
Radial	Spiral groove of humerus after fracture	Wrist, finger, and thumb extensors	Wrist drop, dorsal hand numbness	Distinguish MCPJ extension (radial nerve) from PIP and DIP extension (median, ulnar nerves)
Posterior interosseous (radial tunnel syndrome)	Across radiocapitellar joint Recurrent radial vessels (leash of Henry) Proximal edge of ECRB Proximal supinator (arcade of Frohse) Distal supinator	Finger and thumb extensors	Aching proximolateral forearm pain, weak thumb IP joint or finger MCPJ joint extension	Distinguished from radial nerve palsy by intact wrist extension and absence of dorsal hand numbness
Median nerve at forearm (pronator syndrome)	Supracondylar process of humerus Ligament of Struthers Bicipital aponeurosis Between heads of pronator teres FDS aponeurosis	FDP to index and long fingers, Pronator quadratus, lumbricals to index and long fingers, thumb abduction, and opposition, thumb MCPJ flexion	Aching forearm pain with weakness to thumb, index, and long fine motor function Numbness to the thenar eminence and radial fingers	Reproduction of symptoms with pronosupination or forearm compression
Median nerve at wrist (carpal tunnel syndrome)	Carpal tunnel	Lumbricals to index and long finger, thumb abduction and opposition, thumb MCPJ flexion	Numbness to the tips of thumb through radial ring finger Weakness to thumb, index, and long fine motor function	Reproduction of symptoms with carpal tunnel compression or prolonged wrist flexion/extension Sensation to the thenar eminence is unaffected
Anterior interosseous	As with pronator syndrome	FDP to index and long fingers, pronator quadratus	Aching forearm pain with index and long flexion weakness	No sensory component to patient's symptoms
Ulnar nerve at elbow (cubital tunnel)	Arcade of Struthers Intermuscular septum Osbourne's ligament Fascia of FCU	FDP to ring and small fingers, Intrinsic hand muscles	Medial elbow pain with numbness to dorsal and volar small and ulnar ring fingers Loss of grip strength and fine motor control to the hand	Prolonged elbow flexion and ulnar nerve compression reproduces symptoms Medial forearm sensation remains intact
Ulnar nerve at wrist (Guyon's canal)	Guyon's canal	Intrinsic muscles of hand	Numbness to volar small and ulnar ring fingers Loss of fine motor control to hand	Dorsal ulnar finger sensation and FDP strength remain intact
Dorsal radial sensory nerve (Wartenberg syndrome)	Between brachioradialis and ECRL	None	Pain and numbness to dorsoradial hand	Distinguish from DeQuervain's or intersection syndrome by Tinel's and neurologic symptoms

DIP = distal interphalangeal, ECRB = extensor carpi radialis brevis, ECRL = extensor carpi radialis longus, FCU = flexor carpi ulnaris, FDS = flexor digitorum superficialis, FDP = flexor digitorum profundus, MCPJ = metacarpophalangeal joint, PIP = proximal interphalangeal.

- Pain, if present, is often vague and does not match the full C5 dermatome.
- The Spurling's and shoulder impingement test results are negative.
- Symptoms are unchanged after injection of the subacromial space with local anesthetic.
- Electromyography (EMG) and nerve conduction velocity (NCV) are often helpful at 6 to 8 weeks after the onset of symptoms

Erb's Palsy (Traumatic Upper Brachial Plexus Injury)

- The patient has a history of forceful lateral deviation to the head away from the affected shoulder, most often from a fall on to the head, neck, and shoulder.
- Because the nerve injury is through the upper trunk, both C5 and C6 motor and sensory function are affected.
- "Burners" and "stingers" are paresthesias and the most common signs of injury, but they may be absent with more severe nerve damage.
- Function of the long thoracic nerve is preserved, but function of the suprascapular nerve is variable depending on the level of injury within the upper trunk.
- The Spurling's and shoulder impingement test results signs negative.
- Symptoms are unchanged after injection of the subacromial space with local anesthetic.

Rotator Cuff Tears

- Acutely, there may be a history of a shoulder dislocation/subluxation event. Chronically, patients report progressive pain and weakness with overhead activity.
- Numbness and paresthesias are absent.
- Tears of the supraspinatus most significantly weaken initiation of shoulder abduction. The ability to hold an abducted or flexed shoulder (deltoid) is maintained.
- The patient does not have biceps or other C5-innervated muscle weakness.
- The Spurling's test result is negative.
- Shoulder impingement signs are positive.
- The patient has relief of pain after anesthetic injection of the subacromial space and a repeat of impingement tests (Neer's test).
- Shoulder MRI is useful as a diagnostic tool.

C6 and C7 Radiculopathy Versus Pronator Syndrome and Carpal Tunnel Syndrome

C6 and C7 radiculopathy and compression of the median nerve at the forearm (pronator syndrome) or wrist (carpal tunnel syndrome) each can cause symptoms of numbness to the radial digits of the hand along with thenar weakness and atrophy. As with other cervical levels, radiculopathy may present because of both acute and chronic mechanisms. Pronator syndrome and carpal tunnel syndrome are most often chronic and progressive in presentation, but they may present acutely in association with a neighboring fracture, dislocation, crush, or vascular injury.[15,16]

C6 and C7 Radiculopathy

- The patient has a history of either acute rotational injury to the cervical spine or chronic axial load (e.g., from a spear tackling technique) or no notable inciting event.
- Numbness involves both the thumb and thenar eminence (C6), radial fingers (C6 or C7), and dorsoradial forearm.
- Weakness involves primarily extensors: triceps (C7), brachioradialis and wrist extensors (C6), and finger metacarpophalangeal joint extensors (C7).
- Thenar strength is normal because the thenar motor branch of the median nerve is primarily innervated by C8.
- The Spurling's test result is positive.
- Peripheral nerve compression test results are negative.

Pronator Syndrome (Median Nerve Compression in the Forearm)

- Pronator syndrome is usually chronic and insidious in onset.
- Numbness affects both the radial digits and the palm/thenar eminence.
- Weakness of the muscles innervated by the anterior interosseous nerve (radial flexor digitorum profundus, flexor pollicis longus, and pronator quadratus) along with weakness of the median-innervated hand intrinsics (abductor pollicis brevis, opponens pollicis, flexor pollicis previs, lumbricals 1 and 2).
- The forearm flexors; pronator teres; and elbow, wrist, and finger extensors are unaffected.
- Compression across the forearm and repeated pronosupination can exacerbate symptoms.
- The results of the median nerve compression test, Phalen's test, and Tinel's sign at the wrist are negative.

Carpal Tunnel Syndrome (Median Nerve Compression at the Wrist)

- This is usually chronic and insidious in onset or occurs acutely after wrist trauma. Exacerbations with sleep (from prolonged wrist flexion or extension) are common.

- Numbness affects the radial digits and radial half of the ring finger only. The palm/thenar eminence is spared because the palmar cutaneous branch of the median nerve travels outside the carpal tunnel.
- Weakness affects the median-innervated intrinsic muscles of the hand.
- The median nerve compression test at the wrist is the most sensitive and specific for carpal tunnel syndrome.[17] The results of Phalen's test and Tinel's test may also be positive.
- Injection of corticosteroid in to the carpal tunnel transiently improves symptoms in up to 80% of patients.

C7 Radiculopathy and Posterior Interosseous Nerve Palsy

C7 radiculopathy can also be confused for a radial nerve or posterior interosseous nerve (PIN) palsy if the primary manifestations are motor weakness rather than sensory because all three share symptoms of weakness of the extrinsic finger extensors. Radial nerve palsies are rarely misdiagnosed, however, because they most often occur after fractures of the humerus. PIN injuries can present either acutely after elbow trauma or chronically because of compression within the radial tunnel.[18,19] PIN palsies are distinguished from C7 radiculopathy by preservation of elbow and wrist extension along with an absence of sensory disturbance. Pain and tenderness within the radial tunnel are also unique features of PIN entrapment, absent with C7 radiculopathy. Relief of pain after injection of local anesthetic around the PIN at the point of maximal tenderness can be used as a confirmatory test for PIN entrapment.

C8 Radiculopathy, Lower Brachial Plexus Palsy, and Ulnar Nerve Entrapment

Both C8 radiculopathy, a lower trunk brachial plexus palsy (Klumpke's paralysis), and ulnar nerve entrapment at the elbow can produce medial-sided elbow or forearm pain, numbness of the small finger, and weakness of the hand intrinsics. In athletes, injuries to the C8 nerve root can occur in association with pathology at the cervicothoracic junction or by disk herniation as at other levels.[20,21] Lower brachial plexus palsy commonly results from a traction injury to the arm when held in an abducted position or by compression of the lower trunk against a cervical rib.[13] The ulnar nerve is compressed most often within the cubital tunnel at the elbow, but it can also be compressed within Guyon's canal at the wrist after trauma to the hook of the hamate or ulnar artery.[22]

C8 Radiculopathy

- This is history of trauma or pathology affecting the cervicothoracic junction or no known inciting event.
- Numbness and paresthesias include the small fingers and extend proximal to the elbow along the medial and ulnar wrist and forearm.
- Weakness of the finger flexors (both the flexor digitorum superficialis [FDS] and flexor digitorum profundus [FDP]) is the most unique symptom. Weakness of the median nerve–innervated thumb intrinsic muscles may also occur and distinguishes C8 radiculopathy from ulnar nerve compression.
- Hand intrinsic function is better preserved versus ulnar nerve injury because of intact T1 innervation.
- The results of provocative tests at the cubital tunnel and Guyon's canal are negative.

Lower Brachial Plexus Injury (Klumpke's Paralysis)

- This results from high-energy trauma with traction to an abducted arm or by chronic compression against a cervical rib.
- Numbness and paresthesias affect both the C8 and T1 dermatomes.
- There is more muscle weakness than with either C8 radiculopathy or ulnar nerve injury because the C8 and T1′ contributions to both the median and ulnar nerve are disrupted. Both median- and ulnar-innervated hand intrinsics are affected.
- A Tinel's sign may be present in the axilla.
- The results of provocative tests at the cubital tunnel and Guyon's canal are negative.

Ulnar Nerve Entrapment

- This occurs most commonly at the elbow (cubital tunnel syndrome) or less commonly at the wrist (within Guyon's canal).
- Compression at the elbow in athletes may be idiopathic, caused by compression against the intermuscular septum from triceps hypertrophy, or caused by tension placed across the nerve from repeated valgus strain on the elbow in throwers.[23]
- Compression at the wrist can result from a fracture to the hook of the hamate or a pseudoaneurysm of the ulnar artery after trauma.
- Sensory deficits are typically isolated to the hand because the medial brachial and medial antebrachial nerves are unaffected. The presence of dorsal, ulnar

hand numbness distinguishes compression at the elbow from compression at Guyon's canal.

- Weakness is most notable within the ulnar nerve–innervated intrinsic muscles of the hand. The extrinsic muscles (FDP, flexor carpi ulnaris) are typically not affected.
- Elbow flexion and compression of the ulnar nerve exacerbates cubital tunnel symptoms, and compression of Guyon's canal exacerbates ulnar nerve compression at the wrist.

ADDITIONAL WORKUP

In most cases, a thorough history and physical examination should yield the correct diagnosis. If the diagnosis remains elusive, however, advanced diagnostic studies can be incorporated into the physician's armamentarium. Along with plain radiographs, MRI is used to confirm the level and nature of either spinal cord or nerve root injury. It can also be useful in the diagnosis of brachial plexus injuries because variations in the level and type of injury within the plexus can lead to significant differences in the physical examination findings. MRI is less useful for evaluating peripheral nerve pathology of the upper extremity unless an atypical cause of nerve dysfunction, such as a compressive tumor, is suspected. It is useful for identifying rotator cuff tears or musculoskeletal injuries with a similar presentation to neurologic injuries or if the results of all other study modalities remain inconclusive.[24]

Electrodiagnostic studies can also be valuable in the diagnosis of or monitoring progression of nerve injuries to the extremity while also recognizing that these studies have inherent limitations. Most notable are the skill and reliability of the physician performing the examination. For complex cases, we suggest that the referring surgeon discuss the suspected diagnoses and needs of the study with the physician performing the EMG or NCV to make sure that all potential levels and nerves are adequately tested. In the setting of acute injuries, baseline EMG and NCV studies should not be performed sooner than 3 or 4 weeks after injury. Before this time, Wallerian degeneration of the distal nerve may not have yet occurred, leading to a falsely normal study.[13] The EMG and NCV studies can then also be repeated at a later date to monitor nerve healing. Subsequent studies must be correlated with clinical recovery of function, however. Although electrodiagnostic recovery can predate clinical improvement by weeks or months, if the ultimate clinical recovery of function is insufficient, then the treatment plan may need to be changed.

CLINICAL CASE EXAMPLE

A 45-year-old recreational athlete presented to his primary doctor with complaints of right hand "heaviness," forearm pain, and weakened grip of 1 year's duration without an inciting event. Symptoms were most notable with tennis and weight training, manifesting as early fatigue when performing gripping exercises and when carrying heavy objects at work. Attempts at activity modification and use of over-the-counter medications had no effect on symptoms. On examination, sensation was normal, and no

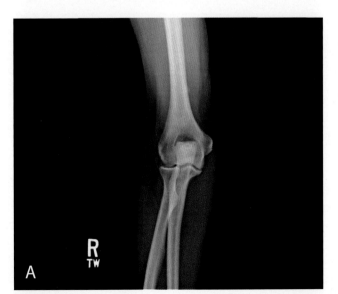
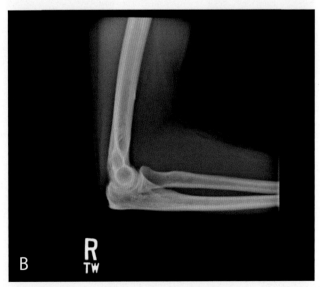

FIGURE 9-2 Anteroposterior (**A**) and lateral (**B**) views of a right elbow demonstrate the subtle presence of a bony supracondylar process present on the distal humerus. This indicates the origin of a ligament of Struthers, which can compress the median nerve at it crosses the elbow.

gross atrophy was noted. The primary doctor ordered an EMG and NCV, interpreted as within normal limits, and an MRI of the cervical spine. The MRI revealed degenerative disk disease at C4 to C5 and C5 to C6 with mild narrowing of the C5 to C6 foramina bilaterally. Based on these results, the patient was referred to a spine specialist.

Examination by the spine surgeon revealed the absence of cervical pain and no clinical signs of either myelopathy or radiculopathy. The patient had maximal tenderness and a reproducible Tinel's sign across the elbow and proximal forearm, with radiation proximally and distally from this point. Grip measured 29 lb on the right versus 55 lb on the left. The patient was then referred to a hand surgeon to evaluate for a peripheral nerve compression. Radiography of the elbow was performed (**Figure 9-2**), demonstrating a small supracondylar process protruding from the distal humerus. An MRI of the elbow was performed next, confirming the presence of a ligament of Struthers arising from the supracondylar process and inserting on to the medial epicondyle (**Figure 9-3**). A diagnostic anesthetic injection was performed to the median nerve under ultrasound guidance at the level of the distal humerus, with which the patient noted substantial relief of his forearm pain. The decision was made to proceed with a surgical release of the ligament of Struthers. Intra-operatively, an anomalous head of the pronator teres was found to

arise from the ligament (**Figure 9-4**), which was believed to be compressing the median nerve. Release of the nerve was performed from the proximal margin of the ligament (**Figure 9-5**) to the level of the tendinous arch of the FDS muscle in the forearm.

Postoperatively, the patient had rapid improvement in the forearm and elbow tenderness present preoperatively. The sensation of heaviness within the hand and weakened grip more slowly improved over the subsequent months. Physical therapy was initiated to assist in recovery of forearm and grip strength. By 4 months after surgery, the patient felt that he was be "back to normal," and he returned to full-duty work and sports.

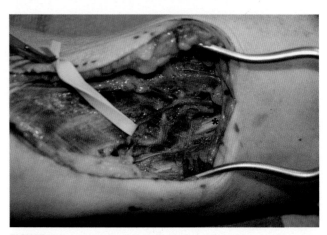

FIGURE 9-4 Intraoperative findings of a ligament of Strutters passing over and compressing the median nerve (*asterisk*) in the upper arm. The upper arm is to the right and the forearm to the left. An anomalous head of the pronator teres muscle can be seen originating from the ligament.

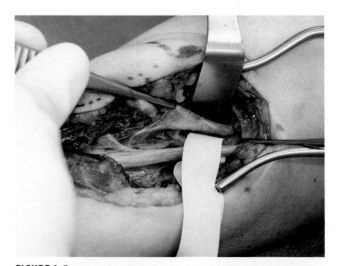

FIGURE 9-5 Full release of the median nerve in the upper arm with no residual crossing fibers from the ligament of Struthers. The neurolysis is typically carried distally through the proximal forearm to ensure no more distal compression of the median nerve or anterior interosseous nerve is present.

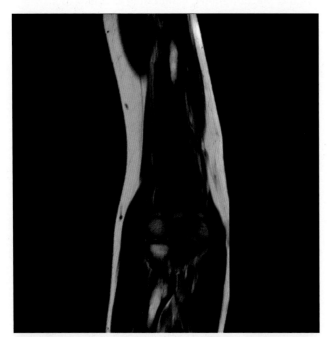

FIGURE 9-3 A T1-weighted coronal MRI of the elbow showing the supracondylar process of the distal humerus, from which a ligament of Struthers is arising and traveling distally towards the medial epicondyle. The median nerve can be seen adjacent to the ligament distally and medially.

● SUMMARY

Pathologies of the cervical spine and upper extremity frequently overlap in their presenting features, and surgeons must be skilled in using the H&P to efficiently and accurately distinguish between the two. Beginning with a sufficiently broad differential and using a systematic physical exam, in most cases a diagnosis can be established based on the H&P alone. With regards to the neurologic examination in particular, a strong understanding of the relationship between the dermatomes and myotomes of the cervical spine in relation to the motor and sensory innervation of the peripheral nerves allows the examiner to correctly locate the source and nature of neurologic injury.

The most common diagnostic dilemmas encountered by spine and upper extremity surgeons alike include differentiating between cervical radiculopathy and peripheral musculoskeletal injury or nerve entrapment. C5 radiculopathy is distinguished from rotator cuff pathology by the presence of upper arm sensory disturbance and potentially more widespread muscle weakness, while there is an absence of pain on active or passive shoulder motion. C6 or C7 radiculopathy can be distinguished from carpal tunnel syndrome by weakness of muscles proximal to the wrist, but with preservation of thenar muscle strength. C8 radiculopathy and ulnar nerve compression are distinguished by forearm numbness and weakness of the FDS muscle in the former, versus predominantly hand numbness and intrinsic weakness in the latter. If the differential cannot be sufficiently narrowed by the H&P, advanced imaging, neurologic studies, or injections can be utilized as additional tools in the diagnostic evaluation.

REFERENCES

1. Boureau F, Doubrère JF, Luu M: Study of verbal description in neuropathic pain. *Pain* 1990;42(2):145–152.

2. Woolf CJ, Mannion RJ: Neuropathic pain: Aetiology, symptoms, mechanisms, and management. *Lancet* 1999;353(9168):1959–1964.

3. Seddon HJ: A classification of nerve injuries. *Br Med J* 1942;2(4260):237.

4. Sunderland S: A classification of peripheral nerve injuries producing loss of function. *Brain* 1951;74(4):491–516.

5. Criado E, Berguer R, Greenfield L: The spectrum of arterial compression at the thoracic outlet. *J Vasc Surg* 2010;52(2):406–411.

6. Sanders RJ, Hammond SL, Rao NM: Thoracic outlet syndrome: A review. *Neurologist* 2008;14(6):365–373.

7. Tong HC, Haig AJ, Yamakawa K: The Spurling test and cervical radiculopathy. *Spine (Phila Pa 1976)* 2002;27(2):156–159.

8. Emery SE: Cervical spondylotic myelopathy: Diagnosis and treatment. *J Am Acad Orthop Surg* 2001;9(6):376–388.

9. Lorei MP, Hershman EB: Peripheral nerve injuries in athletes. *Sports Med* 1993;16(2):130–147.

10. Feinberg JH, Nadler SF, Krivickas LS: Peripheral nerve injuries in the athlete. *Sports Med* 1997;24(6):385–408.

11. Banerjee R, Palumbo MA, Fadale PD: Catastrophic cervical spine injuries in the collision sport athlete, part 1: Epidemiology, functional anatomy, and diagnosis. *Am J Sports Med* 2004;32(4):1077–1087.

12. Cummins CA, Messer TM, Nuber GW: Current concepts review: Suprascapular nerve entrapment. *J Bone Joint Surg* 2000;82(3):415–424.

13. Shin AY, Spinner RJ, Steinmann SP, Bishop AT: Adult traumatic brachial plexus injuries. *J Am Acad Orthop Surg* 2005;13(6):382–396.

14. Markey KL, Di Benedetto M, Curl WW: Upper trunk brachial plexopathy. The stinger syndrome. *Am J Sports Med* 1993;21(5):650–655.

15. Szabo RM: Acute carpal tunnel syndrome. *Hand Clin* 1998;14(3):419–429.

16. Schnetzler KA: Acute carpal tunnel syndrome. *J Am Acad Orthop Surg* 2008;16(5):276–282.

17. Durkan JA: A new diagnostic test for carpal tunnel syndrome. *J Bone Joint Surg* 1991;73(4):535–538.

18. Hirachi K, Kato H, Minami A, Kasashima T, Kaneda K: Clinical features and management of traumatic posterior interosseous nerve palsy. *J Hand Surg Br* 1998;23(3):413–417.

19. Hashizume H, Nishida K, Nanba Y, Shigeyama Y, Inoue H, Morito Y: Non-traumatic paralysis of the posterior interosseous nerve. *J Bone Joint Surg Br* 1996;78(5):771–776.

20. An HS, Vaccaro A, Cotler JM, Lin S: Spinal disorders at the cervicothoracic junction. *Spine (Phila Pa 1976)* 1994;19(22):2557–2564.

21. Post NH, Cooper PR, Frempong-Boadu AK, Costa ME: Unique features of herniated discs at the cervicothoracic junction: Clinical presentation, imaging, operative management, and outcome after anterior decompressive operation in 10 patients. *Neurosurgery* 2006;58(3):497–501; discussion 497–501.

22. Khoo D, Carmichael SW, Spinner RJ: Ulnar nerve anatomy and compression. *Orthop Clin North Am* 1996;27(2):317–338.

23. Del Pizzo W, Jobe FW, Norwood L: Ulnar nerve entrapment syndrome in baseball players. *Am J Sports Med* 1977;5(5):182–185.

24. Filler AG, Kliot M, Howe FA, et al: Application of magnetic resonance neurography in the evaluation of patients with peripheral nerve pathology. *J Neurosurg* 1996;85(2):299–309.

10 Stingers and Burners

Andrew B. Dossett, MD

INTRODUCTION

Stingers are the representation of a neural injury, typically of the cervical nerve root or a portion of the brachial plexus that is injured during athletic participation. The stinger is a symptom complex that is defined by its unilaterality, as opposed to cervical cord neurapraxia (CCN) (discussed separately in this book), which has bilateral symptoms. Stingers are also known as "burners." A stinger is a more commonly used term and is used exclusively for this chapter.

The stinger manifests itself with a unilateral lancinating, burning dysesthesia that radiates down the upper extremity with a variety of sensory and motor findings. There may be pain along the cervical column to include posterior elements, musculoligamentous structures, and the trapezius on the involved side. The participant is usually able to remove him- or herself from the field of play, typically leaving the competition with the arm either dangling at the side or "shaking the arm out." Weakness most commonly involves the deltoid, biceps, and spinati muscles.

MECHANISM OF INJURY

Two classic mechanisms of injury account for the majority of injuries: (1) head contact with extension and rotation to the affected side (**Figure 10-1**), creating dynamic compression of the spinal nerve in the cervical neuroforamen creating a nerve root stinger, and (2) head abduction and shoulder depression (HA/SD) of the affected side, creating a traction injury to the brachial plexus (**Figure 10-2**). Also, to a much lesser degree, a cervical disk herniation may also pose as a nerve root stinger. Persistent neurologic symptoms in a unilateral arm that do not resolve should alert the practitioner to this possibility. Stinger symptoms can last from a few seconds to several weeks. Symptoms that persist for more than 12

Dr. Dossett or an immediate family member has stock or stock options held in Alphatec Spine.

to 24 hours should warrant a more careful imaging evaluation with a cervical spine MRI. A variety of sports are represented in the demographics of the injury. The most common are football, wrestling, rugby, mixed martial arts, rodeo, and hockey. Less common are gymnastics, baseball, body surfing, and cheerleading. The severity of the injury is closely correlated with the amount of initial force that occurred. Subsequent reinjuries require much less energy because the nerve is in a reparative state, as are the supporting musculoskeletal structures.

There are three types of neural injury patterns: (1) neurapraxia, (2) axonotmesis, and (3) neurotmesis, listed in order of severity. In a neurapraxic injury, the myelin sheath of the nerve undergoes degeneration, but the axon wall is intact. This gives a greater motor than sensory component, which is typically seen in the stinger injury pattern. These injuries usually recover in minutes to weeks. Axonotmesis represents an injury to the axon and myelin sheath, but the epineurium and perineurium are still intact. Wallerian degeneration occurs in 2 to 3 weeks, which produces fibrillation and denervation potentials on electromyography (EMG). Both motor and sensory are affected as well. These injuries usually result in motor loss in the deltoid, biceps, and spinati muscles and can last for weeks to months. Last, neurotmesis indicates a complete disruption of the nerve and has a poor prognosis. These are rare and usually involve penetrating trauma or a high-energy, closed injury to the shoulder girdle.

There is no exact pathophysiologic mechanism for this neural injury.[1] Traction/tension and compression are the two predominant mechanisms, but it is usually a combination of these.[2] In the HA/SD mechanism, there is a tensile overload caused by traction of the brachial plexus.[3–5] In the hyperextension-rotation pattern, it is usually a compressive force directed at the spinal nerve root in the neuroforamen. The former (brachial plexus) gives a diffuse, multiroot examination, and the latter (nerve root stinger) is usually a more discreet radiculopathy.

American football has a relatively high incidence of stingers.[5] It is reported that as many as 65% of college players will be affected over a 4-year career.[5] There are

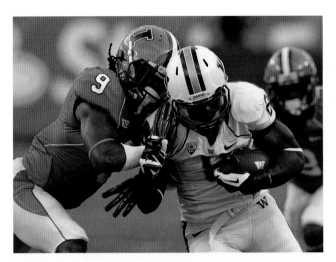

FIGURE 10-1 Head contact with extension and rotation to the affected side creating dynamic compression of the spinal nerve in the cervical neuroforamen creating a nerve root stinger. (Reprinted from the Associated Press.)

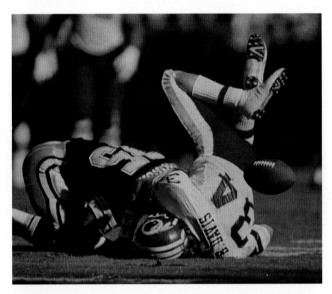

FIGURE 10-2 Head abduction and shoulder depression of the affected side creating a traction injury to the brachial plexus. (Reprinted from Vereschagin KS, Wiens J, Fanton GS, Dillingham MF: The burner: Overview of a common football injury. *Phys Sportsmed* 1991;19(9):96–104.)

trends associated with the type of injuries seen. Younger and less skilled players typically have HA/SD injuries of the brachial plexus. Poor core trunk strength, lack of technique, and perhaps a little less "stick your nose in there" attitude create this situation. Older, more experienced and accomplished players with better technique—"head up, see what you hit"—usually have an extension-rotation injury giving a nerve root or radicular finding. In older, professional players, the repair–injury mechanism seen in the facet and uncovertebral

joints after many years of play can create neuroforaminal stenosis and predisposition to nerve root stinger injuries.

EVALUATION

As in all cases, a thorough history should be taken to determine the likely mechanism, the quality and duration of symptoms, and a history of prior injuries. If bilateral symptoms are encountered, you are not dealing with a stinger but a CCN. Frequently, the athlete is able to articulate the mechanism of injury. At times, an injury video may be available (National Football League sideline injury surveillance). The key differentiating point is that a stinger is always unilateral, and any other pattern (arm/leg, both arms, both arms and legs) represents a more serious CCN.

As a matter of reference, the word "stinger" has several meanings to players. Approximately 30% of the time, a player who presents with isolated neck or trapezial pain without radiation will call it a stinger.[6] This usually represents a musculoligamentous injury to the cervical column.

There are two types of evaluation, the first of which is a game situation when a decision of return to play (RTP) is imminent. The second is a locker room or office evaluation when RTP is less acute. A sideline or in-competition evaluation requires a thorough history, including prior episodes, the likely mechanism of injury, a physical examination, and an RTP decision.

Physical Examination

Physical examination after a stinger injury requires thorough assessment of the cervical column, supporting paraspinal and parascapular musculature, and a neurologic assessment of the upper extremities. The sideline examination is briefer than a locker room or office examination because of the setting. Despite this, ample information can be garnered with a history and thorough examination to make an RTP decision.

Sideline examination requires visual inspection of the cervical column to look for a tilt or paraspinal spasm. This is followed by a manual examination palpating along the cervical column and the facet gutters posteriorly as well as over the parascapular muscles to include the trapezius for identification of trigger points. Provocative maneuvers, namely, Spurling's and HA/SD (**Figure 10-3**), are performed. The examiner should do the unaffected side first to help gauge normal end point of range of motion (ROM). When doing the Spurling's maneuver, I have two preferred modes. The first is after external rotation and

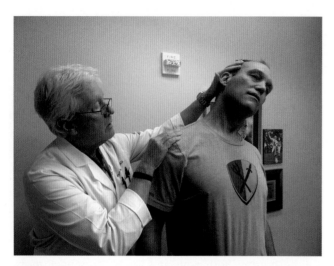

FIGURE 10-3 Head abduction and shoulder depression (HA/SD).

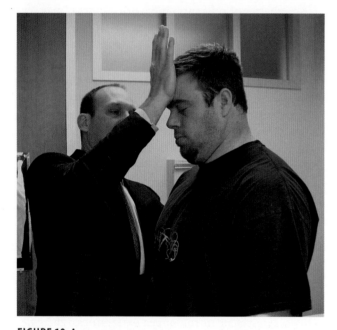

FIGURE 10-4 Examination demonstrating resisted flexion.

extension, and a moderate but meaningful axial load is placed on the head, giving a little "bounce" to see whether a pain response is elicited from either the posterior elements or a nerve root. The second mode is the classic Spurling's maneuver, holding extension-rotation with a small amount of axial load for 15 to 30 seconds.

Notably, a sense of the diagnosis can be achieved with both of these maneuvers. The HA/SD is more consistent with brachial plexus injury, and the Spurling's maneuver is consistent for nerve root compression in the neuroforamen.

Next is the isometric examination of the cervical column. The participant needs to be able to withstand meaningful force in flexion, extension, rotation, lateral flexion, and combinations thereof. The common mode of failure noted at examination is in resisted flexion (**Figure 10-4**). If the player has poor isometric strength, he or she will be unable to protect the cervical column and should not RTP. This examination is particularly meaningful in front of an overengaged parent or coach.

Last, a motor and sensory examination is done. A thorough motor examination of the C5 to T1 myotomes is done. My preference for examination is twofold in that the participant is tested for absolute strength, the first time through the examination, and then repetitively tested to determine fatigability within an isolated muscle group. After the motor examination, a sensory examination is done to both sharp and dull discrimination, with careful notation of deficits.

If it is decided that the participant is not allowed to RTP, a secondary examination in the locker room or office may be done. The patient may have his or her gear removed and shoes off and may disrobe for further visual inspection to look for tone, symmetry, and potentially fasciculations. Deep tendon reflexes are also achieved, as well as the Babinski and clonus examinations. In addition, the original examination done on the sideline is repeated, giving the examiner a second set of data points for this injury and a more comprehensive analysis of the injury.

Diagnostic Testing

Any athlete who presents with a history of significant neck pain or neurologic involvement should undergo cervical spine radiographs. A number of pathological processes may be gleaned from plain films, including fractures of the spinous process, facets, and vertebral bodies or uncovertebral hypertrophy giving rise to foraminal stenosis, disk degeneration, and loss of normal lordosis. Also, on flexion-extension radiographs, you may see splaying of the spinous processes, indicative of an instability pattern.

An athlete who is suspected to have a possible fracture should have a CT scan of the cervical spine. This is discussed in another chapter of this book. This also provides evaluation of the bony elements and secondarily the disk structures as well but not as completely as an MRI of the cervical spine. A cervical MRI is an excellent tool to identify disk pathology; cord pathology; foraminal narrowing; ligamentous injury; and to a lesser extent, fractures. In significant injuries, both an MRI and CT may be performed. In an athlete who presents with a brachial plexus pattern, I rarely go to advanced imaging, but with a nerve root syndrome, MRI can be valuable for persistent symptoms. Symptoms that have persisted longer than 24 hours should warrant further investigation and strong consideration for a cervical spine MRI to rule out most commonly a cervical disk herniation.

Electrodiagnostic studies (EMG or nerve conduction velocity) should not be done until at least 3 weeks after the injury so that result of the needle examination (EMG) will not be falsely negative. I usually defer electrodiagnostic examination because if the participant is still significantly weak at 3 to 4 weeks after injury, it is unlikely the patient will RTP in that season.

DIAGNOSIS

The diagnosis may be achieved through both history and physical examination. Classic findings for a brachial plexus injury are a HA/SD mechanism with reproduction of the symptoms with this maneuver. In addition, trapezial tenderness may be present. In terms of the neurologic findings, there is usually more than one myotome and dermatome involved with a brachial plexus injury.

The nerve root stinger typically has axial neck pain, a positive Spurling's maneuver, and a more discreet dermatomal and myotomal pattern of usually one nerve root.

TREATMENT

Although a single stinger does not increase the risk of more serious injury to the cervical spine, recurrent episodes can lead to delayed or incomplete recovery. Treatment is directed at local structures to decrease inflammation and irritation and creating an environment for neural structures to heal. Initial treatment is directed toward decreasing inflammation, regaining ROM, and settling down the mechanical pain. Institution of anti-inflammatory medicines is indicated for the treatment if the patient still symptomatic 1 or 2 days after the event. Using a nonsteroidal versus a steroid depends on the severity of symptoms. For paracervical pain, including trapezial symptoms, ice is instituted as well as athletic room modalities. Early neuromuscular control of the shoulder girdle and paracervical muscles is initiated. Scapular stabilization, trapezial, and neck strength is normalized. This frequently requires manual training with the therapist or athletic trainer, working the neck through a dynamic range of motion (ROM) with resistance. Chest-out posturing, which involves sticking the chest out, brings the head over the body and limits extension of the neck. This indirect flexion increases the size of the neural foramen and reduces the torque created by the weight of the head on the cervical spine. This posture also opens up the thoracic outlet and reduces pressure on the brachial plexus. This emphasis on chest-out posture is important because many athletes adopt a round shoulder, head-forward posture at baseline as the result of well-developed shoulder musculature, which may irritate the nerve roots.

Finding a neutral, pain-free position allows structures to heal quicker and gives the athlete an early goal with attainable results. If neck pain is severe, a cervical collar is indicated, usually for no longer than 2 weeks. Neck strengthening by the use of midline isometric exercises is important because neck muscle weakness can result from neck and radicular pain. Resistive exercises should commence slowly, and extremes of head flexion should be avoided. As symptoms improve, stretching exercises to improve flexibility and ROM should begin. Athletic trainers and therapists should exercise caution with aggressive stretching in extension because this could lead to recurrent neck pain after a stinger.

For an athlete with a disk herniation or a neuroforaminal stinger that is nonresponsive to these treatments, image-guided corticosteroid injections are an option. Consideration of facet blocks for axial pain and translaminar epidural injections with a steerable catheter to the affected nerve root are efficient means for calming down radicular pain, but this should only be considered after appropriate imaging.

EQUIPMENT MODIFICATIONS AND PREVENTION

Equipment modifications start at the most basic. Make sure helmet and shoulder pads are appropriately fitted. Classic modifications are use of a cowboy collar[7] or a neck roll. Both provide resistance to cervical extension but do little to restrain lateral flexion.[7] The cowboy collar has an added benefit of protection over Erb's point, decreasing direct contact injuries to the brachial plexus. These modifications may also allow the athlete to have greater confidence.

RETURN TO PLAY

A decision to RTP is reached when the examination findings normalize and the player has a pain-free ROM, normal neurologic examination results, negative provocative test results, and a normal isometric examination result. Discussions on RTP, when these criteria are not met, requires judgment, knowledge, experience, and informed consent. In making these decisions, an evaluation of a risk-to-benefit ratio is helpful. Risk is assessed both in real time for reinjury and long-term for sequelae of the injuries. The benefits of athletic participation are seen as lowest for high school athletes, medium for college athletes, and highest for professional or elite amateurs. The general consensus is that both permanent and late neurologic manifestations of weakness and pain may occur. Mild chronic neck pain, trapezial pain, and shoulder girdle weakness are the most common. These are seen in cases of severe injury without recovery and in cases of repetitive injuries over a career. These factors may be part of your informed consent with your player or participant. The risk-to-benefit ratio is another guideline in helping in RTP. For example, a young athlete with two stinger injuries over several weeks and who has recovered, with the exception of mild motor weakness of the shoulder girdle, should not RTP in a freshman football game. However, the same scenario in a professional player in a championship setting, after informed consent, is reasonable. The risk-to-benefit ratio differs considerably. Common sense and judgment prevail. Risk is also different based on your exposure. Certainly, football is high risk, and baseball is a low risk, which changes your management for the same clinical scenario because their risk exposure is different. Also, a superior athlete with the same symptoms has less risk than a less skilled performer doing the same task. The practitioner should have a general understanding of the skill level and goals of the participant along with knowledge of the sport, its demands, and training regimens. Having all of this information guides you in your RTP decisions. The safest and wisest course of action with any athlete is RTP is when the examination findings normalize and the player has a pain-free ROM, normal neurologic examination result, negative provocative test results, and a normal isometric examination result.

Case Example 1

29-year-old fullback: He had lingering neck pain and radiation to the left upper extremity with contact. Over a period of weeks, the pain went from contact related to pain at rest, with significant motor loss. Consultation showed a positive Spurling's maneuver, negative HA/SD, and marked motor weakness in his triceps. MRI showed a large left paracentral herniated nucleus pulposus at C6 to C7. The patient subsequently underwent anterior cervical diskectomy and fusion with iliac crest autograft and

returned to play the next season with normal strength and ROM.

Case Example 2

Professional football player, defensive end: The player had an HA/SD mechanism that gave him a stinger. Initial sideline evaluation showed resolution of symptoms and a normal examination within two series, and the player reentered the game. Late in the game, there was a recurrence but this time with notable motor weakness and both C5 and C6 myotomes. In addition, he had provocation of symptoms with HA/SD and was pulled from the game. After 3 weeks, his isometric strength of the cervical column was normal. Provocative examination results (HA/SD and Spurling's) were negative. There was still mild deltoid and external rotation strength deficits, but he functionally could perform and after informed consent returned to play. After several weeks, his strength returned to normal.

Case Example 3

Saddle bronc rider: This is a 33-year-old saddle bronc rider, on the Professional Rodeo Cowboys Association circuit, with a history of multiple neck injuries. He presented with complaints of stinger symptoms in his left arm (also known as his free arm). During rides, he experienced significant stingers into his left arm, and it would "drop," either causing him to lose his balance or get disqualified by the free arm touching the bronc. Office evaluation showed him to have a positive Spurling's maneuver and subtle C5 myotomal weakness, as well as a normal sensation examination. Diagnostic testing showed C4 to C5 foraminal stenosis. The patient underwent a C4 to C5 laminoforaminotomy after failure to progress with conservative measures. The patient recovered his strength and went on to perform without problems that year; in fact, he won the world championship at the National Finals Rodeo in Las Vegas the same year.

● SUMMARY

Stinger injuries are common in multiple sports. There are two predominant modes of injury. The first is an SA/HD injury that creates a traction injury of the brachial plexus. The second injury is one of extension-rotation mechanism, giving a nerve root stinger. The delineation between the two is seen on a number of levels, the first being that the mechanism is different. Second, the clinical examination for a brachial plexus injury rarely has axial neck pain but typically trapezial pain. Also, the neurologic test shows multiple nerve roots and dermatomes involved.

The nerve root stinger syndrome typically has axial neck pain and usually has a discreet radicular finding in terms of myotomes and dermatomes.

Treatment centers on decreasing inflammation and irritation of the local tissues and normalization of neck strength, ROM, and a neurologic examination results.

Training regimens to increase trunk, shoulder girdle, and neck strength are undertaken. Some modifications may be done in athletic wear.

In a small percentage of patients who have recurring injuries, there can be mild to moderate late sequelae. An RTP decision is based on a normal examination result, and if this criterion is not met, a risk-to-benefit ratio along with informed consent needs to be discussed with the participant.

REFERENCES

1. Watkins RG: Neck Injuries in football players. *Clin Sports Med* 1986;5:215–246.

2. Poindexter, DP, Johnson, EW: Football shoulder and neck injury: A study of the "stinger". *Arch Phys Med Rehabil* 1984;65:601–602.

3. Robertson WC Jr, Eichman PL, Clancy WG: Upper trunk brachial plexopathy in football players. *JAMA* 1979;241:1480–1482.

4. DiBenedetto M, Markey K: Electrodiagnostic localization of traumatic upper trunk brachial plexopathy. *Arch Phys Med Rehabil* 1984;65:15–17.

5. Clancy WG Jr, Brand RL, Bergfield JA: Upper trunk brachial plexus injuries in contact sports. *Am J Sports Med* 1977;5:209–216.

6. Personal communication, Jim Maurer, head athletic trainer, Dallas Cowboys.

7. Gorden JA, Straub SJ, Swanik CB, Swanik KA: Effects of football collars on cervical hyperextension and lateral flexion. *J Athl Train* 2003;38:209–215.

11 Cervical Cord Neurapraxia

Frank H. Valone III, MD • K. Daniel Riew, MD

BACKGROUND

Cervical cord neurapraxia (CCN) is a transient neurologic deficit that occurs after cervical cord trauma in the absence of instability or structural deficiency of the cervical spine. CCN occurs at a rate of 1.3 to 6 per 10,000 athletes.[1] The highest rates of CCN have been found in football players, in whom it is estimated to be as high as 7.3 per 10,000 participants.[2] Torg and coworkers developed the classification system for CCN as defined by the type of neurologic deficit: type 1, "plegia" for episodes with complete paralysis; type 2, "paresis" for episodes with motor weakness; and type 3, "paresthesia" for episodes that involve only sensory changes without motor involvement. CCN is further classified by grade according to the duration of symptoms: grade 1 (<15 minutes), grade II (15 minutes–24 hours), and grade III (>24 hours). Last, CCN can be defined by anatomic distribution of the neurologic symptoms: "quad" for episodes involving all four extremities, "upper" for episodes involving both arms, "lower" for episodes involving both legs, and "hemi" for episodes involving an ipsilateral arm and leg.[2,3]

Dr. Riew or an immediate family member has received royalties from Biomet and Medtronic; is a member of a speakers' bureau or has made paid presentations on behalf of AOSpine, NASS; has stock or stock options held in Amedica, Benvenue, Expanding Orthopedics, Nexgen Spine, Osprey, Paradigm Spine, Spinal Kinetics, Spineology, and Vertiflex; has received research or institutional support from Cerapedics and Medtronic Sofamor Danek; has received nonincome support (such as equipment or services), commercially derived honoraria, or other non-research–related funding (such as paid travel) from Broadwater; and serves as a board member, owner, officer, or committee member of AOSpine and the Global Spine Journal. Neither Dr. Valone III nor any immediate family member has received anything of value from or has stock or stock options held in a commercial company or institution related directly or indirectly to the subject of this article.

SYMPTOMS

In Torg et al's case series of 110 adult patients, the incidence of plegia was 40%, the incidence of paresis was 25%, and the incidence of paresthesia was 35%. The majority of CCN episodes were grade 1 (74%), resolving within 15 minutes, with grade 2 (15%) and grade III (11%) occurring less frequently. Additionally, the CCN pattern was quad extremity involvement in the majority of cases (80%), upper extremity in 15%, lower in 2%, and hemi in 3%.[1] Neck pain and loss of cervical range of motion (ROM) are not frequently experienced in adults at the time of the injury.[4] This is in contrast to children, in whom the deficits were most commonly upper extremity paresis (38%), quadriparesis (31%), hemiparesis (23%), and lower extremity paresis (8%). Additionally, the mean duration of symptoms in children was 26 hours, lasting as long as 5 days in one case, and 77% of pediatric patients experienced neck pain and decreased cervical ROM at the time of their injury.[5]

MECHANISM OF INJURY

The mechanism of injury in CCN involves hyperflexion, hyperextension, or an axial load to the cervical spine causing a temporary derangement in the axonal permeability of the spinal cord.[6,7] In 1962, Penning described the pincer mechanism for cervical spinal cord compression. In extension, the spinal cord becomes pinched between the posterior inferior aspect of the superior vertebral body and the anterior superior aspect of the inferior lamina. Conversely, in flexion, the cervical spine becomes compressed between the lamina of the superior vertebrae and the posterior superior aspect of the inferior vertebral body.[7,8]

Laboratory studies were conducted to quantify these theories. In a system designed to apply uniaxial tension at high strain rates with varying degrees of stretch, Torg and coworkers tested the giant squid axon of the squid *Loligo pealei*. The membrane potential and the cytosolic free calcium concentrations were recorded throughout the experiment. The study demonstrated that rapid stretch resulted in calcium influx. The rise in the calcium concentration was directly proportional to the rate and amount of tension applied to the axon. The calcium influx caused hyperpolarization followed by a prolonged period of depolarization. During this depolarization period, the axon was no longer excitable. Neurologic recovery was inversely proportional to the rise in the calcium concentration. Additionally, this study concluded that local anoxia due to venous spasm did not delay recovery because of the maintenance of the cellular and structural anatomy in the cervical spine.[7]

● RISK FACTORS FOR CERVICAL CORD NEURAPRAXIA

A large epidemiologic study was completed to evaluate the risk factors associated with CCN. The study had five cohorts: cohort 1 ($n = 227$), college football players who did not have a history of CCN; cohort 2 ($n = 97$), professional football players who did not have a history of CCN; cohort 3 ($n = 45$), high school, college, and professional football players with at least one episode of CCN; cohort 4 ($n = 75$), individuals with permanent quadriplegia after a football cohort; and cohort 5 ($n = 105$), a control group of nonathletes without a history of CCN. Cohort 3 had a significantly smaller ratio of diameter of spinal canal to vertebral body (Torg ratio) (**Figure 11-1A**) ($P < 0.05$; C3 ratios: cohort 1, $0.873 + 0.115$ mm; cohort 2, 0.849 ± 0.116 mm; cohort 3: 0.732 ± 0.156 mm; cohort 4, 0.958 ± 0.115 mm; and cohort 5, 0.998 ± 0.123). Additionally, cohort 3 had a significantly smaller mean diameter of the cervical spinal canal (**Figure 11-1B**) ($P < 0.05$; C3 diameter of spinal canal: cohort 1, 18.789 ± 2.031 mm; cohort 2, 18.474 ± 2.323 mm; cohort 3, 15.556 ± 2.704 mm; cohort 4, 19.093 ± 2.188 mm; and cohort 5, 19.025 ± 1.883 mm). The results of this study demonstrated that symptomatic athletes had significantly smaller spinal canals, suggesting an association between stenosis and neurapraxia.[9]

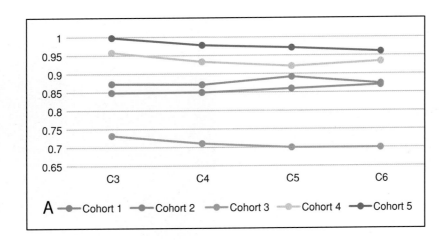

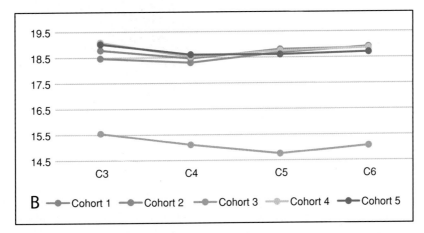

FIGURE 11-1 A, Torg ratio: ratio of the spinal canal diameter to the vertebral body diameter between cohorts. **B,** Spinal canal diameter (in millimeters) among cohorts.

Spinal Stenosis

Cervical spinal stenosis is common in pediatric and adult athletes, with the prevalence in football players reported between 7.6 and 29 cases per 100 players.[9,10] In an evaluation of 104 plain radiographs in adult patients who had experienced an episode of CCN, only 7% had normal findings, and 86% had cervical stenosis, 50% had osteophytic ridging, 21% had loss of cervical lordosis, and 28% had degenerative disk disease. Additionally when MRIs were evaluated in this same group of patients, only 8% of patients had normal findings, but 81% had evidence of disk bulging, 36% had disk protrusion, 55% had osteophytic ridging, and 47% had neuroforaminal compromise.[2] None of the MRIs in this study, nor Maroon et al's study of five professional athletes who had experienced CCN, demonstrated any posttraumatic cord swelling, deformity, or syrinx.[2,3]

Cervical spinal stenosis can be determined by a variety of techniques. In a study of 200 asymptomatic patients, Wolf and coworkers established normative values for the sagittal cervical spine. Measurements were taken from the posterior vertebral body to the site of fusion of the spinous process and laminae (spinolaminar line) (**Figure 11-2**). Wolf and coworkers found the average AP diameter was 22 mm at C1, 20 mm at C2, and 17 mm from C3 to C7. Consensus was that between C3 and C7, sagittal diameters larger than 15 mm were normal, and stenosis was found with sagittal diameters smaller than 13 mm.[11] Similarly, a study of 1066 human cadaveric specimens from the Hamann-Todd collection at the Cleveland Museum of Natural History found an absolute sagittal value of smaller than 13 mm was strongly associated with cervical spinal stenosis at all levels.[12]

The Torg ratio is calculated as the ratio of the spinal canal diameter to the vertebral body diameter at the C3 to C7 levels as measured on a lateral plain radiograph (**Figure 11-3**). A Torg ratio of less than 0.8 is considered evidence of congenital stenosis. They concluded that the low positive predictive value of 0.2% precluded its use as a screening method for participation in contact sports. However, because this method determines a ratio rather than absolute numbers, it is independent of magnification factors caused by differences in target distance and object to field distance.[6] A criticism of this technique is that it does not take into account disproportionate differences in vertebral body size in some patient populations. Herzog and associates demonstrated that football players commonly have larger vertebral bodies relative to other spinal element, and found abnormal Torg ratios in 49% of professional football players they studied.[13]

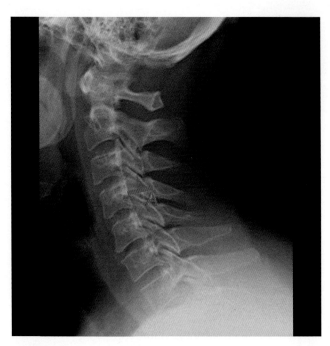

FIGURE 11-2 Lateral cervical spine radiograph with measurement of sagittal spinal cord diameter (A).

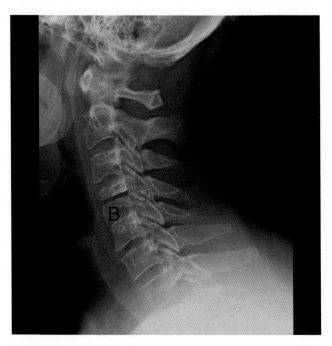

FIGURE 11-3 Lateral cervical spine radiograph with measurement of Torg ratio = A/B.

Additionally, Odor and coworkers observed that one third of asymptomatic professional football players have a Torg ratio of less than 0.8 at one or more levels.[14]

Magnetic resonance imaging is able to demonstrate both bone and soft tissue encroachment on the spinal canal. This allows for the more precise evaluation of the

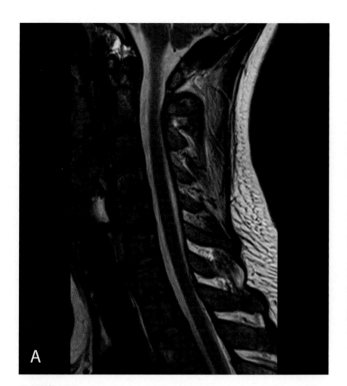
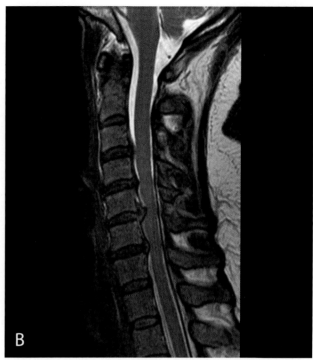

FIGURE 11-4 A, Sagittal T2-weighted MRI with functional reserve. **B,** Sagittal T2-weighted MRI with functional stenosis.

space available for the cord and a determination of the "functional reserve" of the spinal cord. The presence of "functional reserve" or "functional stenosis" is indicated by the presence or absence, respectively, of cerebrospinal fluid signal surrounding the spinal cord (**Figure 11-4**).[15,16] In a study of four athletes who had one episode of CCN, MRI demonstrated maintained functional reserve. None of these athletes had recurrent episodes of CCN after they returned to their sport.[17] Additionally, dynamic flexion and extension cervical MRI would further evaluate for stenosis and the presence of the pincer mechanism; however, this is available only at limited centers.

Treatment

Initial management for the athlete includes immobilization and clinical and radiographic examination. CCN must be differentiated from the more common symptoms after brachial plexus stretch injuries or radiculopathy, and the majority of patients who experience CCN will be treated nonoperatively with supportive care.

However, surgery should be considered in the setting of focal lesions associated with cord compression or instability as demonstrated radiographically. In two series, 8.5% of 142 patients underwent surgery for cord compression or spinal instability.[1,2] Additionally, Maroon and coworkers reported on a series of five professional athletes who underwent anterior cervical decompression

and fusion for focal cord compression after an episode of CCN. All five athletes returned to their prior levels of sport, but two developed career-ending adjacent segment disease.[3]

Return to Play

Return to play (RTP) after CCN remains highly controversial.[18,19] A systematic review of 170 articles showed that the available research lacks prospective randomized trials regarding RTP criteria after CCN.[20] The basis for RTP is primarily based on expert opinion, case series, and retrospective reviews. Generally agreed upon basic requirements for returning to athletics include normal strength, painless ROM, and vertebral stability.[19] Additionally, with the more frequent use of MRI, it is suggested that the player have "functional reserve" around the cord.

Page and Guy recommended absolute contraindications for RTP: ligamentous instability, a single neurapraxic event with evidence of cord damage, and multiple events or symptoms lasting longer than 36 hours.[4] Additionally, the presence of T2 hyperintensity on MRI is considered to be a relative contraindication for RTP.[16,20–22] However, a recent study with a small number of patients ($n = 5$) who were treated operatively concluded that MRI T2 hyperintensity in contact athletes who are symptom free after surgery with normal examination and no evidence of instability may not have contraindications to RTP.[23] However, the numbers in this study were small, and all patients had been surgically stabilized. Additional factors to consider when returning a player to full activity are the specific sport, likelihood of contact and by what mechanism, tackling style, anticipated length of career, and anatomic features particular to the patient.

In Torg and associates' study of 110 athletes who had experienced CCN, 57% of the subjects returned to sports participation at their previous levels of competition. There was no significant difference between the group that returned to play and the group that did not in regards to age, sex, sport, CCN clinical grade, or radiologic findings. Of the athletes who returned to contact sports, 56% (n = 35) experienced a second episode of CCN with an average of 3.1 ± 4 episodes. The subjects who returned to football had the highest recurrence rate of CCN compared with all other sports (P = 0.05). Of the football players who returned to their sport, 62% experienced a recurrent episode of CCN compared with a rate of 27% for all other sports. The athletes who suffered recurrence had a smaller Torg ratio (0.65 ± 0.1) compared with those without recurrence (0.72 ± 0.1; P = 0.05). Participants in this study who experienced recurrence also had smaller disk level canal diameter and had less space available for the cord diameter compared with those with no recurrence (P = 0.05). No permanent neurologic injuries were found in the 35 individuals who returned to their sports and had recurrent episodes of CCN. The athlete's age, level of sports participation, MRI findings, clinical CCN classification, and radiologic CCN classification did not predict which patients would have a recurrence. Furthermore, Torg and coworkers reported that neither disk herniation nor compression or degenerative disk disease were predictors of future episodes of CCN.[1] It is important to counsel the athlete with a CCN that there is a 50% chance that it may occur again.

Bailes retrospectively reviewed MRIs from 10 athletes who experienced episodes of CCN. All subjects had stenosis between 7 and 12 mm over three levels on MRI, but only 3 had no functional reserve at those levels. The 3 athletes with no functional reserve voluntarily retired, and the other 7 returned to their sports without subsequent episodes of CCN.[24,25]

In the single case series with short-term follow-up (14 months) of pediatric CCN and return to sport, the pediatric population showed different prognostic factors for recurrence of CCN. Torg ratios were calculated and noted to be above 0.8 for all patients. Furthermore, MRIs were obtained for each patient and demonstrated no evidence of extra neural pathology, as commonly seen in adults. Additionally, flexion-extension radiographs were taken and demonstrated stability in each patient. Among the 10 subjects with long-term follow-up in the study, each had returned to his or her sport without a subsequent episode of CCN, and no permanent neurologic injury was present throughout the group. This led the authors to conclude that it is the mobility of the pediatric cervical spine, rather than preexisting stenosis, that is the mechanism for CCN in this age group.[5] The mobility of the spine in this age group allows for hyperphysiologic motion and stretches the spinal cord against the bony structures, resulting in transient neurologic symptoms.[5,26]

Cantu reported on three cases of CCN. The third case involved a high school athlete who described an episode of CCN. Radiographs were taken 3 weeks after the injury because of persistent neck pain and stiffness. These radiographs demonstrated a vertebral canal space of 12 mm, consistent with spinal stenosis, and Torg ratios of 0.48 at C4 and 0.5 at C5. The athlete eventually returned to football and made a tackle resulting in an evolving Brown-Séquard syndrome with right-sided hemisensory loss and a flaccid left side. MRI demonstrated a disk herniation and displacement of the spinal cord. Although surgery was performed, the patient remained in a spastic quadriparetic state.[15]

Consequently, some practitioners consider a single episode of CCN as prohibitive for return to sport. However, in a survey of 117 football players who sustained permanent quadriplegia, only 1 (0.9%) had prior sensory symptoms, and none recalled having prior motor symptoms.[1] This is taken as evidence that CCN is not a prelude to permanent quadriplegia. Other practitioners conclude that although a single episode of CCN does not substantially increase the risk of permanent spinal cord injury (SCI), there remains a small but nevertheless present risk of permanent SCI.[25]

● AUTHORS' OPINION

Given the lack of definitive studies on the subject, we are left with small case series and expert opinion on the topic. Hence, what follows is our own interpretation of the literature.

Some may cite Torg et al's finding that none of the 117 players with permanently quadriplegia had a prior history of CCN as evidence that CCN is not predictive of permanent quadriplegia.[1] Based on such data, many physicians will clear a CCN patient to RTP unless they have prolonged or multiple episodes. We agree that Torg and associates' finding reflects the likelihood that the majority of players with CCN will not end up with permanent quadriplegia and that most with quadriplegia will not have a prodromal CCN episode. But to use this argument to say that no intervention is necessary is analogous to concluding, after finding that none of 117 patients with quadriplegia had myelopathy, that myelopathy is not a risk factor for quadriplegia. Most experienced spine surgeons have seen patients with myelopathy who have become quadriplegic and know that myelopathy is indeed a risk factor. However, we also know that the majority of patients with quadriplegia never had myelopathy. Part of the reason for this is that when patients develop myelopathic symptoms, the majority will seek medical attention and get proper treatment. In a similar manner, many players with prolonged or repeat episodes of CCN may, similar to patients with myelopathy, choose an intervention, namely cessation of playing. In fact, in Torg et al's series of 110 players with CCN, 43% quit playing after their very first episode.[1] This suggests that many players with CCN will quit playing, thereby reducing the actual number of CCN players at risk for quadriplegia. What we do not know is what the risk of permanent quadriplegia is in those who continue to play despite a single prolonged or repeat episodes of CCN. Of the remaining players in Torg et al's series, only 35 had recurrent episodes, none of whom sustained a permanent quadriplegic injury. But 35 is such a small number that if the risk of permanent quadriplegia for such patients is only 1 in 36, it could have been missed purely by chance. How many of us would participate in an activity in which the risk of permanent quadriplegia could potentially be as low as 1 in 36 and in which more precise information is lacking? Even if the risk of an untreated patient progressing on to quadriplegia were only 1 in 360, would we not recommend an intervention—even one with inherent risks such as surgery? In patients with CCN, there is no health risk to cessation of play.

Until recently, concussions were considered to be an almost normal part of contact sports and not consequential. Twenty years ago, a surgeon recommending that a player not RTP for the duration of a season after one concussion would likely have been seen as unreasonably cautious. However, we now know that neural tissue is not nearly as resilient as we previously thought and that there are long-term consequences to concussions. We do not know how the spinal cord differs from the brain in terms of its resilience to repeated trauma. At the microscopic level, there may be minor damage to capillaries or neural tissue that remain subclinical. However, with repeated trauma, it is not inconceivable that permanent neural injury might result.

For all of the above reasons, the senior author agrees with the general consensus that the following are *absolute* contraindications to RTP: instability or focal cord compression that cannot be reversed with surgical intervention or residual neurologic symptoms. In addition, we recommend the following criteria after CCN as relative contraindications to RTP. Note that we are referring to weakness in both upper extremities or upper and lower extremities and not a single-limb problem: (1) greater than 24 hours of grade 4 motor loss (able to resist but normally); (2) greater than 60 minutes of grade 3 motor loss (able to move against gravity but not against resistance); (3) greater than 30 minutes of grade 2 motor loss (able to move but not against gravity); (4) greater than 15 minutes of grade 1 or 0 motor loss (minimal to no motion); (5) any episode causing respiratory arrest; (6) second episode of CCN of any degree; (7) T1 or T2 Cord signal change on MRI; (8) any nonprofessional athlete after a first episode of CCN (**Table 11-1**); and (9) despite insufficient data, we believe that players who have a first SCN without a congenitally small canal or any structural lesions may be allowed to RTP, provided that they have normal radiographs, including maximal flexion-extension and lateral flexion

TABLE 11-1	Absolute and relative contraindications to return to play
Absolute contraindications	Instability or focal cord compression not reversed with surgical intervention
	Residual neurologic symptoms
Relative contraindications	>24 hours of grade 4 motor loss
	>60 minutes of grade 3 motor loss
	>30 minutes of grade 2 motor loss
	>15 minutes of grade 1 or 0 motor loss
	Episode causing respiratory arrest
	Second episode of CCN of any degree
	T1 or T2 cord signal change on MRI
	Spear Tackling Techniques
	Any nonprofessional athlete after his or her first episode of CCN

CCN = cervical cord neurapraxia.
Muscle grading: 5, full range of motion (ROM) against full resistance; 4, full ROM against moderate resistance; 3, full ROM against gravity only; 2, full ROM when gravity is eliminated; 1, muscle contraction is noted, but no motion is present; and 0, no muscle contraction or motion is present.

radiographs, along with an MRI and CT that do not show any abnormalities other than normal degenerative changes. We do explain that science is lacking on this topic and that knowledgeable experts do disagree. But it is our opinion that they are putting themselves at risk for further neurologic injury if they RTP. Although the actual risk appears to be relatively low and we agree that the majority of these players who RTP will most likely be fine, we believe that they need to be warned about the risks. An analogous situation might be in recommending intervention to a patient with mild to moderate myelopathy to prevent the small but finite risk of progression to quadriplegia.

The definitive study on this topic is clearly lacking. Ideally, there should be a study that examines the incidence of quadriplegia in a large group of players who suffer CCN but continue to play, compared to those who never had CCN. Until such a study is done, any recommendation that we give to our patients is our own opinion and not based on science.

Economic Considerations

We realize that there may be a strong financial consideration at stake for players who abandon their sports, as well as to the surgeons, who may be seen as being overly cautious and not be consulted again.

For most student athletes, it is the desire to play, rather than economic considerations, that influence RTP decisions. However, elite student athletes may have scholarships or future professional careers at stake. The student, his or her family, or other people in the student's life may be consciously or subconsciously influenced in their decision-making process by economic factors.

For professionals, economic considerations are much more obvious and can play an outsized role in the decision-making process. Professionals often shrug off injury and warning signs in their desire to return. Franchises and agents have a vested interest in seeing them RTP. Team doctors who are perceived as being too cautious compared with generally established opinions (which are simply opinions and not based on science) might find themselves out of a job.

Medicolegal Considerations

Because the lifetime economic consequences of quadriplegia are so enormous, it is common for patients and their families to seek redress for the injury from all possible sources, including the physician who cleared the player to RTP. The treating physician should therefore have a comprehensive and well-documented discussion with the patient, family, agent, franchise, and all other stakeholders. This conversation should warn about the risks of RTP and the fact that the science is not definitive.

● SUMMARY

Cervical cord neurapraxia is a transient neurologic deficit resulting from trauma to the cervical spine. The majority of symptoms resolve in adults within 15 minutes, but they may last much longer in children. The association of CCN with cervical stenosis has been shown in many series in adults, but it has not been well demonstrated in children, in whom cervical spine hypermobility may play a greater role. RTP criteria is greatly based on expert opinion and retrospective case reviews. The literature is without any large series that would allow for recommendations based on meaningful and accurate epidemiologic results. Whereas adults who do return to their sport may have recurrent episodes of CCN, the risk of recurrence in children has not yet been established.

Given that the literature is inadequate to make science-based recommendations, expert-based recommendations have ruled the day. Our recommendations include initial management consisting of immobilization and clinical and radiographic examination. Radiographic examination should include static radiographs as well as MRI, and if instability is suspected, dynamic radiographs or MRI should be undertaken. We believe that absolute contraindications to RTP include instability or focal cord compression that cannot be resolved with an anterior cervical discectomy and fusion (ACDF), as well as any residual weakness in a major motor group, imbalance, loss of dexterity, or other cord-related neurologic deficits, In addition, we recommend the following relative contraindications after CCN (not single-limb neuropraxia) to RTP: (1) greater than 24 hours of grade 4 motor loss (able to resist but normally), (2) greater than 60 minutes of grade 3 motor loss (able to move against gravity but not against resistance), (3) greater than 30 minutes of grade 2 motor loss (able to move but not against gravity), (4) greater than 15 minutes of grade 1 or 0 motor loss (minimal to no motion), (5) any episode causing respiratory arrest, (6) second episode of CCN of any degree, (7) T1 or T2 cord signal change on MRI, and (8) any nonprofessional after the first episode of CCN. Additionally, the physician must consider the specific sport, likelihood of contact and by what mechanism, tackling style, anticipated length of career, and anatomic features particular to the patient.

REFERENCES

1. Torg JS, Pavlov H, Genuario SE, Sennett B, Wisneski RJ, Robie BH, Jahre C: Neurapraxia of the cervical spinal cord with transient quadriplegia. *J Bone Joint Surg Am* 1986;68(9):1354–1370.

2. Torg JS, Corcoran TA, Thibault LE, Pavlov H, Sennett BJ, Naranja RJ Jr, Priano S: Cervical cord neurapraxia: classification, pathomechanics, morbidity, and management guidelines. *J Neurosurg* 1997;87(6):843–850.

3. Maroon JC, El-Kadi H, Abla AA, Wecht DA, Bost J, Norwig J, Bream T: Cervical neurapraxia in elite athletes: evaluation and surgical treatment. Report of five cases. *J Neurosurg Spine* 2007;6(4):356–363.

4. Page S, Guy JA: Neurapraxia, "stingers," and spinal stenosis in athletes. *South Med J* 2004;97(8):766–769.

5. Boockvar JA, Durham SR, Sun PP. Cervical spinal stenosis and sports-related cervical cord neurapraxia in children. *Spine (Phila Pa 1976)* 2001;26(24):2709–2712; discussion 2713.

6. Pavlov H, Torg JS, Robie B, Jahre C: Cervical spinal stenosis: Determination with vertebral body ratio method. *Radiology* 1987;164(3):771–775.

7. Torg JS, Thibault L, Sennett B, Pavlov H: The Nicolas Andry Award. The pathomechanics and pathophysiology of cervical spinal cord injury. *Clin Orthop Relat Res* 1995;(321):259–269.

8. Penning L: Some aspects of plain radiography of the cervical spine in chronic myelopathy. *Neurology* 1962;12:513–519.

9. Torg JS, Naranja RJ Jr, Pavlov H, Galinat BJ, Warren R, Stine RA: The relationship of developmental narrowing of the cervical spinal canal to reversible and irreversible injury of the cervical spinal cord in football players. *J Bone Joint Surg Am* 1996;78(9):1308–1314.

10. Smith MG, Fulcher M, Shanklin J, Tillett ED: The prevalence of congenital cervical spinal stenosis in 262 college and high school football players. *J Ky Med Assoc* 1993;91(7):273–275.

11. Wolf BS, Khilnani M, Malis L: The sagittal diameter of the bony cervical spinal canal and its significance in cervical spondylosis. *J Mt Sinai Hosp N Y* 1956;23(3):283–292.

12. Bajwa NS, Toy JO, Young EY, Ahn NU: Establishment of parameters for congenital stenosis of the cervical spine: an anatomic descriptive analysis of 1,066 cadaveric specimens. *Eur Spine J* 2012;21(12):2467–2474.

13. Herzog RJ, Wiens JJ, Dillingham MF, Sontag MJ: Normal cervical spine morphometry and cervical spinal stenosis in asymptomatic professional football players. Plain film radiography, multiplanar computed tomography, and magnetic resonance imaging. *Spine (Phila Pa 1976)* 1991;16(6 suppl):S178–S186.

14. Odor JM, Watkins RG, Dillin WH, Dennis S, Saberi M: Incidence of cervical spinal stenosis in professional and rookie football players. *Am J Sports Med* 1990;18(5):507–509.

15. Cantu RC: Cervical spine injuries in the athlete. *Semin Neurol* 2000;20(2):173–178.

16. Cantu RC: Return to play guidelines after a head injury. *Clin Sports Med* 1998;17(1):45–60.

17. Veidlinger OF, Colwill JC, Smyth HS, Turner D: Cervical myelopathy and its relationship to cervical stenosis. *Spine (Phila Pa 1976)* 1981;6(6):550–552.

18. Morganti C, Sweeney CA, Albanese SA, Burak C, Hosea T, Connolly PJ: Return to play after cervical spine injury. *Spine (Phila Pa 1976)* 2001;26(10):1131–1136.

19. Morganti C: Recommendations for return to sports following cervical spine injuries. *Sports Med* 2003;33(8):563–573.

20. Dailey A, Harrop JS, France JC: High-energy contact sports and cervical spine neurapraxia injuries: What are the criteria for return to participation? *Spine (Phila Pa 1976)* 2010;35(21 suppl):S193–S201.

21. Vaccaro AR, Watkins B, Albert TJ, Pfaff WL, Klein GR, Silber JS: Cervical spine injuries in athletes: Current return-to-play criteria. *Orthopedics* 2001;24(7):699–703; quiz 704–705.

22. Vaccaro AR, Klein GR, Ciccoti M, Pfaff WL, Moulton MJ, Hilibrand AJ, Watkins B: Return to play criteria for the athlete with cervical spine injuries resulting in stinger and transient quadriplegia/paresis. *Spine J* 2002;2(5):351–356.

23. Tempel ZJ, Bost JW, Norwig JA, Maroon JC: Significance of T2 hyperintensity on magnetic resonance imaging after cervical cord injury and return to play in professional athletes. *Neurosurgery* 2015;77(1):23–30.

24. Bailes JE, Hadley MN, Quigley MR, Sonntag VK, Cerullo LJ: Management of athletic injuries of the cervical spine and spinal cord. *Neurosurgery* 1991;29(4):491–497.

25. Bailes JE: Experience with cervical stenosis and temporary paralysis in athletes. *J Neurosurg Spine* 2005;2(1):11–16.

26. Pang D: Spinal cord injury without radiographic abnormality in children, 2 decades later. *Neurosurgery* 2004;55(6):1325–1342; discussion 1342–1343.

12 Cervical Disk Herniation in Athletes

Andrew C. Hecht, MD • Steven McAnany, MD • Sheeraz Qureshi, MD, MBA

INTRODUCTION

Cervical disk injuries carry with them the risk of prematurely ending an athlete's career with the associated financial ramifications for both the player and the team when at the professional level.[1] Symptoms associated with cervical disk injury in athletes are similar to those seen in the general population with upper extremity radiculopathy (arm pain, paresthesia, or weakness), neck pain, and coordination difficulties being the most common.[2,3] Although the symptoms may be similar between the two groups, Mundt et al[4] found that the symptoms may be more pronounced in athletes given the demands of the specific sport.

Cervical disk injuries in athletes are less common than lumbar disk injuries and tend to affect older athletes. In fact, it has been shown in contact sports such as wrestling and football that there is an age-related increase in the likelihood of sustaining a cervical disk injury over the lifetime of these athletes.[5] Similar findings have not been shown in noncontact athletes, with Mundt et al[4] concluding that athletes in noncontact sports may actually have a conferred protective effect against the development of either cervical or lumbar herniations. The authors hypothesized that improved muscular conditioning protected the disks from the pathological stresses placed on the spine.

In a population-based study, the annual incidence of cervical radiculopathy was found to be 107.3 per 100,000 for men and 63.5 per 100,000 for women.[6] In a more recent study of military personnel, 24,742 people were found to have cervical radiculopathy for an incidence of 1.79 per 1000 person-years.[7] As with nonathletes, the initial treatment for almost all herniated disks should be nonoperative care. Treatment options include rest, activity modification, anti-inflammatory medication, immobilization, cervical traction, and therapeutic injections.[2,3,8,9] Most athletes have complete resolution of their symptoms after nonoperative care. For those who fail to improve, operative intervention should be considered. Potential surgical options include anterior cervical discectomy and fusion (ACDF), a posterior cervical foraminotomy (PCF), and cervical disk replacement (CDR).

Return to play (RTP) after conservative or operative treatment of a cervical disk injury is often the most important question for the athlete and the team (**Figure 12-1**). Comprehensive and definitive guidelines for RTP have yet to be developed, and often the decision to allow an

Dr. Hecht or an immediate family member has received royalties from Zimmer; serves as a paid consultant to Medtronic Sofamor Danek, Stryker, and Zimmer; has stock or stock options held in Johnson & Johnson; and serves as a board member, owner, officer, or committee member of the AAOS, Musculoskeletal Transplant Foundation, the American Journal of Orthopedics, the Global Spine Journal, the Journal of Spinal Disorders and Techniques, the Orthopaedic Knowledge Online Journal, and Orthopedics Today. Dr. Qureshi or an immediate family member has received royalties from Zimmer; is a member of a speakers' bureau or has made paid presentations on behalf of Globus Medical, Medtronic Sofamor Danek, and Stryker; serves as a paid consultant to Medtronic, Orthofix, Stryker, and Zimmer; and serves as a board member, owner, officer, or committee member of the AAOS, the Cervical Spine Research Society, the Clinical Orthopaedics and Related Research, the Contemporary Spine Surgery, the Global Spine Journal, the Musculoskeletal Transplant Foundation, the NASS, the Spine, and the Spine Journal. Neither Dr. McAnany nor any immediate family member has received anything of value from or has stock or stock options held in a commercial company or institution related directly or indirectly to the subject of this article.

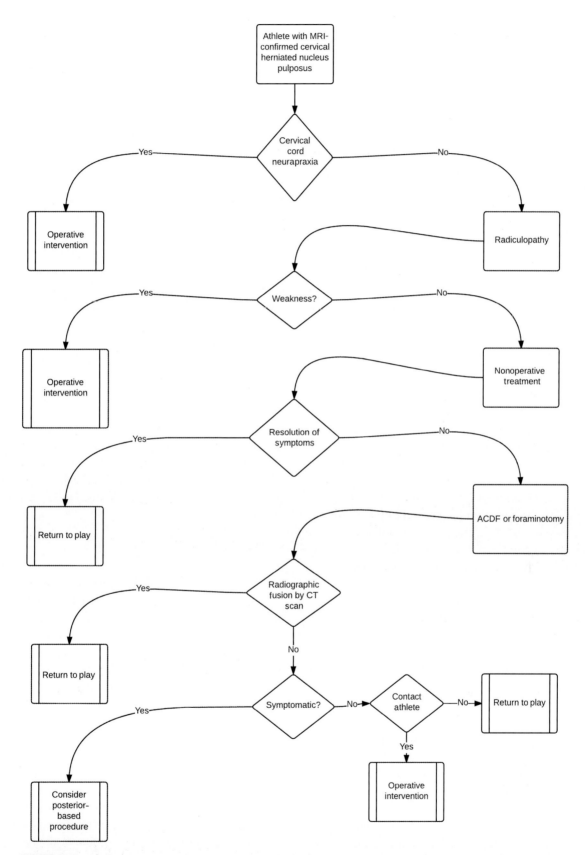

FIGURE 12-1 Flow diagram detailing the return to play guidelines after cervical disk injury in an athlete. ACDF = anterior cervical discectomy and fusion.

athlete to RTP is based on anecdotal evidence and surgeon experience.

NONOPERATIVE MANAGEMENT

Nonoperative management remains the initial standard if care for all patients presenting with symptomatic cervical disk disease without associated neurological deficit, cord signal change, or intractable pain. The natural history of cervical radiculopathy as described by Lees and Turner is considered to be generally favorable with nonoperative management.[10] In their series with long-term follow-up, 45% had only a single episode of pain without recurrence, 30% had mild residual symptoms, and only 25% had persistent or worsening symptoms. Other studies have shown a significant improvement in symptoms in up to 90% of patients with nonoperative care.[11,12] Although nonoperative management remains the standard of care for patients without significant neurologic sequela, there have been no randomized controlled trials (RCTs) comparing the various types of nonoperative with the natural disease history with no intervention. Furthermore, there have been no randomized studies that have shown superior outcomes of nonoperative treatment compared with surgery.

The goals of nonoperative management of an acute cervical disk injury in athletes are to treat the pain and to initiate a treatment plan that can allow the athlete to RTP. The ideal nonoperative treatment algorithm has not been strictly defined in the general population or in competitive elite athletes. The most commonly used medications are anti-inflammatory medications, including nonsteroidal anti-inflammatory (NSAIDs) or corticosteroids (i.e., Medrol dose pack or prednisone taper) and, in severe cases, narcotic analgesics. Additionally, cervical soft collars, ice or heat, cervical traction, narcotics, and muscle relaxants can also be used with variable efficacy. The use of collars in the athletic population has not been directly studied. Caution should be used because a recent study in the general population demonstrated that prolonged collar wear has been associated with atrophy of the cervical musculature.[13]

Physical therapy in the acute setting can often worsen the pain and may prolong the duration of symptoms. Cervical range of motion (ROM) and associated strengthening exercises are generally discouraged while the patient remains acutely symptomatic. After resolution or control of the painful symptoms, the patient can begin these exercises, although there is minimal literature to support the efficacy of these treatments for acute pain.[14,15] Supervised cervical traction has also been advocated as a temporary

adjuvant to help relieve pain. Physical therapy remains a key component to help an athlete regain ROM and strength.

Cervical epidural steroid injections are less commonly used than in the lumbar spine. To date, there are both retrospective and prospective data to support the use of epidural steroid injections in the cervical spine. A recent systematic review suggested that the evidence for cervical pain relief with transforaminal epidural steroid injections was moderate.[16] Two recent studies showed that up to 60% of patients may experience long-term symptomatic relief with an injection.[17,18] A recent RCT assigned 169 patients to one of three arms: cervical epidural injections; physical therapy plus pharmacotherapy; or a combination of injection, physical therapy, and pharmacotherapy.[19] At 3-month follow-up, all groups had improvement with the largest improvement seen in the combination therapy group. By 6 months, however, there was no significant difference between the three groups. To date, there have been no studies that have directly looked at the use of epidural steroid injections in athletes. Furthermore, there is currently no method for determining in which patient the injection will prove to be efficacious. When taken in the context of significant potential risks, including neurologic deficit, epidural hematoma, and possible vascular infarct, cervical epidural injections should be used with caution in the athlete population and only by experienced interventional physiatrists or pain management physicians.

Evidence-Based Review

In a recent study by Hsu,[1] RTP after acute cervical disk herniation was examined in 99 National Football League (NFL) players. Nonoperative treatment was defined as epidural steroid injections, physical therapy, activity modification, or any treatment other than surgical intervention. Overall, at a minimum follow-up of 2 years, only 21 of 46 (46%) players successfully returned to the field to play after treatment for 15 games over a 1.5-year period, which was significantly less than what was seen in the operative group (P <0.04). Hsu concluded that patients treated nonoperatively returned at a lower rate, played fewer games, and had shorter careers posttreatment.

Roberts et al[20] recently published on the outcomes of cervical and lumbar disk herniations in Major League Baseball (MLB) players. Successful RTP was defined as being on the active roster of an MLB team for at least 1 season after treatment. Time to RTP was calculated as the length of time between the last game played before injury and the first game played after treatment at the

MLB level. Overall, 11 pitchers were identified as having an acute cervical disk herniation. The majority of pitchers with cervical disk herniation successfully returned to play (8 of 11; 73%) at an average time of 11.6 months after diagnosis. Pitchers with cervical disk herniation treated with surgery returned to play at a higher rate (7 of 8; 88%) than those treated without surgery (1 of 3; 33%), but the difference was not statistically significant ($P = 0.15$).

Clark et al[21] reported a retrospective case series of five elite wrestlers with an acute cervical disk herniation resulting in cervical radiculopathy. All athletes were treated conservatively with initial activity modification; strengthening; rehabilitation; NSAIDs; and, ultimately, cervical epidural steroid injections. All five athletes were able to successfully return to competition without any negative clinical sequela or the need for operative intervention. The athletes demonstrated a subjective improvement in symptoms and strength, and all were able to return to an elite level of competition. The authors concluded that the epidural steroid injections were safe, efficacious, and well tolerated in this population.

Case Examples

A 28-year-old NFL running back sustained what was thought to be a burner or stinger after sustaining a hit during a game. Symptoms did not resolve, and the patient noted some mild numbness and paresthesias in the C6 distribution that persisted for 1 week after the injury. Radiographs at the time of injury showed no significant spondylosis and a normal cervical canal diameter, with some loss of the normal cervical lordosis (**Figure 12-2**). An MRI was obtained that revealed a C5 to C6 disk herniation with a foraminal disk herniation. The patient was withheld from play, given NSAIDs, and underwent physiotherapy. With these conservative measures, the patient was able to RTP after 6 weeks with a painless arc of cervical spine motion and no neurologic deficits.

Recommendations for Return to Play

Most athletes are able to return to same-level competition after conservation management of a cervical disk herniation. Specific RTP criteria have not yet been established. In general, when a patient becomes asymptomatic and has a painless normal range of cervical spine motion and no corresponding neurologic symptoms, the athlete may be cleared to return. Exceptions to this include patients who have sustained a cervical cord neurapraxia should not RTP until the underlying disk herniation is treated surgically even if asymptomatic over time. The reason

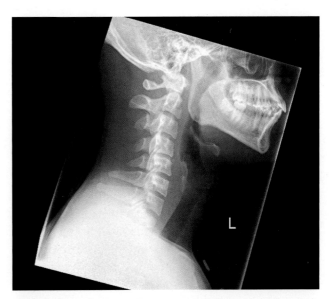

FIGURE 12-2 Lateral cervical radiograph showing loss of cervical lordosis, minimal spondylosis, and a normal cervical canal diameter.

for this is that disk herniation caused a cord level event that must be addressed before return to contact sports. The likelihood of recurrence of symptoms in this setting is more than 50%.

● OPERATIVE MANAGEMENT

Operative management of athletes should follow an appropriate trial of nonoperative treatment, assuming there is no neurologic deficit or cord signal change. For an acute disk injury in an athlete, there are three primary operative interventions that should be considered: ACDF, PCF, and CDR. The decision on which procedure to perform is determined by the location of the pathology, surgeon experience, and the need for the athlete to return to competition and if so, the level of contact required for the given sport.

Anterior Cervical Discectomy and Fusion

Anterior cervical discectomy and fusion for the treatment for the overwhelming majority of cervical disk herniation because it allows for direct access to the pathology without violation of the posterior muscle sleeve. Furthermore, ACDF eliminates the need for direct neural manipulation and also allows for the indirect decompression the neural elements through restoration of foramina height and direct removal of disk fragments. Overall, the anterior approach to the cervical spine is well tolerated by patients. The most common postoperative complication is dysphagia, with rates after

ACDF ranging from 20% to 50%, although this tends to be a transient complication.

Anterior cervical discectomy and fusion is the most commonly performed procedure for acute disk herniation with associated radiculopathy and has the longest track record of proven success. Smith and Robinson first described the procedure in 1955. Multiple studies have shown the efficacy and safety of ACDF in treated acute disk injuries or cervical radiculopathy. The results of ACDF are often reported in terms of achieving a successful fusion. In a landmark study comparing the use of anterior cervical plates versus no plate in single-level ACDFs, Samartzis et al[22] demonstrated fusion rates of 100% with an anterior plate and 90% when no plate was used. There was no difference in clinical outcome between the two groups. Similar fusion results have been seen in the Food and Drug Administration (FDA) trials comparing ACDF and CDR.[23–26]

Clinical outcomes are generally good after ACDF. Gore and Sepic[27] reported an initial improvement in 96% patients, with 64% of patients maintaining this improvement out to 21 years. Pain typically recurred at an average of 7 years from surgery, with only a small percentage of patients requiring a secondary surgery. Similarly, Klein et al[28] reported on the outcomes of 28 patients who underwent ACDF for symptomatic cervical radiculopathy. Statistically significant improvements were found in postoperative scores for bodily pain ($P < 0.001$), vitality ($P = 0.003$), physical function ($P = 0.01$), role function/physical ($P = 0.0003$), and social function ($P = 0.0004$). No significant differences were found before and after surgery for general health, mental health, and role function associated with emotional limitations. Age, educational status, and history of compensation litigation did not appear to affect outcome measures.

Anderson et al[29] recently performed a multivariate analysis to identify predictors of poor outcomes after ACDF. In the full-model logistic analysis for overall success, whereas worker's compensation and weak narcotic use were negative predictors, higher preoperative Neck Disability Index (NDI) score and normal sensory function were positive predictors. For NDI success, only the preoperative NDI scores appeared to have a strong influence on the outcome. In the stepwise regression model, preoperative normal sensory function was a positive predictor, and worker's compensation a negative predictor of overall clinical success. Older age, higher preoperative NDI score, and gainful employment were positive predictors, and spinal litigation was a negative predictor of NDI success.

Several small case-series have been published over the past decade detailing the RTP of contact athletes having undergone ACDF. Although most series demonstrate general favorable RTP rates, significant heterogeneity and bias exist among the studies. The optimum treatment algorithm and criteria for allowing an athlete to RTP has yet to be defined. However, we have a suggested treatment algorithm.

Evidence-Based Review

Maroon et al[30] reported on a consecutive series of 15 professional athletes (7 NFL players, 8 wrestlers) who underwent single-level ACDF for cervical spine pathology. The authors had strict RTP criteria: early bony bridging, absence of segmental motion on flexion-extension radiographs, absence of neurological deficits, and full painless ROM. Seven of the 15 athletes presented with neurapraxia, 8 with cervical radiculopathy, and 2 with hyperintensity of the spinal cord. Thirteen of the 15 players returned to their sport between 2 and 12 months postoperatively (mean, 6 months), with 8 still participating. The RTP duration of the 5 who retired after full participation ranged from 1 to 3 years. All athletes remained asymptomatic for radicular or myelopathic symptoms or signs.

Hsu et al[1] performed a retrospective cohort based on team medical records, newspaper archives, team injury reports, player profiles, and press releases. A total of 99 NFL athletes met the inclusion criteria. In the operative group, on average, 38 of 53 (72%) players successfully returned to play for 29 games over a 2.8-year period, which was significantly greater than that of the nonoperative group, in which only 21 of 46 (46%) players successfully returned to the field to play after treatment for 15 games over a 1.5-year period ($P < 0.04$). Overall, in the operative group, 32 players were confirmed to have had an anterior cervical discectomy and fusion (60.4%); 3 players were treated with a posterior foraminotomy (5.7%); and in 18 patients, the type of surgery was indeterminate from the sources available.

Meredith et al[31] reported a retrospective case series of a single NFL football team from 2000 to 2011. The authors included all athletes with MRI-proven disk herniation with appropriately concordant symptoms. A total of 16 athletes met inclusion criteria. Linemen, linebackers, and defensive backs were the most represented positions (13 of 16 athletes; 81%). The most common presentation was radiculopathy after a single traumatic event (9 of 16 athletes; 56%). Three players had transient paresis. Three players underwent one-level anterior cervical discectomy and fusion. These 3 players had failed nonoperative therapy and had evidence of spinal cord compression with signal change on MRI, but only one returned to sport.

Brigham et al[32] presented a retrospective case series of three professional football players and one professional basketball player. All athletes had documented cervical cord contusions. None of the athletes had an acute disk herniation, fracture, instability, or focal cord compression. The first patient was a 27-year-old NFL safety who sustained a hyperextension injury to his neck. After appropriate nonoperative management of persistent mild myelopathic symptoms, the player underwent a C3 to C4 ACDF. The patient returned to play 5 months after surgery. The second patient was a professional basketball player with a history of multiple cervical contusions. In the first 6 months after being drafted into the National Basketball Association, he presented with his third episode of a cervical cord contusion. His MRI demonstrated a contusion of the cord at the C3 level. He underwent an anterior fusion at the C3 to C4 level and was kept out of competition for the remainder of the year. He returned and played for several more years. The third player was a 27-year-old NFL offensive lineman presenting with a brief episode of neck and shoulder pain. His cervical MRI demonstrated a contusion at the C5 to C6 level. He was allowed to play and finished the season uneventfully. At the end of the season, he underwent an anterior fusion at the C5 to C6 level. The patient was able to RTP the following season but ultimately developed a contusion at C3 to C4. The patient subsequently underwent an ACDF at C3 to C4 and has not returned to play. The fourth player is a 27-year-old defensive tackle who developed bilateral finger tingling after a face-to-face tackle. MRI revealed a cord contusion at C3 to C4. He subsequently underwent a C3 to C4 ACDF and was able to RTP at 6 months.

Andrews et al[33] examined the outcome of 19 professional rugby union players who underwent anterior cervical discectomy and fusion between 1998 and 2003. Their mean age at operation was 28 years (range, 22–37). All patients had experienced neck and radicular pain and had failed to improve with conservative treatment. After surgery, radicular pain was eliminated in 15 patients and improved in 2, and 2 had no improvement in symptoms. Neck pain was eradicated in 8 and improved in 9, and 2 had no change. A total of 13 players returned to their previous level of rugby. One returned to professional rugby but played in a lower division. Nine of the 13 returned to rugby at 6 months after operation (range, 5–17). Only one player took more than 12 months to RTP. Two of the failures had surgery at two levels rather than one.

Maroon et al[34] reported on five elite football players who were evaluated after experiencing episodes of neurapraxia. All patients experienced bilateral paresthesias, three in all four extremities and two in the upper extremities, with symptoms lasting from a few minutes to more than 24 hours. Transient motor deficits occurred in two individuals but caused no permanent sequelae. Imaging confirmed the presence of herniated disks, focal cord compression, and no parenchymal changes in all cases. After aggressive rehabilitation and confirmation of fusion ranging from 9 weeks to 8 months postoperatively, the players were allowed to return to active play. Two of the players developed recurrent career-ending disk herniations, one above and the other below the fusion level. One player required repeated spinal cord decompression.

Case Examples

A 32-year-old NFL safety developed significant back pain and right trapezial and paraspinal muscle spasm as a result of the C3 to C4 disk herniation. After failing appropriate conservative management, the player underwent a C3 to C4 ACDF (**Figure 12-3**). The patient did well after surgery and was asymptomatic. Six months after surgery, the patient was cleared for contact. After

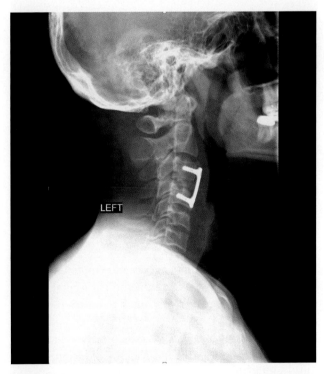

FIGURE 12-3 Lateral cervical radiograph of a National Football League cornerback who underwent C3 to C4 anterior cervical discectomy and fusion for cervical radiculopathy.

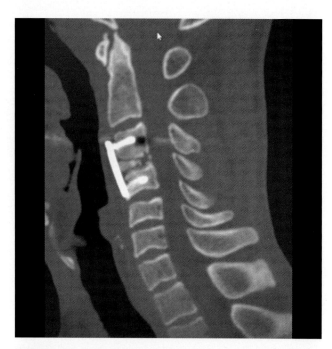

FIGURE 12-4 Sagittal CT scan demonstrating a C3 to C4 pseudoarthrosis.

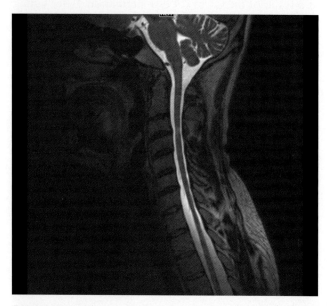

FIGURE 12-5 Sagittal T2 MRI demonstrating a C3 to C4 disk herniation with myelomalacia of the spinal cord.

beginning contact, the patient became symptomatic, noting moderate to severe neck pain and paraspinal muscle spasm. On CT, the player was found to have a pseudoarthrosis (**Figure 12-4**). The player subsequently underwent a posterior spinal fusion. When the patient was asymptomatic and had radiographic evidence of fusion, he was able to RTP.

A 29-year-old NFL linebacker sustained multiple stingers over the course of the season. MRI demonstrated

a C3 to C4 disk herniation, resulting in central stenosis with evidence of cord signal change at this level (**Figure 12-5**). The patient underwent a C3 to C4 ACDF. Six months after surgery, the patient was radiographically healed but continued to demonstrate persistent myelomalacia of the cord and resultant sensory symptoms in his arms. The player was not allowed to RTP and subsequently retired.

Recommendations for Return to Play

Return to play after ACDF remains a controversial topic with multiple factors playing a role in the decision-making process of the physician. In the case of a single-level ACDF achieving a solid, radiographically confirmed fusion with resolution of symptoms and no motor deficit, several authors have supported the RTP, including contact sports such as football and rugby. Pseudoarthrosis, as in the general population, remains a clinical concern. If the patient is a noncontact athlete with a stable, asymptomatic pseudoarthrosis with no motor deficits, it is likely safe to allow for RTP. In contact athletes, a pseudoarthrosis is a contraindication for RTP given the supraphysiological loads that may be experienced and the resultant potential for a catastrophic neurologic injury. Contact athletes should undergo revision surgery to achieve a stable union, and after it has been achieved, may return to competition.

The presence of myelomalacia in the cord presents a difficult challenge to the treating surgeon. Brigham and Meredith both presented evidence that asymptomatic athletes with cord myelomalacia were able to return to contact sports after ACDF. To date, there have been no reports of catastrophic neurologic injury in this patient population. In general, athletes should be allowed to return to contact and noncontact sports if they are asymptomatic with resolution of the neck pain and radicular symptoms. The presence of myelomalacia represents spinal cord damage. If the patient is asymptomatic, this may afford RTP, but most patients with myelomalacia are not asymptomatic and may have some degree of motor or sensory dysfunction. Myelomalacia represents a sign of a "sick spinal cord," and great care and counseling should be provided to the athlete about the implications for his or her long-term health and neurologic status.

Another potential scenario involves performing an ACDF over multiple levels. Meredith et al recommended that fusion at two or more levels is a contraindication for return to football because of an increased risk of sustaining a neurologic injury. The authors note, however, that there is limited data to support this position. Given the lack of evidence-based literature, caution should be used when allowing a contact athlete to RTP when more than one level is addressed surgically. The other issue is that there is an increased rate of degeneration in the adjacent level after ACDF that may be higher in the contact athlete that underwent an ACDF. The focus should be on minimizing risk to the adjacent level after a two-level procedure, and thus this should serve as a relative or absolute contraindication to returning to sports such as football or rugby. In the event of persistent cord myelomalacia, contact athletes should not be allowed to RTP. However, it is important to document that a two-level ACDF is fused and has painless ROM before returning. The RTP must be a careful decision and the risks carefully articulated to the contact athlete. Noncontact athletes can RTP after a two-level ACDF.

Posterior Cervical Foraminotomy

The use of a posterior approach for the treatment of cervical radiculopathy originated more than 65 years ago with Mixter,[35] who reported on the use of a posterior decompression of the neural elements. The PCF or laminoforaminotomy was further pioneered by Frykholm[36] and Scoville et al.[37] Case series presented by Fager[38] and Epstein et al[39] popularized the so-called "keyhole" laminoforaminotomy with a success rate approaching 90%. In a more recent case series of open PCF techniques, Jagannathan et al[40] found a 95% success rate for resolution of radiculopathy.

The open PCF approach allows for excellent visualization and access to lateral disk herniations and bony foraminal compromise secondary to cervical spondylosis. As an alternative to standard open approaches, endoscopic and minimally invasive techniques (MIS) have been developed. Shorter hospital stays, same-day surgery, faster recovery times, and reduced blood loss have been shown using MIS techniques.[41-43] Kim et al[44] performed an RCT of 41 patients, including 19 treated with an open technique and 22 with a MIS approach. The authors found no statistically significant differences in length of hospital stay, analgesic use, length of skin incision, and visual analog scale (VAS) neck pain scores at 1 day, 5 days, and 4 weeks. At 3 months, there was no longer a significant difference in neck pain.

Posterior cervical foraminotomies are typically indicated for patients with cervical radiculopathy caused by foraminal stenosis that is refractory to at least 6 weeks of conservative management. PCF is best used in the treatment of foraminal lesions or cases of posterolateral soft disk herniation that compresses the nerve root while lying lateral to the cord. The primary contraindications to PCF include segmental kyphosis or instability at the operative level. A relative contraindication to PCF is the presence of clinical or radiographic myelopathy or myelomalacia.

Despite its success and proven track record, ACDF remains the more commonly performed procedure. Ruetten el al[45] showed that when patients with treating radiculopathy alone, PCF and ACDF produce clinically equivalent results, as measured by VAS, Hilibrand criteria, and the North American Spine Society Instrument. Similarly, Wirth et al[46] demonstrated similar results, finding no significant differences in surgical complication rates or postoperative symptom relief between the two approaches. The limitation is that most patients are not candidates for cervical foraminotomy based on the location of the pathology. One other misconception is that patients who undergo PCF do not have rates of adjacent segment degeneration. The rate of adjacent segment after PCF is 1.8% per year, but after ACDF, it remains 2.8% per year.[47,48]

Evidence-Based Review

In the only reported case series in athletes treated with an endoscopic PCF, Adamson[49] reported on 10 patients (8 professional football players, 2 race car drivers) who had symptomatic cervical radiculopathy that necessitated operative intervention. Both drivers were treated in the offseason and returned to driving within 4 weeks. The results of the 8 football players were similarly encouraging. Seven players returned to play at full capacity after preoperative motor deficits had cleared. One of these players with multilevel spondylotic disease required additional surgery 1.5 years postoperatively and retired from competition. One football player who had sustained game-related complete C5 deficit secondary to spondylotic foraminal stenosis was unable to RTP because of persistent neurologic deficits. The reoperation rate for the index problem also remains higher with foraminotomy than ACDF.

Case Examples

A 26-year-old NFL offensive lineman developed minimal weakness in his right biceps and pain down his arm to the dorsal aspect of his left thumb. On MRI, the patient was found to have a right C5 to C6 foraminal disk herniation (**Figure 12-6**). The patient had activity modification, ESIs, and NSAIDs without relief. The patient underwent a keyhole laminoforaminotomy with complete resolution of all symptoms. He was able to RTP 8 weeks after surgery.

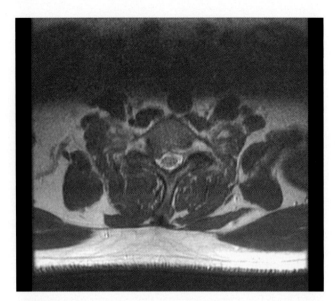

FIGURE 12-6 Axial T2 MRI with a right sided C5 to C6 foraminal disk herniation in a player who underwent a C5 to C6 laminoforaminotomy.

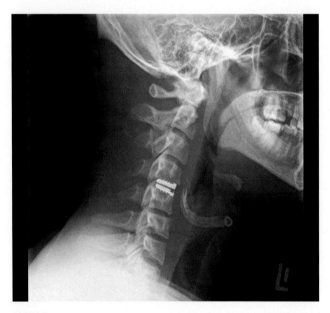

FIGURE 12-7 Lateral cervical radiograph in a patient who underwent a C4 to C5 cervical disk arthroplasty.

Recommendations for Return to Play

An athlete may return to competition when there is complete resolution of pain and no associated neurologic deficit. In Adamson's series,[49] athletes were allowed to begin unrestricted range of motion (ROM) exercises at 3 to 5 days after surgery, with return to aerobic conditioning allowed between 1 to 2 weeks from surgery. Patients may also begin physical therapy approximately 1 week after surgery. Resistance training can begin 2 weeks after surgery if neurologic symptoms have resolved. Full

return to both noncontact and contact sports is allowed after strength has normalized and soreness has resolved. In Adamson's series, this RTP averaged 2.5 to 6 weeks from surgery.

In the event of a persistent motor weakness or other neurologic deficit, the athlete should remain restricted from returning to activity. For an athlete who fails treatment with a PCF, consideration should be given to performing an anterior based surgery to further directly decompress the spinal cord and nerve roots as well as restoring disk height and allowing for indirect decompression. Athletes with arm weakness should strongly consider definitive surgery with ACDF rather than foraminotomy because this may afford a greater decompression and more favorable motor recovery.

Cervical Disk Replacement

Cervical disk replacement was developed because of the concerns over the altered kinematics and adjacent segment disease that may result from ACDF (**Figure 12-7**). Multiple FDA investigational device exemption (IDE) studies have been performed to assess the noninferiority of CDR with respect to ACDF.[26,50,51] The proposed theoretic benefits of CDR include the avoidance on nonunion, preservation of motion segments, reduction in adjacent segment degeneration, and lack of graft-related complications. Reduction of adjacent segment degeneration was initially proposed to be the main benefit of CDR; however, a recent systematic review found no decrease in the rate of degeneration in short- or medium-term follow-up.[52]

In short- and medium-term follow-up, Ziegler et al[26] recently reported the 5-year follow-up comparing CDR and ACDF (ProDisc-C; Synthes, West Chester PA). The study included 209 patients (106 ACDF, 103 CDR) and followed VAS arm pain, NDI, SF-36, patient satisfaction, neurologic examination, and adverse event occurrence for 60 months. Both groups experienced significant clinical improvement at 5 years. There were no device-related failures, and CDR had a significantly lower reoperation rate (2.9%) than ACDF (11.3%).

The goals of the FDA trials, including the establishment of safety, efficacy, and noninferiority of CDR relative to ACDF, have been met in the general population. However, there is a lack of information regarding the level of physical performance attained and the level of restriction that was placed on patients in these studies. This lack of transparency makes it difficult to extrapolate the results of the IDE studies to a young, athletic population. In fact, to date, there are no reports of the use of CDR in athletes.

Evidence-Based Review

Although there are no reports of CDR in competitive athletes. Tumialán et al[53] reported on the use of CDR in military patients. Military patients are similar to athletes in that they have rigorous physical demands that may place supraphysiological stress on the cervical spine. Tumialán et al identified parachute jumps, diving, high-impact water entries, and prolonged runs as representing some of the physical demands required of military patients. Twelve patients were identified who underwent CDR during the study period. All patients in the study were men. The average age at the time of surgery was 36.5 years. The treated levels were C5 to C6 (8 patients) and C6 to C7 (4 patients). All patients returned to unrestricted full duty at an average of 10.3 weeks from surgery. A matched cohort of ACDF patients returned to full active duty at 16.5 weeks, which was statistically significant ($P = 0.008$). In the first 3 months after surgery, there were no self-reported limitations or restrictions. The authors appropriately noted that unlike fusion, there are no radiographic criteria that would indicate when it is safe to allow unrestricted activity. In this study, release to active duty occurred after full resolution of preoperative symptoms resolved.

In a similar study, Kang et al[54] reported on 37 active duty military patients who underwent 41 CDRs. The study found good relief of preoperative symptoms (92%) and the ability to maintain operational readiness with a high rate of return to full unrestricted duty (95%) with an average follow-up period of 6 months. There was a low complication rate related to the anterior cervical approach (5%–8%) with no device- or implant-related complications.

Recommendations for Return to Play

Given the lack of evidence in the athletic population, we cannot currently recommend the routine use of CDR in athletes who want to return to contact sports. CDR could be acceptable for return to noncontact sports. Further studies are required to define the safety and efficacy in this population. Furthermore, investigations should be carried out in both contact and noncontact sports because the RTP criteria may differ. At this time, CDR should be a contraindication to RTP in contact or collision sports despite reports of military experience.

● CONCLUSION

Cervical disk injuries in athletes remain a significant concern with the potential for significant loss of playing time, shortening of career, and loss of revenue for both the player and the team. Most cervical disk injuries can be effectively managed with nonoperative conservative care. In the event that a patient requires operative intervention, good results have been shown with both ACDF and posterior foraminotomy. A comprehensive team approach with athletic trainers, sports medicine physicians, interventional physiatry and pain management, and spine surgery will often serve to help the athlete resume his or her elite level of sport and function and quality of life.

REFERENCES

1. Hsu WK: Outcomes following nonoperative and operative treatment for cervical disc herniations in National Football League athletes. *Spine (Phila Pa 1976)* 2011;36(10):800–805.

2. Scherping SC Jr: Cervical disc disease in the athlete. *Clin Sports Med* 2002;21(1):37–47, vi.

3. Zmurko MG, Tannoury TY, Tannoury CA, Anderson DG: Cervical sprains, disc herniations, minor fractures, and other cervical injuries in the athlete. *Clin Sports Med* 2003;22(3):5/521.

4. Mundt DJ, Kelsey JL, Golden AL, et al: An epidemiologic study of sports and weight lifting as possible risk factors for herniated lumbar and cervical discs. The Northeast Collaborative Group on Low Back Pain. *Am J Sports Med* 1993;21(6):854–860.

5. Albright JP, Moses JM, Feldick HG, Dolan KD, Burmeister LF: Nonfatal cervical spine injuries in interscholastic football. *JAMA* 1976;236(11):1243–1245.

6. Radhakrishnan K, Litchy WJ, O'Fallon WM, Kurland LT: Epidemiology of cervical radiculopathy. A population-based study from Rochester, Minnesota, 1976 through 1990. *Brain* 1994;117(Pt 2):325–335.

7. Schoenfeld AJ, George AA, Bader JO, Caram PM Jr: Incidence and epidemiology of cervical radiculopathy in the United States military: 2000 to 2009. *J Spinal Disord Tech* 2012;25(1):17–22.

8. Dorshimer GW, Kelly M: Cervical pain in the athlete: common conditions and treatment. *Prim Care* 2005;32(1):231–243.

9. Krabak BJ, Kanarek SL: Cervical spine pain in the competitive athlete. *Phys Med Rehabil Clin North Am* 2011;22(3):459–471, viii.

10. Lees F, Turner JW: Natural history and prognosis of cervical spondylosis. *Br Med J* 1963;2(5373):1607–1610.

11. Dillin W, Booth R, Cuckler J, Balderston R, Simeone F, Rothman R: Cervical radiculopathy. A review. *Spine (Phila Pa 1976)* 1986;11(10):988–991.

12. Gore DR, Sepic SB, Gardner GM, Murray MP: Neck pain: A long-term follow-up of 205 patients. *Spine (Phila Pa 1976)* 1987;12(1):1–5.

13. Gavin TM, Carandang G, Havey R, Flanagan P, Ghanayem A, Patwardhan AG: Biomechanical analysis of cervical orthoses in flexion and extension: A comparison of cervical collars and cervical thoracic orthoses. *J Rehabil Res Dev* 2003;40(6):527–537.

14. Tan JC, Nordin M: Role of physical therapy in the treatment of cervical disk disease. *Orthop Clin North Am* 1992;23(3):435–449.

15. Levine MJ, Albert TJ, Smith MD: Cervical radiculopathy: Diagnosis and nonoperative management. *J Am Acad Orthop Surg* 1996;4(6):305–316.

16. Manchikanti L, Nampiaparampil DE, Candido KD, et al: Do cervical epidural injections provide long-term relief in neck and upper extremity pain? A systematic review. *Pain Physician* 2015;18(1):39–60.

17. Bush K, Hillier S: Outcome of cervical radiculopathy treated with periradicular/epidural corticosteroid injections: a prospective study with independent clinical review. *Eur Spine J* 1996;5(5):319–325.

18. Rathmell JP, Aprill C, Bogduk N: Cervical transforaminal injection of steroids. *Anesthesiology* 2004;100(6):1595–600.

19. Cohen SP, Hayek S, Semenov Y, et al: Epidural steroid injections, conservative treatment, or combination treatment for cervical radicular pain: A multicenter, randomized, comparative-effectiveness study. *Anesthesiology* 2014;121(5):1045–1055.

20. Roberts DW, Roc GJ, Hsu WK: Outcomes of cervical and lumbar disk herniations in Major League Baseball pitchers. *Orthopedics* 2011;34(8):602–609.

21. Clark R, Doyle M, Sybrowsky C, Rosenquist R: Epidural steroid injections for the treatment of cervical radiculopathy in elite wrestlers: Case series and literature review. *Iowa Orthop J* 2012;32:207–214.

22. Samartzis D, Shen FH, Lyon C, Phillips M, Goldberg EJ, An HS: Does rigid instrumentation increase the fusion rate in one-level anterior cervical discectomy and fusion? *Spine J* 2004;4(6):636–643.

23. Sasso RC, Smucker JD, Hacker RJ, Heller JG: Clinical outcomes of BRYAN cervical disc arthroplasty: A prospective, randomized, controlled, multicenter trial with 24-month follow-up. *J Spinal Disord Tech* 2007;20(7):481–491.

24. Heller JG, Sasso RC, Papadopoulos SM, et al: Comparison of BRYAN cervical disc arthroplasty with anterior cervical decompression and fusion: Clinical and radiographic results of a randomized, controlled, clinical trial. *Spine (Phila Pa 1976)* 2009;34(2):101–107.

25. Coric D, Nunley PD, Guyer RD, et al: Prospective, randomized, multicenter study of cervical arthroplasty: 269 patients from the KineflexlC artificial disc investigational device exemption study with a minimum 2-year follow-up: clinical article. *J Neurosurg Spine* 2011;15(4):348–358.

26. Zigler JE, Delamarter R, Murrey D, Spivak J, Janssen M: ProDisc-C and anterior cervical discectomy and fusion as surgical treatment for single-level cervical symptomatic degenerative disc disease: Five-year results of a Food and Drug Administration study. *Spine (Phila Pa 1976)* 2013;38(3):203–209.

27. Gore DR, Sepic SB: Anterior discectomy and fusion for painful cervical disc disease. A report of 50 patients with an average follow-up of 21 years. *Spine (Phila Pa 1976)* 1998;23(19):2047–2051.

28. Klein GR, Vaccaro AR, Albert TJ: Health outcome assessment before and after anterior cervical discectomy and fusion for radiculopathy: A prospective analysis. *Spine (Phila Pa 1976)* 2000;25(7):801–803.

29. Anderson PA, Subach BR, Riew KD: Predictors of outcome after anterior cervical discectomy and fusion: A multivariate analysis. *Spine (Phila Pa 1976)* 2009;34(2):161–166.

30. Maroon JC, Bost JW, Petraglia AL, et al: Outcomes after anterior cervical discectomy and fusion in professional athletes. *Neurosurgery* 2013;73(1):103–112; discussion 112.

31. Meredith DS, Jones KJ, Barnes R, Rodeo SA, Cammisa FP, Warren RF: Operative and nonoperative treatment of cervical disc herniation in National Football League athletes. *Am J Sports Med* 2013;41(9):2054–2058.

32. Brigham CD, Capo J: Cervical spinal cord contusion in professional athletes: A case series with implications for return to play. *Spine (Phila Pa 1976)* 2013;38(4):315–323.

33. Andrews J, Jones A, Davies PR, Howes J, Ahuja S: Is return to professional rugby union likely after anterior cervical spinal surgery? *J Bone Joint Surg Br* 2008;90(5):619–621.

34. Maroon JC, El-Kadi H, Abla AA, Wecht DA, Bost J, Norwig J, Bream T: Cervical neurapraxia in elite athletes: Evaluation and surgical treatment. Report of five cases. *J Neurosurg Spine* 2007;6(4):356–363.

35. Mixter WJ: Rupture of the intervertebral disk; a short history of this evolution as a syndrome of importance to the surgeon. *J Am Med Assoc* 1949;140(3):278–282.

36. Frykholm R: Lower cervical vertebrae and intervertebral discs; surgical anatomy and pathology. *Acta Chir Scand* 1951;101(5):345–359.

37. Scoville WB, Whitcomb BB, McLaurin R: The cervical ruptured disc; report of 115 operative cases. *Trans Am Neurol Assoc* 1951;56:222–224.

38. Epstein JA, Janin Y, Carras R, Lavine LS: A comparative study of the treatment of cervical spondylotic myeloradiculopathy. Experience with 50 cases treated by means of extensive laminectomy, foraminotomy, and excision of osteophytes during the past 10 years. *Acta Neurochir (Wien)* 1982;61(1–3):89–104.

39. Fager CA: Posterolateral approach to ruptured median and paramedian cervical disk. *Surg Neurol* 1983;20(6): 443–452.

40. Jagannathan J, Shaffrey CI, Oskouian RJ, Dumont AS, Herrold C, Sansur CA, Jane JA: Radiographic and clinical outcomes following single-level anterior cervical discectomy and allograft fusion without plate placement or cervical collar. *J Neurosurg Spine* 2008;8(5):420–428.

41. Adamson TE: Microendoscopic posterior cervical laminoforaminotomy for unilateral radiculopathy: Results of a new technique in 100 cases. *J Neurosurg* 2001;95(1 suppl):51–57.

42. Fessler RG, Khoo LT: Minimally invasive cervical microendoscopic foraminotomy: An initial clinical experience. *Neurosurgery* 2002;51(5 suppl):S37–S45.

43. Coric D, Adamson T: Minimally invasive cervical microendoscopic laminoforaminotomy. *Neurosurg Focus* 2008; 25(2):E2.

44. Kim KT, Kim YB: Comparison between open procedure and tubular retractor assisted procedure for cervical radiculopathy: Results of a randomized controlled study. *J Korean Med Sci* 2009;24(4):649–653.

45. Ruetten S, Komp M, Merk H, Godolias G: Full-endoscopic cervical posterior foraminotomy for the operation of lateral disc herniations using 5.9-mm endoscopes: A prospective, randomized, controlled study. *Spine (Phila Pa 1976)* 2008;33(9):940–948.

46. Wirth FP, Dowd GC, Sanders HF, Wirth C: Cervical discectomy. A prospective analysis of three operative techniques. *Surg Neurol* 2000;53(4):340–346; discussion 346–348.

47. Clarke MJ, Ecker RD, Krauss WE, McClelland RL, Dekutoski MB: Same-segment and adjacent-segment disease following posterior cervical foraminotomy. *J Neurosurg Spine* 2007;6(1):5–9.

48. Jagannathan J, Sherman JH, Szabo T, Shaffrey CI, Jane JA. The posterior cervical foraminotomy in the treatment of cervical disc/osteophyte disease: A single-surgeon experience with a minimum of 5 years' clinical and radiographic follow-up. *J Neurosurg Spine* 2009;10(4):347–356.

49. Adamson TE: Posterior cervical endoscopic laminoforaminotomy for the treatment of radiculopathy in the athlete. *Oper Tech Sports Med* 2005;13:96–100.

50. Murrey D, Janssen M, Delamarter R, Goldstein J, Zigler J, Tay B, Darden B: Results of the prospective, randomized, controlled multicenter Food and Drug Administration investigational device exemption study of the ProDisc-C total disc replacement versus anterior discectomy and fusion for the treatment of 1-level symptomatic cervical disc disease. *Spine J* 2009;9(4):275–286.

51. Coric D, Cassis J, Carew JD, Boltes MO: Prospective study of cervical arthroplasty in 98 patients involved in 1 of 3 separate investigational device exemption studies from a single investigational site with a minimum 2-year follow-up. Clinical article. *J Neurosurg Spine* 2010;13(6): 715–721.

52. Harrod CC, Hilibrand AS, Fischer DJ, Skelly AC: Adjacent segment pathology following cervical motion-sparing procedures or devices compared with fusion surgery: A systematic review. *Spine (Phila Pa 1976)* 2012;37(22 suppl): S96–S112.

53. Tumialán LM, Ponton RP, Garvin A, Gluf WM: Arthroplasty in the military: A preliminary experience with ProDisc-C and ProDisc-L. *Neurosurg Focus* 2010;28(5):E18.

54. Kang DG, Lehman RA, Tracey RW, Cody JP, Rosner MK, Bevevino AJ: Outcomes following cervical disc arthroplasty in an active duty military population. *J Surg Orthop Adv* 2013;22(1):10–15.

13 Congenital Cervical Anomalies and Special Needs Athletes

Jun Sup Kim, MD • Evan Baird, MD • Lindsay Andras, MD • Nomaan Ashraf, MD, MBA

INTRODUCTION

Sports and exercise is especially essential for the well-being of children with special needs. It promotes psychological and physical well-being. Literature on rehabilitation and therapy of persons with physical disabilities has shown that athletic activity is related to improvements in locus of control, self-image, and life satisfaction.[1-3]

Cervical spine injuries are common in sporting activities and can result in catastrophic impairment if appropriate steps to prevention and treatment are not instituted. Individuals with congenital or developmental anomalies of the cervical spine constitute a unique subset of patients for whom standard return-to-activity guidelines are not wholly applicable. Based on the myriad benefits of sports and exercise in this patient population, these patients should not be globally restricted from these activities. Rather, the clinician must consider the risks and dangers of the sport in question with respect to its therapeutic benefits. Additionally, it is the duty of the clinician to consider the specific congenital spinal anomalies that may pose an increased risk of neurologic injury.

Cervical spine instability should remain a consideration in the workup of the athlete with special needs, especially in the presence of certain anomalies or syndromes, such as Down syndrome, Klippel Feil syndrome, and Morquio syndrome. Instability can lead to compression of the spinal cord, and it often exists in conjunction with other pathology such as spinal stenosis, basilar invagination, and central nervous system (CNS) abnormalities such as Arnold-Chiari malformation.[3]

The majority of literature addressing this population is largely based on case series and level III evidence; however, because of the difficulty in gathering a more expansive body of literature, this information should not be discounted.

CLINICAL EVALUATION

The decision to let an athlete return to play (RTP) should be based on medical history, physical examination, imaging, and the type of sport being played. There are no standardized criteria for RTP because the postinjury management of each individual is unique, especially in athletes with special needs. Children with cervical spine anomalies or instability may present with a variety of complaints, such as head or neck pain, loss of range of motion (ROM), signs of upper motor neuron involvement, or weakness.[4] Many tracts of the spinal cord may be involved, and localizing sites of compression is often difficult. As such, the diagnosis and management of these anomalies are essential for the physician to recognize.

Posterior cord impingement affects the dorsal column, leading to changes or deficits in pain, proprioception, and vibratory sense. Anterior spinal column involvement affects the corticospinal tracts and may lead to muscle weakness and pathologic reflexes such as clonus, Babinski sign, spasticity and hyperreflexia of deep tendon reflexes. Involvement of the cerebellum may manifest as nystagmus, ataxia, and incoordination. Vertebral artery compression compromises blood flow to the posterior cord, which may lead to syncopal episodes, dizziness, and decreased mental acuity. Cranial nerve compression as the nerves exit the medulla may occur from instability or anomalies such as basilar invagination. The more commonly involved cranial nerves include the trigeminal (V), glossopharyngeal (IX), vagus (X), accessory (XI), and hypoglossal (XII) nerves. A thorough neurologic examination should be recorded to evaluate for subtle changes.[4]

Radiographic assessment with plain imaging of the cervical spine should include lateral radiographs in neutral, flexion, and extension; open-mouth odontoid; and anteroposterior views. Compression and instability may occur at the occipitoatlantal and atlantoaxial regions; as such, the clinician should be mindful to examine this area closely to evaluate for basilar invagination, evidence of atlantoaxial instability, congenital anomalies of the cervical vertebrae such as synostosis, and anomalies of the odontoid such as os odontoideum.[4] In the setting of abnormal neurologic examination findings, MRI offers a means of evaluating for signs of cord compression as well as associated CNS anomalies such as hydrocephalus, Chiari malformations, and syringomyelia. CT yields anatomic detail that may help in defining anomalies of the cervical vertebrae such as aplasia, hypoplasia, or os odontoideum as well as congenital synostosis such as that seen in Klippel Feil syndrome.

● CONSIDERATIONS FOR SPECIFIC DISORDERS
Basilar Invagination

Basilar invagination refers to a deformity wherein the odontoid process is located further cephalad than the normal state, violating the foramen magnum, which may be significant enough to encroach on the brainstem. This condition increases the risk of neurologic injury or circulatory compression, especially with contact sports. The etiologies may be basiocciput hypoplasia, occipital condyle hypoplasia, atlas hypoplasia, the presence of an incomplete ring of C1 with subsequent lateral masses diastasis, achondroplasia, or atlanto-occipital assimilation. Additionally, between 25% and 35% of patients with basilar invagination have associated spinal abnormalities such as Chiari malformation, syringomyelia, syringobulbia, and hydrocephalus.[5]

Patients with basilar invagination may exhibit torticollis, restricted neck movements, a low hairline, and a webbed or short neck. Caetano De Barros et al described 66 cases of basilar invagination and found

that the most common clinical symptoms that induced the patient to seek medical attention were weakness in the lower limbs (68%), gait unsteadiness (56%), and headache (53%). Paraesthesias, often localized to the upper limbs, appeared in 43% of cases. Dizziness and dysphagia were described in 37% of patients. The age of presentation in patients without Chiari malformations was commonly in the second decade of life (58%), with 86% presenting within the first 3 decades of life. Notably, a comparative study of symptoms in patients with isolated basilar impression and isolated Arnold-Chiari syndrome has shown that basilar invagination most frequently manifested as weakness and paraesthesias in the limbs, but patients with Arnold-Chiari syndrome presented most often with unsteadiness of gait.[6]

Similarly, Goel et al reported on 190 patients surgically treated with basilar invagination who were divided into two groups—patients with and without Chiari malformations. Symptom presentation was relatively acute in patients without Chiari malformations (group one), but those with Chiari malformations (group two) experienced long-standing and progressive symptomology. Whereas pyramidal symptoms dominated in group one patients, those in group two experienced spinothalamic sensory dysfunction and ataxia as well as motor and deep sensory dysfunction. Trauma was a major factor that influenced acute development of symptoms in those patients without Chiari malformations. The age of presentation in patients with basilar invagination associated with Chiari malformation was reported to be most common in the third decade (44%), with 88% of patients presenting between the second and fourth decades of life. Goel et al postulated that symptoms in the group of patients without Chiari malformations were a result of brainstem compression by the odontoid process, but those with Chiari malformations could be explained by the crowding of neural structures at the foramen magnum.[7]

Numerous radiographic measurements have been described that assess the degree of basilar invagination; these include the lines of Chamberlain, McGregor, and McRae, which gauge the relationship of the odontoid to the foramen magnum (**Figure 13-1**). Chamberlain's line originates from the dorsal margin of the hard palate to the posterior edge of the foramen magnum. It is considered abnormal if the tip of the dens is greater than 5 mm proximal to Chamberlain's line. McGregor's line is drawn from the posterior edge of the hard palate to the most caudal point of the occiput. The odontoid tip should not protrude more than 4.5 mm above the McGregor Line.

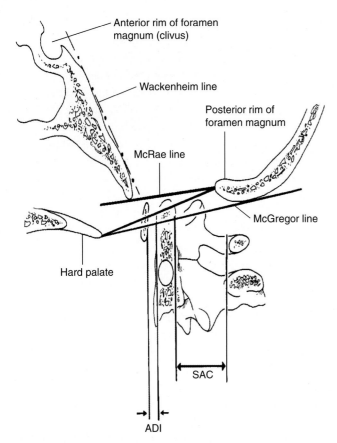

FIGURE 13-1 Lines assessing the degree of basilar invagination: Chamberlain, McGregor, and McRae lines, which gauge the relationship of the odontoid to the foramen magnum. ADI = atlantodens interval, SAC = space available for cord. (Adapted from Copley LA, Dormans JP: Cervical spine disorders in infants and children. *J Am Acad Orthop Surg* 1998;6:204–214.)

McRae's line defines the opening of the foramen magnum, from the basion to the opisthion. If the tip of the dens is below this line, then basilar invagination is not substantial, and the patient is expected to be asymptomatic.[4,5]

Vaccaro and colleagues summarized RTP criteria for athletes with cervical spine injuries.[8] The authors also described congenital anomalies of the spine and placed them in three categories: no contraindications, relative contraindications, and absolute contraindications to RTP. Considering that many of these patients with basilar invagination already present with symptoms of motor weakness and gait instability, there is an extraordinary potential for catastrophic neurologic injury from direct compression of the brainstem by the odontoid. Goel et al showed that many patients presented acutely with symptoms of basilar impression (i.e., motor weakness) after minor trauma.[7] Therefore, radiographic evidence of basilar invagination is an absolute contraindication to participation in contact sports.

Os Odontoideum

Anomalies of the odontoid are a spectrum ranging from aplasia to hypoplasia to os odontoideum. The distinction is better defined in radiologic terms because these anomalies may lead to atlantoaxial instability with similar clinical presentation. In 1886, Giacomini first coined the term *os odontoideum* as a condition in which the dens was separated from the axis body.[9] Although there is debate as to whether the etiology is of a congenital or traumatic nature, sound management requires a thorough appreciation of the natural history of this entity. Given that the transverse atlantal ligament (TAL) may be rendered ineffective at restraining atlantoaxial motion, the secondary ligamentous restraints of the dens become lax over time, leading to instability. The free ossicle of the os odontoideum moves with the anterior arch of the atlas. Over time, this instability becomes multidirectional and may lead to neurologic symptoms.[10]

When initially described, os odontoideum was thought to be the result of a congenital failure of fusion between the dens and the remainder of the axis. However, studies have demonstrated that the failure of fusion of the secondary ossification center of the dens, which normally develops by age 3 years and fuses by age 12 years to the remainder of the axis, is a separate entity known as persistent ossiculum terminale (**Figure 13-2**).[11-13] Persistent ossiculum terminale differs from os odontoideum in that the fragment is smaller in size and located above the TAL. As a result, ossiculum terminale is less likely to result in clinically significant instability, although cases of neurologic deficit resulting from progressive atlantoaxial dislocation have been reported.[11]

Os odontoideum, on the other hand, is theorized to represent either a previous fracture of the odontoid synchondrosis before its closure or the result of excessive motion while the cartilaginous dens is ossifying. Fielding et al reported on 35 patients with os odontoideum and postulated that trauma was the main etiology behind this anomaly.[14] Twenty-six patients had a history of acute injury to the neck, and in nine of these patients, the trauma led to radiographic discovery of the os odontoideum. Fielding and colleagues postulated after the traumatic episode, the alar ligaments, which attach the occiput to the tip of the odontoid, pull the fragment cranially. Over time, the contracted alar ligaments distract the distal odontoid fragment from the proximal body, with blood supply maintained by the proximal arterial arcade from the carotid.[14] Regardless of the etiology, it is critical to differentiate os

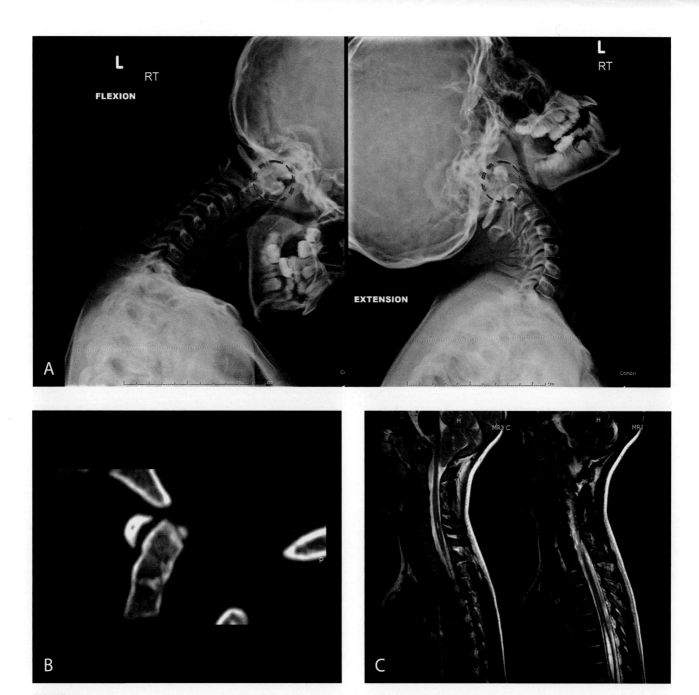

FIGURE 13-2 **A,** Flexion and extension views reveal a stable ADI without evidence of instability in a patient with persistent ossiculum terminale (*red circle*). **B,** Sagittal cut of the odontoid demonstrating a persistent ossiculum terminale. **C,** T2 sagittal MRI demonstrating an associated syrinx involving the cervical and thoracic spinal cord with a Chiari malformation.

odontoideum as a separate entity from the ossiculum terminale because os odontoideum is associated with atlantoaxial instability.

Os odontoideum are classified into two anatomic types: orthotopic and dystopic. In the orthotopic type, the dens remains in its anatomic position and moves with the anterior arch of C1. The dystopic type is located in any other position and may be fused with the clivus

(**Figure 13-3**). Subluxation and instability can be present with either type; however, instability is more commonly associated with the dystopic variant.

Patients may present with a combination of local symptoms and neurologic findings or may be asymptomatic. Local symptoms include high cervical pain, neck stiffness, neck weakness, dizziness, and torticollis, and neurologic symptoms are caused by instability and displacement of

C1 to C2, and minor trauma can be associated with acute symptom onset. Dai et al described neurologic findings in 30 of 44 patients treated for os odontoideum,[15] the most common of which was myelopathy with radicular symptoms (22 patients). Other findings included radiculopathy alone, myelopathy, and cranial nerve palsies.

Os odontoideum can typically be identified and accurately diagnosed with plain radiographs, but CT scans or MRI may be obtained as well when the diagnosis is questionable or neurologic symptoms are present. However, none of these static imaging modalities provides definitive information regarding the degree of instability,

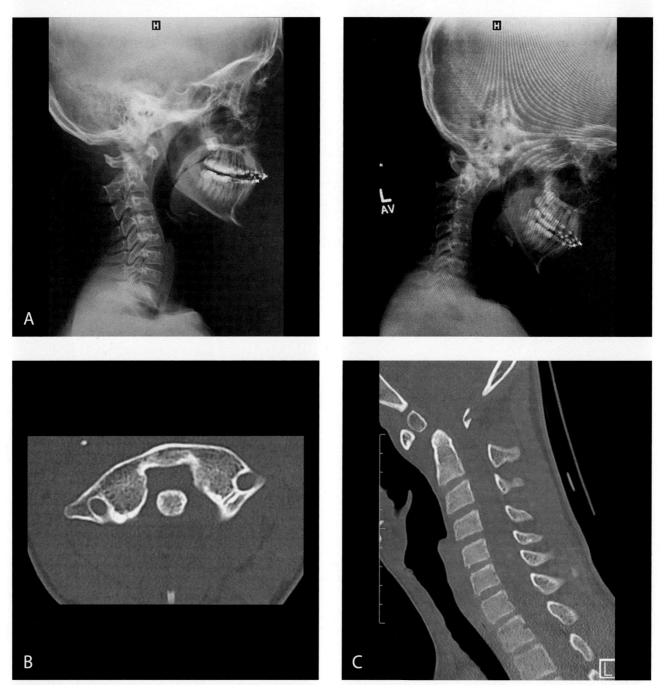

FIGURE 13-3 **A,** A 13-year-old boy who presented with axial neck pain and a sudden onset of paraesthesias and subsequent loss of sensation in his upper extremities and lower extremities after physical activity that subsequently resolved spontaneously. Attempted extension and flexion views demonstrate atlantodens intervals (ADIs) of 7 mm and 11 mm, respectively. **B,** Axial CT cut at the level of the ADI (*dashed line*) showing an abnormal ADI. **C,** Sagittal CT demonstrates that the dens is in close relationship to the atlas, but the distal segment is subluxed and not in line with the dens, suggesting that this is a dystopic os odontoideum. (*continued*)

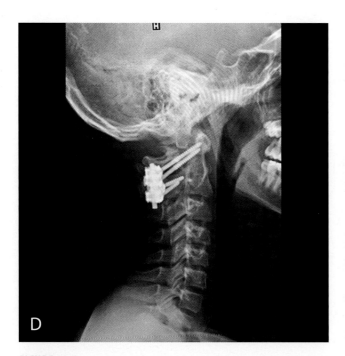
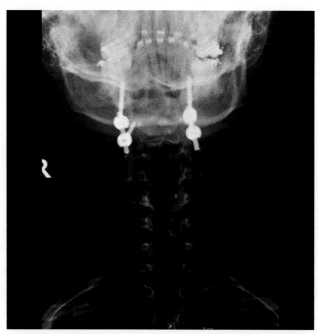

FIGURE 13-3 (*Continued*) **D,** Because of C1 to C2 instability, the patient was indicated for C1 to C2 fusion. Contact and collision sports remain contraindicated in this patient population even after successful fusion.

and even dynamic radiographs taken within physiologic ROM frequently underestimate instability in the absence of appropriate effort.

There are reports of sudden death and major neurologic complications after minor trauma as the initial presentation of patients with previously undiagnosed os odontoideum. In 1989, a high school football player was rendered a ventilator-dependent quadriplegic after a head tackle. Radiographs taken after the trauma demonstrated an os odontoideum with significant C1 to C2 instability. As a result, Torg and Ramsey-Emrhein recommended that any odontoid anomaly (os odontoideum, odontoid hypoplasia, or odontoid agenesis) be considered an absolute contraindication to contact or collision sporting activity.[16] Even after surgical fixation of an os odontoideum, it is still contraindicated that these young athletes return to contact or collision sports.

Klippel-Feil Syndrome

Klippel-Feil syndrome was first described in 1912 with patients demonstrating a characteristic short neck, low hairline, and decreased cervical motion. However, fewer than 50% of patients with congenital fusions of the cervical spine demonstrate all three findings. Associated conditions also include renal disease, congenital heart disease, and congenital scoliosis. As such, a multidisciplinary team approach consisting of a cardiologist, nephrologist, and pediatrician should be taken when

managing these patients. In Klippel-Feil syndrome, a failure in segmentation of cervical somites during gestation results in multiple fused cervical segments (**Figure 13-4**). The spectrum of the disease ranges from fusion of

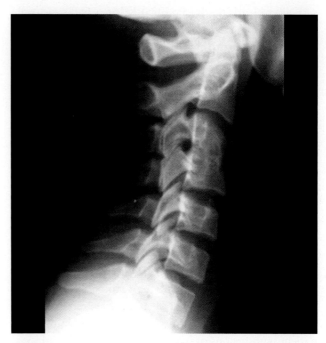

FIGURE 13-4 A patient with Klippel-Feil syndrome demonstrating subaxial congenitally fused C3 and C4 vertebrae. Current recommendations state that isolated two-level deformities may not be an absolute contraindication in return to play but rather depend on factors such as instability.

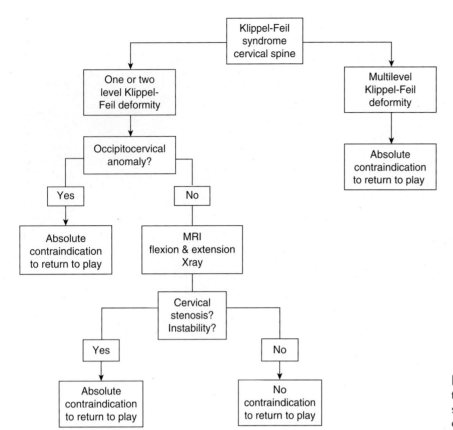

FIGURE 13-5 Return-to-play (RTP) algorithm for patients with Klippel-Feil syndrome and stenosis that can be analyzed via flexion and extension radiographs as well as MRI.

2 cervical vertebrae to a mass fusion of the entire cervical spine and upper thoracic spine.[17]

Feil et al originally classified Klippel-Feil syndrome into three categories.[18,19] In type I, there is a massive fusion of the entire cervical spine. In type II, only two vertebrae are fused. In type III, either type I or type II fusions are associated with thoracic or lumbar spine anomalies. More recently, a new classification system was suggested. In this classification scheme, type I had a single-level fusion, type II includes multiple noncontiguous fused vertebrae, and type III includes multiple contiguous fused segments.[20]

Pizzutillo pointed out that children with congenital cervical spine fusions very rarely develop neurologic sequelae or cervical instability.[21] There are, however, more than 90 cases in the literature of patients with Klippel-Feil with occipitocervical anomalies, instability, and degenerative disk disease who developed neurologic problems, including the development of cervical radiculopathy, pain, spasticity, and quadriplegia. There are even reported cases of sudden death after minor trauma. Interestingly, no patient with fusions of five to seven levels of the subaxial spine had reports of neurologic loss, but several patients with single-level fusions of the upper cervical spine had adverse neurologic sequelae.

Despite the paucity of findings in the literature, a mass fusion of the cervical spine (i.e., fusion of more than two segments) is considered an absolute contraindication to participation in contact sports.[16] It is thought that the marked alteration in spine mechanics predisposes these individuals to unacceptable neurologic risk and increases the propensity to develop degenerative changes. Children with fusion of one or two subaxial segments are allowed to participate in contact sports as long as several criteria are met (**Figure 13-5**). These children must be able to demonstrate full range of cervical motion, have no occipitocervical anomalies, demonstrate no signs of instability, and be free of degenerative changes on radiographs or MRI. The presence of any of these markers for instability or degeneration along with a congenital subaxial fusion is an absolute contraindication to contact sports (**Table 13-1**). Additionally, any occipitocervical fusion in isolation or in conjunction with another cervical abnormality is an absolute contraindication to participation in collision sporting activities.

Atlantoaxial Instability and Down Syndrome

Down syndrome is the most common genetic disorder and cause of developmental disability and mental retardation. Motor development is usually delayed with

TABLE 13-1	Congenital conditions: contraindications to return to athletic activity		
	Contraindications		
Congenital Condition	None	Relative	Absolute
Single-level Klippel-Feil deformity (excluding occipital–C1 articulation) with no evidence of instability or stenosis noted on MRI	X		
Torg ratio <0.8 in asymptomatic individuals	X		
Occipital–C1 assimilation		X	
Radiographic evidence of C1–C2 hypermobility with an anterior dens interval ≥4 mm (i.e., atlanto-axial instability in a patient without Down syndrome)			X
Multiple-level Klippel-Feil deformity			X
Basilar invagination			X
Arnold-Chiari malformation			X
Odontoid anomalies (odontoid aplasia, hypoplasia, os odontoideum)			X

Down syndrome; however, after reaching developmental maturity, highly developed athletic skills are possible. A variety of musculoskeletal problems are associated with Down syndrome, including patellofemoral instability and hip and foot disorders. Cervical spine instability was first described in patients with Down syndrome by Spitzer et al in 1961.[22] Instability and hypermobility at the atlanto-occipital and atlantoaxial level is common, and as such, patients with Down syndrome have certain risk considerations regarding to their cervical spines that must be considered in a RTP evaluation.

Athletes with Down syndrome have a 60% incidence of occipitocervical and atlantoaxial instability caused by extreme ligamentous laxity.[23] The natural history of atlantoaxial instability in people with Down syndrome suggests that neurologic deterioration may not be associated with radiologic findings of atlantoaxial instability. Ferguson et al analyzed flexion and extension radiographs at the C1 to C2 articulation in 84 patients with Down syndrome for the purpose of dividing them into subluxators (atlantodens interval [ADI] ≥4 mm) and non-subluxators.[24] They noted that there was no significant difference in the presence of positive neurologic findings between the two groups, concluding that positive neurologic findings and an abnormal ADI are not adequate to pursue surgical stabilization. In the same way,

an increased ADI in the Down syndrome population has not been correlated with an increased rate of neurologic compromise as it has in the remainder of the population. Instead, it has been shown that in patients with Down syndrome with an ADI of 4 to 10 mm, there are equal rates of neurological injury when compared to patients with Down syndrome who have normal ADIs.

It is important to note that the associated presence of bony anomalies at the base of the skull as well as in the atlas and axis may increase the risk for significant neurologic injury. Osseous anomalies most frequently found in Down syndrome include os odontoideum, atlantal arch hypoplasia, and basilar invagination. Paradoxically, the risk of neurological injury seems to be less if the odontoid process is absent or fractured because the superior fragment is carried with the atlas. In patients with a normal odontoid process and atlantoaxial instability, flexion leads to the atlas sliding forward on the axis and thus decreasing the space available for cord (SAC) while increasing the atlantodens interval.[25]

A large majority of individuals with Down syndrome with atlantoaxial instability are asymptomatic. Pueschel et al reported on 40 patients with Down syndrome and associated atlantoaxial instability (ADI ≥5 mm).[26] A total of 85% of these patients were asymptomatic, and seven patients had positive neurologic findings, which included pyramidal tract signs; quadri-, hemi-, or paraplegia; muscle weakness; gait abnormalities; and difficulty walking. Local symptoms included neck pain, limited neck ROM, and torticollis.

The association between Down syndrome and neurologic injury has been publicized to the lay population through the efforts of the Special Olympics. In the early 1980s, the Special Olympics made the recommendation that every child with Down syndrome who planned to participate required a neurologic evaluation and examination of the cervical spine.[23,27] Unfortunately, national guidelines and protocols have not been established, so each state varies in the frequency with which these examinations are required to be performed. In many states, only one initial examination is required; other states require annual checks. Reevaluation of these patients on an annual basis is preferable because many of these patients are unable to relay subtle complaints secondary to their cognitive deficits.

Occipitoatlantal instability in the general population typically only results after high-energy trauma, such as a motor vehicle collision. However, hypermobility in the occipitocervical junction has been described in the Down syndrome population. The majority of the individuals with

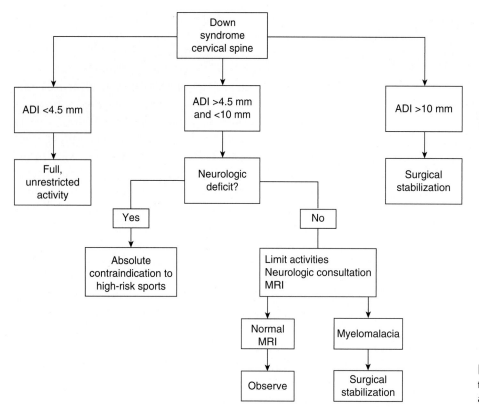

FIGURE 13-6 Return-to-play algorithm for patients with Down syndrome. ADI = atlantodens interval.

this instability are asymptomatic; these anomalies are usually incidental findings discovered on routine examination.

Despite extensive study, interpretation of radiographic findings and determination of the integrity of the cervical spine in patients with Down syndrome remains controversial. Because of patients' impaired cognition and insufficient effort, it is often difficult to obtain technically adequate lateral radiographs, especially in the case of flexion and extension views. Thus, images may underestimate the presence of instability and may incorrectly be interpreted as normal studies.[17] Cineradiography of the cervical spine may be used when adequate radiographs cannot be obtained.

While assessing the occipitocervical junction, ADI, and each cervical level, it is critical to understand that universally accepted radiographic limitations to cervical motion do not apply to athletes with Down syndrome. The cervical spine in patients with Down syndrome does demonstrate hypermobility; however, this does not necessarily imply loss of integrity of the structures that protect neural tissues. About 10% to 30% of patients with Down syndrome demonstrate an increase ADI on lateral radiographs. Fifteen percent of patients with Down syndrome have an ADI greater than 4.5 mm, but fewer than 2% demonstrate any symptoms of neurologic compromise.[27] Although it

is universally agreed that patients with Down syndrome with an ADI greater than 10 mm require surgery, the patient population with ADIs between 4.5 mm and 10 mm requires closer scrutiny; these patients are advised to avoid high-risk sports such as diving and football. Patients with ADIs of less than 4.5 mm are allowed to participate in full, unrestricted activities (**Figure 13-6** and **Table 13-2**).

Steel proposed the "rule of thirds" that helped define a safe zone.[28] He divided the vertebral canal of C1 into one third odontoid, one third spinal cord, and one third uninhabited space. This space represents a safe zone in which displacement can occur without neurologic compromise. He conferred that secondary stability may be attained from the alar ligaments when the TAL had failed. Additionally, Greenberg examined the presence of neurologic signs as related to the sagittal cervical canal diameter behind the dens, also known as the SAC.[29] He determined that cord compression always occurred when the SAC was 14 mm or less, and cord compression was possible when the SAC was between 15 and 17 mm. He noted that neurologic dysfunction never occurred when the SAC was 18 mm or more. Ultimately, in the presence of symptoms and ADI greater than 10 mm, posterior cervical fusion of the atlantoaxial articulation should be considered (**Figure 13-7**). For this, multiple options are

TABLE 13-2 Radiographic guidelines for patients with Down syndrome

I. ADI
  a. ADI
    i. <4.5 mm: full, unrestricted activity
    ii. >4.5 mm and <10 mm + neurologically normal: limit high-risk activities
    iii. >4.5 mm + neurologic deficit
      1. Limit activities
      2. Neurologic consultation
      3. MRI
        a. Normal study: observe
        b. Signal changes within cord: surgical stabilization
    iv. >9.9 mm: surgical fusion
  b. Occipitoatlantal mobility
    i. Normal: full, unrestricted activity
    ii. >2 mm motion + neurologically normal: limit high-risk activities
    iii. >2 mm motion and neurologic deficit
      1. Limit activity
      2. Neurologic consultation
      3. MRI
        a. Normal study: observe
        b. Signal changes within cord: surgical fusion
  c. Subaxial cervical spine degenerative changes
    i. Neurologically normal: observe
    ii. Pain without neurologic deficit: symptomatic treatment
    iii. Neurologic deficit
      1. Neurologic consultation
      2. EMG and NCV studies
      3. MRI
      4. Disk excision and fusion

ADI = atlantodens interval, EMG = electromyography, NCV = nerve conduction velocity. Adapted from Ashraf N, Hecht A: Congenital and developmental abnormalities of the cervical spine encountered in athletes. *Semin Spine Surg* 2010;22:218–221.

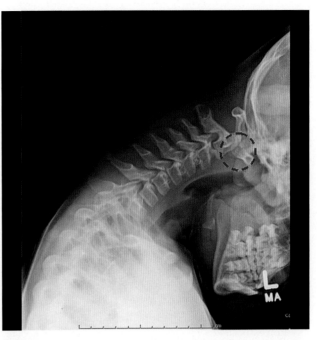

FIGURE 13-7 A patient with Down syndrome demonstrating atlanto-axial instability on flexion views with an atlantodens interval larger than 10 mm and a space available for cord smaller than 14 mm (*red circle*) who is an operative candidate for fusion surgery.

cervical spine should be obtained. Somatosensory evoked potentials may also be necessary to determine the clinical significance of the imaging findings. These patients should be counseled to avoid tumbling, gymnastics, and collision and contact sports but may participate in noncontact sports. If cord compromise on MRI is noted or if there are any abnormalities detected on physical examination, these individuals should be directed toward surgical stabilization.

Young athletes with congenital or developmental disorders benefit greatly from athletic activity, and their participation should be encouraged. Special risk considerations need to be assessed before their participation in sporting activities. Most important, it is critical to judiciously evaluate these patients and not unnecessarily restrict them from the psychological and physical benefits from participating in athletic activities.

available, and they should be based on the patient's anatomy and the surgeon's expertise (e.g., C1–C2 transarticular screws, C1–C2 screw–rod constructs).

If radiography demonstrates hypermobility at the occipitocervical junction, a thorough history and physical examination must be obtained to ensure there has been no change in physical endurance and to assess motor and sensory function. MRI of the brainstem and

REFERENCES

1. Hutzler Y, Bar-Eli M: Psychological benefits of sports for disabled people: A review. *Scand J Med Sci Sports* 1993; 3:217–228.

2. Jackson, RW, Davis GM: The value of sports and recreation for the physically disabled. *Orthop Clin North Am* 1983;14(2):301–315.

3. Wind WM, Schwend RM, Larson J: Sports for the physically challenged child. *J Am Acad Orthop Surg* 2004; 12(2):126–137.

4. Wills BP, Dormans JP: Nontraumatic upper cervical spine instability in children. *J Am Acad Orthop Surg* 2006; 14(4):233–245.

5. Smith JS, Shaffrey CI, Abel MF, Menezes AH: Basilar invagination. *Neurosurgery* 2010;66(3 suppl):39–47.

6. Caetano de Barros M, Farias W, Ataíde L, Lins S: Basilar impression and Arnold-Chiari malformation. A study of 66 cases. *J Neurol Neurosurg Psychiatry* 1968; 31(6):596–605.

7. Goel A, Bhatjiwale M, Desai, K:Basilar invagination: A study based on 190 surgically treated patients. *J Neurosurg* 1998;88(6):962–968.

8. Vaccaro AR1 Klein GR, Ciccoti M, Pfaff WL, Moulton MJ, Hilibrand AJ, Watkins B: Return to play criteria for the athlete with cervical spine injuries resulting in stinger and transient quadriplegia/paresis. *Spine J* 2002; 2(5):351–536.

9. Giacomini C: Sull esistenza dell os odontoideum nelluomo. *Gior Accad Med Torino* 1886;49:24–28.

10. Schuler TC, Kurz L, Thompson DE, Zemenick G, Hensinger RN, Herkowitz HN: Natural history of os odontoideum. *J Pediatr Orthop* 1991;11(2):222–225.

11. Sherk HH, Nicholson JT: Rotatory atlanto-axial dislocation associated with ossiculum terminale and mongolism. A case report. *J Bone Joint Surg Am* 1969;51(5):957–964.

12. Burke SW, French HG, Roberts JM, Johnston CE 2nd, Whitecloud TS 3rd, Edmunds JO Jr: Chronic atlantoaxial instability in Down syndrome. *J Bone Joint Surg Am* 1985;67(9):1356–1360.

13. Liang CL, Lui CC, Lu K, Lee TC, Chen HJ: Atlantoaxial stability in ossiculum terminale. Case report. *J Neurosurg* 2001;95(1 suppl):119–121.

14. Fielding JW, Hensinger RN, Hawkins RJ: Os odontoideum. *J Bone Joint Surg Am* 1980;62(3):376–383.

15. Dai L, Yuan W, Ni B, Jia L: Os odontoideum: Etiology, diagnosis, and management. *Surg Neurol* 2000;53(2): 106–108; discussion 108-109.

16. Torg JS, Ramsey-Emrhein JA: Management guidelines for participation in collision activities with congenital, developmental, or postinjury lesions involving the cervical spine. *Clin J Sport Med* 1997;7(4):273–291.

17. Guille JT Sherk HH: Congenital osseous anomalies of the upper and lower cervical spine in children. *J Bone Joint Surg Am* 2002;84-A(2):277–288.

18. Klippel M, Feil A: Anomalie de la colonne vertebrale par absence des vertebres cervicales; cage thoracique remontant jusqu'a la base du crane. *Bull et Mem Soc Anat de Paris* 1912;LXXXVII:185.

19. Feil A: L'absence et la diminution des vertebres cervicales (etude clinique et pathogenique): le syndrome de reduction numerique cervicale [thesis]. Paris, 1919.

20. Samartzis DD, Herman J, Lubicky JP, Shen FH: Classification of congenitally fused cervical patterns in Klippel-Feil patients: Epidemiology and role in the development of cervical spine-related symptoms. *Spine (Phila Pa 1976)* 2006;31(21):E798–E804.

21. Pizzutillo PD: Klippel-Feil syndrome. The Cervical Spine Research Society Editorial Committee. *The Cervical Spine*, ed 2. St. Louis, CV Mosby, 1991, pp 258–268.

22. Spitze, R, Rabinowitch JY, Wybar KC: A study of the abnormalities of the skull, teeth and lenses in mongolism. *Can Med Assoc J* 1961;84(11):567–572.

23. Pizzutillo PD, Herman MJ: Cervical spine issues in Down syndrome. *J Pediatr Orthop* 2005;25(2):253–259.

24. Ferguson RL, Putney ME, Allen Jr BL: Comparison of neurologic deficits with atlanto-dens intervals in patients with Down syndrome. *J Spinal Disord* 1997;10(3):246–252.

25. Bedi A, Hensinger RN: Congenital anomalies of the cervical spine. *Rothman Simeone The Spine* 2011;6: 524–572.

26. Pueschel SM, Herndon JH, Gelch MM, Senft KE, Scola FH, Goldberg MJ: Symptomatic atlantoaxial subluxation in persons with Down syndrome. *J Pediatr Orthop* 1984;4(6):682–688.

27. Bulletin SO: *Participation by Individuals with Down Syndrome Who Suffer Atlantoaxial Dislocation Condition.* Washington, DC, Special Olympics, 1983.

28. Steel HH: Anatomical and mechanical considerations of the atlanto-axial articulations. *J Bone Joint Surg Am* 1968; 50:1481.

29. Greenberg AD: Atlanto-axial dislocations. *Brain* 1968; 91(4):655–684.

14 Degenerative Disorders of the Cervical Spine and Cervical Stenosis

Kevin L. Ju, MD • John G. Heller, MD

BACKGROUND

Most of the sports medicine and spine literature has focused on acute cervical spine injuries in collegiate and professional sports, especially American football and rugby. However, there is a relative paucity of studies looking at older athletes who have developed degeneration of the cervical spine. Degenerative changes throughout the spine, termed *spondylosis,* become more prevalent with increasing age and create conditions that do not typically affect younger athletes.

Although the development of cervical spondylosis is accepted as a natural consequence of aging, the possible contributory effects and long-term sequelae from repetitive loads and demands placed on a young athlete's neck are less clearly understood. On the one hand, Mundt and colleagues examined weightlifters and other athletes involved in noncollision sports (e.g., baseball, swimming, racquet sports) and found that these activities did not put players at increased risk for developing cervical or lumbar disk herniations.[1] On the other hand, there is literature suggesting that athletes who participate in contact sports hasten the development of cervical degeneration, possibly because of repetitive loads or undiagnosed

Dr. Heller or an immediate family member has received royalties from Medtronic; serves as a paid consultant to Medtronic; has stock or stock options held in Medtronic; and serves as a board member, owner, officer, or committee member of the Cervical Spine Research Society. Neither Dr. Ju nor any immediate family member has received anything of value from or has stock or stock options held in a commercial company or institution related directly or indirectly to the subject of this article.

injuries they may experience.[2-5] Several studies on American football and rugby players have found that the risk of developing low back pain, degenerative disk disease, and facet degeneration increase with the number of years they participate in their sport.[2,6,7] Soccer players have also been shown to be at increased risk of developing early cervical degenerative changes caused by recurrent trauma from heading the ball.[8] Other sports with established risk for cervical spine injuries include rugby, ice hockey, wrestling, skiing, gymnastics, diving, pole vaulting, and cheerleading.[9]

No matter if it is in a previously elite athlete or an individual who is just getting into a new sport, degenerative changes in the cervical spine accumulate over time even if they are initially asymptomatic. Most of the research on cervical spondylosis is in middle-aged or elderly individuals because this is the population in which degenerative changes tend to become symptomatic. By age 65 years, spondylosis is seen in 95% of the population.[10] Boden and colleagues, in their classic study, evaluated 67 individuals who had never had any back pain, sciatica, or neurogenic claudication and found that degenerative changes on lumbar spine MRI scans were present in about 25% of people younger than 60 years old and in about 60% of people older than 60 years.[11] Matsumoto et al performed a similar MRI study involving asymptomatic volunteers but focused specifically on the cervical spine and found that degenerative changes increased linearly with age and was present in nearly 90% of people older than 60 years.[12] Other similar studies have confirmed the pervasiveness of cervical spondylosis on both plain radiographs and MRI.[13,14]

As the human body ages, structural components of the spine naturally wear down. This degenerative process starts with the intervertebral disk, resulting in a loss of disk height that may lead to a bulging annulus, infolding of the ligamentum flavum, arthrosis of the uncovertebral and facet joints, and even loss of normal cervical lordosis and motion.[15–18] These degenerative changes can manifest as axial neck pain, radiculopathy, myelopathy, or a combination of the three. Axial neck pain refers to nonradiating neck pain involving the axial cervical spine or paraspinal region (or both). In addition to being caused by cervical sprains and strains, axial neck pain has been attributed to pathology within cervical disks (innervated by the sinuvertebral nerve) and facet joints (innervated by the medial branches of the cervical dorsal rami).[19,20]

Radiculopathy describes radiating pain that typically begins in the neck and travels into the arm and may be accompanied by sensory or motor deficits in the distribution of the involved nerve root. Radiculopathy is caused by nerve root compression, which can occur with lateral or foraminal stenosis from bulging disks, inflammation of the facet capsule, or osteophyte formation at the facet or uncovertebral joints.

Finally, cervical spondylotic myelopathy (CSM) describes the phenomenon of central cervical stenosis caused by age-related degenerative changes leading to spinal cord compression and dysfunction.[21] When present, developmental stenosis (also known as congenital stenosis) is a critical predisposing condition for developing CSM.[22,23] The normal midsagittal anteroposterior (AP) diameter of the spinal canal from C3 to C7 measures 17 to 18 mm in adults, with the cervical spinal cord itself measuring 10 mm in the same dimension.[24,25] Individuals with a midsagittal canal diameter of less than 13 mm are considered to have developmental cervical stenosis.[26] These individuals have less space available for the spinal cord and thus are more susceptible to the cumulative degenerative factors that further narrow the spinal canal.[27] These contributory degenerative factors can include static elements, such as bulging degenerative disks, osteophytes, and infolded or thickened ligamentum flavum, as well as dynamic factors. Abnormal cervical motion in the setting of a stenotic canal can lead to chronic, repetitive spinal cord trauma from impingement against bony spurs or pathologically subluxed vertebral bodies.[22] It has also been postulated that developmental stenosis reduces the cushioning effect of cerebrospinal fluid during minor trauma, increasing the risk for cord injury.[28]

Cervical stenosis has been quantified using the Torg ratio, which is calculated from plain lateral radiographs by dividing the canal diameter (measured from the anterior aspect of the lamina to the mid-portion of the posterior cortex of the vertebral body) by the AP width of the vertebral body at its midsection.[29] A normal ratio is approximately 1.0, and anything 0.8 or less is indicative of cervical stenosis. However, some studies have called into question how applicable the Torg ratio is for collision sport athletes who have larger vertebral bodies, which can lead to a high false-positive rate and thus poor predictive value.[30,31] Moreover, Torg et al published on the use of the ratio in predicting the likelihood and severity of an athlete's spinal cord injury (SCI) after a fracture or ligamentous instability.[29] This ratio did not predict cases of devastating neurologic injury or quadriplegia. It has mistakenly been thought to be a screening measure for cervical canal stenosis. In fact, Blackley et al demonstrated how poorly the Torg ratio correlated to the actual canal diameter as measured on a CT scan.[32] With the wide availability of MRI today and its ability to directly visualize the neural elements, this is currently the modality of choice for imaging a patient with suspected cervical stenosis.[33]

Stenosis of the cervical spine is thought to be a risk factor for cervical cord neurapraxia (CCN) and SCI.[34,35] CCN results from a compressive or concussive injury to the cervical spinal cord in the absence of a cervical fracture or dislocation and results in a transient complete or partial loss of motor or sensation bilaterally that can last anywhere from a few seconds to 36 hours. The mechanism of CCN is thought to be cord compression between the posteroinferior margin of the vertebral body and the anterosuperior edge of the subjacent lamina,[36] especially with neck extension because this decreases the sagittal diameter of the spinal canal by 2 mm.[37] Therefore, athletes with smaller canal diameters may be at increased risk for sustaining an episode of CCN with trauma, especially if this involves neck hyperextension. A retrospective study consisting of American football players who experienced CCN revealed that all participants had evidence of developmental or acquired spinal stenosis as determined by the Torg ratio.[29]

Although cervical stenosis can place an asymptomatic athlete at risk for CCN, if spinal cord compression is severe enough and present for a long enough time, the individual can develop myelopathy. When the myelopathy is a result of stenosis from cervical spondylosis, it is termed CSM. The clinical findings in early myelopathy are typically subtle, and the insidious onset of symptoms is responsible for lengthy delays in diagnosis. One study reported a 6.3-year average delay in diagnosing myelopathy, with gait abnormalities presenting as the earliest consistent symptom in their cohort.[38] In addition to gait disturbances, patients with myelopathy often complain of hand clumsiness and a decline in their manual dexterity or fine motor skills. Depending on the specific spinal cord tracts that are affected, patients may complain of a constellation of upper extremity weakness or sensory disturbances (or both).

The natural history of CSM has been extensively studied in the literature. Clark and Robinson followed 120 patients and described how 75% deteriorated in a stepwise fashion with episodic periods of stable disease, 20% deteriorated gradually but continuously, and 5% exhibited a rapid onset of symptoms followed by a long period of stable disease.[39] Lees and Turner followed 44 patients for 3 to 40 years and concluded that CSM follows a protracted course with variable periods of stable neurologic function mixed with episodes of disease progression.[40] Nurick's studies on the natural history of CSM reported that mild myelopathy did not significantly worsen over time. However, patients with moderate or severe symptoms and older than 60 years old at symptom onset tended to have a worse prognosis and only had an improvement rate of 30% to 50% with conservative management.[41,42] In general, CSM manifests as a slow stepwise functional deterioration with episodes of stable neurologic function. A recent literature review of the natural history of CSM suggests that 20% to 60% of patients with mild CSM neurologically decline over time in the absence of surgical intervention.[43]

● DIAGNOSIS AND TREATMENT

Patients with degenerative cervical disorders often seek medical attention because of neck pain, arm pain, weakness, or numbness. Their evaluation should begin with a thorough history and physical examination, and although the most common cause is a degenerative condition, if trauma, infection, or a neoplasm is in the differential diagnosis, these should be expeditiously worked up with the appropriate studies. Cervical myelopathy is diagnosed clinically and confirmed through imaging studies that demonstrate a narrowed canal and compromised spinal cord.[44] As a result of the insidious onset of CSM, patients are often unaware of the subtle clinical findings early on in the disease process. When patients do notice functional deterioration, they tend to complain of gait imbalance, difficulty with fine motor skills, and hand clumsiness or loss of manual dexterity (e.g., difficulty manipulating buttons, dropping objects).[15] They can also develop upper extremity weakness or numbness or paresthesias, but the specific constellation of neurologic deficits can vary widely and depend on the specific spinal cord tracts that are affected. Bowel or bladder dysfunction in CSM is rare but may be seen in severe cases. The typical findings on physical examination are lower motor neuron signs (i.e., motor weakness and hyporeflexia) at the levels of cervical stenosis and upper motor neuron signs (i.e., muscle spasticity, hyperreflexia, and clonus) at levels below the stenosis. However, the absence of lower extremity hyperreflexia does not exclude the diagnosis because this can be masked by concomitant lumbar stenosis, diabetic neuropathy, and other conditions. Certain pathological reflexes should be sought in patients with myelopathy, including (1) the Hoffman sign, (2) inverted brachioradialis reflex, (3) extensor plantar reflex (i.e., Babinski sign), (4) finger escape sign, (5) abnormal grip-and-release-test result, and (6) Lhermitte sign.[27,44,45] High cervical myelopathy above the C5 level can lead to "myelopathy hand" in which there is diffuse numbness in the hands that can be confused with a peripheral neuropathy.[45] Even though the presentation of early myelopathy can be subtle, routinely screening athletes for cervical stenosis using radiography or MRI is neither recommended nor cost effective.[46,47] For patients who have a history and physical examination consistent with cervical stenosis and myelopathy, MRI is the imaging modality of choice given its ability to directly visualize neural structures and the degree of central or neuroforaminal stenosis that is present.

A combination of factors goes into deciding whether a patient with CSM should undergo conservative or operative treatment. These factors include the severity and duration of the individual's symptoms, number of levels and degree of cord compression, age, and other medical comorbidities. As shown in the natural history studies on CSM, patients presenting with mild myelopathic symptoms typically have a protracted course of minor impairments without rapid progression and thus may be treated conservatively and observed over time.[39,40,42,48] Poor prognostic factors for conservative treatment include presence of myelopathy for 6 months or longer, compression ratio (determined by dividing the sagittal spinal cord diameter by the transverse diameter) approaching 0.4,[49] and transverse area of the cord less than 40 mm^2.[50] Patients with these factors or moderate to severe myelopathy and dysfunction are unlikely to have their symptoms regress, and thus surgical intervention should be strongly considered.[48,51]

The primary goal of surgical intervention is to prevent further neurologic deterioration by decompressing the spinal cord, which can be accomplished via anterior or posterior approaches. CSM is commonly addressed via an anterior approach for one- or two-level compression and posteriorly if there are three or more levels of compression. When an anterior decompressive procedure is chosen, it typically involves an anterior cervical discectomy and fusion (ACDF) or anterior cervical corpectomy and fusion (ACCF) if there is retrovertebral compression. Posterior decompressive options include laminoplasty or laminectomy and fusion. In addition to the number of levels involved, the sagittal alignment of the cervical spine, specifically the presence and degree of significant cervical kyphosis, is important in deciding whether to undertake an anterior, posterior, or combined procedure.[52]

RETURN TO PLAY

The question of when an athlete should be allowed to return to play (RTP) after sustaining a cervical spine injury or having a cervical spine disorder remains controversial. In fact, no major sporting organization has endorsed any particular guideline regarding RTP after cervical injuries.[53] Furthermore, most of the RTP literature is focused on collegiate and professional athletes involved in collision sports. Given the infrequent nature of CCN (2.05 per 100,000 collegiate athletes),[54] no universally accepted RTP guidelines have been established, and much of the published advice is a based on relatively sparse retrospective studies combined with the expert opinion of practitioners with experience managing cervical spine injuries. Therefore, for the purposes of our discussion on RTP decision making in an individual with stenosis caused by cervical spondylosis, we will have to extrapolate from the available literature involving athletes with developmental stenosis.

A player who sustains an episode of CCN, even with quick return of neurologic function and complete symptom resolution, should be screened for cervical stenosis after appropriate cervical spine clearance protocols have been followed. Plain radiographs of the cervical spine may be obtained for initial screening, but MRI is the study of choice as previously discussed. Although CCN can be caused by the shear concussive energy of an impact or an acute disk herniation, many athletes who sustain a CCN have some underlying component of cervical stenosis, which in the spondylotic spine can be from infolded soft tissue structures or osteophytes. After an episode of CCN without any MRI evidence of cord signal changes or cervical stenosis, the player can RTP when completely asymptomatic and neurologically normal and having regained full range of motion in the neck. However, if the player experiences a second episode of CCN, even in the continued absence of cervical stenosis or cord injury, the player should likely not be allowed to return to collision sports. However, he or she can participate in noncontact sports without restrictions.[46] Furthermore, the presence of any abnormal cord signal on MRI after an episode of CCN is an absolute contraindication for return to contact sports. Similarly, patients with myelopathy, no matter how mild, should not be allowed to participate in contact sports. There is some controversy regarding an athlete who has sustained a CCN in the setting of identifiable stenosis. Some authors advocate that cervical stenosis alone should be a contraindication for collision sports,[46] but others consider it a relative contraindication that should take into account the severity of the initial symptoms, severity of stenosis, and propensity for injury in the sport.[55] Given the seriousness of SCI, our recommendation for patients with degeneration of their cervical spine mirrors that of Torg and colleagues, who suggested that patients who have sustained an episode of CCN and have evidence of either cervical instability, congenital or cervical stenosis, or acute (disk herniation) or chronic degenerative changes in the cervical spine not be allowed to return to collision sports.[29] Examples of collision sports include American football, rugby, wrestling, ice hockey, skiing and snowboarding, pole vaulting, and cheerleading. For noncollision contact sports (e.g., soccer, baseball, basketball, equestrian sports), no good data exist, and thus we recommend counseling the individual on the risks and allow the player to decide whether he or she wishes to assume the risks. Finally, for noncollision, noncontact sports, the risk for catastrophic SCI is low, and thus the player can likely RTP after appropriate counseling, resolution of symptoms, and return of normal neurologic function. If the anatomic condition has been remedied, then the decision about RTP may be revisited (i.e., repair of a disk herniation). The judgment may then be more complicated and will be influenced heavily by both the nature of the surgical treatment and the specific sport in question. Ultimately, the patient-athlete will need to make his or her own decision after thoughtfully weighing the available information and his or her individual tolerance for risk. Second opinions from other qualified physicians are encouraged.

CASE EXAMPLE 1

At age 15 years, a male high school football player was evaluated for recurring "stingers," which caused

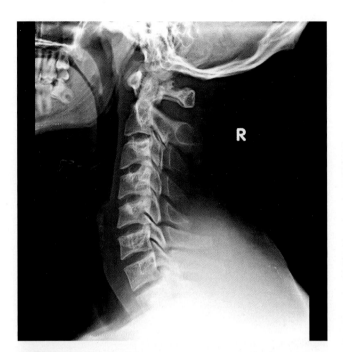

FIGURE 14-1 Lateral cervical radiograph of the 18-year old male patient described in Case 14-1. No plain radiographic abnormalities are noted. Although his Torg ration is less than 0.8, readers are referred to the text for discussion regarding the relevance of this observation.

transient pain, numbness, and weakness in his proximal left arm. Spinal imaging at that time revealed a combination of congenital stenosis and left C3/4 foraminal stenosis caused by uncovertebral osteophytes. He was advised to avoid contact sports and not allowed to RTP. At age 18 years, he returned with the spontaneous onset left proximal arm weakness (deltoid and biceps), with minor amounts of pain and numbness (**Figure 14-1**). MRI (**Figure 14-2**), as well as cervical myelogram and CT images (**Figure 14-3**) confirmed worsening of his left C3 to C4 foraminal stenosis and C4/5 spinal cord compression. He underwent a C3 to C7 laminoplasty with left C3/C4 and C4/C5 foraminotomies to address the combination of congenital spinal canal stenosis and the acquired foraminal stenosis. He has been advised to still avoid collision sports, but he might choose to play recreational basketball or other sports with potential contact now that his stenosis has been addressed.

● CASE EXAMPLE 2

A 30-year-old professional basketball player collided with another player while driving to the basket and hyperextended his neck. He collapsed onto the floor

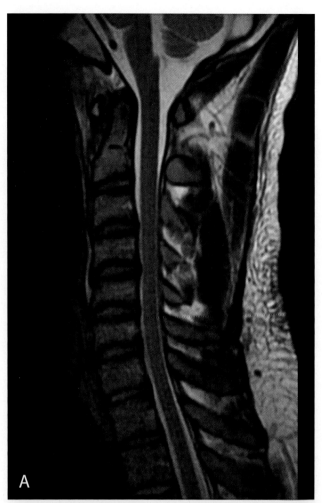

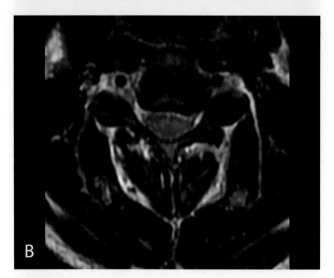

FIGURE 14-2 A, Midsagittal T2 cervical MRI that reveals congenital stenosis, which is best appreciated by the absence of cerebrospinal fluid (CSF) ventral and dorsal to the spinal cord. The spinal cord signal appears unremarkable. **B,** Axial T2 image at C3/C4 reveals severe left foraminal stenosis and C4 root compression. (*continued*)

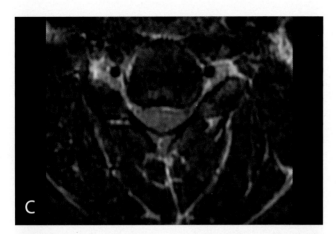

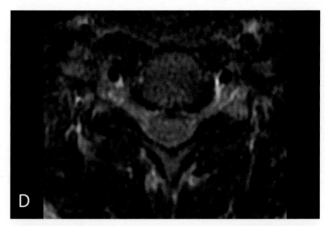

FIGURE 14-2 (*Continued*) **C,** Axial T2 image at C4/C5 revealing mild anterior spinal cord compression caused by the combination of congenital stenosis and disk pathology. **D,** The C5/C6 level has normal disk anatomy but is still congenitally narrow, hence the lack of subarachnoid space (CSF) around the spinal cord.

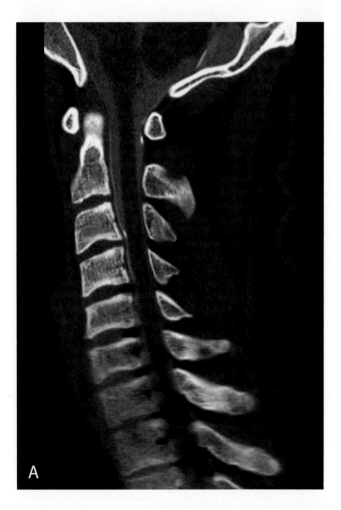

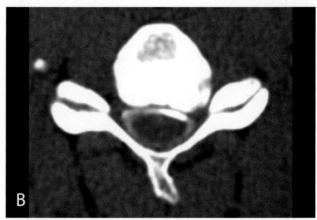

FIGURE 14-3 **A,** Midsagittal cervical myelogram/CT image that reveals congenital stenosis, which is best appreciated by the absence of cerebrospinal fluid (CSF) ventral and dorsal to the spinal cord. **B,** Axial myelogram/CT image at C3/C4 reveals severe left foraminal stenosis and C4 root compression caused by uncovertebral osteophytes rather than a disk herniation. (*continued*)

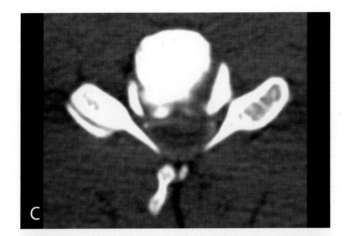

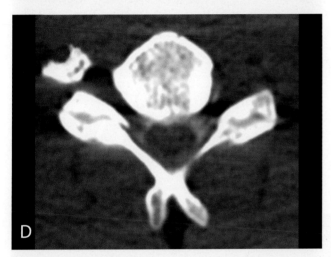

FIGURE 14-3 *(Continued)* **C,** Axial image at C4/C5 revealing mild anterior spinal cord compression caused by the combination of congenital stenosis and disk pathology. **D,** The C5/C6 level has normal disk anatomy but is still congenitally narrow. There is neither spinal cord nor nerve root compression.

appropriate risk counseling and having met the objective criteria for clearance. Before electing this surgical recommendation, RTP criteria were openly discussed. The player understood that he must first be willing to play again given the frightening nature of his spinal cord event. If he was still interested, then he would have to demonstrate healing of all laminoplasty images by CT scan at 6 months after surgery. An MRI would have to document full restoration of adequate space available for his spinal cord (SAC). And flexion-extension lateral radiographs would have to reveal full range of motion compared with preoperative images without any evidence of dynamic instability.

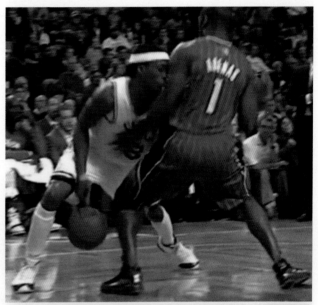

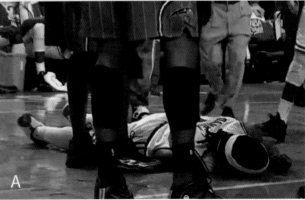

FIGURE 14-4 **A** and **B,** Photographs (with permission) of the player hyperextending his cervical spine at the instant of impact and then on the court immediately after sustaining his cervical cord neurapraxia (CCN). *(continued)*

and was unable to move any of his extremities for approximately 7 minutes before having almost full return of motor function (**Figure 14-4A**). Imaging did not reveal any cervical malalignment or dynamic instability but did show congenital cervical stenosis with spinal cord compression and a Klippel-Feil anomaly consisting of an atlanto-occipital assimilation and failure of segmentation at C2 to C3 (**Figure 14-4B to D**). The player was diagnosed with CCN and mild residual neurologic deficits. He elected to undergo a C2 "dome" laminectomy and C3 to C5 laminoplasty (**Figure 14-5**). Recovery was uneventful, and he was eventually able to RTP 6 months postoperatively with

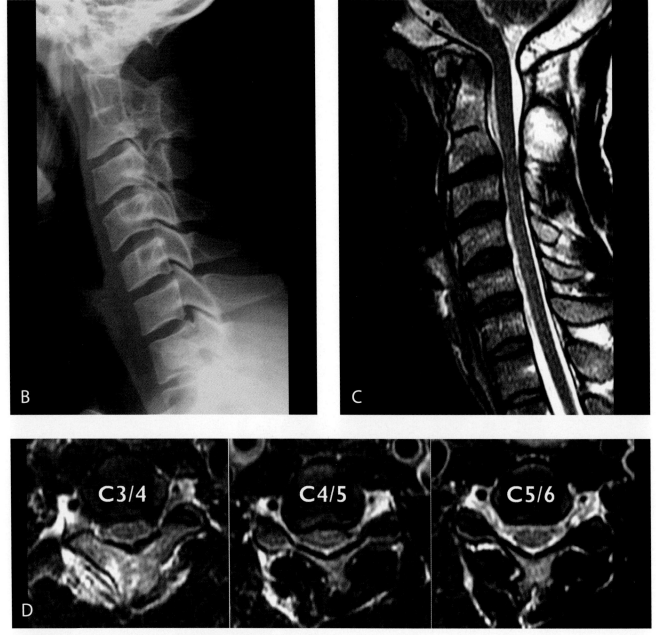

FIGURE 14-4 (*Continued*) **C,** Lateral cervical spine radiograph showing congenital cervical stenosis, as well as the Klippel-Feil constellation of the atlanto-occipital assimilation and C2/C3 failure of segmentation. **D,** Midsagittal T2-weighted MRI and images through disk spaces C3/C4, C4/C5, and C5/C6 illustrating the degree of spinal cord compression caused by his underlying pathology at the time of injury.

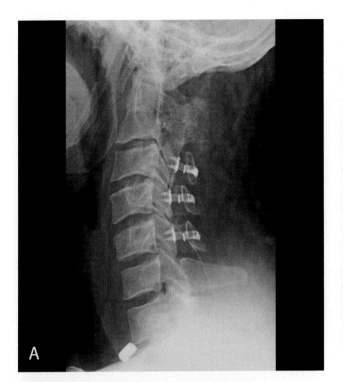

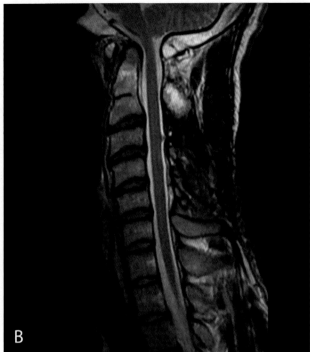

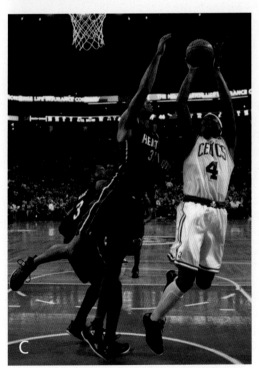

FIGURE 14-5 **A,** Postoperative lateral cervical radiograph after "C3 dome laminectomy" and C4 to C6 laminoplasty. **B,** Midsagittal T2-weighted MRI illustrating the restoration of normal space around the spinal cord. **C,** Photograph (with permission) of the patient playing in the National Basketball Association playoffs after returning to his team.

CONCLUSION

Degeneration of the cervical spine is a natural part of aging, but there is some evidence that contact sports may hasten this process. When advanced enough, this degenerative process can lead to cervical stenosis, which increases one's risk of sustaining a CCN or developing myelopathy. Although the incidental finding of central cervical stenosis is not an absolute contraindication for participation in contact sports, individuals with findings of myelopathy should not RTP. Similarly, patients who have sustained a CCN and have evidence of cervical stenosis should also not return to contact sports. However, these patients can still participate in noncontact sports because the risk of catastrophic SCI is rare in this setting. After appropriate surgical treatment, opportunities may exist for RTP under certain conditions and assumed risk. Thoughtful and informed decisions should be made by well-informed and thoroughly counseled patients about the risks that they will assume.

REFERENCES

1. Mundt DJ, Kelsey JL, Golden AL: An epidemiologic study of sports and weight lifting as possible risk factors for herniated lumbar and cervical discs. *Am J Sports Med* 1993;21(6):854–860.

2. Scher AT: Premature onset of degenerative disease of the cervical spine in rugby players. *S Afr Med J* 1990;77(11):557–558.

3. Albright JP, Moses JM, Feldick HG, Dolan KD, Burmeister LF: Nonfatal cervical spine injuries in interscholastic football. *JAMA* 1976;236(11):1243–1245.

4. Berge J, Marque B, Vital JM, Sénégas J, Caillé JM: Age-related changes in the cervical spines of front-line rugby players. *Am J Sports Med* 1999;27(4):422–429.

5. Hogan BA, Hogan NA, Vos PM, Eustace SJ, Kenny PJ: The cervical spine of professional front-row rugby players: Correlation between degenerative changes and symptoms. *Ir J Med Sci* 2010;179(2):259–263.

6. Gerbino PG, d'Hemecourt PA: Does football cause an increase in degenerative disease of the lumbar spine? *Curr Sports Med Rep* 2002;1(1):47–51.

7. Tall RL, DeVault W: Spinal injury in sport: Epidemiologic considerations. *Clin Sports Med* 1993;12(3):441–448.

8. Kartal A, Yildiran I, Senköylü A, Korkusuz F: Soccer causes degenerative changes in the cervical spine. *Eur Spine J* 2004;13(1):76–82.

9. Swartz EE, Boden BP, Courson RW, et al: National Athletic Trainers' Association position statement: Acute management of the cervical spine–injured athlete. *J Athl Train* 2009;44(3):306–331.

10. Lawrence JS: Disc degeneration. Its frequency and relationship to symptoms. *Ann Rheum Dis* 1969;28(2):121–138.

11. Boden SD, Davis DO, Dina TS, Patronas NJ, Wiesel SW: Abnormal magnetic-resonance scans of the lumbar spine in asymptomatic subjects. A prospective investigation. *J Bone Joint Surg Am* 1990;72(3):403–408.

12. Matsumoto M, Fujimura Y, Suzuki N, et al: MRI of cervical intervertebral discs in asymptomatic subjects. *J Bone Joint Surg Br* 1998;80(1):19–24.

13. Gore DR, Sepic SB, Gardner GM: Roentgenographic findings of the cervical spine in asymptomatic people. *Spine* 1986;11(6):521–524.

14. Nakashima H, Yukawa Y, Suda K, Yamagata M, Ueta T, Kato F: Abnormal findings on magnetic resonance images of the cervical spines in 1211 asymptomatic subjects. *Spine* 2015;40(6):392–398.

15. Heller JG: The syndromes of degenerative cervical disease. *Orthop Clin North Am* 1992;23(3):381–394.

16. Fehlings MG, Tetreault L, Nater A, et al: The aging of the global population: The changing epidemiology of disease and spinal disorders. *Neurosurgery* 2015;77(suppl 4):S1–S5.

17. Baptiste DC, Fehlings MG: Pathophysiology of cervical myelopathy. *Spine J* 2006;6(6 suppl):190S–197S.

18. Nouri A, Tetreault L, Singh A, Karadimas SK, Fehlings MG: Degenerative cervical myelopathy: Epidemiology, genetics, and pathogenesis. *Spine* 2015;40(12):E675–E693.

19. Bogduk N, Windsor M, Inglis A: The innervation of the cervical intervertebral discs. *Spine* 1988;13(1):2–8.

20. Bogduk N, Marsland A: The cervical zygapophysial joints as a source of neck pain. *Spine* 1988;13(6):610–617.

21. Ono K, Ota H, Tada K, Yamamoto T: Cervical myelopathy secondary to multiple spondylotic protrusions: A clinicopathologic study. *Spine* 1977;2(2):109.

22. White AA, Johnson RM, Panjabi MM, Southwick WO: Biomechanical analysis of clinical stability in the cervical spine. *Clin Orthop Relat Res* 1975;(109):85–96.

23. Epstein JA, Carras R, Hyman RA, Costa S: Cervical myelopathy caused by developmental stenosis of the spinal canal. *J Neurosurg* 1979;51(3):362–367. doi:10.3171/jns.1979.51.3.0362.

24. Edwards WC, LaRocca H: The developmental segmental sagittal diameter of the cervical spinal canal in patients with cervical spondylosis. *Spine* 1983;8(1):20–27.

25. Nordqvist L: The sagittal diameter of the spinal cord and subarachnoid space in different age groups: A roentgenographic post-mortem study. *Acta Radiol Diagn (Stockh)* 1964(suppl 227):1–96.

26. Fujiwara K, Yonenobu K, Ebara S, Yamashita K, Ono K: The prognosis of surgery for cervical compression myelopathy. An analysis of the factors involved. *J Bone Joint Surg Br* 1989;71(3):393–398.

27. Bernhardt M, Hynes RA, Blume HW, White AA: Cervical spondylotic myelopathy. *J Bone Joint Surg Am* 1993;75(1): 119–128.

28. Del Bigio MR, Johnson GE: Clinical presentation of spinal cord concussion. *Spine* 1989;14(1):37.

29. Torg JS, Pavlov H, Genuario SE, et al: Neurapraxia of the cervical spinal cord with transient quadriplegia. *J Bone Joint Surg Am* 1986;68(9):1354–1370.

30. Herzog RJ, Wiens JJ, Dillingham MF, Sontag MJ: Normal Cervical spine morphometry and cervical spinal stenosis in asymptomatic professional football players: Plain film radiography, multiplanar computed tomography, and magnetic resonance imaging. *Spine* 1991;16(6S):S178.

31. Odor JM, Watkins RG, Dillin WH, Dennis S, Saberi M: Incidence of cervical spinal stenosis in professional and rookie football players. *Am J Sports Med* 1990;18(5):507–509.

32. Blackley HR, Plank LD, Robertson PA: Determining the sagittal dimensions of the canal of the cervical spine. The reliability of ratios of anatomical measurements. *J Bone Joint Surg Br* 1999;81(1):110–112.

33. Cantu RC: Functional cervical spinal stenosis: a contraindication to participation in contact sports. *Med Sci Sports Exerc* 1993;25(3):316–317.

34. Eismont FJ, Clifford S, Goldberg M, Green B: Cervical sagittal spinal canal size in spine injury. *Spine* 1984;9(7): 663–666.

35. Matsuura P, Waters RL, Adkins RH, Rothman S, Gurbani N, Sie I: Comparison of computerized tomography parameters of the cervical spine in normal control subjects and spinal cord-injured patients. *J Bone Joint Surg Am* 1989; 71(2):183–188.

36. Penning L: Some aspects of plain radiography of the cervical spine in chronic myelopathy. *Neurology* 1962;12:513–519.

37. Murone I: The importance of the sagittal diameters of the cervical spinal canal in relation to spondylosis and myelopathy. *J Bone Joint Surg Br* 1974;56(1):30–36.

38. Sadasivan KK, Reddy RP, Albright JA: The natural history of cervical spondylotic myelopathy. *Yale J Biol Med* 1993;66(3):235–242.

39. Clarke E, Robinson PK: Cervical myelopathy: A complication of cervical spondylosis. *Brain* 1956.

40. Lees F, Turner JA: Natural history and prognosis of cervical spondylosis. *Br Med J* 1963;2(5373):1607.

41. Nurick S: The pathogenesis of the spinal cord disorder associated with cervical spondylosis. *Brain* 1972;95(1):87–100.

42. Nurick S: The natural history and the results of surgical treatment of the spinal cord disorder associated with cervical spondylosis. *Brain* 1972;95(1):101–108.

43. Karadimas SK, Erwin WM, Ely CG, Dettori JR, Fehlings MG: Pathophysiology and natural history of cervical spondylotic myelopathy. *Spine* 2013;38(22 suppl 1): S21–S36.

44. Crandall PH, Batzdorf U: Cervical spondylotic myelopathy. *J Neurosurg* 1966;25(1):57–66.

45. Ono K, Ebara S, Fuji T, Yonenobu K, Fujiwara K, Yamashita K: Myelopathy hand. New clinical signs of cervical cord damage. *J Bone Joint Surg Br* 1987;69(2):215–219.

46. Cantu RC: Stingers, transient quadriplegia, and cervical spinal stenosis: return to play criteria. *Med Sci Sports Exerc* 1997;29(7 suppl):S233–S235.

47. Torg JS, Glasgow SG: Criteria for return to contact activities following cervical spine injury. *Clin J Sports Med* 1991; 1(1):12.

48. LaRocca H: Cervical spondylotic myelopathy: natural history. *Spine* 1988;13(7):854–855.

49. Ogino H, Tada K, Okada K, et al: Canal diameter, anteroposterior compression ratio, and spondylotic myelopathy of the cervical spine. *Spine* 1983;8(1):1–15.

50. Law MD, Bernhardt M, White AA: Cervical spondylotic myelopathy: A review of surgical indications and decision making. *Yale J Biol Med* 1993;66(3):165–177.

51. Tetreault LA, Côté P, Kopjar B, Arnold P, Fehlings MG; AOSpine North America and International Clinical Trial Research Network: A clinical prediction model to assess surgical outcome in patients with cervical spondylotic myelopathy: Internal and external validations using the prospective multicenter AOSpine North American and international datasets of 743 patients. *Spine J* 2015;15(3):388–397.

52. Suda K, Abumi K, Ito M, Shono Y, Kaneda K, Fujiya M: Local kyphosis reduces surgical outcomes of expansive open-door laminoplasty for cervical spondylotic myelopathy. *Spine* 2003;28(12):1258–1262.

53. Kepler CK, Vaccaro AR: Injuries and abnormalities of the cervical spine and return to play criteria. *Clin Sports Med* 2012;31(3):499–508.

54. Boden BP, Tacchetti RL, Cantu RC, Knowles SB, Mueller FO: Catastrophic cervical spine injuries in high school and college football players. *Am J Sports Med* 2006;34(8):1223–1232.

55. Torg JS, Ramsey-Emrhein JA: Management guidelines for participation in collision activities with congenital, developmental, or post-injury lesions involving the cervical spine. *Clin Sports Med* 1997;16(3):501–530.

15 Fractures of the Cervical Spine and Spinal Cord Injuries

Gregory D. Schroeder, MD • Tristan Fried, BS • Christie Stawicki, BA • Peter Deluca, MD • Alexander R. Vaccaro, MD, PhD, MBA

INTRODUCTION

More than 5 million patients seek medical care yearly in the United States after a sports-related injury,[1] and although the most common diagnoses are contusion, sprain or strain,[2] 2.4% of patients admitted to the hospital after a sports-related accident have a spinal cord injury (SCI).[2] Furthermore, sporting accidents are the fourth leading cause (9.2%) of SCIs,[3] behind motor vehicle accidents, falls, and violence, in the United States. Although these injuries are often linked to collision sports, they have been reported in almost all sporting activity, including American football,[4–15] ice hockey,[16,17] diving,[18–20] skiing and snowboarding,[21–23] wrestling,[24] rugby,[25–30] gymnastics,[31] bicycling,[32] basketball,[33] baseball,[33] and equestrian.[34,35] SCIs secondary to sporting activities are particularly devastating because they often occur in patients in the second or third decade of life.[16,33]

Temporary neurologic injuries without damage to the spinal column, such as transient cervical neurapraxia (stingers or burners),[36,37] and transient cervical cord neurapraxia (transient quadriplegia)[5] have been covered in previous chapters, so this chapter focuses solely on cervical spine injuries that result in structural damages to the bony, ligamentous, or neural components of the spinal column.

EPIDEMIOLOGY

Because of the difference in popularity of sports across the globe, the primary sporting activity resulting in cervical spine injuries varies by country. In the United States, American football, wrestling, and gymnastics[33] are common causes of cervical spine injuries; comparatively, a high occurrence of cervical spine injuries occurs from ice hockey in Canada[16] and rugby in Europe.[25–30]

Dr. Schroeder or an immediate family member has received research or institutional support from Medtronic Sofamor Danek; has received nonincome support (such as equipment or services), commercially derived honoraria, or other non-research–related funding (such as paid travel) from AO Spine and Medtronic; and serves as a board member, owner, officer, or committee member of Wolters Kluwer Health. Dr. Vaccaro or an immediate family member has received royalties from Aesculap/B.Braun, Globus Medical, Medtronic, and Stryker; serves as a paid consultant to DePuy, A Johnson & Johnson Company, Ellipse, Expert Testimony, Gerson Lehrman Group, Globus Medical, Guidepoint Global, Innovative Surgical Design, Medacorp, Medtronic, Orthobullets, Stout Medical, and Stryker; has stock or stock options held in Advanced Spinal Intellectual Properties, Avaz Surgical, Bonovo Orthopaedics, Computational Biodynamics, Cytonics, Dimension Orthotics, LLC, Electrocore, Flagship Surgical, FlowPharma,

Gamma Spine, Globus Medical, In Vivo, Innovative Surgical Design, Location Based Intelligence, Paradigm Spine, Prime Surgeons, Progressive Spinal Technologies, Replication Medica, Rothman Institute and Related Properties, Spine Medica, Spinology, Stout Medical, and Vertiflex; has received nonincome support (such as equipment or services), commercially derived honoraria, or other research–related funding (such as paid travel) from Elsevier, Jaypee, Taylor Francis/Hodder and Stoughton, and Thieme; and serves as a board member, owner, officer, or committee member of AO Spine, the Association of Collaborative Spine Research, Clinical Spine Surgery, Flagship Surgical, Innovative Surgical Design, Prime Surgeons, and the Spine Journal. None of the following authors or any immediate family member has received anything of value from or has stock or stock options held in a commercial company or institution related directly or indirectly to the subject of this article: Dr. DeLuca, Mr. Fried, and Dr. Stawicki.

An increased awareness of sports-related SCIs has led to rule changes designed to increase the safety for participants. With the advent of new helmets in the 1960s, American football players began using the crowns of their heads when tackling (spear tackling), and this new technique led to an increase in the number of cervical spine injuries and fatalities.[38] However, in 1976, the rules of American football changed to prohibit spear tackling, and the rate of serious cervical spine injuries dropped dramatically.[38] Despite this, cervical spine injuries are still the most common injury to the axial skeleton in the National Football League (NFL), but fortunately, severe injuries such as cervical fractures and SCIs now account for fewer than 1% of these injuries.[9] Similarly, after the Canadian Amateur Hockey Association (presently Hockey Canada) began penalizing players for pushing or checking other players from behind,[39] the rate of SCIs in ice hockey decreased.[16]

Although injuries from American football and ice hockey often occur in organized practices and games, cervical spine injuries from recreational sporting activities can also occur.[18-20] Across the world, diving is a common cause of SCIs. However, these injuries are rarely seen in high-level competitive divers; rather, they usually occur in recreational divers.[18,20]

COMMON MECHANISM OF INJURIES

Multiple common mechanisms can lead to cervical spine fractures in athletes. A strong contraction of the trapezius and rhomboid muscles can lead to an innocuous avulsion fracture of the spinous process. Comparatively, a high-energy collision may result in the transmission of an axial load across a flexed neck, causing a complete SCI.[5,7,27] The three most common mechanisms leading to significant cervical spine injuries are hyperflexion, axial compression, and hyperextension,[12,39-49] and although these injuries commonly occur in the subaxial cervical spine, upper cervical spine injuries are possible.[5,7,16,17,20,27,30]

Hyperflexion injuries are the most common sports-related cervical spine injury, occurring after a significant axial load is applied to a slightly flexed neck.[5,50] Initially, the posterior ligamentous complex fails under tension followed by the vertebral body fracturing under a compressive load.[51] Comparatively, if the cervical spine is straight when it is exposed to the axial load, a pure compression force is transmitted to the vertebral bodies, leading to a burst fracture.[53] Last, a hyperextension injury occurs when a player's neck is extended and a posterior directed force is applied; this force leads to a tensile failure of the anterior column followed by disruption of the posterior ligamentous complex.[53]

SPINAL PRECAUTIONS

When evaluating an athlete with a possible cervical spine injury, basic spinal precautions must be maintained at all times. Cervical tenderness, pain, or limited motion along with neurologic symptoms necessitates immobilization of the cervical spine in neutral alignment and transfer of the player to a backboard. In a helmeted athlete, the facemask should be promptly removed to allow access to the airway, but the remainder of the helmet should be left in place.[38,50,53] In athletes with properly fitting equipment, the combination of a helmet and shoulder pads will often result in neutral spinal alignment.[54] After the spine has been temporarily stabilized and the on-the-field evaluation is complete, expeditiously transferring the patient to an SCI center is critical because time to decompression of the spinal cord directly affects neurologic recovery related to the spinal cord.[55]

UPPER CERVICAL SPINE FRACTURES

Although the majority of cervical spine fractures caused by athletic activities occur in the subaxial cervical spine, many different upper cervical spine fractures have been reported.[23,27,32] Boden et al reported on 196 cervical spine injuries in high school and college American football players, and nine athletes were diagnosed with an isolated C1 or C2 injury. Although neurologic injuries are less common in these fractures than fractures of the subaxial cervical spine, one third of these injuries resulted in quadriplegia.[5] Furthermore, an SCI at this level is particularly devastating because it may limit the patient's ability to breathe without mechanical assistance.

Compared with other sporting activities, mountain bicycling has a high risk of upper cervical spine fractures. Dodwell et al reported on 79 cervical spine injuries associated with mountain bicycling and found that 17.7% of fractures were located in the upper cervical spine, with almost half the injuries being odontoid fractures.[32] Similar to football players, 28% of cyclists with an upper cervical spine fracture presented with a neurologic injury.[32]

The treatment of upper cervical spine fractures varies by the specific injury, with all atlanto-occipital dissociations requiring surgery; conversely, the majority of C1

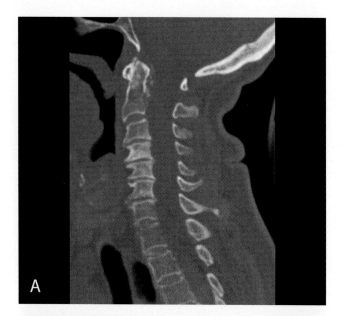

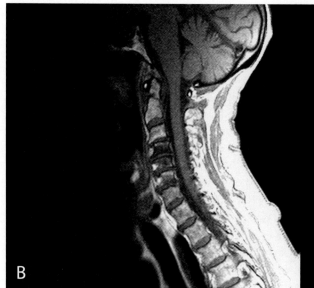

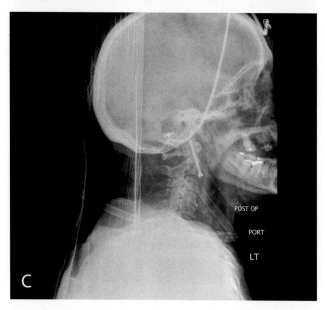

FIGURE 15-1 Preoperative sagittal CT (**A**) and MRI (**B**) and a postoperative lateral radiograph (**C**) of a 45-year-old man who was injured in a mountain bicycling accident.

arch fractures can be managed nonoperatively. Treatment of odontoid fractures varies by the location and displacement of the fracture. Type 1 (avulsion of the tip) and type 3 (fractures extending into the body of the axis) fractures are commonly treated in a hard cervical collar.[56] Similarly, because the vast majority of athletes who sustain cervical spine injuries are younger than 30 years of age, nonoperative treatment of type 2 fractures (fractures at the base of the dens) in a hard collar or halo vest is appropriate;[56] however, in young athletes with neurologic injuries or whose fractures are more than 5-mm displacement or 11° angulated, surgery with either an odontoid screw (**Figure 15-1**) or a posterior C1 to C2 arthrodesis is indicated.[56]

HYPERFLEXION INJURIES

Hyperflexion injuries are the most commonly reported cervical spine injuries from sporting activity.[5,50] With the neck slightly flexed, a significant axial load causes hyperflexion of the cervical spine, resulting in a tensile failure of the posterior column. Although anteroinferior fragmentation of the cranial vertebral body results in the classic "teardrop fragment,"[5,50,51] the severity of the injury is determined by the involvement of the posterior column, which varies from an isolated ligamentous injury to a complete bilateral facet dislocation.[27]

In athletes with bilateral facet dislocation, the risk of an SCI dramatically increases. MacLean and Hutchinson reported SCIs in 90% of athletes with bilateral facet dislocations compared with 58% of athletes with other cervical spine fractures.[27] Some authors have postulated that the high occurrence of SCIs in this fracture pattern is because the intact articular processes prevents spontaneous reduction of the injury, thus resulting in prolonged compression of the spinal cord.[1]

When these injuries occur, it is paramount that the patient be quickly taken to an SCI center. Patients with facet dislocations need to be urgently reduced either via traction and Gardner-Wells tongs or surgically[55] (**Figure 15-2**). Although all patients with hyperflexion injuries with a neurologic deficit require a decompression and fusion, the decision to operate on patients without a neurologic deficit is based on the integrity of the posterior ligamentous structures. Whereas neurologically intact patients with disruption of the posterior ligamentous complex should undergo surgical stabilization, patients with only an anterior compression fracture without a neurologic injury or a posterior ligamentous injury may be treated in a hard collar or halo vest depending on the nature of the bony injury.[57] Patients with vertebral body injuries with residual kyphotic alignment may benefit from surgical intervention, especially those fractures involving the C7 vertebral body.

Although not an acute fracture, the same mechanism responsible for a hyperflexion injury can cause "spear tackler's spine" in American football players who repeatedly lead with their helmets while tackling.[51] The repeated axial load through the flexed cervical spine leads to a loss of normal cervical lordosis, vertebral body abnormalities, and cervical stenosis.[13] Athletes with spear tackler's spine need to be identified because continued participation in collision sporting activity places them at high risk for future catastrophic neurologic injuries.[12,13,58]

BURST FRACTURES

Cervical burst fractures are the second most common cervical spine fracture reported in athletes.[27,32,50] These injuries occur after a pure axial load is applied to a neutrally aligned cervical spine,[53] and as the intradiscal pressure rises, the anterior and middle columns of the vertebral body fail under compression.[50] If the injury is severe, retropulsion of the fragments can lead to compression of the spinal cord.

The prevalence of neurologic injuries in athletes with cervical burst fractures varies in the literature. MacLean and Hutchinson reported on 36 rugby players with cervical spine fractures. Although only four had a burst fracture, none had a neurologic injury.[27] Comparatively, Dodwell et al reported on 13 bicyclists with cervical burst fractures; 11 had a neurologic injury.[32]

Because it is possible for athletes to have a cervical burst fracture leading to spinal instability without neurologic symptoms, spinal precautions are mandatory for all athletes who sustain a significant axial loading injury; furthermore, these athletes should be transported to the nearest SCI center for a complete radiographic evaluation. All athletes with a cervical burst fracture associated with an SCI should expeditiously undergo a decompression and fusion to increase the chances of neurologic recovery[55] (**Figure 15-3**). Similar to hyperflexion injuries, treatment of cervical burst fractures without a neurologic injury is dependent on the integrity of the posterior ligamentous complex. In the majority of cervical burst fractures without neurologic injury, the posterior ligamentous complex is intact, and the patient can be treated without surgery.[59] However, if the posterior ligamentous structures are damaged, significant spinal instability is present, and surgery is warranted.[57] Again, burst injuries involving the C7 level often drift into kyphosis, and early surgical intervention may be preferable over nonoperative treatment.

HYPEREXTENSION INJURIES

Hyperextension injuries are rare but potentially devastating cervical spine injuries in athletes.[11,30] In these injuries, a posterior applied force to the front of the head results in a tensile failure of the anterior column, resulting in disruption of the anterior longitudinal ligament and the anulus fibrosus with or without an accompanying anteroinferior avulsion fracture of the superior vertebra.[53] In severe injuries, the force is sufficient to disrupt the posterior ligamentous complex, and posterior displacement of the superior body into the spinal canal can lead to devastating SCIs.[60]

Although the literature on hyperextension injuries in athletes is limited, Shelly et al reported a hyperextension mechanism in 3 of 12 rugby players who sustained SCIs. Two athletes were able to make a complete recovery after surgical decompression and fusion, but the third sustained a permanent complete SCI.[30]

All athletes who sustain a significant hyperextension injury of the cervical spine should be treated with standard spine precautions and transferred to an SCI center immediately. Although an injury associated with spinal cord compression necessitates a decompression and

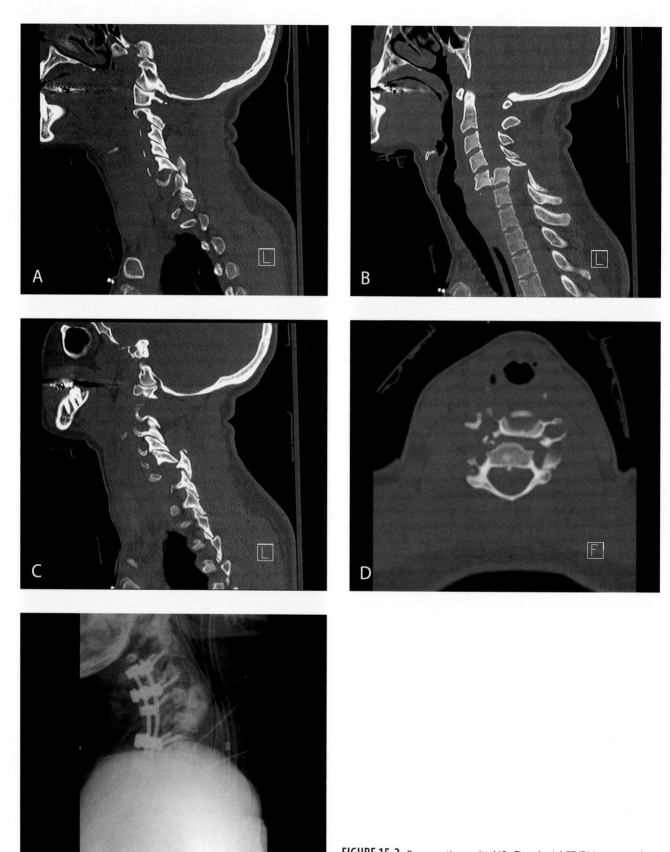

FIGURE 15-2 Preoperative sagittal (**A–C**) and axial CT (**D**) images and a postoperative lateral radiograph (**E**) of a 20-year old man who sustained a complete spinal cord injury during an American football game.

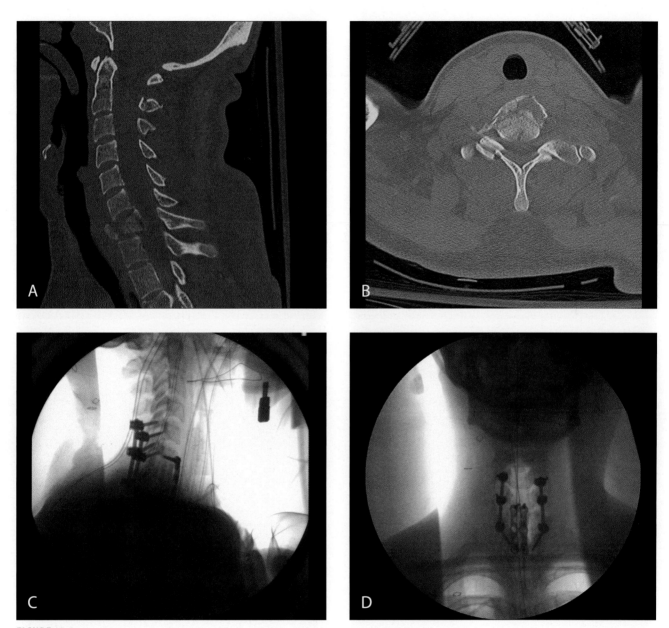

FIGURE 15-3 Preoperative sagittal (**A**) and axial CT (**B**) images and postoperative radiographs (**C** and **D**) of a 25-year-old ice hockey player who sustained an incomplete spinal cord injury after falling head first into the boards.

fusion (**Figure 15-4**), the ideal treatment for hyperextension injuries without a neurologic injury is controversial. A ligamentous injury to the anterior tension band even without posterior involvement is often stabilized surgically.[60]

● RETURN TO PLAY

Despite many publications in which respected spine surgeons have opined on the safety of returning to sporting activity after cervical spine injuries,[1,33,61–65] no high-level evidence is available to guide athletes or treating physi-

cians on when it is safe to return to play after a cervical spine fracture. Furthermore, the decision to return to athletic activities should be individualized based on the demands of the sport, as well as individual patient factors such as the location and severity of the injury and the presence of cervical stenosis or Klippel-Feil anomalies.

Although all patients with ongoing neurologic deficits from SCIs should not return to competitive athletic activities, a cervical spine fracture without an SCI does not necessarily prevent patients from returning to sporting activity (**Table 15-1**). Before returning to athletic activities, radiographic evidence of fracture healing or spinal

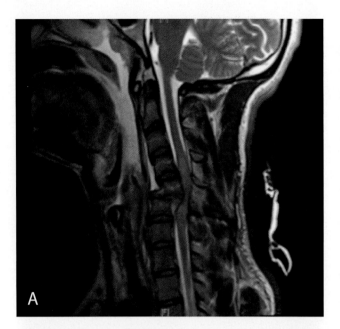

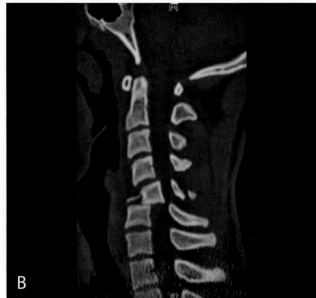

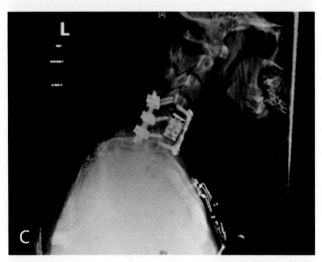

FIGURE 15-4 Preoperative sagittal MRI (**A**) and CT (**B**) images and a postoperative lateral radiograph (**C**) of a 19-year-old American football player who sustained a complete spinal cord injury during practice.

fusion should be evident.[1] Additionally, athletes should have complete, painless range of motion of the cervical spine and preinjury muscles strength in the neck.[1] Even if the aforementioned criteria are met, some patients should be advised against returning to sports. Kepler and Vaccaro proposed nine absolute contraindications to returning to athletic activity after a cervical fracture which are widely supported. These are an atlanto-occipital fusion, atlantoaxial rotatory fixation or instability, spear tackler's spine, persistent instability of the subaxial spine, residual sagittal malalignment, the continued presence of retropulsed bone in the spinal canal, incomplete neurologic recovery, decreased cervical spine range of motion, and a fusion of three or more levels.[1] Similarly, other contraindications mentioned by the authors and widely supported by others include all healed but displaced

upper cervical spine injuries excluding C1 posterior arch fractures, mild C2 body compression fractures, and stable avulsion and spinous process fractures. Ligamentous injuries to the craniocervical region with continued instability is a contraindication to return to contact sports. Patients who undergo a two-level cervical fusion have a relative contraindication for return to contact activity.[1] In a similar note, a patient with a congenital abnormality to the upper cervical spine such as an os odontoideum should be excluded from contact sports.

CONCLUSION

Cervical spine injuries are relatively common injuries in athletes, but thankfully, the number of serious fractures and SCIs has decreased over previous decades.[8,9,16]

TABLE 15-1 Absolute and relative contraindications to returning to play after a cervical spine injury

Injury	Contraindication to Return to Play	Criteria for Return to Play
Any fracture associated with a residual neurologic deficit	Absolute	None
Any fracture in a patient with congenital stenosis	Absolute	None
Any fractures requiring an occipital fusion	Absolute	None
Any fractures requiring a C1–C2 fusion	Absolute	None
Any fracture requiring a fusion of three or more levels	Absolute	None
Spear tackler's spine	Absolute	None
Minimally displaced C1 ring fracture	Relative	Solid union demonstrated on CT; no residual instability on flexion/extension radiographs; complete, painless range of motion of the cervical spine; and preinjury muscles strength in the neck
C2 compression fracture	Relative	Solid union demonstrated on CT; no residual instability on flexion/extension radiographs; complete, painless range of motion of the cervical spine; and preinjury muscles strength in the neck
All other upper cervical spine fractures treated without surgery	Relative	Solid union demonstrated on CT; no bony elements narrowing the spinal canal; no residual instability on flexion/extension radiographs; complete, painless range of motion of the cervical spine; and preinjury muscles strength in the neck
Upper cervical spine fracture requiring surgical stabilization excluding a C1–C2 arthrodesis	Relative	Solid union or arthrodesis demonstrated on CT; no bony elements narrowing the spinal canal; no residual instability on flexion/extension radiographs; complete, painless range of motion of the cervical spine; and preinjury muscle strength in the neck
Isolated compression fracture of the subaxial cervical spine	Relative	Solid union demonstrated on CT; no residual instability on flexion/extension radiographs; complete, painless range of motion of the cervical spine; and preinjury muscle strength in the neck
Isolated stable burst fracture of the subaxial cervical spine	Relative	Solid union demonstrated on CT; no retropulsion of the fracture; no significant sagittal malalignment (>11° compared with adjacent non-injured levels); no residual instability on flexion/extension radiographs; complete, painless range of motion of the cervical spine; and preinjury muscle strength in the neck
Fracture disrupting the posterior bony (lateral mass or articular processes) or ligamentous tension band (excluding spinous or transverse process fractures) of the subaxial cervical spine	Relative	Solid union or arthrodesis demonstrated on CT; no bony fragments in the canal; no significant sagittal malalignment (>11° compared with adjacent noninjured levels); surgical treatment involved fusing less than three segments; no residual instability on flexion/extension radiographs; complete, painless range of motion of the cervical spine; and preinjury muscle strength in the neck
Subaxial spinous process fracture	No	Complete, painless range of motion of the cervical spine and preinjury muscle strength in the neck; the presence of multiple contiguous spinous process fractures is not a further contraindication, but the presence of multiple fractures will likely necessitate a longer recovery time until the patient has complete, painless range of motion
Transverse process fracture in the subaxial spine	No	Complete, painless range of motion of the cervical spine and preinjury muscle strength in the neck

Despite the decreasing number of serious injuries, physicians covering sporting events should remain vigilant, and any player who sustains an injury in which a significant force is transmitted through the cervical spine should be treated with spine precautions, placed in a cervical collar, and transferred to an SCI center for a prompt complete evaluation.

REFERENCES

1. Kepler CK, Vaccaro AR: Injuries and abnormalities of the cervical spine and return to play criteria. *Clin Sports Med* 2012;31(3):499–508.

2. Nalliah RP, Anderson IM, Lee MK, Rampa S, Allareddy V, Allareddy V: Epidemiology of hospital-Based emergency department visits due to sports injuries. *Pediatr Emerg Care* 2014;30(8):511–515.

3. National Spinal Cord Injury Statistical Center: *Spinal Cord Injury: Facts and Figures.* Available at: http://www.spinalcord.uab.edu. Accessed August 2014.

4. Albright JP, Moses JM, Feldick HG, Dolan KD, Burmeister LF: Nonfatal cervical spine injuries in interscholastic football. *JAMA* 1976;236(11):1243–1245.

5. Boden BP, Tacchetti RL, Cantu RC, Knowles SB, Mueller FO: Catastrophic cervical spine injuries in high school and college football players. *Am J Sports Med* 2006;34(8):1223–1232.

6. Brigham CD, Adamson TE: Permanent partial cervical spinal cord injury in a professional football player who had only congenital stenosis. A case report. *J Bone Joint Surg Am* 2003;85-A(8):1553–1556.

7. Drakos MC, Feeley BT, Barnes R, Muller M, Burruss TP, Warren RF: Lower cervical posterior element fractures in the National Football League: A report of 2 cases and a review of the literature. *Neurosurgery* 2011;68(6):E1743–1748; discussion E1748–1749.

8. Gill SS, Boden BP: The epidemiology of catastrophic spine injuries in high school and college football. *Sports Med Arthrosc* 2008;16(1):2–6.

9. Mall NA, Buchowski J, Zebala L, Brophy RH, Wright RW, Matava MJ: Spine and axial skeleton injuries in the National Football League. *Am J Sports Med* 2012;40(8):1755–1761.

10. Olson D, Sikka RS, Labounty A, Christensen T: Injuries in professional football: Current concepts. *Curr Sports Med Rep* 2013;12(6):381–390.

11. Rihn JA, Anderson DT, Lamb K, et al: Cervical spine injuries in American football. *Sports Med* 2009;39(9):697–708.

12. Torg JS, Guille JT, Jaffe S: Injuries to the cervical spine in American football players. *J Bone Joint Surg Am* 2002;84-A(1):112–122.

13. Torg JS, Sennett B, Pavlov H, Leventhal MR, Glasgow SG: Spear tackler's spine. An entity precluding participation in tackle football and collision activities that expose the cervical spine to axial energy inputs. *Am J Sports Med* 1993;21(5):640–649.

14. Waninger KN: On-field management of potential cervical spine injury in helmeted football players: Leave the helmet on! *Clin J Sport Med* 1998;8(2):124–129.

15. Watkins RG: Neck injuries in football players. *Clin Sports Med* 1986;5(2):215–246.

16. Tator CH, Provvidenza C, Cassidy JD: Spinal injuries in Canadian ice hockey: An update to 2005. *Clin J Sport Med* 2009;19(6):451–456.

17. Wennberg RA, Cohen HB, Walker SR: Neurologic injuries in hockey. *Neurol Clin* 2008;26(1):243–255; xi.

18. Aito S, D'Andrea M, Werhagen L: Spinal cord injuries due to diving accidents. *Spinal Cord* 2005;43(2):109–116.

19. Cusimano MD, Mascarenhas AM, Manoranjan B: Spinal cord injuries due to diving: A framework and call for prevention. *J Trauma* 2008;65(5):1180–1185.

20. Tator CH, Edmonds VE, New ML: Diving: A frequent and potentially preventable cause of spinal cord injury. *Can Med Assoc J* 1981;124(10):1323–1324.

21. Hubbard ME, Jewell RP, Dumont TM, Rughani AI: Spinal injury patterns among skiers and snowboarders. *Neurosurg Focus* 2011;31(5):E8.

22. Kary JM: Acute spine injuries in skiers and snowboarders. *Curr Sports Med Rep* 2008;7(1):35–38.

23. Tarazi F, Dvorak MF, Wing PC: Spinal injuries in skiers and snowboarders. *Am J Sports Med* 1999;27(2):177–180.

24. Boden BP, Lin W, Young M, Mueller FO: Catastrophic injuries in wrestlers. *Am J Sports Med* 2002;30(6):791–795.

25. Andrews J, Jones A, Davies PR, Howes J, Ahuja S: Is return to professional rugby union likely after anterior cervical spinal surgery? *J Bone Joint Surg Br* 2008;90(5):619–621.

26. Fuller CW, Brooks JH, Kemp SP: Spinal injuries in professional rugby union: A prospective cohort study. *Clin J Sport Med* 2007;17(1):10–16.

27. MacLean JG, Hutchison JD: Serious neck injuries in U19 rugby union players: An audit of admissions to spinal injury units in Great Britain and Ireland. *Br J Sports Med* 2012;46(8):591–594.

28. Quarrie KL, Cantu RC, Chalmers DJ: Rugby union injuries to the cervical spine and spinal cord. *Sports Med* 2002;32(10):633–653.

29. Scher AT: Rugby injuries to the cervical spine and spinal cord: A 10-year review. *Clin Sports Med* 1998;17(1):195–206.

30. Shelly MJ, Butler JS, Timlin M, Walsh MG, Poynton AR, O'Byrne JM: Spinal injuries in Irish rugby: A ten-year review. *J Bone Joint Surg Br* 2006;88(6):771–775.

31. Momaya A, Rozzelle C, Davis K, Estes R: Delayed presentation of a cervical spine fracture dislocation with posterior ligamentous disruption in a gymnast. *Am J Orthop (Belle Mead NJ)* 2014;43(6):272–274.

32. Dodwell ER, Kwon BK, Hughes B, et al: Spinal column and spinal cord injuries in mountain bikers: A 13-year review. *Am J Sports Med* 2010;38(8):1647–1652.

33. Bailes JE, Hadley MN, Quigley MR, Sonntag VK, Cerullo LJ: Management of athletic injuries of the cervical spine and spinal cord. *Neurosurgery* 1991;29(4):491–497.

34. Ball JE, Ball CG, Mulloy RH, Datta I, Kirkpatrick AW: Ten years of major equestrian injury: Are we addressing functional outcomes? *J Trauma Manag Outcomes* 2009;3:2.

35. Hamilton MG, Tranmer BI: Nervous system injuries in horseback-riding accidents. *J Trauma* 1993;34(2):227–232.

36. Clancy WG Jr, Brand RL, Bergfield JA: Upper trunk brachial plexus injuries in contact sports. *Am J Sports Med* 1977;5(5):209–216.

37. Shannon B, Klimkiewicz JJ: Cervical burners in the athlete. *Clin Sports Med* 2002;21(1):29–35, vi.

38. Bailes JE, Petschauer M, Guskiewicz KM, Marano G: Management of cervical spine injuries in athletes. *J Athl Train* 2007;42(1):126–134.

39. Tator CH, Provvidenza CF, Lapczak L, Carson J, Raymond D: Spinal injuries in Canadian ice hockey: Documentation of injuries sustained from 1943–1999. *Can J Neurol Sci* 2004;31(4):460–466.

40. Burke DC: Hyperextension injuries of the spine. *J Bone Joint Surg Br* 1971;53(1):3–12.

41. Carvell JE, Fuller DJ, Duthie RB, Cockin J: Rugby football injuries to the cervical spine. *Br Med J (Clin Res Ed)* 1983;286(6358):49–50.

42. Dolan KD, Feldick HG, Albright JP, Moses JM: Neck injuries in football players. *Am Fam Physician* 1975;12(6):86–91.

43. Edeiken-Monroe B, Wagner LK, Harris JH Jr: Hyperextension dislocation of the cervical spine. *AJR Am J Roentgenol* 1986;146(4):803–808.

44. Funk FF, Wells RE: Injuries of the cervical spine in football. *Clin Orthop Relat Res* 1975(109):50–58.

45. Melvin WJ, Dunlop HW, Hetherington RF, Kerr JW: The role of the faceguard in the production of flexion injuries to the cervical spine in football. *Can Med Assoc J* 1965;93(21):1110–1117.

46. Paley D, Gillespie R: Chronic repetitive unrecognized flexion injury of the cervical spine (high jumper's neck). *Am J Sports Med* 1986;14(1):92–95.

47. Silver JR: Injuries of the spine sustained in rugby. *Br Med J (Clin Res Ed)* 1984;288(6410):37–43.

48. Tator CH, Edmonds VE: National survey of spinal injuries in hockey players. *Can Med Assoc J* 1984;130(7):875–880.

49. Wu WQ, Lewis RC: Injuries of the cervical spine in high school wrestling. *Surg Neurol* 1985;23(2):143–147.

50. Banerjee R, Palumbo MA, Fadale PD: Catastrophic cervical spine injuries in the collision sport athlete, part 1: Epidemiology, functional anatomy, and diagnosis. *Am J Sports Med* 2004;32(4):1077–1087.

51. Torg JS, Pavlov H, O'Neill MJ, Nichols CE Jr, Sennett B: The axial load teardrop fracture. A biomechanical, clinical and roentgenographic analysis. *Am J Sports Med* 1991;19(4):355–364.

52. Allen BL Jr, Ferguson RL, Lehmann TR, O'Brien RP: A mechanistic classification of closed, indirect fractures and dislocations of the lower cervical spine. *Spine (Phila Pa 1976)* 1982;7(1):1–27.

53. Anderson A, Tollefson B, Cohen R, Johnson J, Summers RL: A comparative study of American football helmet removal techniques using a cadaveric model of cervical spine injury. *J Miss State Med Assoc* 2011;52(4):103–105.

54. Banerjee R, Palumbo MA, Fadale PD: Catastrophic cervical spine injuries in the collision sport athlete, part 2: Principles of emergency care. *Am J Sports Med* 2004;32(7):1760–1764.

55. Fehlings MG, Vaccaro A, Wilson JR, et al: Early versus delayed decompression for traumatic cervical spinal cord injury: Results of the Surgical Timing in Acute Spinal Cord Injury Study (STASCIS). *PLoS One* 2012;7(2):e32037.

56. Hsu WK, Anderson PA: Odontoid fractures: Update on management. *J Am Acad Orthop Surg* 2010;18(7):383–394.

57. Vaccaro AR, Hulbert RJ, Patel AA, et al: The subaxial cervical spine injury classification system: A novel approach to recognize the importance of morphology, neurology, and integrity of the disco-ligamentous complex. *Spine (Phila Pa 1976)* 2007;32(21):2365–2374.

58. Torg JS, Sennett B, Vegso JJ, Pavlov H: Axial loading injuries to the middle cervical spine segment. An analysis and classification of twenty-five cases. *Am J Sports Med* 1991;19(1):6–20.

59. Dvorak MF, Fisher CG, Fehlings MG, et al: The surgical approach to subaxial cervical spine injuries: An evidence-based algorithm based on the SLIC classification system. *Spine (Phila Pa 1976)* 2007;32(23):2620–2629.

60. Vaccaro AR, Klein GR, Thaller JB, Rushton SA, Cotler JM, Albert TJ: Distraction extension injuries of the cervical spine. *J Spinal Disord* 2001;14(3):193–200.

61. Cantu RC, Bailes JE, Wilberger JE Jr: Guidelines for return to contact or collision sport after a cervical spine injury. *Clin Sports Med* 1998;17(1):137–146.

62. Morganti C: Recommendations for return to sports following cervical spine injuries. *Sports Med* 2003;33(8):563–573.

63. Torg JS, Ramsey-Emrhein JA: Management guidelines for participation in collision activities with congenital, developmental, or postinjury lesions involving the cervical spine. *Clin J Sport Med* 1997;7(4):273–291.

64. Vaccaro AR, Klein GR, Ciccoti M, et al: Return to play criteria for the athlete with cervical spine injuries resulting in stinger and transient quadriplegia/paresis. *Spine J* 2002;2(5):351–356.

65. Zmurko MG, Tannoury TY, Tannoury CA, Anderson DG: Cervical sprains, disc herniations, minor fractures, and other cervical injuries in the athlete. *Clin Sports Med* 2003;22(3):513–521.

SECTION 3

Lumbar Spine

16 Incidence of Low Back Pain in Athletes and Differential Diagnosis and Evaluation of Athletes with Back or Leg Pain

Kenneth Nwosu, MD • Christopher M. Bono, MD

INTRODUCTION

Low back pain (LBP) is nearly universal in the general population with a documented lifetime prevalence of 65% to 80%; 15% of the U.S. population reports frequent or persistent episodes.[1] The economic impact in this country has ranged from $84.1 to $624.8 billion annually.[2] Similarly, a high prevalence has been cited in other countries as well, with Biering-Sørensen and Hilden[3] reporting that 405 to 60% of individuals aged 30 to 40 years in Denmark had a history of LBP. Considering the causes of LBP, frequent bending and twisting were the most frequent cause of back injuries in one study.[4] Such movements are pervasive in most sports, and thus it is no surprise that low back injuries are exceedingly common in athletes. Sudden unexpected maximum efforts as well as lifting in combination with lateral bending and

Dr. Bono or an immediate family member has received nonincome support (such as equipment or services), commercially derived honoraria, or other nonresearch–related funding (such as paid travel) from United HealthCare and Wolters Kluwer Health—Lippincott Williams & Wilkins; and serves as a board member, owner, officer, or committee member of AAOS, Journal of the American Academy of Orthopaedic Surgeons, and North American Spine Society. Neither Dr. Nwosu nor any immediate family member has received anything of value from or has stock or stock options held in a commercial company or institution related directly or indirectly to the subject of this article.

twisting are found to be particularly injurious.[5] Overall, the static and dynamic forces exerted on the low back are exponentially magnified by the intense power generated during a golf or baseball swing, gymnast's landing, power-lifter's squat, boxer's punch, cycler's tuck, or a ballerina's arabesque.[6] In fact, LBP is the most common cause of lost playing time among professional athletes.[7]

In a discussion of LBP in athletes, it is important to delineate LBP as a symptom rather than a diagnosis, which may be influenced by many factors, including athleticism.[6] In nonathletes, a variety of nonmechanical factors can predispose to LBP such as anxiety, depression, and stressful life events.[8] Supportively, case-control studies have indicated that psychosocial factors are more influential than mechanical factors. In athletes, however, mechanical factors are more often implicated because they are modifiable via technique and training alterations. Furthermore, athletes, particularly those at the professional or competitive level, have a strong drive and vested interest in returning to play despite pain. Notwithstanding, the psychological and emotional burden of LBP in athletes should not be overlooked or underestimated.

INCIDENCE

The published prevalence of LBP in athletes widely ranges, being influenced heavily by sports type; gender; and training intensity, frequency, and technique.[9–11] Observing a 10-year period of time, Keene et al reported that 7% of 4790 varsity college athletes had LBP,[12] with rates highest in football players, gymnasts, and wrestlers. Diagnosis of acute muscle strain occurred most frequently (59%) compared with overuse injuries (2%), which were the least common.

Influence of Sports Type

From review of a variety of studies, it appears that the incidence of LBP is not equivalent among all sports and athletes. Among athletes participating in a variety of sports, Keene and Drummond found the highest incidence of LBP in football players, gymnasts, and wrestlers.[13] Granhed and Morelli[11] found a higher prevalence of LBP in wrestlers (59%) compared with weight lifters (23%) and a control population (31%). There is a common perception that running, because of the repetitive axial loading, can be injurious to the lumbar spine. In reality, the incidence of LBP in runners is comparatively low, ranging from 1.1% to 22.5%.[14] Furthermore, runners do not have a higher prevalence of radiographic degenerative changes than nonrunners.[15]

Ferguson et al[16] reported a high incidence of LBP in collegiate interior linemen, citing that 50% sought consultation for this complaint during a 1-year period. Of these, half were found to have spondylolysis, and 16.5% had spondylolisthesis. This group postulated that this was likely the result of repetitive posterior element loading during tackles. Others sports that require repeated hyperextension, such as gymnastics, diving, and volleyball, may be associated with a high incidence of LBP.[17] Rossi et al[14] documented 32% and 63% incidences of spondylolysis among competitive gymnasts and divers, respectively.

Hyperextension is not the only mechanism by which LBP is thought to develop. High rates of LBP have also been commonly reported with sports requiring repetitive rotation of the torso such as tennis, badminton, squash, and golf. Spencer and Jackson et al[18] found that 90% of tournament golfers have had back injuries. Specifically, in professional golfers, Tall and Devault et al[19] reported a 29% incidence of LBP.

Although LBP is quite prevalent in athletes while competing, it does not seem to be a permanent complaint despite longstanding radiographic changes. For example, in a study of former athletes, wrestlers had a high prevalence of old, healed fractures, and weight lifters had substantially decreased intervertebral disk heights. However, none of the wrestlers and only 5% of the weight lifters reported that they were disturbed by LBP during work compared with 70% of nonathlete control participants.[11]

Low Back Pain with Associated Leg Pain

In both athletes and nonathletes, LBP often concomitantly presents with radicular leg pain. Because it can be a part of the degenerative cascade, disk herniations can lead to lumbar root compression and irritation. The prevalence of LBP with associated leg pain (LBPLP) in the general population has varied from 1.2% to 43%.[20] The literature is sparse regarding the prevalence of LBPLP in athletes. One study reported a 58% prevalence of one or more disk herniations in Olympic athletes with LBP, some of whom had leg pain.[21] Of note, the L5 to S1 disk was most commonly affected in this study.

Although not helpful in estimating incidence or prevalence, recent reports of treatment outcomes in athletes with lumbar disk herniations and associated leg pain implicitly support that it occurs with at least some frequency.[22] Furthermore, Hsu et al reported that perception of a positive outcome in athletes may be different than nonathletes.[22] This group found that age was a negative predictor of career length, and experience was a positive predictor of clinical outcome in athletes with disk herniations and LBPLP. Of note, National Football League (NFL) athletes were more likely to have a positive outcome compared with those in other sports when treated surgically.[22]

● EVALUATION

History

Evaluation of athletes with LBP begins with a thorough history. The onset and duration of symptoms must be noted. Whereas sudden onset of acute symptoms can suggest an acute fracture or disk herniation, a slow, indolent presentation is more consistent with pain from disk degeneration, spondylolysis, or stress fracture. The location of pain is an important feature to note. Pain that is localized to one midline point without radiation is consistent with dysfunction of a single motion segment. Symptoms that diffusely involve multiple levels are more suggestive of muscular pain. Directionality of pain provocation can be helpful in distinguishing disk-related pain, which is aggravated by bending forward, and posterior element pain (e.g., pars interarticularis or facet joints), which is worsened with extension and often relieved with flexion. The type of sport, position played, and volume of training should be recorded because these can be factors in the onset of LBP. So-called red flag symptoms such as fever, malaise, weight loss, neurologic abnormalities, or night pain can indicate serious conditions such as

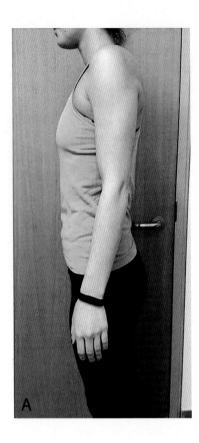
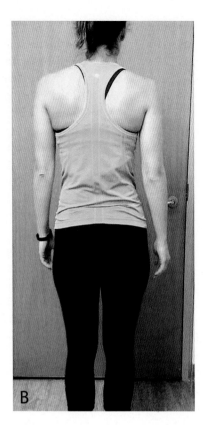

FIGURE 16-1 Clinical photographs of normal static coronal (**A**) and sagittal (**B**) posture.

infection or tumor that require more aggressive diagnostic imaging workup.

Physical Examination

Athletes often develop side-to-side musculoskeletal asymmetry. The spinal column is no exception. Thus, gait and static posture should be observed for abnormalities (**Figure 16-1**). Posterior inspection should note the presence of shoulder, trunk, or pelvic asymmetry. Lateral inspection should confirm normal spinal curvature, including moderate lumbar lordosis without thoracic hyperkyphosis.

Next, the athlete should be observed flexing, extending, and rotating through the lumbar spine. Importantly, the pelvis should be kept fixed during rotation so as to isolate movement to the lumbar spine. Distinction should be made between painless limitation of motion, which suggests loss of flexibility, and painful motion, indicating that the motion is loading a pain generator.

Routinely, provocative nerve tension maneuvers should be performed, including straight leg and femoral stretch tests. The straight leg raise should be performed in the supine position; the femoral stretch test should be performed in the prone position. A single-legged hyperextension test can be performed to assess for possible injury to the posterior elements (**Figure 16-2**). Specific tests, such as the flexion abduction external rotation (FABER), Gaenslen, and compression tests, should be performed to assess the sacroiliac joint as this may be an extraspinal origin of LBP.

The spinous processes and paraspinal muscles should be systematically palpated for tenderness. Tenderness that can be elicited by direct palpation of a one spinous process is suggestive of a localized pain generator at a motion segment, such as a stress fracture or degenerated disk. Multilevel, paraspinal pain with palpation is more consistent with pain originating from the muscles. A detailed neurologic examination of both the upper and lower extremities is requisite. This must include assessment of strength, sensation, and reflexes. Pathological signs such as a Babinski or Hoffman's or more than four beats of clonus suggest upper motor neuron involvement warranting advanced imaging of the cervical or thoracic spine or brain.

Imaging

Barring red flags, an athlete with a LBP episode lasting more than a few weeks should initially undergo plain radiographs of the lumbar spine. Admittedly of low yield because it only shows gross bony changes, it can demonstrate acute or chronic fractures or alignment

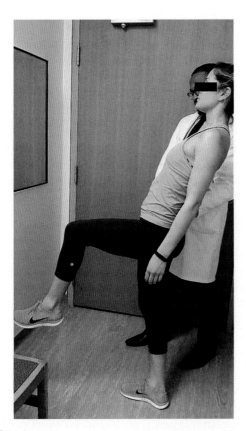

FIGURE 16-2 Clinical photo of single-legged hyperextension test.

abnormalities, such as a spondylolisthesis. Flexion-extension views can be helpful in revealing dynamic instability or spondylolytic defects (**Figure 16-3**).

Advanced imaging should be obtained if pain persists beyond 6 weeks and is recalcitrant to initial nonoperative treatment. MRI is the advanced imaging modality of choice because it can demonstrate a wide range of underlying conditions that can be associated with LBP, including stress reactions, disk herniations, disk degeneration, and spondylolisthesis. A CT scan can also be useful in cases of back or leg pain. It is more sensitive in detecting an established spondylolysis. However, because of the substantial amount of radiation exposure, it should be reserved for cases in which an MRI is inconclusive or contraindicated. Studies have reported that MRI fails to diagnose fewer than 10% of suspected cases of spondylolysis.

The detection of a stress reaction can be more difficult. Stress reactions represent the intraosseous bony changes from repetitive loading before fracturing. This is not detectable on a standard CT or plain radiograph. An MRI or bone scan are sensitive in detecting stress reactions. A single-photon emission computed tomography (SPECT) scan is a radionuclide-enhanced CT scan. This is the most sensitive test for stress reactions in the lumbar spine. Detecting a stress reaction before a frank stress fracture occurs is important. Early treatment with orthotic immobilization and restriction of activity can potentiate bone healing. Failure to do so can result in fracture and chronic nonunion (i.e., spondylolysis).

Intertwined with the decision to obtain imaging in an athlete with LBP is consideration that many asymptomatic individuals can have degenerative changes in the lumbar spine. Thus, the coexistence of lumbar degeneration and LBP does not imply causality. Similarly, disk degeneration

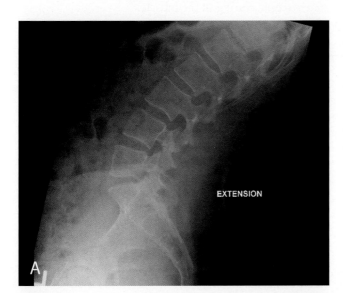

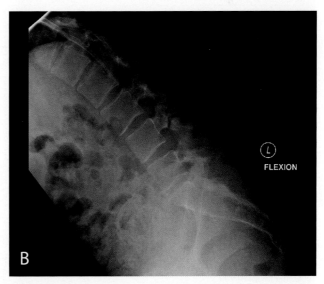

FIGURE 16-3 Extension radiograph (**A**) of a 29-year-old competitive diver with a complaint of low back pain, which does not clearly demonstrate any identifiable structural abnormality. However, a flexion radiograph (**B**) clearly reveals a spondylolytic defect at the L4 level.

is common in athletes but often has little correlation to the presence or intensity of LBP. Videman et al[9] found that LBP was less common in former elite athletes than nonathletes despite more degenerative disk changes. Swärd et al reported radiographic abnormalities in 36 to 55% of athletes.[23] Of athletes with no pain, 36% had signs of degeneration. However, in those with moderate and severe pain, 42% and 57% had degenerative changes.

DIFFERENTIAL DIAGNOSIS

The differential diagnosis of LBP with or without associated leg pain in athletes includes a number of conditions. These are outlined in **Table 16-1**. A discussion of the most common is detailed here. It is important to rule out serious spinal issues, such as neoplasm and infection, based on a detailed history and imaging when indicated. Furthermore, one must not overlook nonspinal orthopaedic issues that can present as back or leg pain (or both). This is particularly true for hip issues, which can be ruled out with a detailed examination of hip range of motion. Nonorthopaedic diagnoses must also be considered, such as kidney or ovarian pathology, because they can often present as back pain with or without radiation.

TABLE 16-1	Differential diagnoses of persistent low back pain in athletes

Spinal Diagnoses	Non-Spinal Orthopaedic Problems	Nonorthopaedic Diagnoses
Muscle strain or ligament sprain	Sacroiliac joint dysfunction	Intrapelvic, gynecologic issues (e.g., ovarian cysts)
Degenerative disk disease	Trochanteric bursitis	
Disk herniation (with radiculopathy)	Intraarticular hip issues (e.g., labral tears, femoroacetabular impingement)	Renal disease
Isthmic spondylolysis (with no slip)		
Isthmic spondylolisthesis		
Facet syndrome	Muscular tears (e.g., gluteus, proximal hamstring)	
Ring apophyseal injury (adolescents)		
Referred LBP secondary to pelvic injuries		
Sacral stress fracture		
Facet stress fracture		
Acute traumatic lumbar fracture		
Discitis or osteomyelitis		
Spinal neoplasm		

LBP = low back pain.

Muscle Strains and Ligament Sprains

Strains are a result of muscle fiber disruptions that most often occur during eccentric contraction.[6] Muscle strains and interspinous ligament sprains are the most common causes of LBP in athletes and can occur at any age and in any sport.[24] A retrospective study of 4790 varsity athletes who sustained back injuries reported 60% of all injuries were muscle strains, which was significantly greater than all other types of injuries.[13] Of note, it occurred most often in football and gymnastics compared with other sports. Predictably, most injuries (64%) were not associated with any radiographic abnormalities.

Acute strains often present as localized or diffuse pain that is most intense 48 hours after injury. There can be associated muscle spasm, which after a few days may be localized to a so-called trigger point.[13] Chronic strains are characterized by persistent pain attributable to a muscle injury. On examination, athletes may have localized tenderness over the affected muscle and pain exacerbated by flexion. Neurologic examination results are typically normal.

Low back strains and sprains are usually self-limiting. Because of the high demands of competitive athletes and the availability of trainers, nonoperative care can start soon after injury. This includes a short period rest followed by stretching and muscular rehabilitation. If pain persists beyond 3 weeks, plain radiographs can be obtained to rule out an underlying structural issue. Advanced imaging such as MRI is unlikely to change management; it can be helpful in the rare instance where severe pain persists because it may reveal edema or hemorrhage at the myotendinous junction with or without macroscopic tearing of the muscle.[25]

Degenerative Disk Disease

Degeneration of the lumbar spine can lead to a spectrum of conditions. Although an in-depth discussion regarding the pathogenesis is beyond the scope of this chapter, it is important to note the high prevalence of degenerative changes in athletes. There is an association between participation in competitive sports and a higher prevalence of degenerative changes in the lumbar spine.[21,23] However, the causality of degeneration in leading to LBP is not clear.[9,23,26,27] Regardless, disk degeneration continues to be assigned culpability for chronic, unremitting LBP (with minimal lower extremity radiation) in both athletes and nonathletes. Without a universally agreed upon definition, this is commonly termed *degenerative disk disease* or so-called *discogenic LBP*.

The incidence or prevalence of true discogenic LBP in athletes is not well characterized. It is the authors' opinion that it probably represents a very small proportion of athletes with chronic or recurrent LBP. The role of discography in determining which (if any) degenerative disks are the cause of LBP is entangled in controversy.[28] The history and physical examination features that suggest degenerative disk disease include pain worse with flexion and sitting, localized tenderness with palpation of the spinous processes, and an absence of nerve root tension signs.

Disk Herniation

Symptomatic disk herniation in athletes commonly result in both back and leg pain. It is generally accepted that leg pain is a result of mechanical or chemical irritation of a nerve root (or both), which can progress to sensory and motor deficits in some cases.[29-31] Classically, pain and paresthesias radiate in a discrete dermatomal pattern[24] (**Figure 16-4**). In general, leg pain is often more troublesome than LBP. Similar to that from degenerative disk disease, back pain is typically characterized as midline, exacerbated by lumbar flexion, and relieved with extension.[32] In distinction from degenerative disk disease, athletes with lumbar disk herniations have positive neural tension signs during straight leg (L4–S1 nerve roots) or femoral stretch (L1–L3 nerve roots) testing.[33] A contralateral straight leg raise test is highly specific for a disk herniation.[33]

Magnetic resonance imaging is the diagnostic modality of choice for detecting lumbar disk herniations. CT myelography may be useful in patients with a pacemaker or other MRI incompatible implants. Similar to the high prevalence of degenerative changes in asymptomatic individuals, disk herniations can also be present in those without symptoms.[34] Thus, it is critically important to relate the laterality, dermatome, and myotome involvement with imaging findings, particularly before invasive treatments such as injections or surgery.

Spondylolysis and Spondylolisthesis

As discussed previously, *spondylolysis* refers to a defect in the pars interarticularis that is the sequelae of a chronic, unhealed stress fracture. It is widely believed that repetitive extension and torsion of the spine, as commonly seen in football linemen, dancers, figure skaters, and gymnasts, is a predisposing factor.[35] *Isthmic spondylolisthesis* refers to anterolisthesis of the vertebral body at the level with the lytic defect in relation to the infradjacent vertebra. In addition to complaints of LBP, radicular (leg) symptoms are common, usually localized to the L5 dermatome. High-grade slips can present with an obvious deformity of the low back.[36,37]

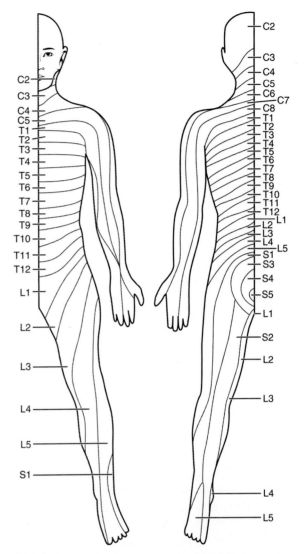

FIGURE 16-4 Diagram illustrating the dermatomes of the upper and lower extremities. (Reproduced from Rydevik B, Brisby H, Myers RR: The Pathophysiology of Cervical and Lumbar Radiculopathy, in: Rao RD, Smuck M (eds): *Orthopaedic Knowledge Update Spine 4*. Rosemont, IL, American Academy of Orthopaedic Surgeons, 2012, pp 44.)

Spondylolysis with or without slippage has been reported to be present in as many as 47% of athletes with back pain.[38] Affected athletes often have a hyperlordotic lumbar spine and complaints of an insidious onset extension-related LBP and hamstring tightness.[39] On examination, pain is reproduced with lumbar hyperextension and further exacerbated by the single-leg extension test (Figure 16-2).[40]

Sacral Stress Fractures

Athletes with sacral stress fractures can present with pain in the low back region. Although these fractures have been reported in male athletes, they more typically present in female athletes, particularly those involved in long-distance running sports.[41,42] Sacral stress fractures are associated with the so-called terrible triad in women athletes, characterized by amenorrhea, an eating disorder, and osteoporosis. Physical examination features include a positive FABER test result and tenderness to palpation just medial to the posterior superior iliac spine. A "hopping test" has been described, which can reproduce pain on the side of the stress fracture while hopping on the ipsilateral leg.[42] MRI or a radionuclide study is usually diagnostic because it has been demonstrated to be as sensitive as bone scan.[41] Furthermore, it avoids the radiation exposure of a bone scan. Initial treatment consists of rest and protected weight bearing. When symptoms begin to subside, the athlete can gradually return to full weight bearing and, after an ample period of rehabilitation, can return to sport.

● SUMMARY

Low back pain with or without leg pain is a common cause of impaired performance and lost play time in competitive athletes. The incidence and prevalence are influenced by a number of factors, such as sport type, training intensity, and position played. When evaluating an athlete with LBP, a number of common causes should be included in the differential diagnosis. The importance of the history and physical examination cannot be underestimated because it helps distinguish among the common causes of back pain. This is highlighted in light of the high prevalence of structural abnormalities on imaging, such as degenerative changes and spondylolysis, which may or may not be the culprit. If possible, a discrete disorder with an identifiable pain generator should be determined to best direct treatment.

REFERENCES

1. Lawrence RC, Helmick CG, Arnett FC, et al: Estimates of the prevalence of arthritis and selected musculoskeletal disorders in the United States. *Arthritis Rheum* 1998;41;778–799.

2. Dagenais S, Caro J, Haldeman S: A systematic review of low back pain cost of illness studies in the United States and internationally. *Spine J* 2008;8:8–20.

3. Biering-Sørensen F, Hilden J: Reproducibility of the history of low-back trouble. *Spine* 1984;9:280–286.

4. Troup JD: Causes, prediction and prevention of back pain at work. *Scand J Work Environ Health* 1984;10:419–428.

5. Brown JR: Factors contributing to the development of low back pain in industrial workers. *Am Ind Hyg Assoc J* 1975;36:26–31.

6. Bono CM: Low-back pain in athletes. *J Bone Joint Surg Am* 2004;86(suppl A):382–396.

7. Bernstein RM, Cozen H: Evaluation of back pain in children and adolescents. *Am Fam Physician* 2007;76:1669–1676.

8. Frymoyer JW, Pope MH, Costanza MC, Rosen JC, Goggin JE, Wilder DG: Epidemiologic studies of low-back pain. *Spine* 1980;5:419–423.

9. Videman T, Sarna S, Battié MC, Koskinen S, Gill K, Paananen H, Gibbons L: The long-term effects of physical loading and exercise lifestyles on back-related symptoms, disability, and spinal pathology among men. *Spine* 1995;20:699–709.

10. Hickey GJ, Fricker PA, McDonald WA: Injuries to elite rowers over a 10-yr period. *Med Sci Sports Exerc* 1997;29:1567–1572.

11. Granhed H, Morelli B: Low back pain among retired wrestlers and heavyweight lifters. *Am J Sports Med* 1988;16:530–533.

12. Keene JS, Albert MJ, Springer SL, Drummond DS, Clancy WG: Back injuries in college athletes. *J Spinal Disord* 1989;2:190–195.

13. Keene JS, Drummond DS: Mechanical back pain in the athlete. *Compr Ther* 1985;11:7–14.

14. Rossi F: Spondylolysis, spondylolisthesis and sports. *J Sports Med Phys Fitness* 1978;18:317–340.

15. Hangai M, Kaneoka K, Hinotsu S, et al: Lumbar intervertebral disk degeneration in athletes. *Am J Sport Med* 2009;31:149–155.

16. Ferguson RJ, McMaster JH, Stanitski C: L. Low back pain in college football linemen. *J Sports Med* 1974;2:63–69.

17. Curtis C, d' Hemecourt P: Diagnosis and management of back pain in adolescents. *Adolesc Med State Art Rev* 2007;18:140–164, x.

18. Spencer CW, Jackson DW: Back injuries in the athlete. *Clin Sports Med* 1983;2:191–215.

19. Tall RL, DeVault W: Spinal injury in sport: Epidemiologic considerations. *Clin Sports Med* 1993;12:441–448.

20. Konstantinou K, Dunn KM: Sciatica: Review of epidemiological studies and prevalence estimates. *Spine* 2008;33:2464–2472.

21. Ong A, Anderson J, Roche J: A pilot study of the prevalence of lumbar disc degeneration in elite athletes with lower back pain at the Sydney 2000 Olympic Games. *Br J Sports Med* 2003;37:263–266.

22. Hsu WK, McCarthy KJ, Savage JW, et al: The Professional Athlete Spine Initiative: Outcomes after lumbar disc herniation in 342 elite professional athletes. *Spine J* 2011;11:180–186.

23. Swärd L, Hellstrom M, Jacobsson B, Pëterson L: Back pain and radiologic changes in the thoraco-lumbar spine of athletes. *Spine* 1990;15:124–129.

24. Deyo RA, Rainville J, Kent DL: What can the history and physical examination tell us about low back pain? *JAMA* 1992;268:760–765.

25. Bennett DL, Nassar L, DeLano MC: Lumbar spine MRI in the elite-level female gymnast with low back pain. *Skeletal Radiol* 2006;35:503–509.

26. Lundin O, Hellström M, Nilsson I, Swärd L: Back pain and radiological changes in the thoraco-lumbar spine of athletes. A long-term follow-up. *Scand J Med Sci Sports* 2001;11:103–109.

27. Kujala UM, Salminen JJ, Taimela S, Oksanen A, Jaakkola L: Subject characteristics and low back pain in young athletes and nonathletes. *Med Sci Sports Exerc* 1992;24:627–632.

28. Carragee EJ, Don AS, Hurwitz EL, Cuellar JM, Carrino JA, Herzog R: 2009 ISSLS Prize Winner: Does discography cause accelerated progression of degeneration changes in the lumbar disc: A ten-year matched cohort study. *Spine* 2009;34:2338–2345.

29. Miyoshi S, Sekiguchi M, Konno S, Kikuchi S, Kanaya F: Increased expression of vascular endothelial growth factor protein in dorsal root ganglion exposed to nucleus pulposus on the nerve root in rats. *Spine* 2011;36:E1–6.

30. McCarron RF, Wimpee MW, Hudkins PG, Laros GS: The inflammatory effect of nucleus pulposus. A possible element in the pathogenesis of low-back pain. *Spine* 1987;12:760–764.

31. Murphy DR, Hurwitz EL, Gerrard JK, Clary R: Pain patterns and descriptions in patients with radicular pain: Does the pain necessarily follow a specific dermatome? *Chiropr Osteopat* 2009;17:9.

32. Young S, Aprill C, Laslett M: Correlation of clinical examination characteristics with three sources of chronic low back pain. *Spine J* 2003;3:460–465.

33. Vroomen PC, de Krom MC, Knottnerus JA: Diagnostic value of history and physical examination in patients suspected of sciatica due to disc herniation: A systematic review. *J Neurol* 1999;246:899–906.

34. Herzog RJ: The radiologic assessment for a lumbar disc herniation. *Spine* 1996;21(suppl):19S–38S.

35. Watkins RG: Lumbar disc injury in the athlete. *Clin Sports Med* 2002;21:147–165, vii.

36. Tsirikos AI, Garrido EG: Spondylolysis and spondylolisthesis in children and adolescents. *J Bone Joint Surg Br* 2010;92:751–759.

37. Smith JA, Hu SS: Management of spondylolysis and spondylolisthesis in the pediatric and adolescent population. *Orthop Clin North Am* 1999;30:487–499, ix.

38. Micheli LJ, Wood R: Back pain in young athletes. Significant differences from adults in causes and patterns. *Arch Pediatr Adolesc Med* 1995;149:15–18.

39. Weiker GG: Evaluation and treatment of common spine and trunk problems. *Clin Sports Med* 1989;8:399–417.

40. Kraft DE: Low back pain in the adolescent athlete. *Pediatr Clin North Am* 2002;49:643–653.

41. Johnson AW, Weiss CB, Stento K, Wheeler DL: Stress fractures of the sacrum. An atypical cause of low back pain in the female athlete. *Am J Sports Med* 2001;29:498–508.

42. Delvaux K, Lysens R: Lumbosacral pain in an athlete. *Am J Phys Med Rehabil* 2001;80:388–391.

17 Spondylolysis and Spondylolisthesis in Immature and Adult Athletes

Rahul Basho, MD • Andre M. Jakoi, MD • Jeffrey C. Wang, MD

● INTRODUCTION

Athletes place increased demands and repetitive stresses on their musculoskeletal systems. Studies have shown that almost 30% of athletes experience low back pain referable to athletic participation.[1,2] In professional sports, lower back pain is the most common cause of lost playing time.[3] Lower back injuries differ in adult and adolescent athletes; whereas nearly 70% of lumbar injuries in adolescents occur in the posterior elements of the spine, adult athletes are more likely to have muscle strains and discogenic disease.[4]

The anatomic region of the spine particularly susceptible to injury is the pars interarticularis (**Figure 17-1**). Also referred to as the isthmus (Greek for narrow), it is the thin region of bone that connects the superior and inferior articular processes of a vertebral body. A defect in the pars, termed *spondylolysis,* can result in pain and sometimes lead to instability within the spine. This instability, termed spondylolisthesis, refers to slippage of one vertebral body (*spondylos* in Greek) relative to another (**Figure 17-2**). When spondylolisthesis occurs because of a defect in the pars, it is termed *isthmic spondylolisthesis.*

Spondylosis has been extensively studied and is one of the few spinal conditions with follow-up data long enough to give insight into its natural history. In the early 1950s, Dr. Baker initiated a prospective study to determine the natural history of spondylolysis and spondylolisthesis. A study population of 500 children was enrolled and followed, with the last reported follow-up being at 45 years. The data showed an incidence of pars defects of 4.4% at age 6 years, which rose to 6% in adulthood.[5] The majority of lesions occurred at the L5 level. The study also attempted to delineate the likelihood of pars defects progressing to symptomatic spondylolisthesis. Of the 30 children with pars defects, 8 had unilateral pars defects and never developed spondylolisthesis. In the 22 children with bilateral defects, all but 4 developed some degree of spondylolisthesis over their lifetimes. However, only 1 patient was found to have symptomatic slip progression in adulthood; the authors concluded that the likelihood of this occurring was 5%. Progression of the spondylolisthesis decreased with each decade of life, with the greatest progression occurring early in life. No patient developed a slip beyond 40 years. The authors stated that there was "no justification for generally advising children and adolescents with spondylolysis and low grade spondylolisthesis not to participate in competitive sports."[5]

Dr. Wang or an immediate family member has received royalties from Aesculap/B. Braun, Amedica, Biomet, Seaspine, and Synthes; has stock or stock options held in Alphatec Spine, Amedica, Benevenue, Bone Biologics, Corespine, Electrocore, Expanding Ortho, Fziomed, Nexgen, Paradigm Spine, Pearl Diver, Promethean Spine, Surgitech, and Vertiflex; and serves as a board member, owner, officer, or committee member of AO Spine International, the Cervical Spine Research Society, the Evidence-Based Spine-Care Journal, the Global Spine Journal, Spine, *the* Spine Journal, *the* Journal of Spinal Disorders and Techniques, *the* North American Spine Foundation, the North American Spine Society, and the Journal of the American Academy of Orthopaedic Surgeons. *Neither Dr. Basho nor any immediate family member has received anything of value from or has stock or stock options held in a commercial company or institution related directly or indirectly to the subject of this article.*

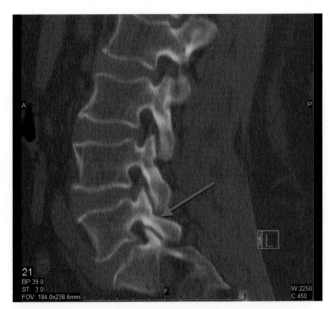

FIGURE 17-1 Depiction of the pars interarticularis. (Reprinted from Oatis CA: *Kinesiology*, ed 2. Philadelphia, PA, Lippincott Williams & Wilkins, 2008.)

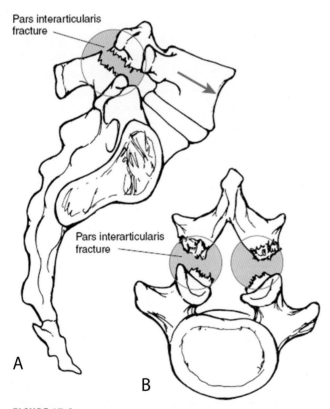

FIGURE 17-2 Progressive displacement of a pars interarticularis fracture. (Reprinted from Egol K, Koval KJ, Zuckerman JD: *Handbook of Fractures*, ed 4. Philadelphia, PA, Lippincott Williams & Wilkins, 2010.)

Although the prevalence of pars fractures in the general population is between 4% and 6%, a higher incidence is seen among athletes involved in sports requiring repetitive hyperextension, such as weight lifting, wrestling, gymnastics, and football.[6–8] Some studies have found that up to 15% of college football players and 11% of female gymnasts have spondylolysis.[9,10] Different theories have been postulated in regards to the etiology of pars fractures. Among athletes, the most widely accepted is one of repetitive stress resulting in fracture. Extension of the lumbar spine results in the inferior articular process of the cranial vertebrae impacting the pars of the caudal vertebrae.[11] Shear stresses of 400 to 600 N caused by this motion are concentrated across the pars, an area calculated to be only 0.75 cm² at L5.[12] This repetitive stress results in a pars "stress reaction," which if untreated can progress to a fracture.[13] The stress reaction, microfracture, overt fracture, and spondylolisthesis are viewed as progressive stages of an overuse injury at the pars interarticularis.[14]

HISTORY

Pars defects account for a much larger percentage of lumbar spine injuries in skeletally immature athletes compared with adults.[15] Hunter et al showed that 47% of patients younger than the age of 18 presenting to a sports medicine clinic with back pain had spondylolysis compared with 5% of adults older than the age of 21 years presenting with similar symptoms.[16] Skeletally immature athlete typically describes a history of activity related pain and 40% will recall a specific inciting even.[17] Adult athletes usually complain of lower limb pain greater than back pain.[18]

PHYSICAL EXAMINATION

A gait examination and detailed neurologic examination should be performed. The typical presentation is one of back pain exacerbated by extension. Hyperlordosis and hamstring tightness can be present. Radicular symptoms are usually not present but can occur secondary to nerve root irritation from fibrocartilaginous tissue overgrowth at the defect narrowing the foramen. Younger patients with higher grade subluxations can present with a palpable step-off. The only "pathognomonic" finding in the literature is the stork test, in which the patient extends his or her lumbar spine while in a single-limb stance; recreation of pain in the lumbar region is indicative of a pars lesion (**Figure 17-3**). This test, however, has been shown to have a low sensitivity and specificity.[19,20]

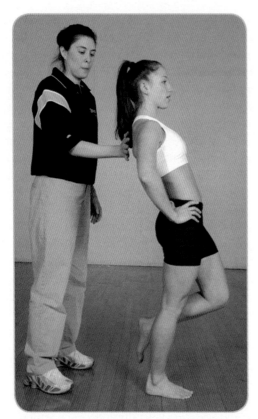

FIGURE 17-3 Depiction of the stork test. (Reprinted from Anderson MK: *Foundations of Athletic Training.* Philadelphia, PA: Wolters Kluwer, 2017.)

● IMAGING STUDIES

Plain Radiography

Imaging studies are used to diagnose spondylolysis, differentiate acute and chronic lesions, guide treatment, and assess healing. Initial imaging studies have traditionally consisted of six views (anteroposterior, lateral, flexion, extension, and oblique views of the lumbar spine). On oblique views, the pars appears as the neck of the "Scotty dog," and visualized fractures show a radiolucency through this region. Whereas acute fractures typically present as narrow and irregular, chronic fractures are smooth and rounded.[1,22]

Amato et al demonstrated that the single best view for detecting spondylosis was the collimated lateral view; 84% of cases were diagnosed with this view alone.[23] However, 19% of the cases were only visible on the oblique view. In a review of 1743 soldiers, Libson et al demonstrated that 20% of all cases of spondylolysis were visible only on oblique views.[24] Based on these studies, 45° oblique views have been long regarded as necessary when screening for a pars defect. However, they can be insensitive because the pars is obliquely oriented to all three orthogonal planes.[21] Fractures are only well visualized when the radiographic beam is tangential to the plane of the fracture. This fact, coupled with increasing concerns about radiation exposure, have called into question the utility of the oblique view as a screening modality for spondylosis. Beck et al demonstrated no significant difference between the sensitivity and specificity of two-view versus four view radiographs in detecting a pars defect in the pediatric population.[25] They emphasized that the addition of oblique views increased the radiation dose to the patient by 75%, from 0.72 mSV for a two-view study to 1.26 mSV for a four-view study. Although the authors thought that oblique views did add some diagnostic value in patients with unilateral pars defects, they concluded that "the increased radiation and costs associated with the use of oblique views are not outweighed by their diagnostic value." It is important that the clinician consolidate findings from both the history and physical examination before ordering oblique films on adolescent patients. If two view studies do not show evidence of a pars defect and it is clinically suspected, advanced imaging is warranted.

Magnetic Resonance Imaging

There is a lack of consensus on which advanced imaging studies to obtain and in which order. Traditionally, CT scans and single-photon emission computed tomography (SPECT) have been used. Concerns about radiation dosage, especially among the pediatric population, have led to interest in MRI as an initial screening modality after plain radiography. In addition to the lack of radiation exposure, MRI allows detailed evaluation of the disks and neural elements and can provide prognostic data about fracture healing. Hollenberg et al developed a MRI classification system for stress injuries to the pars[26] (**Table 17-1**). They divided the findings into five grades, with grade 0 being a normal pars with no signal change, grade 1 showing edema of the pars without spondylolysis, grade 2 showing edema and irregularity at the pars, grade 3 showing edema at the pars with cortical disruption, and grade 4 demonstrating cortical disruption with no edema at the pars. Grades 1 to 3 represent progressive stages of injury to the pars, with grade 4 injuries indicative of chronic injuries with pseudarthrosis at the pars.

Sairyo et al also used the ability of MRI to detect cortical edema but focused on the pedicle adjacent to the pars in cases of spondylosis.[27] In an elegant study, they used CT scans to classify spondylolysis into one of four categories: early, late early, progressive, and terminal. MRI

TABLE 17-1	Hollenberg et al[26] classification of stress injuries to the pars interarticularis	
Grade	Description	MRI Features
0	Normal	Normal marrow signal Intact cortical margins
1	Stress reaction	Marrow edema Intact cortical margins
2	Incomplete fracture	Marrow edema Cortical fracture extending incompletely through the pars
3	Complete active fracture	Marrow edema Cortical fracture extending completely through the pars
4	Fracture nonunion	No marrow edema Cortical fracture extending completely through the pars

Adapted from Viroslav AB: Acute injuries of the lumbar neural arch in adolescents. *MRI Web Clinic,* March 2011. Available at: http://radsource.us/lumbar-neural-arch. Accessed September 16, 2016.

scans were then performed and evaluated for the presence of high signal changes (HSCs) within the pedicles adjacent to the spondylolysis. A total of 100% of patients in the early and late-early groups had HSC on the ipsilateral pedicle, 50% of the progressive stage, on 0% in the terminal stage. Of the patients treated conservatively, 79% with HSC on the MRI showed bony healing, but none of the HSC-negative patients showed healing. The authors concluded that the presence of HSC on the pedicles adjacent to a spondylolysis can help determine the acuity and thus healing potential of the injury. Sakai et al demonstrated that the disappearance of HSC on T2-weighted MRI imaging of pedicles adjacent to spondylosis was indicative of fracture healing.[28] They performed monthly MRIs on patients with spondylosis and found that in compliant patients, HSC within the pedicle disappeared at 3 months. They recommended MRI at the third month of conservative treatment to evaluate the efficacy of conservative treatment. Other studies have shown favorable results for the use of MRI as a first-line imaging modality but acknowledge the superiority of CT scans to delineate fracture size and extent.[29,30]

Single-Photon Emission Computed Tomography

In patients with persistent pain despite normal radiographs, SPECT has been traditionally used because of its high sensitivity. Images are acquired in multiple projections as the gamma scintillation camera moves in an axial orbit about the patient, allowing creation of a cross-sectional image[31] (**Figure 17-4**). No additional radiation from traditional scintigraphy is needed. Increased isotope uptake in the region of a metabolically active fracture can identify a lesion not seen on plain radiographs because of its anatomic orientation or because it may be in the early stages of the stress process.[32] In addition, SPECT allows differentiation between acute lesions and chronic nonunions.

The shortcomings of SPECT lie in its low specificity. Positive SPECT findings have been documented in asymptomatic athletes, and it is unable to differentiate among spondylolysis, facet arthropathy, and osteoid osteoma.[32] In addition, the radiation dose of 5 mSV is substantial, especially in the pediatric population. These facts, coupled with the advances seen in MRI, render SPECT obsolete as a screening investigation for spondylolysis. In cases when MRI is contraindicated, it still can provide valuable diagnostic data.[26]

Computed Tomography Scans

Computed tomography scans, long regarded as the "gold standard" in diagnosing spondylolysis, provide excellent anatomic detail and can help confirm bony healing. Traditionally used in conjunction, the combination of SPECT and CT scans provide high specificity and sensitivity and give insight into prognosis. A patient with a positive lesion on SPECT with a negative CT scan likely has a stress reaction at the pars, which carries a favorable prognosis for healing. In contrast, a negative SPECT scan with a positive CT scan is likely indicative of a chronic nonunion with poor healing potential. Despite these advantages, the radiation doses seen with these two examinations is of concern, especially in adolescent athletes. Rush et al compared MRI and CT in their ability to diagnose spondylosis in adolescents.[33] Their data showed a 92% sensitivity for MRI in detecting pars injuries. In addition, MRI identified 11 lesions in 9 patients with negative CT scans. Of these, 7 were stress reactions (grade 1), and 4 were frank fractures (grade 4). The authors recommended that MRI should be strongly considered as the advanced imaging modality of choice in evaluating adolescents for spondylolysis.

No definitive algorithm exists when ordering imaging studies to evaluate patients for spondylolysis. Physicians must be familiar with the available imaging modalities in their communities and be aware of the limitations. Initial studies evaluating MRI in diagnosing spondylosis showed low sensitivity and positive predictive value.[34] Over time, many of these limitations have been overcome and the ability of MRI to visualize the neural elements,

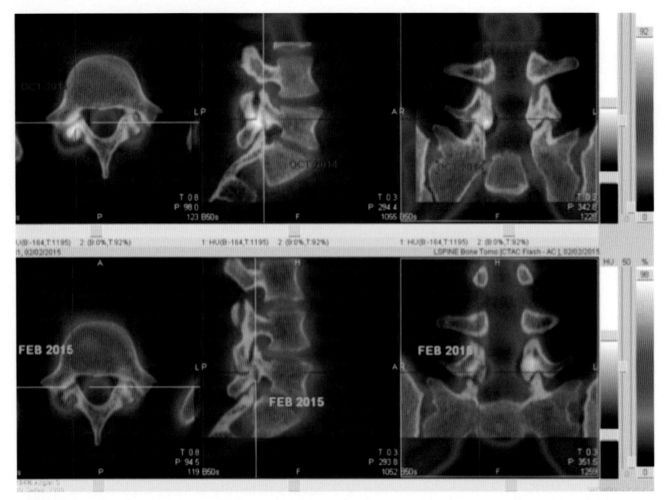

FIGURE 17-4 Single-photon emission computed tomography images showing an acute pars lesion. (From Birch N, Harrison D: Minimally invasive surgical treatment of spondylolysis in sportsmen and sportswomen. *Spinal Surgery News*, March 23, 2016.)

assess healing, detect stress reactions, and provide prognostic data all without radiation make it the advanced imaging modality of choice. It is the authors' opinion that MRI should be the first-line advanced imaging modality in diagnosing pars defects. CT scans should be used in patients whom MRI is contraindicated, in those with persistent symptoms and equivocal findings on the MRI, or when there is a need to confirm fracture healing. The role for SPECT scanning has become limited; when MRI in contraindicated and there is a need to differentiate an acute lesion from a chronic pseudarthrosis, SPECT remains the only option.

● TREATMENT AND RETURN TO PLAY

After the diagnosis of a pars fracture or spondylolisthesis is made in a symptomatic athlete, athletic activity should be ceased and conservative treatment begun. The initial goal of conservative management is alleviation of pain.

This is accomplished with a period of rest from athletic participation, and in acute lesions, a period of bracing. No consensus exists on the type of brace to use or the duration of conservative measures. Despite the lack of definitive protocols, evidence-based recommendations can be made based on the available literature. Each athlete must be evaluated individually because pars injury represent a spectrum of disease. Treatments may need to be modified based on the age of the athlete and acuity of the injury. Adolescent patients with an acute pars injury are much more likely to respond to conservative measures. Sairyo et al performed a prospective study evaluating the healing potential of pars defects with a hard trunk brace.[35] The authors indicated that in their institution, they found superior healing rates of pars fractures using a hard brace instead of a soft corset. Based on these findings, they placed patients in a hard trunk brace. The patients were divided into four groups based on CT and MRI findings: early, progressive with HSC on

MRI, progressive with low signal on MRI, and terminal. Along with bracing, the patients were instructed to cease any athletic activity. CT scans were performed every 3 months to evaluate healing. The authors found union rates of 94% in the early group (3.2 months), 64% in the progressive group with HSC (5.4 months), 27% in the progressive group with low signal intensity (5.7 months), and 0% in the terminal group. The importance of early diagnosis and initiation of treatment was highlighted by the results of this study. In addition, it provides insight into duration of treatment: Progressive stage defects needed to be braced almost twice as long (~6 months) as early stage defects (3 months).

It should be made clear that the duration of treatment may be lengthy but that the majority of patients will respond to conservative treatment and return to play (RTP) at a high level. Also, the final end point is pain control; even if a pars fracture does not heal, a fibrous union can still lead to a good clinical result.[14]

Acute Lesions

Although randomized studies comparing bracing and activity restriction are lacking, multiple studies have demonstrated successful outcomes with a dedicated period of bracing.[14,35,36] Patients with grade 1 lesions based on advanced imaging should begin a 3-month period of bracing for 23 hours per day. Patients with grade 2 or 3 defects on advanced imaging studies should brace for 6 months for 23 hours per day. Studies with antilordotic and lordotic bracing have both shown successful outcomes,[14,37] so compliance is more important than the type of brace. At the conclusion of 3 or 6 months of bracing, the brace should be weaned and the patient examined for pain with daily activities and pain with extension of the lumbar spine. If pain is still present, bracing should be continued for another month and the patient reexamined. If absent, physical therapy with an emphasis on lumbar core strengthening should be initiated. After 1 month of therapy, asymptomatic patients should be transitioned into sport-specific noncontact drills followed by full participation in sports (**Figure 17-5**).

Chronic Lesions

Chronic fractures (stage 4 on advanced imaging) will not heal with conservative measures, but pain relief and return to athletic activity can be achieved. Patients should begin a dedicated period of rest and activity cessation, typically for 4 to 6 weeks. When pain is absent, physical therapy with an emphasis on lumbar core strengthening is begun. The patient should be progressed to sport-specific noncontact drills after 1 month followed by return to full participation in

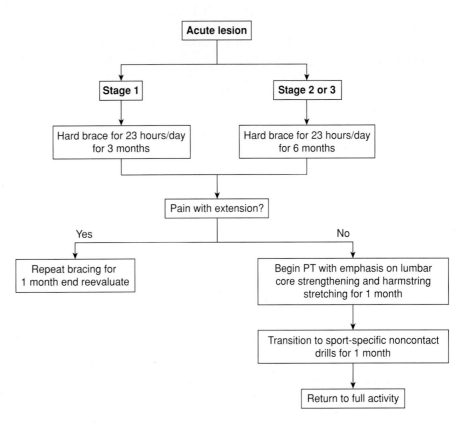

FIGURE 17-5 Treatment algorithm for acute pars lesions. PT = physical therapy.

sports. If during the course of treatment there is a recurrence of pain, activity should be restricted and a trial of bracing begun. The goal of bracing is to alleviate pain by limiting motion at the site of the spondylolysis. The brace should be worn for 3 months before beginning physical therapy and resuming the aforementioned protocol.

Surgical Intervention

Patients with persistent pain despite 6 months of conservative treatment, a neurologic deficit, or progressive worsening of a symptomatic spondylolisthesis are candidates for operative fixation. Direct repair of a pars defect is precluded if there is a grade 2 or higher spondylolisthesis, a dysplastic lamina, significant disk degeneration at the level of the lysis, or patient age older than 20 years.[15] Ivanic et al showed a higher pseudarthrosis rate and poorer clinical outcomes in patients older than the age of 20 years who underwent direct pars repair.[38] Various techniques have been described ranging from lag screw fixation and cerclage wiring to hybrid constructs combining pedicle screws and hooks. Regardless of the technique chosen, meticulous grafting of the pars defect and solid fixation are necessary for a successful postsurgical outcome. Although the data are limited, available studies examining RTP in athletes after a pars repair show favorable outcomes.[39-43] No consensus exists on when to return these athletes to sport, but most studies have athletes returning to full athletic activity 6 months after a pars repair.

Patients undergoing fusion to stabilize a spondylolisthesis typically have a longer rehabilitation period and can expect to return to athletic activity at approximately 12 months. Data on this subset of patients are even more limited than for those undergoing a pars repair. Rubery and Bradford's survey of the Scoliosis Research Society demonstrated that 51% to 56% of surgeons permitted return to contact sports, such as basketball and soccer, at 1 year after surgery regardless of slip grade.[44] The most important factors that influenced decision making on RTP were radiographic appearance and time from surgery. Football and hockey were placed into a separate category defined as collision sports in this study, and only 27% to 36% of surgeons allowed return at 1 year postoperatively. A total of 49% of surgeons surveyed recommended against or disallowed collision sports for low-grade slips, and 58% made the same recommendation for high-grade slips. The most common sports listed by surgeons disallowing patients to return to after fusion for spondylolisthesis were gymnastics, football, rugby, wrestling, weight lifting, skydiving, and bungee jumping.[44] Burnett et al published an article on their current practice paradigm of returning athletes to play that had been successfully used for more than 20 years at their institution.[45] The authors stated that after a lumbar fusion, athletes may return to contact sports when they are pain free and have no disabling neurologic deficit and when their radiographs demonstrate evidence of fusion. Any athlete requiring a repeated operation or additional spinal surgery at the spinal region was prohibited from returning to contact sports[45] (Figure 17-6).

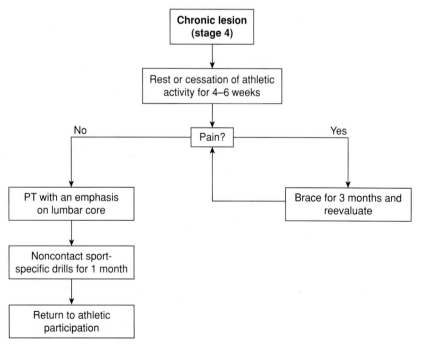

FIGURE 17-6 Treatment algorithm for chronic pars lesions.

Surgeons must examine the unique requirements of each athlete: the nature of their injury, the requirements of the sport, and the type of surgery required to address the pathology. No level 1 studies exist to facilitate these decisions, but a skilled clinician should be able to formulate a treatment plan based on the available data that gives the athlete the best chance of returning to his or her preinjury level of athletic participation.

REFERENCES

1. Muschik M, Hahnel H, Robinson PN, et al: Competitive sports and the progression of spondylolisthesis. *J Pediatr Orthop* 1996;16:364–369.

2. Recknagel S, Witte H: Landing after jumps: Wrong technique promotes spondylolysis. *Z Orthop Ihre Grenzgeb* 1996;134:214–218.

3. Daniels JM, Pontius G, El-Amin S, Gabriel K: Evaluation of low back pain in athletes. *Sports Health* 2011;3(4):336–345.

4. Micheli LJ, Wood R: Back pain in young athletes. Significant differences from adults in causes and patterns. *Arch Pediatr Adolesc Med* 1995;149:15–18.

5. Beutler W, Fredrickson BE, Murtlan A, et al: The natural history of spondylolysis and spondylolisthesis—45 year follow up evaluation. *Spine* 2003;28:1027–1035.

6. Rossi F: Spondylolysis, spondylolisthesis and sports. *J Sports Med Phys Fitness* 1978;18:317–340.

7. Wiltse L, Cirincione R: Spondylolysis in the female gymnast. *Clin Orthop Relat Res* 1976;117:68–74.

8. Soler T, Calderon C: The prevalence of spondylolysis in the Spanish elite athlete. *Am J Sports Med* 2000;28:57–62.

9. Jackson DW: Low back pain in young athletes: Evaluation of stress reaction and discogenic problems. *Am J Sports Med* 1979;7:364–366.

10. McCarroll JR, Miller JM, Ritter MA: Lumbar spondylolysis and spondylolisthesis in college football players. A prospective study. *Am J Sports Med* 1986;14:404–406.

11. Farfan HF, Osteria V, Lamy C: The mechanical etiology of spondylolysis and spondylolisthesis. *Clin Orthop Relat Res* 1976;117:40–55.

12. Kocher MS, Andersen J: Injuries and conditions of the adolescent athlete, in Fischgrund J, ed: *Orthopaedic Knowledge Update 8*. Rosemont IL, American Academy of Orthopaedic Surgeons, 2008.

13. Wiltse LL, Widell EH, Jackson DW: Fatigue fracture: the basic lesion in isthmic spondylolisthesis. *J Bone Joint Surg Am* 1975;57(1):17–22.

14. Sys J, Michielsen J, Bracke P, et al: Nonoperative treatment of active spondylolysis in elite athletes with normal x-ray findings: Literature review and results of conservative treatment. *Eur Spine J* 2001;10:498–504.

15. Dunn IF, Proctor MR, Day AL: Lumbar spine injuries in athletes. *Neurosurg Focus* 2006;21:1–5.

16. Hunter JS, Guin PD, Theiss SM: Acute lumbar spondylolysis in intercollegiate athletes. *J Spinal Disord Tech* 2012;25:422–425.

17. el Rassi G, Takemitsu M, Woratanarat P, Shah SA: Lumbar spondylolysis in pediatric and adolescent soccer players. *Am J Sports Med* 2005;33:1688-1693.

18. Friberg S: Studies on spondylolisthesis. *Acta Chir Scan* 1939;(suppl):55.

19. Kobayashi A, Kobayashi T, Kato K, Higuchi H, Takagishi K: diagnosis of radiographically occult lumbar spondylolysis in young athletes by magnetic resonance imaging. *Am J Sports Med* 2013;41:169–176.

20. Sundell CG, Jonsson H, Ådin L, Larsén KH: Clinical examination, spondylosis and adolescent athletes. *Int J Sports Med* 2013;34:263–267.

21. Dunn AJ, Campbell RS, Mayor PE, Rees D: Radiological findings and healing patterns of incomplete stress fractures of the pars interarticularis. *Skeletal Radiol* 2008;37:443–450.

22. Foreman P, Griessenauer C, Watanabe K, et al: L5 Spondylosis/spondylolisthesis: A comprehensive review with an anatomic focus. *Childs Nerv Sys* 2013;29:209–226.

23. Amato M, Totty WG, Gilula LA: Spondylolysis of the lunar spine: Demonstration of defects and laminal fragmentation. *Radiology* 1984;153(3):627–629.

24. Libson E, Bloom RA, Dinari G, Robin GC: Oblique lumbar spine radiographs: Importance in young patients. *Radiology* 1984;151(1):89–90.

25. Beck NA, Miller R, Baldwin K, et al: Do oblique views add value in the diagnosis of spondylosis in adolescents? *J Bone Joint Surg Am* 2013;95:e65(1–7).

26. Hollenberg GM, Beattie PF, Meyers SP, et al: Stress reactions of the lumbar pars interarticularis: The development of a new MRI classification system. *Spine* 2002;27:181–186.

27. Sairyo K, Katoh S, Takata Y, et al: MRI signal changes of the pedicle as an indicator for early diagnosis of spondylolysis in children and adolescents: A clinical and biomechanical study. *Spine* 2006;31:206–211.

28. Sakai T, Sairyo K, Mima S, et al: Significance of magnetic resonance imaging signal change in the pedicle in the management of pediatric lumbar spondylolysis. *Spine* 2010;14:641–645.

29. Masci L, Pike J, Malara F, Phillips B, Bennell K, Brukner P: Use of the one-legged hyperextension test and magnetic resonance imaging in the diagnosis of active spondylolysis. *Br J Sports Med* 2006;40:940–946.

30. Campbell RS, Grainger AJ, Hide IG, Papastefanou S, Greenough CG: Juvenile spondylosis: A comparative

analysis of CT, SPECT, and MRI. *Skeletal Radiol* 2005; 34:63–73.

31. Zukotynski K, Curtis C, Grant FD, Micheli L, Treves ST: The value of SPECT in the detection of stress injury to the pars interarticularis in patients with low back pain. *J Orthop Surg Res* 2010;5:13.

32. Papanicolaaou N, Wilkinson RH, Emans JB, Treves S, et al: Bone scintigraphy and radiography in young athletes with low back pain. *AJR Am J Roentgenol* 1985; 145:1039–1044.

33. Rush JK, Astur N, Scott S, et al: Use of magnetic resonance imaging in the evaluation of spondylolysis. *J Pediatric Orthop* 2015;35(3):271–275.

34. Leone A, Cianfoni A, Cerase A, et al: Lumbar spondylolysis: A review. *Skeletal Radiol* 2011;40:683–700.

35. Sairyo K, Sakai T, Yasui N, et al: Conservative treatment of pediatric lumbar spondylolysis to achieve bone healing using a hard brace: What type and how long? *J Neurosurg Spine* 2012;16:610–614.

36. Kurd MF, Patel D, Norton R, et al: Nonoperative treatment of symptomatic spondylolysis. *J Spinal Disord Tech* 2007;20:560–564.

37. Blanda J, Bethem D, Moats W, Lew M. Defects of pars interarticularis in athletes: A protocol for nonoperative treatment. *J Spinal Disord* 1993;6(5):406–411.

38. Ivanic GM, Pink TP, Achatz W, et al: Direct stabilization of lumbar spondylolysis with a hook screw: Mean 11-year follow-up period for 113 patients. *Spine* 2003;28: 255–259.

39. Brennan RP, Smucker PY, Horn EM: Minimally invasive image-guided direct repair of bilateral L-5 pars interarticularis defects. *Neurosurg Focus* 2008;25(2):E13.

40. Debnath UK, Freeman BJ, Gregory P, de la Harpe D, Kerslake RW, Webb JK: Clinical outcome and return to sport after the surgical treatment of spondylolysis in young athletes. *J Bone Surg Joint Br* 2003;85:244–249.

41. Hardcastle PH: Repair of spondylolysis in young fast bowlers. *J Surg Joint Bone Br* 1993;75:398–402.

42. Ranawat VS, Dowell JK, Heywood-Waddington MB: Stress fractures of the lumbar pars interarticularis in athletes: A review based on long-term results of 18 professional cricketers. *Injury* 2003;34:915–919.

43. Reitman CA, Esses SI: Direct repair of spondylolytic defects in young competitive athletes. *Spine J* 2002;2: 142–144.

44. Rubery PT, Bradford DS: Athletic activity after spine surgery in children and adolescents: results of a survey. *Spine (Phila Pa 1976)* 2002;27(4):423–427.

45. Burnett MG, Sonntag VK: Return to contact sports after spinal surgery. *Neurosurg Focus* 2006;21(4):E5.

18 Lumbar Disk Herniation in Immature and Adult Athletes

Tyler J. Jenkins, MD • Wellington Hsu, MD

INTRODUCTION

The prevalence of back pain can be as high as 30% in competitive athletes.[1,2] Lumbar disk herniation (LDH) should be considered when an athlete is presenting for evaluation of radiating leg or back pain.[3] Athletes may be predisposed to a higher incidence of LDH than the general population because of the rigorous demands of their sports.[4] Although extensively studied in the general population, the evaluation and management of LDH in this patient population is still evolving. This chapter highlights the pathoanatomy, clinical evaluation, and management of LDH in athletes using the best literature available to date.

PATHOANATOMY

Lumbar disk herniations occur when the gel-like nucleus pulposus ruptures through the fibrous outer annulus, causing a displacement of disk contents beyond the circumferential border of the intervertebral disk. Because of the relative weakness of the posterior longitudinal ligament (PLL) at the posterolateral disk space, herniations occur most commonly at this location.[5,6] The disk herniation then leads to irritation of an adjacent nerve root.

Disk herniations vary considerably, and the terminology associated with LDH has also evolved over time. Disk bulges are ubiquitous throughout the population and are commonly seen in MRIs of asymptomatic patients.[7,8] Asymptomatic herniations discovered with the increased use of advanced imaging have led to a paradigm shift in the nomenclature associated with LDH. LDH today primarily describes symptomatic pathology and not the common disk bulge.[5]

After childhood development, intervertebral disks receive a limited nutrient supply via diffusion through vertebral vasculature.[5,6] The inherent avascularity allows the accumulation of irreparable disk degeneration over time.[5,6] Recurrent torsional strain causes fissure development in the outer annulus, combined with increased intradiscal pressure from axial loading and forward flexion, can culminate in the herniation of the nucleus pulposus.[5,6] The lumbosacral spine is particularly susceptible to herniation because of its mobility in flexion, extension, and torsion.[9]

The most clinically relevant LDH classifications describe the location and anatomic characteristics of the fragment. The anatomic location describes the disk fragment relationship to the thecal sac and includes central, posterolateral (paracentral), foraminal, and extraforaminal (i.e., far lateral) (**Figure 18-1**).[5] Anatomic descriptions of LDH can include protrusions, extrusions, and sequestrations. Another important factor to consider when describing a LDH is the size of the annular defect. A larger annular defect is associated with a higher risk of recurrent LDH after lumbar discectomy.[10]

Symptoms associated with LDH occur secondary to nerve root irritation. The nerve root irritation is initiated

Dr. Hsu or an immediate family member has received royalties from Stryker; is a member of a speakers' bureau or has made paid presentations on behalf of AONA; serves as a paid consultant to AONA, Bacterin, Bioventus, CeramTec, Globus, Graftys, Lifenet, Medtronic Sofamor Danek, Relievant, Rti, SI Bone, and Stryker; has received research or institutional support from Medtronic; and serves as a board member, owner, officer, or committee member of the AAOS, the Cervical Spine Research Society, the Journal of Spinal Disorders and Techniques, the Lumbar Spine Research Society, and the North American Spine Society. Neither Dr. Jenkins nor any immediate family member has received anything of value from or has stock or stock options held in a commercial company or institution related directly or indirectly to the subject of this article.

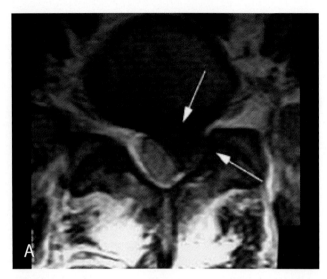 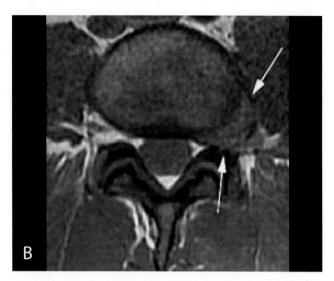

FIGURE 18-1 L4 to L5 lumbar disk herniation. **A,** Axial T2-weighted MRI illustrating a common posterolateral L4 to L5 herniation. The patient presented with a L5 radiculopathy caused by irritation of the traversing L5 nerve root. **B,** Axial T1-weighted MRI illustrating a far-lateral L4 to L5 herniation. The patient presented with L4 radiculopathy caused by irritation of the exiting L4 nerve root. (Reprinted from Hsu WK: Lumbar degenerative disease, in: *Orthopaedic Knowledge Update, Update 10.* Rosemont, IL: American Academy of Orthopaedic Surgeons, 2011.)

by two intertwined pathways: chemical inflammation and mechanical compression. Many studies have looked at which pathway is the predominate factor in symptomatology, but they are inconclusive to date.[11–15] Nucleus pulposus extracts have been shown to set off an inflammatory cascade when exposed to nerve roots, causing the release of several cytokines.[11–14] This inflammatory cascade leads to priming of the nerve root and secondary hypersensitivity from mechanical compression, which in turn cases local ischemia and irritation, further propagating the cascade.[5,11–15] The cytokines most prevalent in this inflammation cycle include tumor necrosis factor alpha, osteoprotegerin, interleukin-6, prostaglandin E_2, and phospholipase A2.

● CLINICAL PRESENTATION

Lumbar disk herniations classically result in dermatomal radicular pain with patients complaining of pain, paresthesias, and weakness of the lower extremities. The unique pattern of pain experienced by the patient depends on the level and location of the herniation. Up to 95% of LDHs occur at the L4 to L5 and L5 to S1 levels.[16,17] Axial back pain and sclerotomal pain are also commonly present. These symptoms of low back, buttock, and posterior thigh pain occur secondary to irritation of local mesodermal tissue (i.e., muscle and ligaments) and can also indicate dorsal rami involvement.

Evaluation of the athlete presenting with a combination of leg and back pain should include a broad differential diagnosis. Evaluation of common lower extremity sports injuries should be excluded, including primary hip pathology, knee pathology, muscle sprains, and ligament tears. Common back injuries that athletes present with include muscle strains, aggravation of degenerative disk disease, and spondylolysis.[18] The predominance of leg pain over back pain, dermatomal distribution of pain, and pain that increases with Valsalva maneuver and forward flexion are more specific signs for LDH.[19,20]

Complete neurologic evaluation should be performed on all patients, including sensation, muscle strength, and reflex testing. Abnormal sensation in a dermatomal pattern, muscle weakness, and decreased reflexes are all associated with LDH (**Table 18-1**). A positive ipsilateral straight-leg raise (SLR) result is sensitive but not specific for LDH; a positive contralateral SLR test result is more specific but less sensitive.[19,20] For herniations affecting the L1 to L4 nerve roots, the femoral-nerve stretch test may alternatively be used. A reproduction of anterior thigh radiculopathy is a positive test result.

Evaluation should also exclude the two surgical urgencies associated with LDH: cauda equina and conus medullaris syndrome. Both conditions cause saddle anesthesia, autonomic nervous system dysfunction (i.e., overflow incontinence, impotence), and leg pain. Concern for either diagnosis should lead to prompt advanced imaging. The urgency of these two conditions is largely justified by the poor outcomes seen with delays in surgical decompression.[21]

TABLE 18-1	Findings in lumbar disk herniations			
Level	**Nerve Root**	**Sensory Loss**	**Motor Loss**	**Reflex Loss**
L1–L3	L2, L3	Anterior thigh	Hip flexors	None
L3–L4	L4	Medial calf Medial foot	Quadriceps Tibialis anterior	Patellar
L4–L5	L5	Lateral calf Dorsum of foot	Extensor digitorum longus Extensor hallucis longus	None
L5–S1	S1	Posterior calf Plantar foot	Gastrocnemius	Ankle
S2–S4	S2, S3, S4	Perianal	Bowel and bladder	Cremasteric

⬤ CASE PRESENTATION 1 (FIGURE 18-2)

Imaging

Plain radiographs of the lumbosacral spine can rule out associated pathology in athletes presenting with radicular pain.[22] Nonspecific findings such as loss of disk height, loss of lumbar lordosis, and vacuum phenomena can identify preexisting conditions.[5,22] A noncontrast MRI scan allows for unparalleled evaluation of nerve roots and soft tissues.[23] The high rate of asymptomatic LDH illustrates the importance of correlating presenting symptoms and physical examination findings to the pathology observed on MRI.[7,24] If MRI is contraindicated, then a CT myelogram may be performed to visualize neural element compression.[5,23]

In more complex cases, intervertebral disk avascularity may be used to distinguish pathologies. Intravenous contrast in conjunction with MRI or CT myelogram will cause enhancement in vascular structures. In patients with recurrent radiculopathy after operative treatment, MRI with contrast can help distinguish a recurrent disk herniation (no enhancement) with postsurgical scar tissue (enhancement). Contrast can also be used to illustrate rare causes of nerve compression such as tumors and vascular malformations.[4,21]

Management

Nonoperative Treatment

The natural history of LDH is favorable for the general population with more than 90% of patients improving

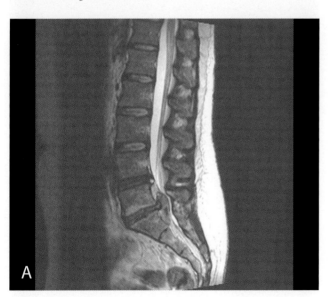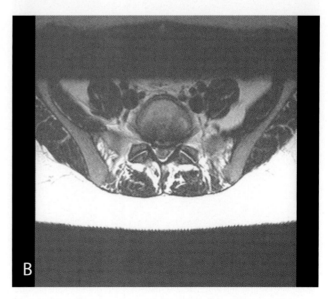

FIGURE 18-2 Case presentation 1. A 31-year-old active woman with no significant medical history presented to the emergency department (ED) with a 2-day history of severe low back pain and left buttock numbness after a run. After performing a cycling class the next day, she developed vaginal numbness and had an episode of fecal incontinence, which prompted her visit to the ED. Physical examination reveals decreased perianal sensation, absent rectal tone, but 5 of 5 strength in the lower extremity muscle bilaterally. MRI without contrast was performed. Sagittal (**A**) and axial (**B**) T2-weighted MRI demonstrated a large L5 to S1 disk extrusion. She was taken urgently to the operating room for laminotomy and diskectomy. Follow-up showed a resolution of the bowel incontinence and radicular pain. Saddle anesthesia was still present but improving.

within 6 weeks of symptom onset after conservative treatment.[25] Professional athletes of basketball, American football, baseball, and hockey treated for LDH are able to return to their sport 82% of the time.[4] Conservative treatment options focuses on early mobilization, psychological support, anti-inflammatory medications, physical therapy, and epidural steroid injections. None of these conservative measures alters the natural history of LDH symptoms but instead provides symptom relief while radiculopathy resolves naturally.

Psychological support can be provided by explaining the natural history and favorable prognosis of LDH symptoms. Setting an expectation for recovery and reaffirming the rehabilitation process has proven beneficial.[5] Anti-inflammatory medications can provide relief by decreasing the production of inflammatory cytokines. Although oral corticosteroids have long been advocated to treat acute radiculopathy, there may be no benefit over placebo from a recent randomized clinical trial.[26] However, oral steroids may be effective agents in helping the acute symptoms of radicular pain. They are far less effective for athlete's with axial back pain as the only symptom. Management with narcotics is reserved for patients with severe pain that limits patient mobilization. The potential for abuse must be weighed by the treating physician.

Physical therapy is also commonly prescribed during the conservative management of LDH.[27,28] Therapy regimens mainly focus on core strengthening, back muscle strengthening, and flexibility. A phased rehabilitation protocol for athletes with LDH has been described that correlates with the natural history of disk herniation resolution.[29] Specifically, movements that increase intradiscal pressure (rotation and flexion) are gradually incorporated into the routine as symptoms regress.[29]

Epidural steroid injections (ESIs) provide an alternative to surgical treatment for patients with severe symptoms. The temporary symptom improvement can be experienced for months in certain patients[30] and may avoid surgery in up to 50% of cases.[31] A study of National Football League (NFL) athletes with LDH treated with ESI showed a return to play (RTP) rate of 89% and an average loss of only 0.6 games played.[32]

● CASE PRESENTATION 2 (FIGURE 18-3)
Operative Treatment

Laminotomy combined with diskectomy is the surgical treatment of choice for LDH. Clinical outcomes after LDH in the general population are excellent with a 90% satisfaction rate and 75% return-to-work rate.[31,33] Extrapolating these data to high-level athletes is more

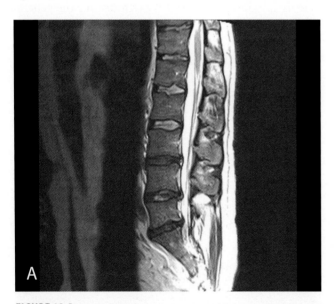
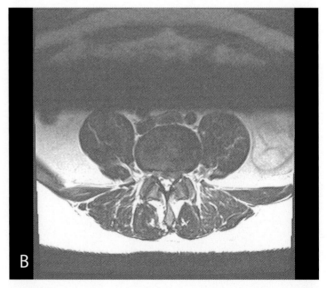

FIGURE 18-3 Case presentation 2. A 33-year-old man, cross-fit athlete, presented to clinic with 2 weeks of left lower extremity pain. The pain was worse with sitting and with Valsalva maneuver. His primary care provider gave him a Medrol dose pack, which failed to relieve his pain. He has started physical therapy but states that he cannot work with his current pain. Physical examination reveals 4 of 5 strength with left foot dorsiflexion and pain radiating to the dorsum of his left foot. He has a positive ipsilateral and contralateral straight-leg raise. Sagittal (**A**) and axial (**B**) T2-weighted MRI illustrate a posterolateral disk protrusion at the left L4-5 lateral recess compressing the L5 nerve root. Note that other disk bulges seen on sagittal MRI do not correlate with his presentation. The patient was prescribed an epidural steroid injection and had near resolution of his symptoms at follow-up 2 weeks later. After demonstration of pain-free full range of motion of his lumbar spine, resolution of his neurologic deficit, and elimination of pain, he returned to his cross-fit regimen.

difficult because of the physical demands and schedule restraints of their sports. When considering operative treatment in athletes, the treating physician must consider the unique situations specific to each case. Minimally invasive techniques may provide a quicker return to sport, but no studies have shown this to date.

A systematic review of the literature revealed that on average, 75% to 100% of athletes successfully returned to play after lumbar diskectomy.[34] RTP after diskectomy on average ranged from 2.8 to 8.7 months. Athletes that successfully returned to play had career longevity that ranged from 2.6 to 4.8 years.[34] The Professional Athlete Spine Initiative concluded that there were no differences in RTP, career games, and years played after operative or conservative management in players of all sports. Performance-based outcomes were better in younger and more experienced athletes. Watkins et al published the largest single series of professional athletes treated with lumbar microdiskectomy for symptomatic LDH by a single surgeon.[35] Professional athletes from this study were able to RTP after microdiskectomy in 89% of cases, with 72% returning to play by 6 months.[35] A recent meta-analysis assessing elite athletes' RTP after microdiskectomy for symptomatic LDH included 558 athletes.[36] This study showed that elite athletes were able to RTP 83.5% of the time after undergoing a single-level lumbar microdiskectomy.[36] Furthermore, the meta-analysis showed no difference in RTP rates between lumbar microdiskectomy and nonoperative treatment, suggesting that a more aggressive approach to treatment may be used to benefit timing for an athletic season.[36]

The inherent difference in specific sports and positions should also be considered when treating athletes. Linemen in American football have a higher perceived risk for LDH because of the flexion and axial loads experienced by their spines due to the nature of the position. A cohort study demonstrated that surgical treatment for LDH in NFL linemen yielded a higher rate of RTP (80.8%) than their nonoperative cohort (28.6%).[36] Of note, 13.5% (7 of 52) of the surgically treated linemen required revision decompression with 85.7% of these reoperations (6 of 7) successfully returning to play.[37] Similar results have been reported in National Hockey League athletes with 82.1% returning after LDH with no differences in RTP games played, or statistical performance between operatively and conservatively treated cohorts.[38]

Notably, professional baseball players appear to demonstrate a different course compared with athletes of other sports. Baseball athletes have significantly longer recovery times (8.7 months vs. 3.6 months) after

operative treatment for LDH compared with nonoperative cohorts.[38] Furthermore, career length after LDH was shorter in operative versus conservative cohorts (233 vs. 342 games, respectively; $P = 0.08$).[39] One potential explanation for these differences is the daily rotational torque demands from throwing and hitting that are unique to this sport. In a biomechanical study using reflective motion markers, axial rotation values for both pitchers and batters exceeded 45° per motion, which translates to at least 1.5° per lumbar disk level.[40]

Postoperative rehabilitation focusing on a stepwise protocol of primarily trunk strengthening can improve recovery time.[41,42] Studies have shown that a more vigorous and intense postoperative therapy can reduce disability and pain while increasing outcome measures.[41,42] The athlete's commitment to rehabilitation is as critical as the surgery itself if not more so. RTP criteria vary widely throughout the literature and should be individualized to the athlete, injury, and sport. Generally, athletes must demonstrate resolution of preoperative symptoms, regain full range of motion, and successfully complete a structured rehabilitation program before returning to play.[43]

● CASE PRESENTATION 3 (FIGURE 18-4)
Central Disk Herniation

Although LDH is typically associated with a clinical presentation of radicular symptoms, a large central disk herniation can produce a variation in presentation. In this scenario, athletes may present with only axial back pain. These patients have unique challenges for the treating physician because discogenic pain has an unpredictable natural history. Nonoperative therapy should be the mainstay of treatment, and many physical therapy protocols exist for long-term axial back pain treatment in athletes. The combination of core strengthening, lumbar mobilization, and biopsychosocial support yields good outcomes.[44]

Operative treatment for the management of axial back pain in athletes with a central disk herniation should be used only in very select patients who have failed conservative management and cannot return to sport. Strict criteria would include mechanical low back pain with evidence of a single-level degenerative disk on imaging studies, failure of at least 12 months of nonoperative treatment, and localized midline spinal tenderness that corresponds to the radiographic level of disease. Narcotic abuse, smoking, and unrealistic patient expectations are relative contraindications to operative treatment. Even with selective indications, RTP at preoperative

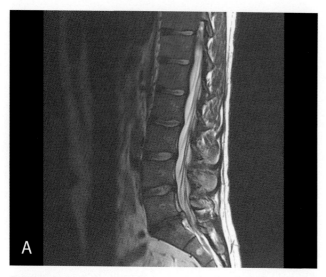
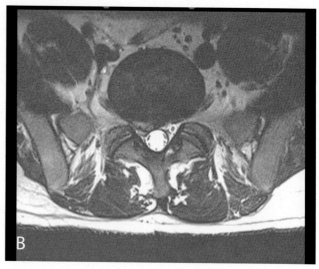

FIGURE 18-4 Case presentation 3. A 21-year-old collegiate wrestler presented to the clinic with 2 months of right lower extremity radicular symptoms. He stated that his team physician has prescribed him two Medrol dose pack courses, physical therapy, and an epidural steroid injection. His symptoms prevented him from training. He is 6 months from starting his last collegiate season. On physical examination, he has decreased sensation on the plantar aspect of his right foot but 5 of 5 muscle strength in all lower extremity muscles. T2-weighted sagittal (**A**) and axial (**B**) MRI demonstrates a right-sided L5 to S1 posterolateral disk protrusion compressing the right S1 nerve root. Because of the timing of the season and inability to train with failure of conservative treatment, the patient underwent L5 to S1 microdiscectomy. He was able to return for his final collegiate season after completing formalized physical therapy and demonstrating pain-free full range of motion of his lumbar spine.

performance levels after operative treatment of axial back pain is unpredictable at best.

Few studies have investigated the outcomes after operative treatment of axial back pain in athletes. The outcomes of eight professional hockey players who underwent single-level fusion for lumbar disk herniation was reported by Schroeder and coworkers.[45] All eight players returned to play and were still active after 4 years. The study also showed no significant difference in number of games played per season or performance scores before or after the procedure, but the authors did note their small sample size made conclusions difficult.[45] In another study, Schroeder and associates reported on two NFL players with productive careers despite undergoing lumbar fusion.[46] Further studies are needed to identify the appropriate indications and long-term outcomes of operatively treated axial back pain in elite athletes; however, the current literature does illustrate that lumbar fusion is not necessarily a contraindication to RTP.

CASE PRESENTATION 4 (FIGURE 18-5)
Adolescent Lumbar Herniation

Lumbar disk herniation is a rare condition in the pediatric and adolescent population.[47] The diagnosis should be considered in any child presenting with back and radiating

leg pain. A delay in diagnosis is common because the diagnosis is often not considered by treating physicians. Disk herniations in this population are often not amenable to conservative treatment, but a trial of nonoperative treatment should still be attempted.[48] Laminotomy and sequestrectomy is again the treatment of choice in patients who fail conservative treatment.[47] Ninety percent of pediatric patients have excellent outcomes defined by minimal or no pain 1 year postoperatively.[48] However, long-term data predict that only 80% of surgically treated pediatric patients will be able to avoid additional surgery at 10 years.[49]

CONCLUSION

The diagnosis of LDH should be considered in athletes presenting with a combination of leg and back pain. Symptoms are due to nerve root irritation from the herniated nucleus pulposus expanding beyond the circumferential border of the intervertebral disk space. The natural history of LDH is favorable with most athletes experiencing an improvement of symptoms within 6 weeks. Conservative treatment should be the mainstay of initial management using anti-inflammatory medications, physical therapy, and epidural steroid injections. In athletes who fail to improve with conservative measures or present with a progressive neurologic deficit, surgical

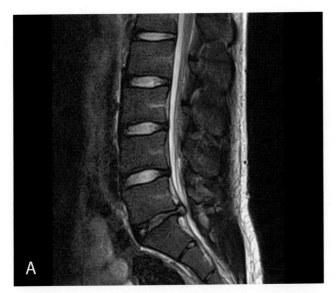
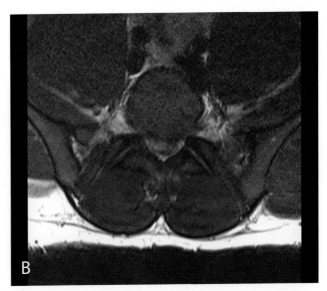

FIGURE 18-5 Case presentation 4. A 19-year-old collegiate basketball player presented to the clinic with 2 weeks of acute-onset low back pain. He stated that his symptoms were limiting him from peak performance. On physical examination, he had midline spinal tenderness that was worse with axial loading. He had 5 of 5 muscle strength throughout his lower extremities with no evidence of radicular pain. **A,** Radiographs of the lumbar spine showed early disk degenerative changes at L5 to S1. He was managed conservatively for 1 month with no improvement in symptoms. **B,** MRI of the lumbar spine showed a large central disk herniation at L5 to S1 with degenerative disk changes. He was managed conservatively with aggressive physical therapy and had near-full resolution of symptoms 4 months after his initial presentation.

treatment is a viable option. Studies of professional athletes demonstrate that athletes who require surgical management can have favorable outcomes compared with their conservatively managed peers. RTP should be assessed on a case-by-case basis with the athlete demonstrating a resolution of symptoms, full range of motion, and successful completion of a rehabilitation program before return.

REFERENCES

1. Clinical Standards Advisory Group: *Back Pain and Epidemiology Review: The Epidemiology and Cost of Back Pain.* London:, Her Majesty's Stationary Office, 1994.

2. Dreisinger TE, Nelson B: Management of back pain in athletes. *Sports Med* 1996;21(4):313–320.

3. Baker RJ, Patel D: Lower back pain in the athlete: Common conditions and treatment. *Primary Care* 2005; 32(1):201–229.

4. Hsu WK, McCarthy KJ, Savage JW, et al: The Professional Athlete Spine Initiative: Outcomes after lumbar disc herniation in 342 elite professional athletes. *Spine J* 2011;11(3):180–186.

5. Herkowitz HN, International Society for Study of the Lumbar Spine: *The Lumbar Spine,* ed 3. Philadelphia, PA, Lippincott Williams & Wilkins, 2004.

6. Herkowitz HN, Rothman RH, Simeone FA: *Rothman-Simeone, The Spine,* ed 5. Philadelphia, Saunders Elsevier, 2006.

7. Boos N, Rieder R, Schade V, Spratt KF, Semmer N, Aebi M: 1995 Volvo Award in clinical sciences. The diagnostic accuracy of magnetic resonance imaging, work perception, and psychosocial factors in identifying symptomatic disc herniations. *Spine* 1995;20(24):2613–2625.

8. Fraser RD, Sandhu A, Gogan WJ: Magnetic resonance imaging findings 10 years after treatment for lumbar disc herniation. *Spine* 1995;20(6):710–714.

9. Weinstein PR: *Anatomy of the Lumbar Spine,* ed 2. New York, Raven Press, 1993.

10. McGirt MJ, Eustacchio S, Varga P, et al: A prospective cohort study of close interval computed tomography and magnetic resonance imaging after primary lumbar discectomy: factors associated with recurrent disc herniation and disc height loss. *Spine* 2009;34(19):2044–2051.

11. Brisby H, Olmarker K, Larsson K, Nutu M, Rydevik B: Proinflammatory cytokines in cerebrospinal fluid and serum in patients with disc herniation and sciatica. *Eur Spine J* 2002;11(1):62–66.

12. Nishimura K, Mochida J: Percutaneous reinsertion of the nucleus pulposus. An experimental study. *Spine* 1998;23(14):1531–1538; discussion 1539.

13. Olmarker K, Brisby H, Yabuki S, Nordborg C, Rydevik B: The effects of normal, frozen, and hyaluronidase-digested nucleus pulposus on nerve root structure and function. *Spine* 1997;22(5):471–475; discussion 476.

14. Olmarker K, Rydevik B: Selective inhibition of tumor necrosis factor-alpha prevents nucleus pulposus-induced thrombus formation, intraneural edema, and reduction of nerve conduction velocity: possible implications for future pharmacologic treatment strategies of sciatica. *Spine* 2001;26(8):863–869.

15. Yabuki S, Kikuchi S, Olmarker K, Myers RR: Acute effects of nucleus pulposus on blood flow and endoneurial fluid pressure in rat dorsal root ganglia. *Spine* 1998;23(23):2517–2523.

16. Deyo RA, Weinstein JN: Low back pain. *N Engl J Med* 2001;344(5):363–370.

17. Weinstein JN, Lurie JD, Tosteson TD, et al: Surgical versus nonoperative treatment for lumbar disc herniation: Four-year results for the Spine Patient Outcomes Research Trial (SPORT). *Spine* 2008;33(25):2789–2800.

18. d'Hemecourt PA, Gerbino PG, 2nd, Micheli LJ: Back injuries in the young athlete. *Clin Sports Med* 2000; 19(4):663–679.

19. Andersson GB, Deyo RA: History and physical examination in patients with herniated lumbar discs. *Spine* 1996;21(24 suppl):10S–18S.

20. Gregory DS, Seto CK, Wortley GC, Shugart CM: Acute lumbar disk pain: Navigating evaluation and treatment choices. *Am Fam Physician* 2008;78(7):835–842.

21. Srikandarajah N1 Boissaud-Cooke MA, Clark S, Wilby MJ: Does early surgical decompression in cauda equina syndrome improve bladder outcome? *Spine* 2015; 40(8):580–583.

22. Scientific approach to the assessment and management of activity-related spinal disorders. A monograph for clinicians. Report of the Quebec Task Force on Spinal Disorders. *Spine* 1987;12(7 suppl):S1–S59.

23. Jarvik JG, Deyo RA: Diagnostic evaluation of low back pain with emphasis on imaging. *Ann Intern Med* 2002;137(7):586–597.

24. Jensen MC, Brant-Zawadzki MN, Obuchowski N, Modic MT, Malkasian D, Ross JS: Magnetic resonance imaging of the lumbar spine in people without back pain. *N Engl J Med* 1994;331(2):69–73.

25. Lively MW, Bailes JE Jr: Acute lumbar disk injuries in active patients: making optimal management decisions. *Phys Sportsmed* 2005;33(4):21–27.

26. Goldberg H, Firtch W, Tyburski M, et al: Oral steroids for acute radiculopathy due to a herniated lumbar disk: A randomized clinical trial. *JAMA* 2015;313(19): 1915–1923.

27. Luijsterburg PA, Verhagen AP, Ostelo RW, van Os TA, Peul WC, Koes BW: Effectiveness of conservative treatments for the lumbosacral radicular syndrome: A systematic review. *Eur Spine J* 2007;16(7):881–899.

28. Luijsterburg PA, Lamers LM, Verhagen AP, et al: Cost-effectiveness of physical therapy and general practitioner care for sciatica. *Spine* 2007;32(18):1942–1948.

29. Vangelder LH, Hoogenboom BJ, Vaughn DW: A phased rehabilitation protocol for athletes with lumbar intervertebral disc herniation. *Int J Sports Phys Ther* 2013; 8(4):482–516.

30. Pinto RZ, Maher CG, Ferreira ML, et al: Epidural corticosteroid injections in the management of sciatica: a systematic review and meta-analysis. *Ann Intern Med* 2012;157(12):865–877.

31. Buttermann GR: Treatment of lumbar disc herniation: Epidural steroid injection compared with discectomy. A prospective, randomized study. *J Bone Joint Surg Am* 2004;86-A(4):670–679.

32. Krych AJ, Richman D, Drakos M, et al: Epidural steroid injection for lumbar disc herniation in NFL athletes. *Med Sci Sports Exerc* 2012;44(2):193–198.

33. Weinstein JN, Lurie JD, Tosteson TD, et al: Surgical vs nonoperative treatment for lumbar disk herniation: The Spine Patient Outcomes Research Trial (SPORT) observational cohort. *JAMA* 2006;296(20):2451–2459.

34. Nair R, Kahlenberg CA, Hsu WK: Outcomes of lumbar discectomy in elite athletes: The need for high-level evidence. *Clin Orthop Relat Res* 2015;473(6):1971–1977.

35. Watkins RG, Hanna R, Chang D, Watkins RG: Return-to-play outcomes after microscopic lumbar diskectomy in professional athletes. *Am J Sports Med* 2012;40(11): 2530–2535.

36. Overley SC, McAnany SJ, Andelman S, et al: Return to play in elite athletes after lumbar microdiskectomy: A meta-analysis. *Spine (Phila Pa 1976)* 2016;41(8):713–718.

37. Weistroffer JK, Hsu WK: Return-to-play rates in National Football League linemen after treatment for lumbar disk herniation. *Am J Sports Med* 2011;39(3):632–636.

38. Schroeder GD, McCarthy KJ, Micev AJ, Terry MA, Hsu WK: Performance-based outcomes after nonoperative treatment, discectomy, and/or fusion for a lumbar disc herniation in National Hockey League athletes. *Am J Sports Med* 2013;41(11):2604–2608.

39. Earhart JS, Roberts D, Roc G, Gryzlo S, Hsu W: Effects of lumbar disk herniation on the careers of professional baseball players. *Orthopedics* 2012;35(1):43–49.

40. Fleisig GS, Hsu WK, Fortenbaugh D, Cordover A, Press JM: Trunk axial rotation in baseball pitching and batting. Sports biomechanics. *Sports Biomech* 2013; 12(4):324–333.

41. Danielsen JM, Johnsen R, Kibsgaard SK, Hellevik E: Early aggressive exercise for postoperative rehabilitation after discectomy. *Spine* 2000;25(8):1015–1020.

42. Manniche C, Skall HF, Braendholt L, et al: Clinical trial of postoperative dynamic back exercises after first lumbar discectomy. *Spine* 1993;18(1):92–97.

43. Li Y, Hresko MT: Lumbar spine surgery in athletes: Outcomes and return-to-play criteria. *Clin Sports Med* 2012;31(3):487–498.

44. Stuber KJ, Bruno P, Sajko S, Hayden JA: Core stability exercises for low back pain in athletes: A systematic review of the literature. *Clin J Sport Med* 2014;24(6):448–456.

45. Schroeder GD, McCarthy KJ, Micev AJ, Terry MA, Hsu WK: Performance-based outcomes after nonoperative treatment, discectomy, and/or fusion for a lumbar disc herniation in National Hockey League athletes. *Am J Sports Med* 2013;41(11):2604–2608.

46. Schroeder GD, Lynch TS, Gibbs DB, et al: Pre-existing lumbar spine diagnosis as a predictor of outcomes in National Football League athletes. *Am J Sports Med* 2015; 43(4):972–978.

47. Lavelle WF, Bianco A, Mason R, Betz RR, Albanese SA: Pediatric disk herniation. *J Am Acad Orthop Surg* 2011; 19(11):649–656.

48. Kumar R, Kumar V, Das NK, Behari S, Mahapatra AK: Adolescent lumbar disc disease: Findings and outcome. *Childs Nerv Syst* 2007;23(11):1295–1299.

49. Papagelopoulos PJ, Shaughnessy WJ, Ebersold MJ, Bianco AJ Jr, Quast LM: Long-term outcome of lumbar discectomy in children and adolescents sixteen years of age or younger. *J Bone Joint Surg Am* 1998;80(5):689–698.

19 Lumbar Degenerative Disk Disease and Spinal Stenosis in Athletes

Heath P. Gould, BS • Colin M. Haines, MD • William J. Kemp, MD • Timothy T. Roberts, MD • Thomas Mroz, MD

EPIDEMIOLOGY

Participation in sports is an independent risk factor for the development of lumbar disk degeneration at an early age.[1] Multiple studies have demonstrated that degenerative changes of the spine are more common in athletes than in nonathletes.[2-6] Furthermore, disk degeneration in athletes tends to be more severe than in nonathletes, with 58% of all degenerative disks in athletes being categorized as severely degenerated.[7] Much of the increased risk for lumbar disk degeneration in athletes can be attributed to the repetitive stress placed on their lumbar spines over extended periods. Athletes are routinely subject to supraphysiologic loads in positions not routinely experienced by the general population. Thus, these individuals are uniquely susceptible to lumbar disk degeneration, with L4 to L5 and L5 to S1 being the most commonly affected levels.[8,9] Still, the epidemiologic data comparing athletes with nonathletes must be cautiously interpreted. Whereas the general population may overreport pain and injury for various reasons, athletes have been shown to underreport symptoms.[10,11] Prevalence statistics in athletes may also be skewed by the "healthy worker effect," which is the phenomenon in which epidemiologic investigations typically study only the *active* athletes while neglecting to capture individuals who have ended participation because of injury.[12]

Both injury type and severity vary based on age in athletes.[13] Whereas the majority of lumbar injuries in adult athletes are related to muscle strain and diskogenic disease, 70% of lumbar injuries in adolescent athletes occur in the posterior elements. Micheli and Wood examined several possible causes of low back pain in 100 young athletes and 100 nonathlete adults.[13] Only 11 adolescent participants had low back pain attributable to degenerative disk disease compared with 48 adult participants. In the same study, no adolescents had low back pain attributable to spinal stenosis compared with 6 adults. Orchard et al later corroborated this finding when they reported a correlation between lumbosacral impingement of the L5 and S1 nerves and increasing athlete age.[14]

Sports involving repetitive hyperextension, axial loading or jumping, twisting, or direct contact are associated with a higher incidence of lumbar disk degeneration.[15,16] Gymnastics, in particular, has been strongly associated with degenerative changes of the lumbar spine. A landmark MRI study by Swärd et al showed a 75% prevalence of disk degeneration in male gymnasts compared with 31% in control participants.[17] Goldstein et al conducted a subsequent MRI study that further

Dr. Mroz or an immediate family member has received royalties from Stryker; is a member of a speakers' bureau or has made paid presentations on behalf of AO Spine; serves as a paid consultant to Ceramtec and Stryker; has stock or stock options held in Pearl Diver; and serves as a board member, owner, officer, or committee member of the AO Spine North America Education, NASS, and SpineLine. Dr. Roberts or an immediate family member has received nonincome support (such as equipment or services), commercially derived honoraria, or other non-research–related funding (such as paid travel) from McGraw-Hill Education. None of the following authors or any immediate family member has received anything of value from or has stock or stock options held in a commercial company or institution related directly or indirectly to the subject of this article: Mr. Gould, Dr. Haines, and Dr. Kemp.

stratified gymnasts into pre-elite, elite, and Olympic-level groups.[18] The study reported prevalence rates of lumbar spine abnormality as 9%, 43%, and 63%, respectively, suggesting that an increased level of competition may be associated with an increased risk of lumbar spine abnormality.

In addition to gymnastics, elite weight lifting has also been strongly associated with lumbar disk degeneration. MRI evidence of disk degeneration presents early in weight lifters, typically in the first decade in men and the second decade in women. By age 40 years, degenerative changes are present in 80% of male weight lifters and 65% of female weight lifters.[19] Weight lifters also claim the highest prevalence of degenerative disk changes from L1 to L3; soccer players have the highest prevalence of disk pathology from L4 to S1.[20]

Several groups have examined the effect of American football on the lumbar spine. Semon and Spengler reported axial back pain in 27% of American football players, including 50% of interior lineman.[21] In a biomechanical investigation, Gatt et al concluded that average loads to the lumbar spine during American football blocking maneuvers exceed the minimum threshold necessary to cause pathologic changes in the intervertebral disk.[22] With these studies in mind, Gerbino and d'Hemecourt conducted a review of the literature and definitively concluded that playing American football increases an athlete's risk of developing degenerative changes in the lumbar spine.[23]

In addition, other sports associated with increased prevalence of lumbar disk degeneration include waterski jumping, golf, tennis, and diving.[2,24–26] In contrast, dancing and distance running have been associated with a lower prevalence of lumbar disk degeneration compared with control participants.[12,27]

● DISK PATHOLOGY

Mechanism of Disk Degeneration

The process of intervertebral disk degeneration occurs gradually and varies widely in severity (**Figures 19-1 to 19-3**). Initially, the inner layers of the disk begin to weaken and separate. This can produce a concentric annular tear that places increased stress on the outer layers. Under this increased stress, the outer layers may separate and create a radial tear of the intervertebral disk. When the outer layers tear, the nerve endings in these layers may convert nociceptive input into discogenic back pain. The inner layers then separate with portions of the nucleus pulposus. Subsequent axial

loads displace the nucleus to the weakest area of the annulus with the least resistance.[25] If this sequence is completed, the disk will herniate at this weakest location. This can initiate an inflammatory response that

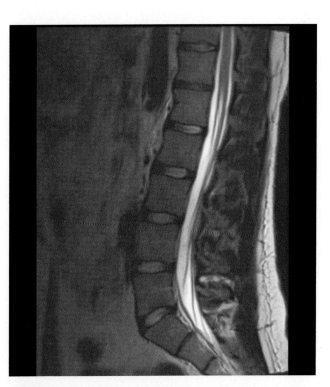

FIGURE 19-1 T2-weighted MRI showing mild degeneration of the L5 to S1 disk. A dark disk is also present at T12 to L1.

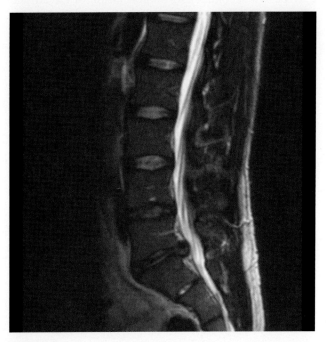

FIGURE 19-2 T2-weighted MRI showing moderate degeneration of the L5 to S1 disk.

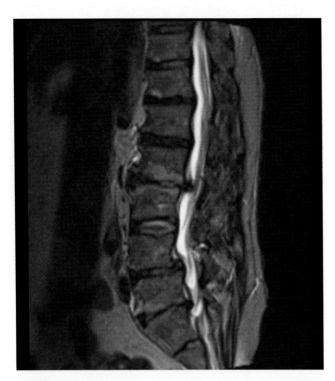

FIGURE 19-3 T2-weighted MRI showing severe degeneration of the L5 to S1 disk.

can irritate the dura, posterior longitudinal ligament, and nerve roots.[28] In most cases, the annular tear will heal with time. Despite healing, the disk will not regain the same biomechanical functionality. Discogenic pain may persist secondary to the formation of intradiscal granulation tissue.

It is also pertinent to understand the biomechanics behind disk degeneration. Three predominant forces act on the spine: compression, shear, and torque. The combination of compression and shear forces produces tensile stress on the annulus fibrosus and shear stress on the neural arch. During athletic activity, the vertical compressive force on the L3 to L4 disk can reach 7500 N in golf[29] and 6100 N in rowing.[30] On the L4 to L5 disk, the vertical compressive force can reach 8600 N during football blocking[22] and 17000 N while lifting weights.[31] Because the body's center of gravity lies anterior to the vertebral column, the spine is also subjected to torque.[25] The torque (τ) can be calculated by the equation $\tau = rF\sin\theta$, where F is the body weight, r is the distance from the body's center of gravity to the spine, and θ is the angle of axial force with respect to the spine (typically 90°). The erector spinae muscles and the lumbodorsal fascia normally resist this torque. With abnormal stresses added to the equation, annular tears of the intervertebral disk are more likely to occur.

Disk Degeneration in Aging Athletes

As the intervertebral disk ages, it undergoes a series of compositional changes. With increasing age, the nucleus pulposus loses water; the water content begins at 90% in infancy and diminishes to 70% by age 70 years.[32] This parallels the age-related loss of proteoglycans and an increase in density of type 2 collagen fibers, leading to decreased tensile strength and a corresponding inability to distribute loads uniformly. After age 12 years, the disk becomes avascular, and nutrition occurs via diffusion from the end plates.[33] As the cartilaginous end plates calcify with aging, diffusion to the nucleus center becomes increasingly difficult. Additionally, the oxygen content of the disk is lower in older individuals. This leads to increased lactate formation and a corresponding decrease in intradiscal pH.[34]

Changes in disk composition such as loss of hydration, decreased proteoglycans, and increased type 2 collagen are characteristic of normal aging.[35-37] Normal aging is distinct from the degenerative process (**Table 19-1**), which may be described as a spectrum that ranges from degenerative disk disease to facet joint arthritis and spinal stenosis. This degenerative process is the most common source of low back pain and leg pain in the aging population and is often accelerated in athletes.[38]

The intervertebral disk is part of a three-joint complex that comprises the motion segment of the spine. Damage to the intervertebral disk, in the form of annular tears that occur in degenerative disk disease, leads to alterations in the mechanics of the motion segment. This results in increased force distribution to the facets, rendering the joints vulnerable to the onset of osteoarthritis.[34] In an MRI study examining 41 vertebral levels with facet degeneration, Butler et al found evidence of disk degeneration in all but one, suggesting that degenerative disk disease precedes facet joint osteoarthritis in older athletes.[39]

As athletes age, degenerative disk disease may also progress to spinal stenosis. As noted previously, degenerative disk disease can lead to disk desiccation and a profound loss of proteoglycans. These changes are especially severe in the nucleus pulposus, resulting in a decreased ability of the nucleus to absorb pressure. Even in the absence of nuclear herniation, degenerative disk disease and associated facet joint arthritis can independently lead to stenosis via hypertrophy of the ligamentum flavum, facet joint capsule, and inferior articular process. The result of this degenerative

TABLE 19-1   Normal aging versus disk degeneration

Type of Change (Reference)	Normal Aging	Disk Degeneration
Biochemistry (Oegema[34])	Decreased proteoglycans Loss of hydration Increased type 2 collagen	Decreased proteoglycans Loss of transition zone (between inner annulus fibrosus and nucleus pulposus)
Histology (Boos et al,[63] Coventry et al[64])	Major cell proliferation as indicated by hypertrophic chondrocytes Mucoid degeneration of extracellular matrix Granular change Edge neovascularity	Annulus: invasion of blood vessels along tears and clefts; connective tissue meshwork replaced by hyalinized collagen fibers Nucleus: residues of notochordal cell aggregates replaced by proliferating chondrocytes; replacement of nucleus by fibrous tissue
Gross pathology (Hadjipavlou et al[65])	Division between nucleus and annulus becomes less distinct Nucleus becomes more solid, dry, and granular Collagen lamellae of annulus increase in thickness, become increasingly fibrillated	Narrowing of intervertebral disks Radial tears of annulus (fissures) Osteophyte formation Collapse of intervertebral space
Radiology (Shao et al,[66] Sether et al,[67] Modic et al[48])	Radiograph: increased disk height, decreased concavity of vertebrae, increased number of osteophytes MRI: decreased signal intensity in central area of disk	Radiograph: disk space narrowing, sclerosis of adjacent vertebral bodies, disk calcification, gas accumulation (vacuum disk) MRI: type 1, type 2, and type 3 Modic changes

progression is encroachment on the spinal dura centrally and the nerve roots laterally.[40]

DIAGNOSIS

Clinical Presentation

Lumbar disk degeneration follows a three-stage clinical progression: degenerative disk disease, facet joint arthritis, and spinal stenosis. Degenerative disk disease is characterized by pain caused by tearing of the annulus fibrosus and desiccation of the nucleus pulposus. Athletes classically present with back spasm and pain, which tends to worsen with flexion maneuvers as this places the highest pressure on the disk.[41] This initial pain is often attributed to the sinuvertebral nerves that innervate the outer layers of the disk.[38] Affected individuals may also complain of referred leg pain on straight-leg raise and paraspinal tenderness from spasm. Pain may be more common in the morning because of the discal swelling that occurs while sleeping in an extended supine position.[42]

The second stage of disk degeneration is distinguished by facet joint injury, classically osteoarthritis. In contrast to the flexion-induced pain observed in degenerative disk disease, pain caused by facet joint injury occurs on extension and rotational maneuvers.[41] Athletes may also report tenderness in the paraspinous area over the facet joint, slightly lateral to midline. Referred leg pain often becomes a particular concern at this stage of degeneration. Athletes complain of a deep, dull, aching pain that is poorly localized to the lumbosacral area, buttocks, and upper thighs. Affected individuals may report an increased incidence of referred leg pain in response to abnormal stimuli such as excessive stretching.

Spinal stenosis is the final stage of disk degeneration. Although often coexistent with axial back pain, athletes now typically present with radicular complaints localized in a dermatomal distribution, with the L5 and S1 nerve roots most commonly affected.[38] Spinal stenosis may be acquired via the disk degeneration pathway or it may arise congenitally (**Figure 19-4**). Congenital stenosis of the lumbar spine is an important prognostic factor for disk injury. Athletes with preexisting congenital stenosis are less likely to achieve symptomatic resolution in response to nonoperative treatment protocols. These individuals are more likely to require operative intervention and more likely to experience postoperative complications, such as epidural hematoma.[41] Symptoms from stenosis classically worsen on extension maneuvers that narrow the spinal canal and neural foramina. In addition to the radicular pain, neurogenic claudication can also arise secondary to spinal stenosis. Neurogenic claudication represents the strongest indication to perform surgery on elite athletes; every effort should be made to avoid operative intervention in this population unless claudicatory symptoms are present.

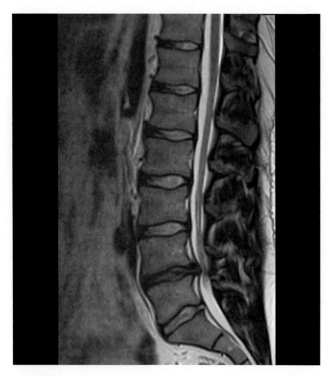

FIGURE 19-4 T2-weighted MRI showing congenital stenosis and mild degeneration of the L4 to L5 disk.

Physical Examination

Although no single maneuver is pathognomonic for lumbar disk degeneration, a thorough physical examination is indicated.[43] On examination, the athlete's gait may be antalgic, and if a disk herniation is present, the athlete may lean away from the affected side to open the neuroforamen and decrease pressure on the nerve root. Palpation near the symptomatic level may elicit pain, and referred hyperesthesia may also be present over the iliac crest, iliolumbar ligaments, or sacroiliac joints. If the degenerative process is advanced, the athlete may report tenderness over the facet joints that can be exacerbated with spinal extension.

A thorough neurologic examination is mandatory. All lower extremity myotomes must be graded and any dermatomal pain patterns or decreases in sensation recorded. Patellar and Achilles deep tendon reflexes should be assessed and compared with the opposite sides. If any signs of claudication are present, especially in aged athletes, differentiating a neurogenic from vascular origin is paramount. In neurogenic claudication, pain and paresthesias begin proximally and move distally with improvement in spinal flexion, which may take 30 minutes or more.[38] Vascular claudication, by contrast, is distinguished by pain that spreads from distal to proximal and is quickly relieved by rest. Dyck and Doyle's bicycle test is able to differentiate between the two possible etiologies of claudication.[44] Patients with spinal stenosis tend to ride longer before symptomatic onset.

Radiologic Manifestations

Radiologic studies play a critical role in the evaluation of athletes with suspected disk degeneration. Plain radiographs may reveal traction osteophytes, loss of disk space, and bone sclerosis of the vertebral bodies adjacent to the affected disk.[45,46] The "vacuum phenomenon" may also appear on radiographs because of the accumulation of predominantly nitrogen gas within the affected disk and adjacent vertebral bodies.[47]

Magnetic resonance imaging can also be highly informative, both in diagnosing disk degeneration as well as in staging the degenerative process. T2-weighted images allow for direct visualization of the annular fissure and any associated tissue hypertrophy. These images typically have a "dark disk" appearance owing to the loss of hydration that accompanies disk degeneration.[46] Bone marrow and end plate changes, classified by Modic and coworkers, may also be evident on T2-weighted films (**Table 19-2**).[48] Type 1 Modic changes, shown by hypointensity on T1-weighted MRI and hyperintensity on T2-weighted MRI because of increased water content, indicate inflammation and edema. Type 2 changes refer to fatty infiltration into the vertebral bodies, shown by hyperintensity on T1- and T2-weighted MRI. Type 3 changes denote bone sclerosis and are characterized by hypointensity on T1- and T2-weighted MRI. Sagittal and axial images become particularly useful as the disk degeneration progresses to its later stages. These views can reveal characteristic signs of spinal stenosis, including decreased patency of the neural foramina, decreased spinal canal size, and hypertrophy of the ligamentum flavum and facet joint capsule.[40]

Discography has historically been used as a supplement to plain radiographs and MRI. However, this

	TABLE 19-2	Modic changes	
Type	**Key Characteristic**	**Signal Intensity on T1-Weighted MRI**	**Signal Intensity on T2-Weighted MRI**
1	Inflammation and edema of fibrous tissue	Low	High
2	Deposition of fat within and below endplate	High	High or Equivalent
3	Bone sclerosis	Low	Low

procedure is controversial because of its invasive nature and its high rate of false-positive results, as well as increased progression toward disk degeneration at the tested level.[49]

● TREATMENT

Nonoperative Management

Nonoperative management is the mainstay of treatment for disk degeneration since most athletes achieve symptomatic resolution. Acutely, the athlete may need to abstain from practice and competition. Oral nonsteroidal anti-inflammatory drugs (NSAIDs) should be used as needed, and stronger analgesics may be required on a short-term basis, particularly if the athlete is experiencing sleep disruptions because of pain. Early physical therapy to maintain core strengthening and flexibility should be initiated as tolerated. Lumbosacral corsets and orthoses have not shown benefit for discogenic pain.[50,51] Although these devices are successful in limiting extremes of motion, they can also lead to muscle wasting, which can be a significant hurdle to the competitive athlete.

DePalma and Bhargava outlined a therapeutic protocol for athletes with discogenic back pain.[52] First-line treatment consisted of physical therapy, namely dynamic stabilization and core conditioning. These practices decrease anterior shear and torsional strain across the affected disk. Second-line treatment included transforaminal epidural steroid injection, which should be administered shortly after symptomatic onset to maximize the likelihood of a positive outcome. Third-line treatment comprised surgical intervention.

Operative Management

Surgery for spinal stenosis should be reserved for athletes with lumbar disk degeneration who have failed conservative treatment. Indications for operative management include mechanical low back pain with positive findings on imaging, continuous symptoms over a period of 4 to 6 months despite nonoperative efforts, and localized midline spinal tenderness that corresponds to the radiographic level of disk degeneration.[15]

When considering surgical intervention in an athlete, several preoperative variables must be taken into account. Both the age and the level of athlete must be taken into consideration. A professional athlete may be managed differently than a middle-aged, recreational one. Both short- and long-term gains must also be addressed and treated differently in recreational versus professional athletes, whose professional and financial futures are reliant on returning to the field. Last, quality of life gains in athletes are different than in the general population. Although a "good" surgical outcome is often enough to improve quality of life in the general population, it may not be sufficient for satisfactory return to play (RTP) in a competitive athlete.[53]

If surgery is warranted, surgical decompression is preferable. This can be done via a standard open approach with laminectomy or laminotomies at the affected levels. Over the past decade, less invasive approaches have been developed to achieve the same decompressive goals but with less theoretical morbidity and better outcomes. Comparative trials between less invasive and open approaches generally demonstrate less narcotic use, shorter hospitalizations, and less narcotic usage. Long-term clinical outcomes, however, have been shown to be the same. There is a lack of literature currently to define the optimal approach in athletes. Regardless of the technique, care to avoid overresection is vital to prevent iatrogenic instability, particularly in high-level athletes. Decompression is typically well tolerated in athletes because of its relatively short period of immobilization and earlier RTP. Spine stability is not in jeopardy with an appropriate decompression, but there may be an increased risk of back pain or acceleration of degenerative changes with return to competitive sports compared with population norms.[54] Postoperative follow-up is critically important in athletes undergoing decompression for lumbar degenerative disk disease and spinal stenosis. If an athlete with a surgical history of decompression presents with acute-onset low back pain, he or she should be evaluated for disk herniation as well as the presence of a pars defect.

Spinal fusion and decompression may be considered in the treatment of athletes if certain findings are present, most commonly spondylolisthesis.[55] The course of rehabilitation after fusion is longer and often not well tolerated by athletes.[46] Few studies have examined postoperative outcomes in athletes after a fusion procedure. Schroeder et al reported performance-based outcomes in 87 professional hockey players who had fusion procedures.[56] In this study, 31 athletes underwent nonoperative care, 48 underwent discectomy, and 8 underwent single-level fusion. When able to RTP, the lumbar fusion group did not show a decrease in games played per season or in performance score. Importantly, all athletes included in the study had lumbar disk herniation. Therefore, the external validity of these results to degenerative disk disease is uncertain.

Reporting postfusion outcomes drawn from a survey of 450 spine surgeons, Wright et al reported that 80% and 62% of high school and collegiate athletes, respectively, returned to play after spinal fusion.[57] However, only 18% of professional athletes successfully returned to their preoperative level of competition after lumbar fusion.

The use of total disk arthroplasty in both the general population and athletes remains controversial in the United States. The indication for lumbar disk arthroplasty is isolated discogenic pain, which may be a difficult diagnosis. Siepe et al reported postoperative outcomes in 39 athletes after total disk arthroplasty.[58] Compared with the data collected preoperatively, postoperative scores on both the Visual Analogue Scale and the Oswestry Disability Low Back Pain Questionnaire were significantly improved. In this study, 94.9% of the athletes returned to play, and athletic performance was significantly improved from injury state in 84.6% of these individuals. However, more high-quality studies need to be conducted before using lumbar disk arthroplasty in athletes becomes universally accepted by surgeons.

RETURN TO PLAY

Rehabilitation

Cooke and Lutz detailed a five-stage rehabilitation protocol widely used in athletes with low back pain.[59] Stage I entails a brief period of rest, usually spanning 48 to 72 hours, during which NSAIDs and early, protected mobilization should be initiated. Stage II involves dynamic spinal stabilization exercises that emphasize the abdominal musculature and lumbar extensors. Isometric exercises may also be performed at this time. When neutral position of the spine can be reliably attained and maintained, the athlete may graduate to stage III. This stage begins with extension exercises and steadily progresses to flexion exercises. Stage IV entails plyometric exercises and sport-specific drills, and stage V consists of maintenance exercises to prevent recurrence of pain after RTP.

Return to Play After Surgery

Return-to-play guidelines are highly debated among physicians. Despite a lack of standardized criteria, most experts agree that an injured athlete should not return to competitive sports before a series of milestones have been reached.[60] First, the athlete must have had adequate time to recover with reasonable assurance that a recurrent injury will not occur. Second, the athlete must be pain

free with preinjury range of motion and strength. Third, the athlete should be able to demonstrate sport-specific maneuvers and compete at or near the preinjury level of performance.[61,62]

Depending on the severity of degeneration and the treatment modality used, the physician must consider other variables. If a fusion was performed, osseous healing should be either symptomatically or radiographically confirmed, and the athlete must have sufficient residual flexibility before athletic activity.[40] When discussing RTP with the affected athlete, the physician must inform the athlete that the disk degeneration process may be accelerated by participation in competitive sports.[54]

Prevention

Although it is impossible to halt the progression of disk degeneration, the recurrence of symptoms can be delayed or prevented. Upon RTP, a comprehensive evaluation of the athlete's training regimen and individual technique should occur. Athletes who have been diagnosed with disk degeneration should maintain a regular program of core strengthening and flexibility exercises. The athlete should be especially diligent in stretching the paraspinous, quadriceps, hamstrings, calves, and hip flexors, and extensors. Importantly, the athlete must be cognizant and receptive to his or her own body. These patients must be taught to recognize the warning signs of injury and to scale down their levels of training appropriately.[38] For athlete-patients with lumbar disk degeneration and subsequent treatment, these steps exist to ensure the best possible outcome and increase the likelihood of patients' return to their preinjury states.

SUMMARY

Lumbar disk degeneration and spinal stenosis can have a profound detrimental impact on the career of an athlete. Affecting young and old athletes, this disease is prevalent throughout sports. With a sufficient history and by using effective physical examination and radiologic imaging, the surgeon can recognize the disease and discern the proper treatment. Additionally, the physician can educate the patient about the proper course to delay disease progression. If conservative treatment is unsuccessful, spinal decompression and fusion may be necessary for adequate relief of symptoms and return to baseline activity. Equipped with an understanding of the disease, the surgeon can better care for these patients and safely return them to the playing field through effective conservative and surgical treatment.

REFERENCES

1. Barile A, Limbucci N, Splendiani A, Gallucci M, Masciocchi C: Spinal injury in sport. *Eur J Radiol* 2007; 62(1):68–78.

2. Baranto A, Hellstrom M, Nyman R, Lundin O, Sward L: Back pain and degenerative abnormalities in the spine of young elite divers: A 5-year follow-up magnetic resonance imaging study. *Knee Surg Sports Traumatol Arthrosc* 2006;14:907–914.

3. Bennett DL, Nassar L, Delano MC: Lumbar spine MRI in the elite-level female gymnast with low back pain. *Skeletal Radiol* 2006;35:503–509.

4. Hangai M, Kaneoka K, Hinotsu S, et al: Lumbar intervertebral disk degeneration in athletes. *Am J Sports Med* 2009;37(1):149–155.

5. Hellström M, Jacobsson B, Swärd L, Peterson L: Radiologic abnormalities of the thoraco-lumbar spine in athletes. *Acta Radiologica* 1990;31(2):127–132.

6. Sward L, Hellstrom M, Jacobsson BO, et al: Back pain and radiologic changes in the thoraco-lumbar spine of athletes. *Spine (Phila Pa 1976)* 1990;15:124–129.

7. Ong A, Anderson J, Roche J: A pilot study of the prevalence of lumbar disc degeneration in elite athletes with lower back pain at the Sydney 2000 Olympic Games. *Br J Sports Med* 2003;37:263–266.

8. Baker RJ, Patel D: Lower back pain in the athlete: common conditions and treatment. *Prim Care Clin Office Pract* 2005; 32:201–229.

9. Sassmannshausen G, Smith BG: Back pain in the young athlete. *Clin Sports Med* 2002;21:121–132.

10. Trainor TJ, Trainor MA: Etiology of low back pain in athletes. *Curr Sports Med Rep* 2004;(3):41–46.

11. Lundin O, Hellström M, Nilsson I, Swärd L: Back pain and radiological changes in the thoraco lumbar spine of athletes. A long term follow up. *Scand J Med Sci Sports* 2001;11(2):103–109.

12. Capel A, Medina FS, Medina D, Gómez S: Magnetic resonance study of lumbar disks in female dancers. *Am J Sports Med* 2009;37(6):1208–1213.

13. Micheli LJ, Wood R: Back pain in young athletes. Significant differences from adults in causes and patterns. *Arch Pediatr Adolesc Med* 1995;149:15–18.

14. Orchard JW, Farhart P, Leopold C: Lumbar spine region pathology and hamstring and calf injuries in athletes: Is there a connection? *Br J Sports Med* 2004;38(4):502–504.

15. Bono CM: Low-back pain in athletes. *J Bone Joint Surg Am* 2004;86:382–396.

16. Trainor TJ, Wiesel SW: Epidemiology of back pain in the athlete. *Clin Sports Med* 2002;21:93–103.

17. Swärd L, Hellström M, Jacobsson B, Nyman R, Peterson L: Disc degeneration and associated abnormalities of the spine in elite gymnasts: A magnetic resonance imaging study. *Spine (Phila Pa 1976)* 1991;16(4):437–443.

18. Goldstein JD, Berger PE, Windler GE, Jackson DW: Spine injuries in gymnasts and swimmers. An epidemiologic investigation. *Am J Sports Med* 1991;19(5):63–468.

19. Miller JA, Schmatz C, Schultz AB: Lumbar disc degeneration: correlation with age, sex, and spine level in 600 autopsy specimens. *Spine (Phila Pa 1976)* 1988;13(2):173–178.

20. Videman T1, Sarna S, Battié MC, Koskinen S, Gill K, Paananen H, Gibbons L: The long-term effects of physical loading and exercise lifestyles on back-related symptoms, disability, and spinal pathology among men. *Spine (Phila Pa 1976)* 1995;20(6):699–709.

21. Semon RL, Spengler D: Significance of lumbar spondylolysis in college football players. *Spine (Phila Pa 1976)* 1981;6(2):172–174.

22. Gatt CJ Jr, Hosea TM, Palumbo RC, Zawadsky JP: Impact loading of the lumbar spine during football blocking. *Am J Sports Med* 1997;25(3):317–321.

23. Gerbino PG, d'Hemecourt PA: Does football cause an increase in degenerative disease of the lumbar spine? *Curr Sports Med Rep* 2002;1(1):47–51.

24. Horne JW, Cockshott P, Shannon HS: Spinal column damage from water ski jumping. *Skeletal Radiol* 1987; 16(8):612–616.

25. Watkins RG, Dillin WH: Lumbar spine injury in the athlete. *Clin Sports Med* 1990;9(2):419–448.

26. Alyas, Faisal, Michael Turner, and David Connell. MRI findings in the lumbar spines of asymptomatic, adolescent, elite tennis players. *Br J Sports Med* 2007;41(11):836–841.

27. Schmitt H, Dubljanin E, Schneider S, Schiltenwolf M: Radiographic changes in the lumbar spine in former elite athletes. *Spine (Phila Pa 1976)* 2004;29(22):2554–2559.

28. Kang JD, Stefanovic-Racic M, McIntyre LA, Georgescu HI, Evans CH: Toward a biochemical understanding of human intervertebral disc degeneration and herniation: Contributions of nitric oxide, interleukins, prostaglandin E2, and matrix metalloproteinases. *Spine (Phila Pa 1976)* 1997;22(10):1065–1073.

29. Hosea TM, Gatt CJ, McCarthy KE, Langrana NA, Zawadsky JP: Analytical computation of rapid dynamic loading of the lumbar spine. *Trans Orthop Res Soc* 1989; 14:358.

30. Hosea TM, Hannafin JA: Rowing injuries. *Sports Health* 2012;4(3):236–245.

31. Cholewicki J, McGill SM, Norman RW: Lumbar spine loads during the lifting of extremely heavy weights. *Med Sci Sports Exerc* 1991;23(10):1179–1186.

32. Lees A, McCullagh PJ: A preliminary investigation into the shock absorbency of running shoes and shoe inserts. *J Hum Move Stud* 1984;10(2):95–106.

33. Hassler O: The human intervertebral disc. A microangiographical study on its vascular supply at various ages. *Acta Orthop Scand* 1969;40(6):765.

34. Oegema TR Jr: Biochemistry of the intervertebral disc. *Clin Sports Med* 1993;12(3):419–439.

35. Adams P, Eyre DR, Muir H: Biochemical aspects of development and ageing of human lumbar intervertebral discs. *Rheumatol Rehabil* 1977;16(1):22–29.

36. Eyre DR: Biochemistry of the intervertebral disc. *Int Rev Connect Tissue Res* 1979;8:227–291.

37. Gower WE, Pedrini V: Age-related variations in protein-polysaccharides from human nucleus pulposus, annulus fibrosus, and costal cartilage. *J Bone Joint Surg Am* 1969;51(6):1154–1162.

38. Hackley,DR, Wiesel SW: The lumbar spine in the aging athlete. *Clin Sports Med* 1993;12(3):465–468.

39. Butler D, Trafimow JH, Andersson GB, McNeill TW, Huckman MS: Discs degenerate before facets. *Spine (Phila Pa 1976)* 1990;15(2):111–113.

40. Graw BP, Wiesel SW: Low back pain in the aging athlete. *Sports Med Arthrosc Review* 2008;16(1):39–46.

41. Watkins RG: Lumbar disc injury in the athlete. *Clin Sports Med* 2002;21(1):147–165.

42. Nachemson A: Towards a better understanding of low-back pain: A review of the mechanics of the lumbar disc. *Rheumatol Rehabil* 1975;14(3):129–143.

43. Schwarzer AC, Aprill CN, Derby R, Fortin J, Kine G, Bogduk N: The prevalence and clinical features of internal disc disruption in patients with chronic low back pain. *Spine (Phila Pa 1976)* 1995;20(17):1878–1883.

44. Dyck P, Doyle JB Jr: "Bicycle test" of van Gelderen in diagnosis of intermittent cauda equina compression syndrome: Case report. *J Neurosurg* 1977;46(5):667–670.

45. Swärd L. The thoracolumbar spine in young elite athletes. Current concepts on the effects of physical training. *Sports Med* 1992;13(5):357–364.

46. Lawrence JP, Greene HS, Grauer JN: Back pain in athletes. *J Am Acad Orthop Surg* 2006;14(13):726–735.

47. Resnick D, Niwayama G, Guerra J Jr, Vint V, Usselman J: Spinal vacuum phenomena: Anatomical study and review. *Radiology* 1981;139(2):341–348.

48. Modic MT, Steinberg PM, Ross JS, Masaryk TJ, Carter JR. Degenerative disk disease: Assessment of changes in vertebral body marrow with MR imaging. *Radiology* 1988;166(1 Pt 1):193–199.

49. Carragee EJ, Tanner CM, Khurana S, et al: The rates of false-positive lumbar discography in select patients without low back symptoms. *Spine (Phila Pa 1976)* 2000;25(11):1373–1380; discussion 1381.

50. Deyo RA:. Conservative therapy for low back pain: Distinguishing useful from useless therapy. *JAMA* 1983;250(8):1057–1062.

51. Million R, Nilsen KH, Jayson MI, Baker RD: Evaluation of low back pain and assessment of lumbar corsets with and without back supports. *Ann Rheum Dis* 1981;40(5):449–454.

52. DePalma MJ, Bhargava A: Nonspondylolytic etiologies of lumbar pain in the young athlete. *Curr Sports Med Rep* 2006;5(1):44–49.

53. Day AL, Friedman WA, Indelicato PA: Observations on the treatment of lumbar disk disease in college football players. *Am J Sports Med* 1987;15(1):72–75.

54. Micheli LJ: Sports following spinal surgery in the young athlete. *Clin Orthop Relat Res* 1985;(198):152–157.

55. Herkowitz HN, Kurz LT: Degenerative lumbar spondylolisthesis with spinal stenosis. A prospective study comparing decompression with decompression and intertransverse process arthrodesis. *J Bone Joint Surg* 1991;73(6):802–808.

56. Schroeder GD, McCarthy KJ, Micev AJ, Terry MA, Hsu WK: Performance-based outcomes after nonoperative treatment, discectomy, and/or fusion for a lumbar disc herniation in National Hockey League athletes. *Am J Sports Med* 2013;41(11):2604–2608.

57. Wright A, Ferree B, Tromanhauser S: Spinal fusion in the athlete. *Clin Sports Med* 1993;12(3):599–602.

58. Siepe CJ1 Wiechert K, Khattab MF, Korge A, Mayer HM: Total lumbar disc replacement in athletes: clinical results, return to sport and athletic performance. *Eur Spine J* 2007;16(7):1001–1013.

59. Cooke PM, Lutz GE: Internal disc disruption and axial back pain in the athlete. *Phys Med Rehabil Clin North Am* 2000;11(4):837–865.

60. Burgmeier RJ, Hsu WK: Spine surgery in athletes with low back pain—considerations for management and treatment. *Asian J Sports Med* 2014;5(4):e24284.

61. Eddy D, Congeni J, Loud K: A review of spine injuries and return to play. *Clin J Sport Med* 2005;15(6):453–458.

62. Krabak B, Kennedy DJ: Functional rehabilitation of lumbar spine injuries in the athlete. *Sports Med Arthrosc* 2008;16(1):47–54.

63. Boos N, Weissbach S, Rohrbach H, Weiler C, Spratt KF, Nerlich AG: Classification of age-related changes in lumbar intervertebral discs: 2002 Volvo Award in basic science. *Spine (Phila Pa 1976)* 2002;27(23):2631–2644.

64. Coventry MB, Ghormley RK, Kernohan JW: The intervertebral disc: Its microscopic anatomy and pathology. *J Bone Joint Surg* 1945;27(3):460–474.

65. Hadjipavlou AG, Tzermiadianos MN, Bogduk N, Zindrick MR: The pathophysiology of disc degeneration. *Bone Joint J* 2008;90(10):1261–1270.

66. Shao Z, Rompe G, Schiltenwolf M: Radiographic changes in the lumbar intervertebral discs and lumbar vertebrae with age. *Spine (Phila Pa 1976)* 2002;27(3):263–268.

67. Sether LA, Yu S, Haughton VM, Fischer ME: Intervertebral disk: Normal age-related changes in MR signal intensity. *Radiology* 1990;177(2):385–388.

20 Piriformis Syndrome, Sacral Stress Fractures, and Hip Labral Disorders

Diana Patterson, MD • Brian Neri, MD • Alexis Chiang Colvin, MD

● INTRODUCTION

Pain in the low back, either chronic or acute, is one of the most common orthopedic complaints seen by physicians ranging from surgical specialists to primary care physicians. In an adult or adolescent athlete presenting with lumbar back pain, the pathology may not be found in the spine or surrounding musculature itself. Pathology of the hip can commonly present with referred pain to the spine, confounding the root source of symptoms, prolonging the period without appropriate treatment, and preventing return to activity or sport. Several conditions of the pelvic girdle and hips can refer pain to the low back and present as though they were lumbar spine pathology. Of these, stress fractures, piriformis syndrome, and femoroacetabular impingement (FAI) syndrome are a few of the more frequent diagnoses seen in the young athlete.

● PIRIFORMIS SYNDROME

Case Presentation

A 35-year-old woman presents to the office complaining of right-sided low back and buttock pain intermittently radiating down the posterior aspect of her right leg. It

---

---

started a few months prior, initially during certain rotational yoga poses. She stopped yoga, and it improved, but then she began noticing the pain and radiculopathy after walking prolonged distances. She recently changed jobs to one where she spends more time at a desk and is having increasingly difficulty sitting for long periods of time because of pain in the back and leg. She denies any symptoms on the contralateral side, fevers, chills, and weight loss. She has not tried any intervention or medications for the pain. On examination, she has tenderness over the greater sciatic notch, mildly positive straight-leg-raise, and significant reproduction of her symptoms with hip external rotation and abduction but no motor or sensory deficits. Radiographs taken in the office are normal.

Etiology

For decades, piriformis syndrome has posed a clinical conundrum. The earliest mention of the piriformis muscle as a source of radicular low back pain was 1928, by Yeoman, who theorized fibrosis of the muscle could cause sciatica.[1] In 1947, Robinson formally established "piriformis syndrome," setting forth six diagnostic features: a history of trauma to the sacroiliac or gluteal region, pain in the sciatic notch and piriformis muscle that extends down the leg and hinders walking, exacerbation with stooping or lifting that is relieved by traction, presence of a palpable and tender mass over the piriformis, a positive Lasègue sign, and gluteal atrophy.[2]

The piriformis muscle originates from the anterior aspect of S2 to S4, exits through the sciatic notch, and inserts on the posteromedial corner of the superior edge of the greater trochanter (**Figure 20-1**). With the hip extended, it acts as an external rotator; when in flexion, it acts as an abductor. The sciatic nerve (L4–S1) exits the

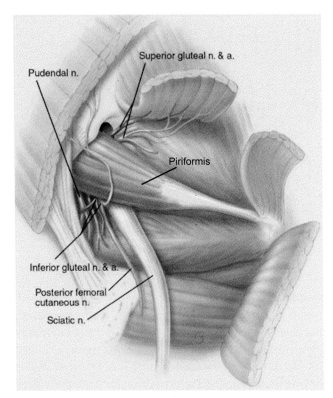

FIGURE 20-1 Normally, the sciatic nerve exits the sciatic notch under the piriformis. The superior gluteal nerve and artery exit above the piriformis. The inferior gluteal nerve and artery and pudendal nerve exit below with the sciatic. Not shown are the internal pudendal artery, nerve to obturator internus, posterior femoral cutaneous nerve, and nerve to quadrates femurs, all exiting below the piriformis. (Reprinted from Byrd JWT: Piriformis syndrome. *Op Tech Sports Med* 2005;13:71–79.)

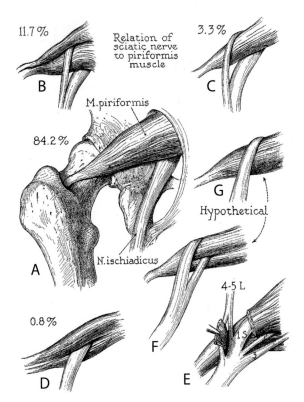

FIGURE 20-2 **A-G,** Six variations on the arrangement of the sciatic nerve, or of its subdivisions, in relation to the piriformis muscle. Arranged in the order of frequency; the percentage is incidence in a study of 120 examples. **F** and **G** are hypothetical; others are actual cases. **E,** Pelvic view, others gluteal views. **A,** Nerve undivided passes out of the greater sciatic foramen, below the piriformis muscle. **B,** The divisions of the nerve pass between and below the heads of the muscle. **C,** Divisions above and below the undivided piriformis muscle. **D,** Nerve undivided between the heads of the piriformis muscle. **E,** A variation of the arrangement in **D. F,** Hypothetical divisions of the nerve between and above the heads of the piriformis. **G,** Hypothetical undivided nerve above an undivided piriformis muscle. (Reprinted from Beaton LE, Anson BJ: The relation of the sciatic nerve and its subdivisions to the piriformis muscle. *Anat Rec* 1934:70:1–5.)

sciatic notch, most commonly, anterior to, or "under," the piriformis. Anatomic studies identified variations on this normal anatomy, such as a high division of the nerve splitting above and below the muscle or a single nerve piercing a bifid muscle.[3] A cadaveric study cadavers showed that 94% of the time, the piriformis and sciatic nerve follow the expected course, but that the most common variation, occurring in 4% of subjects, was a high-dividing nerve with the common peroneal division passing through and the tibial division below a bifid piriformis muscle[4] (**Figure 20-2**). Other structures exiting the sciatic notch can potentially also be affected by piriformis pathology, including the superior gluteal artery (above the piriformis), the inferior gluteal artery and nerve, the pudendal nerve and internal pudendal vessels, and the posterior femoral cutaneous nerve.

Symptoms are thought to be due to compression of the sciatic nerve by the piriformis muscle, although some physicians attribute any sciatica without a clear discogenic cause to be piriformis syndrome. Any lesion or mass causing compression of the proximal sciatic nerve,

such as endometriosis, hematoma, myositis ossificans, tumors, or aberrant vascular formations, can lead to symptoms of piriformis syndrome.[5] Reports in the literature indicate that it may be simultaneously overdiagnosed and overlooked, causing between 0.33% and 6% of all low back pain and radicular symptoms.[6,7] Across all etiologies, there is a greater incidence among women, with the ratio in some studies reported as high as 6:1.[8]

Piriformis syndrome is most commonly attributed to trauma, either from acute hematoma or posttraumatic scar formation, as well as overuse syndromes or variant anatomy.[2,9] Benson and Schutzer presented a series of patients with piriformis syndrome, all of whom had symptoms only after a confirmed blow to or fall on the gluteal muscles. In this series, all patients had electromyographic (EMG) abnormalities in the muscles supplied by the sciatic nerve that resolved with surgical release.[9] Overuse theorists believe the gait cycle, during which the piriformis muscle is under strain throughout the entirety of a stride, leads to hypertrophy or spasm.[10] Similarly, Fishman and Schaefer proposed it to be a functional entrapment of the sciatic nerve, occurring only when the leg or hip was in specific positions.[11] In more sedentary individuals, prolonged sitting on hard surfaces has been blamed, hence the nickname "wallet neuritis."[12] Variant anatomy may make the nerve more susceptible to compression, but the incidence of piriformis syndrome in patients with documented anatomic aberrations is no higher than that in those with normal anatomy.[13]

Diagnosis and Decision Making

Piriformis syndrome may present acutely, particularly if traumatic, or insidiously, as in the overuse or compression types. Patients describe buttock or posterior hip pain (or both), variable patterns of radiculopathy, and intolerable pain with prolonged sitting. In one study, buttock pain occurred in 95% of patients, more common than low back pain, and pain aggravated by sitting occurred in 97% of subjects.[14] Distal radicular symptoms generally follow a pattern consistent with sciatic nerve distributions, but motor or reflex deficits are uncommon. Additionally, some have pain with bowel movements, and women have complained of dyspareunia.

No single physical examination finding is pathognomonic. Palpation of the muscle belly can cause focal tenderness or recurrence of radicular symptoms; a sausage-shaped mass may be present. Pain at this site is distinct from pathology at the insertion of the gluteus maximus on the greater trochanter or the sacroiliac joint.[15] Palpation of the piriformis should be performed directly posterior to the hip joint, which is close to the sciatic notch. This is distinct from the location pain of greater trochanteric pain syndrome (GTPS), which is found overlying the greater trochanter on the lateral aspect of the thigh just distal and lateral to the hip joint (**Figure 20-3**).

Many studies advocate palpating the sciatic notch internally via a rectal or pelvic examination.[8] Reproduction of symptoms is often quite obvious, and the absence of pain during these examinations should cause reconsideration of the diagnosis.

Some patients may report positive findings with straight-leg raise, but these are more likely seen because of a lumbar nerve root irritation. In a systemic review of piriformis syndrome, only 31% had a positive straight-leg raise.[14] The cross straight-leg raise test is not reported

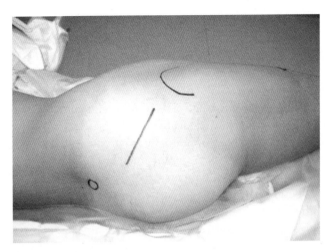

FIGURE 20-3 Markings illustrating location of incision for piriformis and its relation to the greater trochanter and posterior superior iliac spine. (Reprinted from Byrd JWT: Piriformis syndrome. *Op Tech Sports Med* 2005; 13:71–79.)

in the piriformis syndrome population.[16] The Freiberg sign, resisted external rotation of the hip with it in extension and internal rotation, is positive in 63% of patients.[10] The Pace test,[7] resisted abduction and external rotation of hip in flexion or in a seated position, is positive in 30% to 74% of patients.[14] The piriformis stretch, passive adduction with internal rotation in 90° of flexion, may cause symptoms. The Beatty test, pain with flexion and elevation of the symptomatic side while the patient lies on the asymptomatic side, has also been described.[10] These tests may be held for up to 1 minute before symptoms appear, similar to the Phalen test for carpal tunnel syndrome.[5]

There are no unique radiographic findings of piriformis syndrome. Plain films are recommended to rule out other pathology. MRI can be performed to rule out lesions causing mass effect. A full workup of the lumbar spine for possible source should be performed as well, particularly if there are motor deficits. Neurodiagnostic studies have revealed that a prolonged H-reflex latency can be indicative of piriformis syndrome.[13] These are accentuated with the hip is tested in flexion, abduction, and internal rotation.[14] If conductive abnormalities are seen, there should still be preservation of the superior gluteal nerve as it exits the notch above the piriformis muscle.[9]

Treatment

Conservative treatment is the initial recommendation for suspected piriformis syndrome. Lifestyle and activity modifications and anti-inflammatory medications are principal. A general back and hip physical therapy program, with attention paid to specific piriformis stretches, is beneficial. If there is limited or no response to these nonoperative measures, then an injection of local anesthetic agent, corticosteroids, or both is a next step. It can be done with ultrasound or computed tomography guidance or by gross palpation. There are several described techniques for injecting via anatomic landmarks,[13,15] but a cadaver study showed that only 30% of injections via any landmark technique for piriformis syndrome were accurate compared with 95% accuracy for ultrasound-guided.[17] In studies, 79% of patients experience at least a 50% reduction in pain after a corticosteroid injection combined with therapy.[12] In some studies, this diagnostic injection was curative.[15] Recently, data are available on Botox injections, particularly for persistent cases.[18–20] In a study by Michel et al, 77% of patient who did not respond to rehabilitation in 6 weeks experienced good to very good pain relief after three injections of botulinum toxin A.[19] A small trial comparing Botox with corticosteroid injections in refractory patients showed superior improvement in pain and function with Botox A at 12 weeks.[20]

Surgical release of the piriformis muscle can also be performed for recalcitrant symptoms. The diagnosis must be convincingly proven without confounding sources. The response can be excellent, but it can also be incomplete if there is other involved pathology. Through the posterior approach, the piriformis attachment on the greater trochanter is released, the course of the muscle is explored, the nerve is decompressed if necessary, and the proximal stump of the tendon is amputated. Improvement in symptoms can be immediate or appear gradually over several weeks. The published results from this intervention are, overall, good, but they are generally from small case series or case reports[9,13,15] without uniform criteria or outcomes scores. Most report somewhere between 59% to 69% with good to excellent results.[16,21] Future research includes standardization of outcomes scores in the operative and nonoperative groups to be better able to interpret and compare data on diagnosis, etiology, and outcomes.

● SACRAL STRESS FRACTURES

Case Presentation

A 40-year-old woman presents to the office with complaints of increasing low back pain. She reports that it worsens throughout the day with activity, particularly when she tries to go running. She has always been a recreational runner but decided recently to run a marathon and has increased her training. She denies any radicular symptoms. She has tried massage therapy and notes that her back is sometimes so tender that she cannot tolerate the massage. She has not tried any further treatment. She denies trauma, fevers, and weight loss. Radiographs of her pelvis and lumbar spine are grossly normal.

Etiology

Stress fractures account for a significant percentage of diagnosed overuse injuries and up to 15% of all injuries to runners.[22] Stress fractures of the sacrum are being diagnosed in the athletic population with increasing frequency. They can occur in both high-level competitive athletes and "weekend warriors," and a high clinical suspicion should be maintained. Most commonly seen in the tibia, fibula, and metatarsals, stress fractures of the pelvis are reported to account for only 1% to 7% of stress fractures.[23] The most prevalent sport is track and long-distance runners, but they have also been reported in tennis, gymnastics, and other sports with repetitive high-impact movements. Military trainees, particularly female recruits, constitute up to 22% of all stress fractures.[24]

Stress fractures are skeletal defects caused by repeated application of lower intensity stress than is required to cause an outright fracture.[25] The first description of one in the sacrum was by Volpin et al in 1989.[26] The underlying cause of stress injuries is still debated. The overload theory is that repetitive contractions of muscles leads to stress at osseous insertions and impairs the bone's ability to resist mechanical forces.[27] This theory is strongly advocated in stress fractures from non–weight-bearing activities. Second, the fatigue theory is that progressive exhaustion during activity reduces the ability of the muscles to function as shock absorbers, leading to abnormal load distributions and stress concentrations in bone.[28] The accumulation of microdamage to the bone cannot be repaired before new additional stress is placed. In the "female athlete triad"—disordered eating, amenorrhea, and osteoporosis—it is theorized that the decrease of estrogen and resulting loss of bone mineral density heighten risk for repetitive stress injuries.

The sacrum is the keystone arch of the pelvis, and it receives repetitive loading to the axial skeleton from ground reactive forces and muscle contraction.[29] Leg length discrepancies predisposing to uneven stride length and asymmetrical motion of the hips and lumbar spine have been proposed to potentiate these fractures, but they have not been shown in biomechanic studies.[30] Muscular imbalances may cause abnormal load transfer and increased risk of stress fracture.[31] Many studies describe diagnosis after an increase of intensity or change in type of training.[32,33] Women presenting with pelvic stress fractures have been shown to have an average body mass index of 21, an average age of 20 years old, and an average weekly running mileage of 25 to 33 miles per week.[29] In both populations, a history of amenorrhea[24,33] or prior stress fractures[34] are significant risk factors.

Sacral stress fractures have been classified to occur in one or more of three anatomic zones. Zone I is lateral to the foraminal line and involves the sacral ala. Zone II consists of one or several sacral foramina. Zone III is the central sacral canal. Zone I fractures can cause irritation of the L5 nerve root as it runs over the pelvic brim; this occurs in 6% of zone I fractures. The risks of neurologic symptoms with zone II and III fractures are 28% and 57%, respectively. Zone III fractures can present with symptoms of cauda equina syndrome.[35]

Diagnosis and Decision Making

Commonly, patients complain of nonspecific low back, buttock, or hip pain. It is important to ask the patient about any changes in intensity or type of activity. Women must be asked about any intervals of amenorrhea and be screened for nutritional deficiencies.[33,34] Rarely, though possible, if there is foraminal involvement, patients may complain of radicular symptoms in the posterior and distal leg. On examination, many have point tenderness paramedian to the sacrum or around the sacroiliac joints. The FABER test, placing the leg in flexion-abduction-external rotation, can be positive on the injured side, but it can also be an indicator of sacroiliac joint pathology.[36] The "hopping" test reproduces pain on the ipsilateral side with single-leg bouncing,[37] and the "flamingo" test does so with standing on the ipsilateral leg.[36] The time to presentation varies widely among patients, from immediately after a specific, localized onset of pain, to after months of vague complaints and indistinct symptoms. The differential diagnoses for this presentation includes muscle injury, degenerative disk disease, spondylolisthesis, sacroiliac joint injury, infection, or referred pain from the hip or genitourinary or gastrointestinal tract.

Radiographs typically lack the sensitivity to detect early stress fractures, especially if the symptoms are recent.[32] If present, radiographic changes include subtle radiolucency in the early stages or periosteal reactions in the later stages.[38] Radiographs repeated after some weeks of rest can reveal callus formation or vertical bands of sclerotic bone involving the sacral ala running parallel to sacroiliac joints.[39] Currently, MRI is the gold-standard imaging test. It allows visualization of a wide spectrum of injury, from soft tissue swelling, edema of the cortex or trabecular bone, or the presence of a distinct fracture line.[38] MRI is an excellent modality to stage these fractures and monitor for resolution. The Fredericson et al[40] MRI grading scale for tibial stress fractures has been applied to the sacrum. A grade 1 injury is visible only as mild marrow or periosteal edema on fat-suppressed T2 but not on T1. Grade 2 is moderate marrow or cortical edema on fat-suppressed T2 but not T1. Grade 3 injuries are severe marrow or periosteal edema visible on both T2 and T1 sequences. Grade 4 injuries are a grade 3 injuries with the additional of a visible fracture line.[40] Nuclear bone scans are highly sensitive for areas of bone turnover and can be positive within 72 hours after symptoms. However, increased uptake does not definitively diagnose fracture and can be seen with tumors, infection, arthritis, or metabolic defects. CT is more specific than bone scan, but the findings are more subtle,[41] and they are not endorsed by all physicians.[22] If there is a suspicion of metabolic bone disease or the "female athlete triad" as a contributing factor, additional workup may include laboratory tests such as thyroid-stimulating hormone, calcium, phosphate, alkaline phosphatase, parathyroid hormone, and vitamin D levels as well as liver function.[22]

Treatment

Treatment of these injuries is largely nonoperative, consisting of rest periods without activity, nonsteroidal anti-inflammatory drugs (NSAIDs), and a progressive but conservative return to activity or sport. In the initial stages, weight bearing can be limited until pain free. Activity modifications should be made to unload the affected bone. After a few weeks of rest, low or no impact activity, such cycling or swimming, may be allowed. Physical therapy with a stronger emphasis on core and hip strengthening can then begin. Total recovery and rehabilitation time is usually approximately 4 to 8 weeks.[42] After treatment, the same level of athletic participation is often reached, sometimes requiring alterations in training regimens to prevent recurrence such as increasing the proportion of cross-training activities or changing techniques.

Pelvic and Acetabular Stress Fractures

Stress fractures in other anatomic sites of the pelvis, such as the pubic rami and acetabulum, should also be considered, particularly in ballet dancers and gymnasts. As in the sacrum, abnormal loading leads to weakened bone, which is unable to completely heal because of repetitive impact. Both male and female athletes who participate in

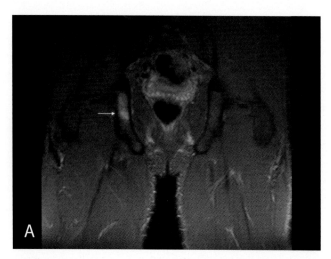
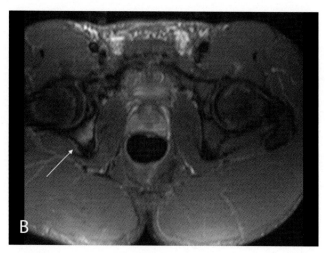

FIGURE 20-4 **A,** T2-weighted coronal view of the pelvis showing bony edema consistent with a stress fracture of the posterior acetabulum (*arrow*). **B,** T2-weighted axial view of the same lesion; arrow indicates bony edema of stress fracture.

these sports commonly have nutritional deficiencies secondary to maintaining a certain body type.

Patients with stress fractures of the pubic symphysis report chronic pain in the symphysis pubis or groin, which is exacerbated with running or kicking.[43] Male subjects may complain of abdominal pain, scrotal pain, or perineal pain. Weakness or imbalance of the rectus abdominis, the adductors, and the gracilis muscles is thought to contribute to development of this injury, placing abnormal stress at their insertion sites on the pubic symphysis. On examination, patients have distinct tenderness to palpation of the pubic symphysis or muscle insertion.

Stress fractures of the pubic rami or acetabulum also present with prolonged insidious pain over the groin, perineum, buttock, or thigh, with direct tenderness over the involved site. There may be a visible limp with weight bearing and potentially a reduced range of motion (ROM) of the ipsilateral hip.

As in the sacrum, MRI is typically required for diagnosis of an acetabular stress fracture (**Figure 20-4**). The usual course of treatment is conservative, with return to participation ranging from 7 to 12 weeks.[44]

● FEMOROACETABULAR IMPINGEMENT AND ACETABULAR LABRAL TEARS
Case Presentation

A 24-year-old male elite ice hockey player presents to the office for evaluation of lower back pain that is limiting his ability to compete. He reports pain in his low back and groin area since high school, needing to take time off from play for periods of pain and what was thought to be recurrent groin muscle strains. He recalls being told by trainers

and strength coaches that he had "tight hips." In addition, he reports a specific game a few months prior in which the pain worsened significantly after he was checked into the boards. He has tried physical therapy and core strengthening over the years, but the pain continues to return. He now has pain during all skating activities and finds that even prolonged sitting or standing is uncomfortable.

Etiology

Injury to the acetabular labrum can occur in isolation or with underlying pathology. The labrum, which is key to hip stability and force distribution in load bearing, can be injured in hip dysplasia and instability, sports activities, or trauma or can develop atraumatically through degeneration.[45-47] Disruption of the labrum increases cartilage compression and contact stresses, alters joint forces, and theoretically accelerates osteoarthritis.[45,48] FAI, a pathological abutment of a bony overgrowth on the femoral head–neck junction with the acetabular rim (cam impingement), a conflict between acetabular overcoverage and the femur (pincer impingement), or both (mixed impingement), is a well-acknowledged etiology of hip and groin pain. Cam impingement causes a shearing force at the chondrolabral junction, leading to pathologic delamination. Pincer impingement, secondary to coxa profunda, acetabuli protrusio, or acetabular retroversion, crushes the labrum, leading to tears[49] (**Figure 20-5**).

Femoroacetabular impingement is usually attributed to an idiopathic anatomic variant[50] in adolescent and adult athletes. In part, it has been attributed to a developmental process causing irregular bony growth around the femoral head epiphysis.[51] Prospective studies show an increase in the alpha angle, a radiographic measurement overgrowth

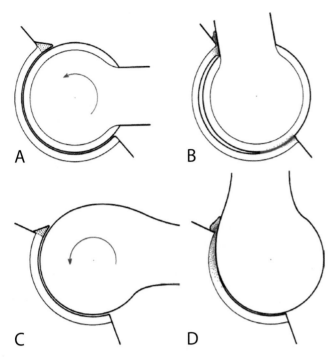

FIGURE 20-5 Illustrations of the joint damage patterns in femoroacetabular impingement (FAI). **A,** The persistent anterior over coverage of pincer FAI causes linear impact, which leads to (**B**) labral crushing and posterior contrecoup chondral injury. **C,** In cam FAI, the femoral head–neck junction abuts the acetabulum, causing (**D**) shearing the labrum and damage to peripheral cartilage. (Reprinted from Lavigne M, Parvizi J, Beck M, Siebenrock KA, Ganz R, Leunig M: Anterior femoroacetabular impingement. Part I. Techniques of joint pre-serving surgery. *Clin Orthop Relat Res* 2004;418:71.)

of the femoral head–neck junction representing the loss of sphericity of the femoral head, with increasing age in young athletes.[52,53] With more participation in sports at higher levels at younger ages, FAI must be included on the differential diagnosis of any patient with low back pain. Among elite athletes, FAI has been diagnosed in up to 72% of male and 50% of female soccer players on radiographic imaging; the diagnoses were made on anteroposterior (AP) pelvis and frog-leg lateral radiographs.[54]

Diagnosis and Decision Making

The clinical presentation of FAI is an athletic patient who participates in sports involving repetitive deep flexion, flexion-adduction, or extension-abduction movements, which bring the cam lesion on the femoral head or the pincer lesion on the acetabulum into conflict, placing excessive stress on the hip and surrounding soft tissues.

A patient with FAI may describe an injury leading to pain but is more likely to detail a prolonged course over months to years. The classic description of the pain

localizes to the anterior groin or thigh but can also be experienced at the lateral hip or buttock region.[49,55] Most report that it is worse with prolonged sitting or deep flexion maneuvers. Occasionally, the patient may complain of mechanical symptoms such as clicking and locking. The range of motion, particularly internal rotation of the hip, is often restricted in patients with FAI and labral pathology.[56] The anterior impingement test (Ganz test) is positive when flexion-adduction-internal rotation (FLAIR) elicits anterior groin pain. The FABER test for FAI, slightly different from the FABER for sacroiliac joint pathology or piriformis syndrome, evaluates restrictions in motion by measuring the distance between the lateral aspect of the knee and the examination table with the involved ankle placed on top of the contralateral knee.[57] An intraarticular lidocaine injection can help differentiate between intra- and extraarticular pathology. One study found that therapeutic alleviation of symptoms in response to an intraarticular injection of anesthetic was 90% accurate in predicting intraarticular pathology.[58]

Diagnostic imaging routinely includes a standardized AP pelvis, cross-table or Dunn lateral, and faux (false) profile views. The AP pelvis is used to measure the joint space at the level of the sourcil, the center edge, and Sharp's angles (**Figure 20-6**). Pincer impingement is diagnosed if this view shows coxa profunda, protrusio acetabuli, or a cross-over sign of acetabular retroversion. The cross-table lateral roughly assesses the alpha angle, which is diagnostic of a head–neck offset discontinuity.[59] Classically described on an axial MRI, it has been extrapolated and acceptably used on the lateral hip radiograph; an alpha angle greater than 42° is suggestive of a head–neck deformity. MRI, with or without arthrography, is the study of choice to diagnose a labral tear and

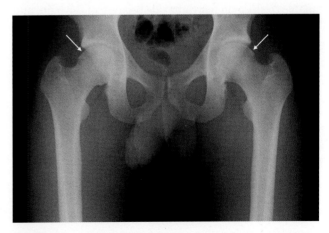

FIGURE 20-6 Anteroposterior hip radiograph showing bilateral cam lesions (*arrows*) at the femoral head–neck junction.

other periarticular or soft tissue pathology. However, meta-analyses reveal that MRI has only a 66% sensitivity and a 79% specificity for diagnosis of labral tears. MR arthrography, which has superior diagnostic accuracy, has an 87% sensitivity and 64% specificity for acetabular labral pathology.[60]

Treatment

Initial treatment can consist of 6 weeks of conservative therapy, including NSAIDs, physical therapy, and activity modification.[61] Patients can become surgical candidates if they have clinical and radiographic evidence of labral tears or FAI and fail a conservative treatment program.[52] Osteoplasty and acetabular rim-trimming for FAI lesions can be performed via open surgical dislocation or arthroscopic approach. Although both approaches have been found to be successful in the treatment of FAI and labral tears, arthroscopic management has gained popularity because of lower morbidity. Other procedures, such as lengthening of the iliopsoas/iliotibial tendon, excision of the greater trochanteric bursa, or repair of gluteal pathology, can be performed as well. Postoperatively, early ROM has been shown to reduce the formation of adhesions. Rehabilitation progresses from regaining ROM, to gentle strengthening and, eventually, to functional activities.[52,62] Sport-specific activities may be initiated as early as 6 weeks with most athletes returning to sport 3 to 6 months postoperatively.[62]

● GREATER TROCHANTERIC PAIN SYNDROME

Case Presentation

A 50-year-old woman presents with 3 months of ongoing right lateral hip pain. She cannot remember any inciting event, but the pain has been worsening. She is unable to sleep on her right side because of the pain, and it worsens with ambulating. Radiographs were negative for arthritis. She has tried a round of physical therapy. She presents for evaluation in the office because of lateral pain that is causing her to limp.

Etiology

The incidence of GTPS, a chronic lateral hip pain and tenderness of the greater trochanter region, has been reported to range between 1.8 to 5.6 per 1000 per year.[63,64] Women are diagnosed more frequently than men, with ratios as high as 3 or 4 to 1.[64–66] Historically, lateral hip pain was universally diagnosed as greater trochanteric bursitis, but recent research has shown there to be a wider spectrum of underlying causes, including

abductor (gluteus medius and minimus) tendinopathy or tears, thickening of the iliotibial band (ITB), and external coxa saltans. In fact, lateral-sided pain may have as debilitating effect on quality of life as hip osteoarthritis.[67]

The superficial layer of the peritrochanteric space is a fibromuscular sheath formed by the tensor fascia lata (TFL), gluteus maximus, and ITB. The maximus inserts into the posterior aspect of the ITB and the posterolateral femur via a thick expansion, the gluteal sling (**Figure 20-7**). The TFL inserts into the superoanterior aspect of the ITB. Deep to this, there are three or four bursae peripheral to the greater trochanter, which cushion and provide smooth motion of the overlying structure or underlying medius and minimus.[68] The largest of these fluid-filled sacs, the subgluteus maximus (trochanteric) bursa, lies between the gluteus maximus muscle and underlying gluteus medius tendon; it is a common pain source in GTPS.[69] Because of this, the gluteus medius tendon has two distinct insertions on the greater trochanter, the lateral facet, and the superoposterior facet. The thick, main portion inserts at the posterosuperior facet, and a thin lateral lamina attaches to the lateral trochanter, lateral to the bald spot.[70] The minimus tendon is deep to the medius, inserting to the lateral facet. The gluteus medius and minimus have been called the "rotator cuff of the hip."[71] Together, they stabilize the femoral head in the acetabulum during motion and gait, and the vertical pull force of the medius tendon helps initiate abduction.[72]

Greater trochanteric bursitis, inflammation of one or more of the peritrochanteric bursae, is thought to be caused by repetitive friction over the greater trochanter and ITB secondary to overuse, altered gait patterns, or trauma. However, recent imaging studies have revealed that few patients with symptoms have true bursitis. Tears, partial undersurface and full thickness; tendinosis; degeneration; and thickened ITBs are more commonly seen on imaging. Causes of these tears are thought to be analogous to the chronic attritional tendinopathy similar to degenerative tears of the rotator cuff.[71,73] Calcific tendinitis or calcium deposits, which can be seen on radiographs or ultrasound imaging, can also be sources of pain. Despite recent attention and improved diagnosis and treatment options, GTPS remains frequently missed, ignored, or untreated.

Diagnosis and Decision Making

Patients present with complaints of lateral hip pain, which can radiate into the groin, the lateral leg, or proximally into the buttock of low back. Patients with coexisting lumbar spine pathology may have weakness, paresthesias, radiculopathy distal to the knee, or positive

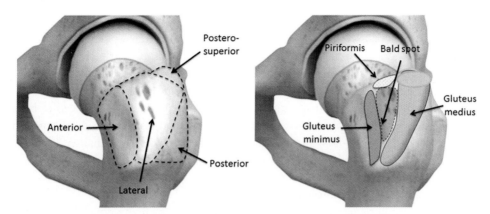

FIGURE 20-7 Peritrochanteric anatomy. The footprint of the gluteus medius includes the posterior aspect of the tendon, which inserts on the posterosuperior part of the greater trochanter, and the lateral aspect, which inserts on the lateral greater trochanter at the proximal bald zone. The gluteus minimus tendon inserts on the anterior aspect of the greater trochanter. The fascia lata covers the gluteus medius and trochanteric bursa. The gluteus medius and minimus bursae are appended to their respective tendons. (Reprinted from Thaunat M, Noel E, Nove-Josserland L, et al.: Endoscoping management of gluteus medius tendon tears. *Sports Med Arthrosc Rev* 2016;24:11–18.)

straight-leg raise. For patients with GTPS, the pain is mechanical, worsens with weight bearing, and is reproducible with direct pressure of the tendon or provocative maneuvers. Aggravating factors can include side bending, pain with sleeping on the affected side, and pain with prolonged sitting. Any prior surgeries on the hip or prior treatments should be queried. On examination, pain can be elicited with abduction of the symptomatic hip in 0° or 45° of flexion while the patient lies on the contralateral side.[74] Stretching the abductors with forced external rotation in flexion can also produce symptoms. The Lequesne test assesses pain with resisted internal rotation with the hip in 90° of flexion.[75] Many patients, particularly if there is injury of the abductor tendons, will have a Trendelenburg gait—the trunk tilts toward the painful side while the contralateral pelvis sags, compensating for the ipsilateral abductor weakness.[76]

The differential diagnosis for lateral hip pain includes intraarticular sources, such as labral tears, FAI, hip dysplasia, ligamentum trees injury, chondral damage, or loose bodies. Extraarticular possibilities include pelvic or ischial tuberosity stress fractures and piriformis syndrome. Outside the hip, meralgia paresthetica, lumbar radiculopathy, or spondylosis can be to blame.[77]

Standard radiographs of the hip are necessary to rule out intraarticular bony pathology, such as degenerative arthritis, FAI, or hip dysplasia. A trochanter that protrudes more lateral than the lateral aspect of the iliac crest may be a predisposing risk factor for GTPS.[78] In an MRI comparison study, surface irregularities of the trochanter on radiographs had a 90% correlation with abductor tendon

changes.[79] MRI has historically been the study of choice to evaluate intra- and extraarticular soft tissue structures. True bursitis is seen with inflammation surrounding the greater trochanter. A thickened tendon with increased signal on T2 series is characteristic of tendinosis.[80] Tendon retraction is evidence of a full-thickness tear, and partial-thickness tears show a focal discontinuity, usually on the undersurface side of the tendon.[77] Gluteus medius tendon pathology is frequently seen along with hypertrophy of tendon fascia lata, significantly enlarged compared with the contralateral side.[81] MRI is also excellent for assessing muscle quality; similar to the shoulder, fatty degeneration and atrophy portend poor surgical outcomes. Nevertheless, there are cases of tears missed on MRI, and it can be difficult to differentiate partial-thickness tear from simple tendinopathy in some cases.[75,82]

Increasingly, MRI is joined by ultrasonography as an imaging option and is certainly the most cost effective. In 877 trochanters ultrasounds, Long et al showed that true bursitis was only seen in 20%. Fifty percent had gluteal tendinosis, 0.5% had tendon tears, and 28.5% had a thickened ITB.[83] Ultrasound can allow for dynamic exam if the pain is positional, palpation of specific areas for focal pathology, or simultaneous administration of a therapeutic injection. A systematic review showed ultrasonography to have a 79% to 100% sensitivity and 95% to 100% positive predictive value for abductor tendon pathology.[84]

Treatment

Traditionally, treatment for GTPS has been nonsurgical. Anti-inflammatory medications, physical therapy, and corticosteroid injections are the mainstays. More recently, ultrasound and extracorporeal shock-wave therapy have been tried. Results are usually good with this regimen. In a small group treated with therapy, injections, ice, heat, and ultrasound, 66% were able to return to sports and 83% were able to return to labor-heavy employment at 3 months.[85,86] A systematic review of the use of corticosteroid injections showed improvement between 49% and 100% compared with baseline activities. Standard and ultrasound-guided injections are similarly efficacious.[24] Extracorporeal shock-wave therapy has shown improved pain and function at 1, 3, and 12 months from treatment in comparison with rest, therapy, NSAIDs, and injections.[86] In a direct comparison of shock-wave, injection only with therapy only, the steroid injection recipients performed best at 1 month, but the shock-wave and therapy patients had superior results at 15 months.[64] Other injections, just as platelet rich plasma (PRP), are still under study. The usefulness of PRP is theorized because of its prior uses in other chronic tendinopathies, but results are limited.

Surgical treatment options are a more recent appearance and only recommended in patients who have failed 6 to 12 months of nonoperative treatment.[85] In those with isolated trochanteric bursitis, open bursectomy with or without ITB release was described by Brooker in 1978.[87] More recently, bursectomy can be performed endoscopically; ITB release can also be performed.[64] In a small studies, patients do well at 1 year with few recurrences at longer follow-up.[88]

For patients with partial- or full-thickness abductor tears, open or endoscopic repair can be performed. Open suture anchor repair with drill holes in the trochanter has shown excellent improvement in Harris hip scores at 1 and 5 years postoperatively; the mean improvement was comparable to total hip arthroplasty.[89] Endoscopic repair has also had good outcomes, with decreased pain and improved strength in small case series.[90] If the tendon is retracted and cannot be repaired back to the trochanter primarily, allograft tendon can be used to reattach and augment the medius remnant.[89,91] Alternatively, the vastus lateralis can be advanced to bridge the defect in abductor tendons,[92] or the gluteus maximus and TFL can be transferred to the trochanter.[93]

● SUMMARY

In conclusion, many conditions refer pain to the low back and can confound diagnosticians, particularly if an incomplete history, physical examination, or radiologic evaluation is performed. Sacral or pelvic stress fractures, piriformis syndrome, and FAI can be observed in young athletes with back pain. A complete physical examination leads providers to appropriate imaging or other studies to ensure diagnosis. Initially, normal radiographs with persistent or specific symptoms require further investigation. Piriformis syndrome can present with persistent buttock pain and radiculopathy without an identifiable discogenic cause. Stress fractures of the sacrum, pelvis, and acetabulum similarly can present with localized or vague pain, usually worsening with increasing exercise. Labral pathology or FAI is seen in patients complaining of groin and back pain initially with activity and then with standing or rising from a chair. Greater trochanteric pain syndrome can cause pain on the lateral aspect of the hip radiating into the lower aspect of the back. All have excellent outcomes when they are expediently diagnosed and specifically treated, both surgically and conservatively. It is important that spine specialists, general orthopaedists, and the primary care physicians consider that the underlying cause of symptoms can, in fact, be found apart from the spine.

REFERENCES

1. Yeoman W: The relation of arthritis of the sacroiliac joint to sciatica, with an analysis of 100 cases. *Lancet* 1928; 212(5492):1119–1123.

2. Robinson DR: Pyriformis syndrome in relation to sciatic pain. *Am J Surg* 1947;73(3):355–358.

3. Beaton LE, Anson BJ: The relation of the sciatic nerve and of its subdivisions to the piriformis muscle. *Anat Rec* 1937;70(1):1–5.

4. Natsis K, Totlis T, Konstantinidis GA, et al: Anatomical variation between the sciatic nerve and piriformis muscle: A contribution to surgical anatomy in piriformis syndrome. *Surg Radiol Anat* 2014;36(3):273–280.

5. Cass SP: Piriformis syndrome: A cause of nondiscogenic sciatica. *Curr Sports Med Rep* 2015;14(1): 41–44.

6. Bernard TN Jr, Kirkaldy-Willis WH: Recognizing specific characteristics of non-specific low back pain. *Clin Orthop Relat Res* 1987;(217):266–280.

7. Pace JV, Nagle D: The piriformis syndrome. *West J Med* 1976;124(6):435–439.

8. Durrani Z, Winnie AP: Piriformis muscle syndrome: an underdiagnosed cause of sciatica. *J Pain Symptom Manage* 1991;6(6):374–379.

9. Benson ER, Schutzer SF: Posttraumatic piriformis syndrome: Diagnosis and results of operative treatment. *J Bone Joint Surg Am* 1999;81(7):941–949.

10. Jankovic D, Peng P, van Zundert A: Brief review: Piriformis syndrome: Etiology, diagnosis and management. *Can J Anaesth* 2013;60(10):1003–1012.

11. Fishman LM, Schaefer MP: The piriformis syndrome is underdiagnosed. *Muscle Nerve* 2003;28(5):646–649.

12. Parziale JR, Hudgins TH, Fishman LM: The piriformis syndrome. *Am J Orthop (Belle Mead NJ)* 1996;25(12):819–823.

13. Fishman LM, Dombi GW, Michaelsen C, et al: Piriformis syndrome: Diagnosis, treatment, and outcome—a 10-year study. *Arch Phys Med Rehabil* 2002;83(3):295–301.

14. Hopayian K, Song F, Riera R, et al: The clinical features of the piriformis syndrome: A systematic review. *Eur Spine J* 2010;19(12):2095–2109.

15. Byrd JWT: Piriformis syndrome. *Op Tech Sports Med* 2005;13:71–79.

16. Deville WL, Van Der Windt DA, Dzafcragic A, et al: The test of Lasegue: Systematic review of the accuracy in diagnosing herniated discs. *Spine (Phila Pa 1976)* 2000;25(9):1140–1147.

17. Finnoff JT, Hurdle MFB, Smith J: Accuracy of ultrasound-guided versus fluoroscopically guided contrast-controlled piriformis injections: a cadaveric study. *J Ultrasound Med* 2008;27(8):1157–1163.

18. Lang AM: Botulinum toxin type B in piriformis syndrome. *Am J Phys Med Rehabil* 2004;83(3):198–202.

19. Michel F, Decavel P, Toussirot E, et al: Piriformis muscle syndrome: Diagnostic criteria and treatment of a monocentric series of 250 patients. *Ann Phys Rehabil Med* 2013;56(5):371–383.

20. Yoon SJ, Ho J, Kang HY, et al: Low-dose botulinum toxin type A for the treatment of refractory piriformis syndrome. *Pharmacotherapy* 2007;27(5):657–665.

21. Miller TA, White KP, Ross DC: The diagnosis and management of piriformis syndrome: Myths and facts. *Can J Neurol Sci* 2012;39(5):577–583.

22. Hosey RG, Fernandez MM, Johnson DL: Evaluation and management of stress fractures of the pelvis and sacrum. *Orthopedics* 2008;31(4):383–385.

23. Snyder RA. Koester MC. Dunn WR: Epidemiology of stress fractures. *Clin Sports Med* 2006;25(1):37–52, viii.

24. Shaffer RA. Rauh MJ. Brtxlinc SK, et al: Predictors of stress fracture susceptibility in young recruits. *Am J Sports Med* 2006;34(1):108–115.

25. Martin AD, McCulloch RG: Bone dynamics: stress, strain, and fracture. *J Sports Sci* 1987;5(2):155–163.

26. Volpin G, Milgrom C, Goldsher D, et al: Stress fractures of the sacrum following strenuous activity. *Clin Orthop Relat Res* 1989;(243):184–188.

27. Stanitski CL, McMaster JH, Scranton PE: On the nature of stress fractures. *Am J Sports Med* 1978;6(6):391–396.

28. Puddu GC, Guglielmo C, Alberto S, et al: Stress fractures, in: Harries M, Williams C, Standish W, et al, eds: *Oxford Textbook of Sports Medicine*, ed 2, vol. Oxford, Oxford University Press, 1998, pp 650–657.

29. Lin JT, Lane JM: Sacral stress fractures. *J Womens Health (Larchmt)* 2003;12(9):879–888.

30. Micheli LJ, Curtis C: Stress fractures in the spine and sacrum. *Clin Sports Med* 2006;25(1):75–88, ix.

31. Hameed F, McInnis K: Sacral stress fracture causing radiculopathy in a female runner: A case report. *PM R* 2011;3(5):489–491.

32. Fredericson M, Salamancha L, Bealieu C: Sacral stress fractures, tracking nonspecific pain in distance runners. *Phys Sportsmed* 2003;31(2):31–42.

33. Yeager KK. Agostini R, Nauiv A, et al: The female athlete triad: disordered eating, amenorrhea, osteoporosis. *Med Sci Sports Exerc* 1993;25(7):775–777.

34. Miller C, Major N, Toth A: Pelvic stress injuries in the athlete: Management and prevention. *Sports Med* 2003;33(13):1003–1012.

35. Jones JW: Insufficiency fracture of the sacrum with displacement and neurologic damage: A case report and review of the literature. *J Am Geriatr Soc* 1991;39(3):280–283.

36. Bono CM: Low-back pain in athletes. *J Bone Joint Surg Am* 2004;86-A(2):382–396.

37. Delvaux K, Lysens R: Lumbosacral pain in the athlete. *Am J Phys Med Rehabil* 2001;80(5):388–391.

38. Fredericson M, Moore W, Biswal S: Sacral stress fractures: Magnetic resonance imaging not always definitive for early stage injuries: A report of 2 cases. *Am J Sports Med* 2007;35(5):835–839.

39. Cooper KL, Beabout JW, Swee RG: Insufficiency fractures of the sacrum. *Radiology* 1985;156(1):15–20.

40. Fredericson M, Bergman AG, Hoffman KL, et al: Tibial stress reaction in runners: correlation of clinical symptoms and scintigraphy with a new magnetic resonance imaging grading system. *Am J Sports Med* 1995;23(4):472–481.

41. Haun DW, Kettner NW, Yochum TR, et al: Sacral fatigue fracture in a female runner: A case report. *J Manipulative Physiol Ther* 2007;30(3):228–233.

42. Raasch WG, Hergan DJ: Treatment of stress fractures: The fundamentals. *Clin Sports Med* 2006;25(1):29–36, vii.

43. Miller C, Major N, Toth A: Pelvic stress injuries in the athlete: Management and prevention. *Sports Med* 2003;33(13):1003–1012.

44. Kahanov L, Eberman LE, Games KE, et al: Diagnosis, treatment and rehabilitation of stress fractures in the lower extremity in runners. *Open Access J Sports Med* 2015;6:87–95.

45. Ferguson SJ, Bryant JT, Ganz R, et al: The influence of the acetabular labrum on hip joint cartilage consolidation: A poroelastic finite element model. *J Biomech* 2000;33(8):953–960.

46. Ferguson SJ, Bryant JT, Ganz R, et al: An in vitro investigation of the acetabular labral seal in hip joint mechanics. *J Biomech* 2003;36(2):171–178.

47. Kelly BT, Weiland DE, Schenker M, et al: Arthroscopic labral repair in the hip: surgical technique and review of the literature. *Arthroscopy* 2005;21(12):1496–504.

48. McCarthy JC, Noble PC, Schuck MR, et al: The role of labral lesions to development of early degenerative hip disease. *Clin Orthop Relat Res* 2001;(393):25–37.

49. Ganz R, Parvizi J, Beck M, et al: Femoroacetabular impingement: A cause for osteoarthritis of the hip. *Clin Orthop Relat Res* 2003;(417):112–120.

50. Philippon M, Schenker M: Arthroscopy for the treatment of femoroacetabular impingement in the athletes. *Clin Sports Med* 2006;25(2):299–308, ix.

51. Siebenrock K, Wahab K, Werlen S, et al: Abnormal extension of the femoral head epiphysis as a cause of cam impingement. *Clin Orthop Relat Res* 2004;(418): 54–60.

52. Philippon M, Ejnisman L, Ellis H, et al: Outcomes 2 to 5 years following hip arthroscopy for femoroacetabular impingement in the patients aged 11 to 16 years. *Arthroscopy* 2012;28(9):1255–1261.

53. Philippon M, LaPrade R, Briggs K, et al: Screening of asymptomatic elite youth hockey players: clinical and MRI exam. *Br J Sports Med* 2011;45:322.

54. Gerhardt MB, Romero AA, Silve HJ, et al: The prevalence of radiographic hip abnormalities in elite soccer players. *Am J Sports Med* 2012;40(3):584–588.

55. Philippon MJ: New frontiers in hip arthroscopy: The role of arthroscopic hip labral repair and capsulorrhaphy in the treatment of hip disorders. *Instr Course Lect* 2006;55:309–316.

56. Martin RL, Enseki KR, Draovitch P, et al: Acetabular labral tears of the hip: Examination and diagnostic challenges. *J Orthop Sports Phys Ther* 2006;36(7):503–515.

57. Philippon MJ, Briggs KK, Johnston TL, et al: Clinical presentation of femoroacetabular impingement. *Knee Surg Sports Traumatol Arthrosc* 2007;15(8):1041–1047.

58. Byrd JW, Jones KS: Diagnostic accuracy of clinical assessment, magnetic resonance imaging, magnetic resonance arthrography, and intra-articular injection in hip arthroscopy patients. *Am J Sports Med* 2004;32(7):1668–1674.

59. Clohisy JC, Carlisle JC, Beaule PE, et al: A systematic approach to the plain radiographic evaluation of the young adult hip. *J Bone Joint Surg Am* 2008;90(suppl 4): 47–66.

60. Smith TO, Hilton G, Toms AP, et al: The diagnostic accuracy of acetabular labral tears using magnetic resonance imaging and magnetic resonance arthrography: a meta-analysis. *Eur Radiol* 2011;21(4):863–874.

61. Philippon M, Yen Y-M, Briggs K, et al: Early outcomes after hip arthroscopy for femoroacetabular impingement in the athletic adolescent patient: A preliminary report. *J Pediatr Orthop* 2008;28(7):705–710.

62. Wahoff M, Ryan M: Rehabilitation after hip femoroacetabular impingement arthroscopy. *Clin Sports Med* 2011;30(2):463–482.

63. Lievense A, Bierma-Zeinstra S, Schouten B, et al: Prognosis of trochanteric pain in primary care. *Br J Gen Pract* 2005;55(512):199–204.

64. Rompe JD, Segal NA, Cacchio A, et al: Home training, local corticosteroid injection, or radial shock wave therapy for greater trochanter pain syndrome. *Am J Sports Med* 2009;37(10):1981–1990.

65. Anderson TP: Trochanteric bursitis: diagnostic criteria and clinical significance. *Arch Phys Med Rehabil* 1958;39(10):617–622.

66. Segal NA, Felson DT, Torner JC, et al: Greater trochanteric pain syndrome: epidemiology and associated factors. *Arch Phys Med Rehabil* 2007;88(8):988–992.

67. Fearon AM, Cook JL, Scarvell JM, et al: Greater trochanteric pain syndrome negatively affects work, physical activity and quality of life: a case control study. *J Arthroplasty* 2014;29(2):383–386.

68. Williams BS, Cohen SP: Greater trochanteric pain syndrome: A review of anatomy, diagnosis and treatment. *Anesth Analg* 2009;108(5):1662–1670.

69. Woodley SJ, Mercer SR, Nicholson HD: Morphology of the bursae associated with the greater trochanter of the femur. *J Bone Joint Surg Am* 2008;90(2):284–294.

70. Robertson WJ, Gardner MJ, Barker JU, et al: Anatomy and dimensions of the gluteus medius tendon insertion. *Arthroscopy* 2008;24(2):130–136.

71. Bunker TD, Esler CN, Leach WJ: Rotator-cuff tear of the hip. *J Bone Joint Surg Br* 1997;79(4):618–620.

72. Gottschalk F, Kourosh S, Leveau B: The functional anatomy of tensor fasciae latae and gluteus medius and minimus. *J Anat* 1989;166:179–189.

73. Kagan A: Rotator cuff tears of the hip. *Clin Orthop Relat Res* 1999;(368):135–140.

74. Lequesne M: From "periarthritis" to hip "rotator cuff" tears: Trochanteric tendinobursitis. *Joint Bone Spine* 2006;73(4):344–348.

75. Thaunat M, Noël E, Nové-Josserand L, et al: Endoscopic management of gluteus medius tendon tears. *Sports Med Arthrosc* 2016;24(1):11–18.

76. Domb BG, Brooks AG, Byrd JW: Clinical examination of the hip joint in athletes. *J Sport Rehabil* 2009;18(1):3–23.

77. Redmond JM, Chen AW, Domb BG: Greater trochanteric pain syndrome. *J Am Acad Orthop Surg* 2016; 24(4):231–240.

78. Viradia NK, Berger AA, Dahners LE: Relationship between width of greater trochanters and width of iliac wings in tronchanteric bursitis. *Am J Orthop (Belle Mead NJ)* 2011;40(9):E159–E162.

79. Steinert L, Zanetti M, Hodler J, et al: Are radiographic trochanteric surface irregularities associated with abductor tendon abnormalities? *Radiology* 2010;257(3):754–763.

80. Kingzett-Taylor A, Tirman PF, Feller J, et al: Tendinosis and tears of gluteus medius and minimus muscles as a cause of hip pain: MR imaging findings. *AJR Am J Roentgenol* 1999;173(4):1123–1126.

81. Sutter R, Kalberer F, Binkert CA, et al: Abductor tendon tears are associated with hypertrophy of the tensor fasciae latae muscle. *Skeletal Radiol* 2013;42(5):627–633.

82. Cvitanic O1, Henzie G, Skezas N, et al: MRI diagnosis of tears of the hip abductor tendons (gluteus medius and gluteus minimus). *AJR Am J Roentgenol* 2004;182(1):137–143.

83. Long SS, Surrey DE, Nazarian LN: Sonography of greater trochanteric pain syndrome and the rarity of primary bursitis. *AJR Am J Roentgenol* 2013;201(5):1083–1086.

84. Westacott DJ, Minns JI, Foguet P: The diagnostic accuracy of magnetic resonance imaging and ultrasonography in gluteal tendon tears: A systematic review. *Hip Int* 2011;21(6):637–645.

85. Lustenberger DP, Ng VY, Best TM, et al: Efficacy of treatment of trochanteric bursitis: A systematic review. *Clin J Sport Med* 2011;21(5):447–53.

86. Furia JP, Rompe JD, Maffulli N: Low-energy extracorporeal shock wave therapy as a treatment for greater trochanteric pain syndrome. *Am J Sports Med* 2009;37(9):1806–1813.

87. Brooker AF Jr: The surgical approach to refractory trochanteric bursitis. *Johns Hopkins Med J* 1979;145(3):98–100.

88. Fox JL: The role of arthroscopic bursectomy in the treatment of trochanteric bursitis. *Arthroscopy* 2002;18(7):E34.

89. Davies JF, Stiehl JB, Davies JA, et al: Surgical treatment of hip abductor tendon tears. *J Bone Joint Surg Am* 2013;95(15):1420–1425.

90. McCormick F, Alpaugh K, Nwachukwu BU, et al: Endoscopic repair of full-thickness abductor tendon tears: Surgical technique and outcome at minimum of 1-year follow- up. *Arthroscopy* 2013;29(12):1941–1947.

91. Fehm MN, Huddleston JI, Burke DW, et al: Repair of a deficient abductor mechanism with Achilles tendon allograft after total hip replacement. *J Bone Joint Surg Am* 2010;92(13):2305–2311.

92. Betz M, Zingg PO, Peirrmann CW, Dora C: Advancement of the vastus lateralis muscle for irreparable hip abductor tears: Clinical and morphological results. *Acta Orthop Belg* 2012;78(3):337–343.

93. Whiteside LA: Surgical technique: Transfer of the anterior portion of the gluteus maximus muscle for abductor deficiency of the hip. *Clin Orthop Relat Res* 2012;470(2):503–510.

21 Lumbar Spine Disorders in Aging Athletes

Gordon R. Bell, MD

Although physical decline is part of the aging process, the rate of decline varies and may be adversely affected by long-standing disuse and a sedentary lifestyle.[1] Between 1900 and 1988, the average life expectancy in industrialized Western countries increased by more than 60%, from 47 years to 75 years. Furthermore, the percentage of older individuals has accelerated more rapidly than other segments of the population, with those 85 years of age and older increasing 232% between 1960 and 1990 compared with a 39% overall growth in population during that 30-year period.[2] Currently, more than 25% of the population is older than 55 years.

There are many physiologic musculoskeletal manifestations of aging (**Table 21-1**). With muscle strength, for example, peak muscle strength occurs at 30 years of age and decreases by approximately 15% per decade between ages 50 and 70 years, such that by age 70 years, it is reduced by 30%. The spine contains all of the musculoskeletal anatomic structures listed in Table 21-1 and is therefore subject to a host of potential abnormalities as it ages.

Anatomically, spinal degenerative changes begin anteriorly in the disk (annulus fibrosus and nucleus pulposus) and secondarily involve the posterior elements (facet joints). As the annulus develops fissures and the nucleus pulposus undergoes reduction of its proteoglycan content, the disk space narrows. The ligamentum flavum is then under less tension and buckles, and secondary degenerative changes occur in the facet joints. The net effect of these changes is that the spinal canal undergoes progressive narrowing as a result of the infolding and thickening of ligamentum flavum anteriorly and facet arthropathy posteriorly.

The narrowing of the canal may or may not be accompanied by symptoms. When symptoms do occur, they can manifest as low back pain, radiculopathy, or both. The radicular symptoms are partially mechanical as a result of neural compression from the circumferential degenerative changes that narrow the spinal canal. Although symptoms from aging with degeneration of the lumbar spine can have a significant effect on everyone, they can have a profound effect on those accustomed to a very active lifestyle, such as former athletes.

Discussion of *lumbar spine disorders in aging athletes* comprises a myriad of potential concepts and issues. First, there is the gamut of conditions that may be included under *lumbar spine disorders*. These include intrinsic low back pain, low back pain from other nonspinal causes (e.g., hip disease and other organ causes), radicular syndromes (e.g., disk herniation and spinal stenosis), and vertebral compression fractures (VCFs).

Second, there is a whole separate discussion regarding the definition of *aging*. It is known, for example, that aging is associated with reduced activity and sarcopenia, particularly a reduction in type II (fast-twitch) muscle fibers.[3] Muscle mass has been shown to decrease by approximately 1.25% per year after age 35 years, with further acceleration after age 70 years.[4] In addition, women tend to deteriorate with age more than men. With regard to the spine, spinal disorders are generally more common as individuals age, regardless of whether or not they are athletes, former athletes, or nonathletes. This is due to both development of degenerative changes and a reduction in bone mass.

Third, there is the concept of what is meant by the term *athlete*. Does this mean those actively involved with athletics or merely former athletes? Does the term *aging athlete*, therefore, refer to an active professional athlete entering

Dr. Bell or an immediate family member serves as a paid consultant to American Medical Foundation for Peer review & Education and Pfizer; and has received nonincome support (such as equipment or services), commercially derived honoraria, or other non-research–related funding (such as paid travel) from Saunders/Mosby-Elsevier.

TABLE 21-1 Musculoskeletal manifestations of aging

Area	Effects of Aging	Protective Modifications or Treatments
Bone	Progressive loss of mineral density "Tubularization" of diaphyseal bone	Regular exercise Well-balanced diet Vitamin D and calcium supplementation Hormone therapy (women) Medical therapy (e.g., bisphosphonates)
Ligaments and tendons	Decreased fiber compliance Stiffness of ligaments and tendons Increased susceptibility to catastrophic failure Decreased glycosaminoglycan concentration Decreased collagen fiber bundle thickness Decreased vascularity	Regular exercise Preexercise stretching
Meniscus	Intrasubstance degeneration Loss of ability to dissipate stress Increased propensity to degenerative tears	Débridement of unstable degenerative tears*
Articular cartilage	Decreased concentration of chondroitin sulfate; relative increase in keratan sulfate (nonosteoarthritic) Relative increase in chondroitin sulfate (osteoarthritic) Chondromalacia (cumulative damage)	Microfracture for selected full-thickness chondral lesions Débridement of unstable chondral lesions* Glucosamine and chondroitin sulfate* Hyaluronate viscosupplementation*
Skeletal muscle	Sarcopenia Decreased type I and II muscle fiber loss Volumetric loss of individual fiber size Progressive muscle denervation Decreased mitochondrial volume Increased collagen content Degenerative ultrastructural changes Decreased muscle flexibility	Regular exercise, muscle training Preexercise stretching Hormonal supplementation* Nutritional supplementation*

*Routinely used with anecdotal success, but long-term benefits have not been clearly established.
Reproduced from: Chen AL, Mears SC, Hawkins RJ: Orthopaedic Care of the aging athlete. *JAAOS* 2005;13(6):407–416.

the twilight of his or her career? Or does it refer to a still athletically active individual who is either a "weekend warrior" or is a physically active septuagenarian engaging in moderate aerobic activities? The term *master* is commonly used to designate athletes older than 35 years of age and typically older than 50 years.[4] In addition, there is a wide variety of sports, and it may not be reasonable to assume that spine disorders encountered later in life in a former professional hockey player are the same as those encountered by a former long-distance runner. Furthermore, weight training is a common part of conditioning and training for many sports. It can be difficult, if not impossible, to determine if clinical symptoms or radiographic changes are due to the effect of such weight training for a sport or are due to the actual sport itself.

Finally, one must make a distinction between *radiographic* evidence of spinal degeneration and *clinical* symptomatology. Degenerative changes in the lumbar spine are ubiquitous with aging, regardless of the presence or absence of symptoms and regardless of whether or not the individual is or was athletic. In the general population, there is little, if any, correlation between such radiographic findings and symptoms because such findings relate more to age than to the presence or absence of symptoms. Although some data suggest that athletes in some sports have more degenerative changes and back pain than the general population, such information is hard to obtain in former and aging athletes. In addition to the issue of radiographic degenerative changes in the spines of athletes, there is also the issue of spinal bone mineral density (BMD) and whether or not BMD values correlate with risk of VCF in aging athletes.

Finally, no discussion of back pain and spinal disorders would be complete without consideration of other, nonspinal, conditions that can mimic back pain. This is particularly true of older individuals, including aging athletes, in whom other musculoskeletal conditions, such as hip arthritis, may mimic back pain (**Table 21-2**).[5] It

● TABLE 21-2 Differential diagnosis of low back pain in athletes

Diagnosis	Presentation
Low back strain	Belt-line or paravertebral pain with motion
Degenerative disk disease	Midline pain with sitting or loading
Lumbar transitional vertebra	Midline low back pain
Facet mediated pain	Midline and paramedian pain with extension
Spondylolisthesis	Mechanical midline and paramedian pain
Traumatic fracture	Midline pain at the level of injury
Disk herniation	Pain, numbness and weakness radiating into the leg
Lumbar spinal stenosis	Low back, buttock, and leg pain, improved with flexion
Cauda equina syndrome	Radicular symptoms with bowel and bladder dysfunction and saddle anesthesia
Spinal infection	Constant low back pain with fevers, chills, night sweats, recent infection or dental procedure
Tumor	Night pain, fever, older age (>60 years), weight loss
Intraabdominal or intrapelvic processes	Boring nonmechanical pain, GI disturbance
Renal disease or stones	Colicky pain, GI disturbance
Hip pathology	Groin pain, pain with rotation or weight bearing
Sacroiliac pathology	Buttock and posterior superior iliac spine area pain, pain with loading
Abdominal aortic aneurysm	Constant boring front to back pain

GI = gastrointestinal.
Reproduced from Truumees E: Low back pain in the aging athlete. *Semin Spine Surg* 2010;22(4):222–233.

should be noted that not all of the diagnoses listed in Table 21-2 are universally accepted as causing symptoms, such as a lumbar transitional vertebra causing midline low back pain.

● EPIDEMIOLOGY OF LOW BACK PAIN IN ATHLETES

It is important to remember that low back pain is a symptom and not a diagnosis. In many cases, the actual pathology responsible for back pain is unknown, and no specific diagnosis can be discerned.[6] This is generally of little consequence because back pain is often a self-limited condition. In Western civilizations, low back pain occurs in approximately 80% to 90% of the adult population. An association has been shown between heavy physical loading and back symptoms and degenerative changes, although most studies have focused on occupational loading rather than that associated with athletics. There are many obvious differences between occupational loading and athletic loading of the spine, and one significant factor may be the duration and frequency of loading between the two types of activities. As noted by Lundin et al, comparisons between back pain in athletes and back pain in the general population are difficult for

many reasons.[7] These include differences in motivation, pain perception, susceptibility, and physical activity between the two groups. In addition, relatively minor pain might be significantly more important in an athlete than a nonathlete because an athlete's performance could be hampered by even a small degree of pain. Conversely, some athletes might be able to ignore some pain that would otherwise hamper daily activities in a nonathlete.[8] In general, there are conflicting reports on the association between athletics and low back pain.[9]

The protective effect of strenuous physical activity in seniors was demonstrated in a population-based study of Danish twins 70 years of age and older.[10] Although this study did not look specifically at senior athletes, it found that more frequent and strenuous physical activity, defined as more than 30 minutes of walks or bike rides, sports, or dancing, was associated with a significantly lower risk of developing back pain than no physical activity or less strenuous activity. In athletes, the data on back pain are inconclusive, with some studies reporting increased rates of low back pain ranging up to 75% in young athletes.[11-17] The risk of developing low back pain is influenced by gender, age, type of sport, type and intensity of training techniques, and other factors. For example, low back pain has been reported to be more common in certain sports than others, particularly in sports associated with heavier loads, such as wrestling and gymnastics. Swärd et al reported that radiographic abnormalities in the thoracolumbar spine occurred in 36% to 55% of a group of 142 elite athletes representing gymnastics, wrestling, soccer, and tennis.[12] When compared with control participants, wrestlers and elite gymnasts were found in one study to have back pain at frequencies of 69% and 85%, respectively.[12,18] Other studies have also reported an increased incidence of low back pain ranging from 25% to 75% in gymnastics[13,15] and in other sports, such as football[16,17] and wrestling.[7] These studies generally represented findings of active athletes, and whether or not they would hold true for aging athletes is unknown.

A contrary view of the relationship between athletics and back pain was reported by Videman et al, who generally found a lower risk of low back pain in a retrospective questionnaire study of former elite athletes compared with a control group, 29% versus 44%, respectively.[19] The mean age of the former athletes in that study ranged from 55.3 years (former soccer players) to 59.8 years (shooting athletes). This difference was statistically significant for endurance sports, sprinting and game sports, wrestling, and boxing. In addition, there was no association found between former athletes in the various sporting groups and sciatica. This study concluded that there was no evidence to support an association between sciatica or disk herniation and heavy physical loading from athletics.

Similar results were reported in a case-control epidemiologic study of 287 athletic patients with lumbar disk herniation.[20] This study looked at the relative risk of developing a lumbar disk herniation in multiple sports, including baseball or softball, golf, swimming, aerobics, diving, jogging, racket sports, weight lifting, and bowling. It did not look specifically at older athletes, with only 38% of the participant being older than 40 years of age. The study found that all the sports, with the sole exception of bowling, had a relative risk for the development of a lumbar disk herniation of approximately 1.0 or less. Bowling showed a weak positive association (relative risk, 1.27) for developing a lumbar disk herniation, perhaps because of the combination of bending and torsion required in the sport. That study represents one of the few studies to look at the association between sports and disk herniation.

● RADIOGRAPHIC ABNORMALITIES IN ATHLETES

Radiographic spinal abnormalities by MRI are common in the asymptomatic population and increase with age.[21,22] It is against this background that radiographic abnormalities in aging athletes must be viewed and evaluated. One small study of asymptomatic, active men older than age 40 years found that the incidence of degeneration was similar to that reported in other populations.[23] It should also be noted that most studies report on active athletes rather than older athletes. It is presumed, however, that the degenerative findings noted in younger athletes remain, and likely advance, throughout life and that their increased frequency compared with control participants is likely to persist into later life. With that in mind, several studies have documented a higher risk of radiographic abnormalities in active athletes. The previously cited study by Videman et al, which reported less back pain in former elite athletes than in control participants, found that degenerative changes in the spine were more common in some athletes.[19] This included increased focal changes in the lower lumbar levels of soccer players and throughout the spine in weight lifters. Runners and athletes involved in shooting sports had the least degenerative findings by MRI. Similar findings were reported by Granhed and Morelli, who reported increased degenerative findings but no increase in back pain in a cohort of retired heavyweight power lifters.[24] Swärd et al reported a strong correlation between Schmorl's nodes, disk height reduction, and abnormal configuration of vertebral bodies with back pain.[12] These radiographic findings were consistent with Scheuermann's disease, although the locations of the Schmorl's nodes in athletes were more frequent in the anterior portion of the end plates than in the control group of nonathletes. The authors concluded that such radiographic findings were highly suggestive of a causative relationship between athletic activity and back pain.

In a separate study, Swärd et al reviewed MRI findings in 24 elite male gymnasts and compared them with 16 nonathlete control participants and noted significantly more radiographic disk degeneration in the athletes (75%) than in the control population (31%).[18] The authors believed that their findings of abnormal configuration of the vertebral bodies in the gymnasts represented disturbed vertebral growth, and the predominantly anterior degeneration of the disks suggested a traumatic etiology. Back pain was also found to be more frequent in the gymnasts (79%).

One study looked at lumbar spine radiographic changes in 70 former professional soccer players, stratified by position, and compared them with a control group of 59 men.[25] The former soccer players were found to have a decreased functional outcome and increased lumbar osteophytes compared with control participants, and forward position players were found to have decreased disk height, suggesting that such changes were due to increased load on the spine in forward position players.

Some sports appear to have a more significant effect on spinal degenerative changes than others. In a study of 159 former elite male athletes from seven different track and field disciplines, athletes in throwing sports (shot putters, discus throwers, and javelin throwers) and high jumpers were found to have a significantly higher prevalence of degenerative changes, especially at L5 to S1, compared with marathoners and race walkers.[26,27] Of interest, however, no significant differences were found among the various groups with regard to subjective assessment of low back pain. The authors hypothesized that extreme hyperextension and rotation of the lumbar spine was responsible for these changes and further speculated that this could also explain the observed high risk of pars defects noted in throwers.

One radiographic abnormality that is well documented to be more common in athletes than in the general population is isthmic spondylolysis and spondylolisthesis. The incidence of spondylolisthesis in the general population is approximately 6%, with the risk being approximately two to three times that in large population studies of athletes.[28,29] Pars defects are even more common in some sports such as gymnastics, wrestling, and diving.[13,14] In weight lifting, for example, the incidence ranges from 15% to 31%.[24,30] In that vein, it must also be remembered that training for many sports includes weight training, and it is therefore possible that the incidence of pars defects in some sports, such as American football, might reflect the contribution from such weight training activities. What long-term effect spondylolisthesis has in aging athletes is not completely known. As with nonathletes, however, disk collapse associated with a slip causes foraminal narrowing and places the individual at risk for radicular symptoms.

The relationship between radiographic changes and symptoms in athletes is not entirely clear. In a 12- to 15-year follow-up of 173 athletes and nonathletes comprising wrestling, gymnastics, soccer, and tennis, athletes were found to have significantly more radiographic abnormalities, but no more back pain, than control participants.[7] On the other hand, there was no correlation found between the number of radiographic abnormalities and back pain. This included a lack of correlation between back pain and spondylolysis or spondylolisthesis.

A 15-year follow-up of 71 male athletes (weight lifters, wrestlers, ice hockey players, and orienteers) and 21 nonathlete control participants found that 78% of athletes and 38% of control participants reported current or previous history of back pain at the beginning of the study.[31] At final follow-up, 71% of athletes and 75% of nonathletes reported back pain. Back pain was more common in ice hockey players both at the beginning and end of the observation period. Of interest, high rates of degenerative findings by MRI were found in all athletes, particularly in weight lifters and ice hockey players. Although progression of degenerative changes was nearly universal, development of new MRI findings was uncommon during the 12- to 15-year interval.

One of the confounding issues in aging athletes that can also affect younger athletes is the coexistence of a hip disorder and a spinal disorder. In an aging athlete, it could be signs and symptoms of hip osteoarthritis and spinal stenosis or in a younger athlete of a hip labral tear and lumbar disk process. There is a great deal of overlap of the signs and symptoms. Even groin pain, one of the key symptoms of hip arthritis, can be prevalent in 40% of patients with lumbar stenosis. The key issue is sorting out which problem is the true source of symptoms because degenerative disorders are so common as patients age. Even physical findings and history can be source of frustration for even the most experienced clinicians. **Figure 21-1** is a case of a 58-year-old female former professional tennis player with low back pain, buttock and groin pain, and thigh pain radiating to her knee. The patient had radiographic evidence of lumbar spondylolisthesis and spinal stenosis (**Figure 21-1A** and **21-1B**) and hip osteoarthritis (**Figure 21-1C**). After failing a short course of anti-inflammatory medication, she underwent a fluoroscopically guided anesthetic arthrogram of her right hip (**Figure 21-1D**) that produced immediate relief of her symptoms. The hip anesthetic injection is 100% specific and more than 90% sensitive for diagnosing the hip as the source of the pain. The injection lasted only 6 days, and the patient then underwent total hip replacement with a complete return to tennis. The key point was to identify the source of her pain by anesthetizing the joint and not via spinal injections or spine surgery. If the anesthetic arthrogram had produced no relief, attention could then have been focused on a spinal source of her pain. The same paradigm often holds true for cervical spine and shoulder disorders.

● BONE MINERAL DENSITY IN ATHLETES

There are conflicting reports on the effect of athletic physical activity on BMD. Although it is true that bone responds the mechanical stresses placed upon it (Wolff's

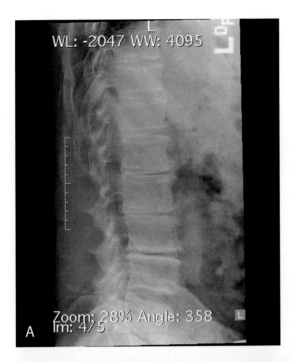

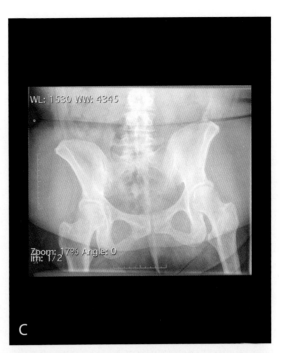

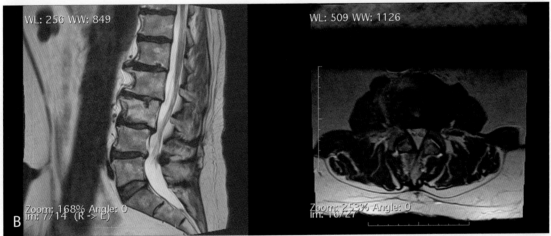

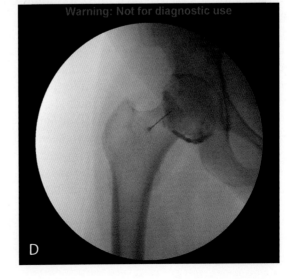

FIGURE 21-1 A, Sagittal radiograph revealing extensive degenerative changes. **B,** Sagittal (*left*) and axial (*right*) T2-weighted MRI revealing mild to moderate spinal stenosis worst at L3 to L4. **C,** Pelvis anteroposterior radiograph revealing mild to moderate osteoarthritis in the right hip. **D,** Anesthetic arthrogram confirming intraarticular spread of dye and medication.

law), it is unclear which activities have the most beneficial effect on vertebral bone strength, whether or not the effect of such activities translates to a reduced risk of VCFs, and whether or not such effects have a continued positive effect in older athletes after such physical activities have ceased.[32,33] Most studies have examined the effect of certain activities on BMD in active, rather than former, athletes. Several studies, for example, have reported that lumbar spine BMD is higher in throwers, pole vaulters, long jumpers, and triple jumpers than in endurance athletes such as marathon runners or race walkers.[34,35] This may reflect the higher mechanical stresses to the spine with certain sports or the higher muscle strength associated with those sports because higher muscle strength is associated with stronger bones. One study compared the BMD at nine different anatomic sites in 106 athletes from nine sports with 15 age-matched control participants and found both a site-specific (loaded) and generalized (unloaded peripheral or axial sites) beneficial effect of activity on BMD.[35] Site-specific benefits included greater BMD in the upper extremity of throwing athletes and in the legs of runners. However, rugby players were found to have the greatest BMD of all sports studied, which was greater than control participants at all nine sites. Of note, some activities (keepfit, cycling, and rowing) failed to demonstrate increased BMD compared with age-matched control participants. The conclusion of the study was that high impact, physical contact, and rotational sports produced higher BMD at both the loaded sites and at other unloaded axial and peripheral sites.

The protective effect of strenuous physical activity on BMD after retirement from sports has also been shown in some studies.[36-39] In a study of former soccer players who had been retired for at least 10 years, BMD was found to be significantly higher in the lumbar spine and other weight-bearing areas such as femoral neck and trochanter, distal tibia, and calcaneus.[36] This effect was related to time after retirement but not to age per se. Similar findings were noted in a study of active and senior female soccer players.[40] In that study, total-body, lumbar spine, and proximal femur BMD of active and senior female soccer players were compared with a control population. A site-specific significant increase in BMD was noted for the players compared with the control participants, with greater differences in BMD for the proximal femur than for the lumbar spine or for total-body BMD. Other studies have also shown that the long-term beneficial effects of sporting activity on BMD are self-limited, dissipating by approximately age 65 years of age.[37,38]

Not all strenuous physical activity produces long-term beneficial effects on BMD. A study of young and older male master cyclists showed a significantly lower BMD in older master cyclists compared with their younger counterparts and control participants.[41] The study concluded that such highly trained athletes might actually be at risk for future osteoporosis despite their high level of fitness. A similar later study by some of the same authors showed that competitive male master cyclists had a consistent and significant pattern of lower BMD than nonathlete control participants.[42] Cyclists who engaged in weight training or some form of impact exercise lost less BMD than those who did not. A significantly greater number of cyclists fulfilled the criteria for osteopenia and osteoporosis than did the nonathlete control participants. The authors issued a warning that the reduced BMD puts the cyclists at a high risk for fracture after cycling-associated falls.

A different study compared both male (65 subjects) and female (44 subjects) endurance runners (3 km to marathon distance) with a control group.[43] Although runners had normal hip BMD, they had lower lumbar spine BMD compared with reference values, with more than one third of the group having low BMD. Twiceweekly resistance training seemed to offer some protection for lumbar spine "T scores" in male runners. A study of 104 elite senior athletes and 79 healthy control participants found that participation in competitive sports was not related to total-body or regional BMD but that age, sex, body weight, and vitamin D and calcium intake were related to BMD.[44]

Another study looked at the effect of long-term regular sports participation on bone size, quality, strength, and BMD in the lumbar spine and midfemur. It concluded that regular sports participation had a beneficial effect on the bone size, quality, and strength but not on BMD.[45] A contrary view was reported in another study of senior running and swimming athletes older than the age of 65 years from the 2005 National Senior Olympic Games.[46] The study found that total-body BMD of runners was significantly greater than that of control participants and was marginally greater than that of swimmers.

Few studies examined the potential clinical effect of increased BMD from physical activity, namely, a reduced fracture risk. One study of former male athletes reported a protective effect of exercise on future fracture risk 5 years after the athletes had retired.[47] In the study, the BMDs of 97 young male athletes and 48 control participants were measured and repeated 5 years later when 55 of the athletes had retired. Although the young athletes who retired lost more BMD than those who were still active, the BMDs of the former athletes were still higher than those of the control population. Furthermore, the former athletes had significantly fewer fractures than the age-matched control participants. In a separate study comparing 400 former athletes with 800 control participants, the former athletes were found to have a lower incidence of fragility fractures and distal radius fractures than the control population.[47] Therefore, although the beneficial effect of exercise on BMD lessened over time, there still appeared to be a protective effect of exercise on the future development of fractures.

In a large 35-year follow-up study of 435,445 Swedish military recruits, it was found that fracture risk was significantly reduced in those in the highest decile of fitness or strength compared with those in the lowest decile.[48] Although that study did not specifically look at athletic activity or BMD, it did confirm the long-term beneficial effect of strength and fitness on bone health, as measured by subsequent reduced fracture risk.

CONCLUSIONS

There appears to be an association between some sports and radiographic degenerative changes in the lumbar and thoracolumbar spine. This is particularly true of track and field throwing sports. What effect such findings have, if any, on back symptoms, particularly back pain, is an entirely different matter. Indeed, most studies seem to suggest that no such correlation exists or is tenuous at best. Few data are available for other back conditions, such as lumbar disk herniation and lumbar spinal stenosis, although there does not appear to be any significant correlation between athletics and lumbar disk herniation.

The effect of sports on BMD is at least partially dependent on the type of sport. BMD is higher in throwers, pole vaulters, long jumpers, and triple jumpers than it is in endurance athletes. The effect of endurance sports on BMD seems to be enhanced by regular (twice-weekly) resistance training. Whether or not increased spine BMD results in reduced fracture risk is unclear, but it seems probable.

In general, therefore, there seems to be no long-term adverse effect of sports on back symptoms, although there may be an association between some sports and the development of future degenerative changes. Indeed, some sports may result in fewer symptoms in older athletes compared with control participants.

REFERENCES

1. Chen AL, Mears SC, Hawkins RJ: Orthopaedic care of the aging athlete. *J Am Acad Orthop Surg* 2005;13(6):407–416.

2. U.S. Department of Commerce, Bureau of the Census: *Current Population Reports. Statistical Abstract of the United States.* Washington, DC, US Government Printing Office, 2001, p 42.

3. Foster C, Wright G, Battista RA, et al: Training in the aging athlete. *Curr Sports Med Rep* 2007;6(3):200–206.

4. Borg-Stein J, Elson L, Brand E: The aging spine in Sports. *Clin Sports Med* 2012;31(3):473–86.

5. Truumees E: Low back pain in the aging athlete. *Semin Sports Surg* 2010;22(4):222–233.

6. Wiesel S, Feffer H, Borenstein D: Evaluation and outcome of low-back pain of unknown etiology. *Spine (Phila Pa 1976)* 1988;13(6):679–680.

7. Lundin O, Hellström M, Nilsson I, et al: Back pain and radiological changes in the thoraco-lumbar spine of athletes. A long-term follow-up. *Scand J Med Sci Sports* 2001;11:103–109.

8. Lawrence JP, Greene HS, Grauer JN: Back pain in athletes. *J Am Acad Orthop Surg* 2006;14(13):726–735.

9. Bono CM: Low-back pain in athletes. *J Bone Joint Surg Am* 2004;86-A(2):382–396.

10. Hartvigsen J, Christensen K: Lifestyle protects against incident low back pain in seniors: A population-based 2-year prospective study of 1387 Danish twins aged 70–100 years. *Spine (Phila Pa 1976)* 2007;32(1):76–81.

11. Graw BP, Wiesel SW: Low back pain in the aging athlete. *Sports Med Arthrosc Rev* 2008;16(1):39–46.

12. Swärd L, Hellström M, Jacobsson B, et al: Back pain and radiologic changes in the thoraco-lumbar spine in athletes. *Spine (Phila Pa 1976)* 1990;15(2):124–129.

13. Jackson D, Wiltse L, Cirincoine R: Spondylolysis in the female athlete. *Clin Orthop Rel Res* 1976;117:68–73.

14. Jackson D: Low back pain in young athletes: Evaluation of stress reaction and discogenic problems. *Am J Sports Med* 1979;7:364–346.

15. Szot Z, Boron Z, Galaj Z: Overloading changes in the motor system occurring in elite gymnasts. *Int J Sports Med* 1985;6:36–40.

16. Ferguson RJ, McMaster JH, Stanitski CL: Low back pain in college football linemen. *J Sports Med* 1974;2:63–69.

17. Semon R, Spengler D: Significance of lumbar spondylolysis in college football players. *Spine (Phila Pa 1976)* 1981;2:172–174.

18. Swärd L, Hellström M, Jacobsson B, et al: Disc degeneration and associated abnormalities of the spine in elite gymnasts: A magnetic resonance imaging study. *Spine (Phila Pa 1976)* 1991;16(4):437–443.

19. Videman T, Sarna S, Crites Battie M, et al: The long-term effects of physical loading and exercise lifestyles on back-related symptoms, disability, and spinal pathology among men. *Spine (Phila Pa 1976)* 1995;20(6):699–709.

20. Mundt DJ, Kelsey JL, Golden AL, et al: An epidemiologic study of sports and weight lifting as possible risk factors for herniated lumbar and cervical discs. *Am J Sports Med* 1993;21(6):854–860.

21. Boden SD, Davis DO, Dina TS, et al: Abnormal magnetic-resonance scans of the lumbar spine in asymptomatic subjects. A prospective investigation. *J Bone Joint Surg* 1990;72:403–408.

22. Jensen MC, Brant-Zawadzki MN, Obuchowski N, et al: Magnetic resonance imaging of the lumbar spine in people without back pain. *N Engl J Med* 1994;331(2):69–73.

23. Healy JF, Healy BB, Wong WHM, et al: Cervical and lumbar MRI in asymptomatic older male lifelong athletes: Frequency of degenerative findings. *J Comput Assist Tomogr* 1996;20(1):107–112.

24. Granhed H, Morelli B: Low back pain among retired wrestlers and heavyweight lifters. *Am J Sports Med* 1988;16:530–533.

25. Ozturk A, Ozkan Y, Ozdemir RM, et al: Radiographic changes in the lumbar spine in former professional football players: A comparative and matched controlled study. *Eur Spine J* 2008;17(1):136–141.

26. Schmitt H, Brocai DRC, Carstens C: Long-term review of the lumbar spine in javelin throwers. *J Bone Joint Surg* 2001;83-B(3):324–327.

27. Schmitt H, Dubljanin E, Schneider S, et al: Radiographic changes in the lumbar spine in former elite athletes. *Spine (Phila Pa 1976)* 2004;29(22):2554–2559.

28. Rossi F: Spondylolysis, spondylolisthesis and sports. *J Sports Med and Phys Fitness* 1978;18(4):317–340.

29. Billings RA, Burry HC, Jones R: Low back injury in sport. *Rheumatol Rehabil* 1977;16(4):236–240.

30. Kotani T, Ichikava N, Wakabayashi W: Studies of spondylolysis found among weight lifters. *Br J Sports Med* 1971;6:4–8.

31. Baranto A, Hellström M, Cederlund CG, et al: Back pain and MRI changes in the thoraco-lumbar spine of top athletes in four different sports: A 15-year follow-up study. *Knee Surg Sports Traumatol Arthrosc* 2009;17(9):1125–1134.

32. Wolff J: *Das Gesetz der Transformation der Knochen (The Law of Bone Transformation)*. Berlin, Hirschwald, 1892.

33. Frost HM: *Bone Remodeling and its Relationship to Metabolic Bone Diseases*. Springfield, IL, Thomas, 1973.

34. Schmitt H, Friebe C, Schneider S, et al: Bone mineral density and degenerative changes of the lumbar spine in former elite athletes. *Int J Sports Med* 2005;26(6):457–463.

35. Nevill AM, Holder RL, Stewart AD: Do sporting activities convey benefits to bone mass throughout the skeleton? *J Sports Sci* 2004;22(7):645–650.

36. Uzunca K, Birtane M, Durmus-Altun G, et al: High bone mineral density in loaded skeletal regions of former professional football (soccer) players: What is the effect of time after active career? *Br J Sports Med* 2005;39(3):154–157.

37. Karlsson MK, Hasserius R, Obrant KJ: Bone mineral density in athletes during and after career: A comparison between loaded and unloaded skeletal regions. *Calcif Tissue Int* 1996;59(4):245–248.

38. Karlsson MK, Johnell O, Obrant KJ: Is bone mineral density advantage maintained long-term in previous weight lifters? *Calcif Tissue Int* 1995;57(5):325–328.

39. Nilsson M, Ohlsson C, Eriksson AL, et al: Competitive physical activity early in life is associated with bone mineral density in elderly Swedish men. *Osteoporos Int* 2008;19(11):1557–1566.

40. Duppe H, Gardsell P, Johnell O, et al: Bone mineral density in female junior, senior and former football players. *Osteoporos Int* 1996;6(6):437–441.

41. Nichols JF, Palmer JE, Levy SS: Low bone mineral density in highly trained male master cyclists. *Osteoporos Int* 2003;14(8):644–649.

42. Nichols JF, Rauh MJ: Longitudinal changes in bone mineral density in male master cyclists and nonathletes. *J Strength Cond Res* 2011;25(3):727–734.

43. Hind K, Truscott JG, Evans JA: Low lumbar spine bone mineral density in both male and female endurance runners. *Bone* 2006;39(4):880–885.

44. McCrory JL, Salacinski AJ, Hunt Sellhorst SE, et al: Competitive athletic participation, thigh muscle strength, and bone density in elite senior athletes and controls. *J Strength Cond Res* 2013;27(11):3132–3141.

45. Daly RM, Bass SL: Lifetime sport and leisure activity participation is associated with greater bone size, quality and strength in older men. *Osteoporos Int* 2006;17(8):1258–1267.

46. Velez NF, Zhang A, Stone B, et al: The effect of moderate impact exercise on skeletal integrity in master athletes. *Osteoporos Int* 2008;19(10):1457–1464.

47. Nordström A, Karlsson C, Nyquist F, et al: Bone loss and fracture risk after reduced physical activity. *J Bone Miner Res* 2005;20(2):202–207.

48. Nordström P, Sievänen H, Gustafson Y, et al: High physical fitness in young adulthood reduces the risk of fractures later in life in men: A nationwide cohort study. *J Bone Miner Res* 2013;28(5):1061–1067.

22 Thoracic Injuries and Pain Syndromes in Athletes

Tanvir Choudhri, MD • Haroon Fiaz Choudhri, MD • Julian E. Bailes, Jr., MD

INTRODUCTION

The evaluation and management of thoracic pain and spinal and paraspinal injuries in athletes requires an understanding of the regional anatomy and injury patterns. Compared with other parts of the spine, thoracic spinal injuries are much less frequent because of the added anatomical support provided by the surrounding thoracic structures. When thoracic spinal injuries do occur, they can range from minor musculoskeletal strains or sprains to serious injuries with fractures, structural compromise, or neurologic deficits from spinal cord compression. Failure to identify and properly evaluate and treat these injuries may result in serious and sometimes permanent disability. The regional pulmonary and cardiovascular structures can provide added challenges. Perhaps as a result of their infrequency and complex regional anatomy, thoracic spinal injuries have few guidelines and treatment algorithms compared with other spinal regions, and management is generally based on treatment pathways adapted from other spinal injuries and the experience of the treating team. This chapter reviews thoracic spinal and paraspinal injuries and pain syndromes in athletes with attention to unique anatomy, injury patterns, evaluation, and management.

OVERVIEW AND EPIDEMIOLOGY

Anatomy

The thoracic spine typically consists of 12 vertebral levels with associated ribs with costovertebral and costotransverse spinal articulations. The rib cage, intercostal ligaments, paraspinal musculature, and sternum provide a "fourth column" of enhanced stability for the thoracic spine.[1-5] This strong thoracic "cage" protects important neurologic, cardiac, pulmonary, and vascular structures, which can be important considerations during the evaluation and management of thoracic spinal injuries.

Because of the relative difference in mobility of the thoracic spine and surrounding spinal segments, the cervicothoracic and thoracolumbar junctional regions have increased susceptibility to injury. The cervicothoracic region includes important neurologic structures (lowest cervical nerve roots and brachial plexus) that can affect upper extremity function. The thoracolumbar junction is susceptible to injury because of reduced stability from the lowest "floating" ribs and because the facet orientation changes from primarily coronal in the midthoracic spine to sagittal in the lumbar spine, providing less resistance to anterior translation.

The normal thoracic spine alignment has a mild to moderate kyphosis (normal range, 20°–45°) in part related to shorter anterior (compared with posterior) vertebral body heights. Increased kyphosis tends to occur with advancing age (especially in women older than 40 years of age), spinal degeneration, and medical conditions such as Scheuermann's disease.[6,7] Thoracic scoliosis, often asymptomatic, is seen in 2% to 3% of the population and may require monitoring, particularly in growing adolescents, and occasionally intervention. These aspects of thoracic anatomy and alignment, as well as overall health and bone density, can factor into management of thoracic spinal injuries in athletes.

Thoracic Pain in Athletes

Thoracic spinal pain commonly occurs in the general population; therefore, when seen in athletes, it does not necessarily represent an injury that needs treatment.[8] There has been little formal evaluation of thoracic pain in athletes compared with the general population. Jonasson et al

Tanvir Choudhri or an immediate family member has received research or institutional support from Pfizer. Neither of the following authors nor any immediate family member has received anything of value from or has stock or stock options held in a commercial company or institution related directly or indirectly to the subject of this article: Dr. Haroon Choudhri and Dr. Bailes.

evaluated the incidence of thoracic pain in high-performance athletes, including divers, weight lifters, wrestlers, hockey players, and orienteers.[9] The study found that athletes had the same rate (33%) of thoracic pain symptoms in the past year compared with nonathlete control participants, although athletes had a mildly higher, but not significant, rate of such symptoms in the past week (22% vs. 17%). As discussed later in this chapter, thoracic pain can be caused by a variety of spinal, paraspinal, and thoracic conditions. In addition, some cervical and lumbar conditions can manifest as thoracic pain for various musculoskeletal reasons. For example, cervical kyphosis often manifests as upper thoracic pain related to compensatory alignment and muscular strain. Similarly, loss of lumbar lordosis can shift the center of balance anteriorly and result in thoracic muscular pain.

Thoracic Spinal Degeneration in Athletes

Participation in sports can cause radiographic changes reflecting accelerated degeneration or accumulation of multiple small injuries over time.[10,11] Increased spinal degeneration has been reported in both contact and noncontact sports. Healy et al found that enhanced degeneration is more common in high-performance athletes than recreational athletes.[12] Degenerative changes in the thoracic spines of athletes have been evaluated in several studies, often focusing on the lower thoracic spine in combination with the lumbar spine. In a study of thoracolumbar spines in elite skiers, Rachbauer et al found that almost 50% of ski jumpers and alpine skiers and 36% of cross-country skiers had radiographic vertebral end plate lesions compared with fewer than 20% of age-matched control participants.[13] Similarly, Daniels et al found twice the rate of degenerative abnormalities in the thoracic spine of adolescent motocross racers compared with age-matched control participants.[14] Baranto et al evaluated back pain and thoracolumbar degenerative changes in elite athletes.[15,16] Not surprisingly, they found increased rates of thoracolumbar pain and degenerative findings in athletes compared with nonathlete control participants. Interestingly, follow-up radiographic studies 15 years later (mean age, 40 years) revealed that the vast majority of radiographic findings were present on the earlier studies (mean age, 26 years). The authors suggest that athletes may be more susceptible to developing degenerative spinal changes earlier in life during or near growth spurts.

Thoracic Injury Patterns

In athletes, the majority of thoracic injuries are related to blunt force or repetitive impacts. Penetrating trauma,

although much less common, can occur in certain sports, including fencing, javelin, pole vaulting, and skiing (from poles).[17-21] As part of the evaluation of thoracic pain, the clinician should remember that the symptoms may be the related to spinal, paraspinal, or surrounding structures (e.g., cardiac, pulmonary, vascular). After injury or during workup for potential injury, serious life-threatening or fatal conditions including commotio cordis, myocarditis, myocardial infarction, and pulmonary embolism, have been reported in athletes from a wide range of sports.[22-29] In their study of pediatric sports-related pneumothorax, Soundappan et al found that the presentation may be atypical with minimal to no signs.[30]

Thoracic spinal and paraspinal injuries can be defined by the structure(s) and region(s) of involvement as well as the injury characteristics such as instability or neurologic dysfunction. Thoracic spinal injuries can be categorized by specific sites or types of anatomic injury, although clearly some injuries involve multiple structures. Paraspinal injuries are very common and generally represent soft tissue injuries such as superficial bruises or contusions and muscular injuries along the spectrum from strains to tears.[31,32] Thoracic spinal ligamentous injuries (e.g., intraspinous, supraspinous, and costovertebral ligaments) can be painful and when extensive can compromise stability. Excessive demands on the paraspinal muscles as well as the rhomboids and latissimus dorsi muscles can result in trigger points or enthesopathy.

Thoracic disk herniations can cause regional pain or radiculopathy from nerve root compression or neurologic deficits from spinal cord impingement. Published reports on the prevalence of thoracic disk herniations range from 1 in 1000 to 1 in 1,000,000 individuals. The incidence of asymptomatic thoracic disk herniations on imaging was found to be 11% to 13% in an autopsy study and 13% to 15% in a CT myelography study but as high as 37% in an MRI study.[33-35] Symptomatic thoracic disk herniations are relatively rare compared with cervical and lumbar herniations. In a retrospective review of disk herniation in National Football League (NFL) players, Gray et al found that only 1.5% (4) of 275 disk herniations were in the thoracic spine compared with 22.2% (61) in the cervical and 76.4% (210) in the lumbar spine.[36]

Although thoracic disks can present acutely after an athletic injury, they are commonly associated with a chronic presentation (**Figure 22-1**).[32-40] Repetitive injuries to the thoracic spine, especially with excessive loads and forces, can injure the disk annulus and result in thoracic disk herniation. Similarly, chronic microinstability can result in thoracic spondylosis, which encompasses a

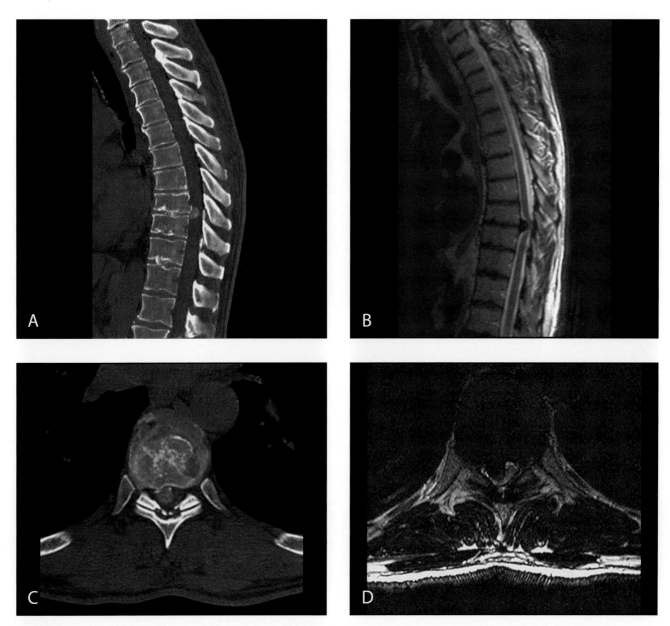

FIGURE 22-1 Chronic calcified thoracic disk. A former male elite (Olympic) gymnast in his 60s presented with myelopathy from calcified T9 to T10 herniated disk eccentric to the right. After discussing the options, he was treated with a posterolateral decompression with right transpedicular decompression. **A,** Sagittal CT scan. **B,** Sagittal T2-weighted MRI. **C,** Axial CT. **D,** Axial T2-weighted MRI.

variety of degenerative findings, including disk bulges, osteophyte formation, and hypertrophy of the posterior longitudinal ligament. Thoracic disk herniations and spondylosis can result in effacement of the cerebrospinal fluid spaces and nerve root or spinal cord impingement.

Thoracic fractures can involve anterior elements (vertebral body), posterior elements (e.g., spinous process, transverse process, lamina, facets), or both.[41] Thoracic fracture patterns include compression fractures; burst fractures; and complex injuries producing deformity with subluxation, kyphosis, rotation, or distraction

(**Figure 22-2**).[42] Compression fractures are usually associated with forced flexion and involve compromise of the anterior vertebral body with preservation of the middle column and posterior elements. With middle column compromise as well, the fracture is considered a burst fracture. With some burst fractures, the posterior part of the vertebral body can retropulse into the spinal canal, resulting in neurologic compromise.

With any spinal fracture, it is important to assess for the presence or potential for instability or neurologic compromise. With kyphosis, the forward spinal

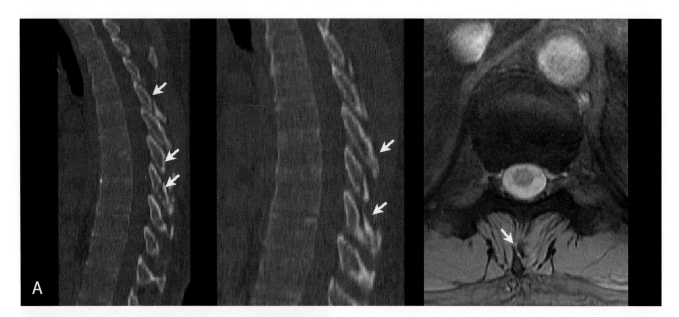

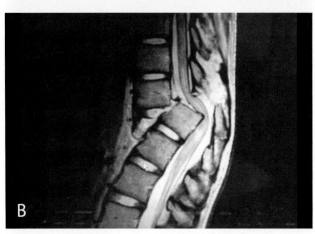

FIGURE 22-2 Thoracic fractures can range from spinous process fractures to fracture dislocations with spondyloptosis. **A,** Sagittal CT and axial MRI of a male cyclist in his 40s who presented with multiple injuries after a bicycle accident. **B,** Sagittal MRI from a teenage gymnast who developed a spinal injury after gymnastic trauma.

angulation can cause the spinal cord to drape over retropulsed bone or disk herniation in the spinal canal. Fractures associated with rotation and distraction injuries are more likely to be associated with ligamentous compromise. Chance fractures, often seen with distraction injuries, involve a three-column injury through the anterior and posterior elements, generally in one plane (**Figure 22-3**).[43] Identification of these structural fracture patterns is important in guiding management as discussed later in this chapter.

● EVALUATION

After thoracic trauma, the initial assessment should evaluate for serious life-threatening conditions and injuries that have caused (or have the potential to cause) instability or neurologic injury. As with other injuries, the evaluation of thoracic injuries should assess both the region of known

symptomatic trauma as well as the surrounding regions that could harbor potential occult injuries. After the history and physical examination, appropriate diagnostic studies are used to characterize the injury (**Table 22-1**).

Approach to Acute Thoracic Injuries

The initial evaluation of acute thoracic injuries, often in the field, should follow standard trauma protocols (e.g., advanced trauma life support [ATLS]). Spinal precautions for potential spinal injury and spinal instability (e.g., immobilization, log rolling) are required throughout the evaluation and transportation process until the patient has been "cleared" for spinal instability with clinical or radiographic evaluation. Athletes who are unresponsive or not breathing require attention to maintain or restore adequate ventilation and circulation. Rarely, blunt force injuries to the anterior chest region can cause commotio cordis, a serious cardiac condition

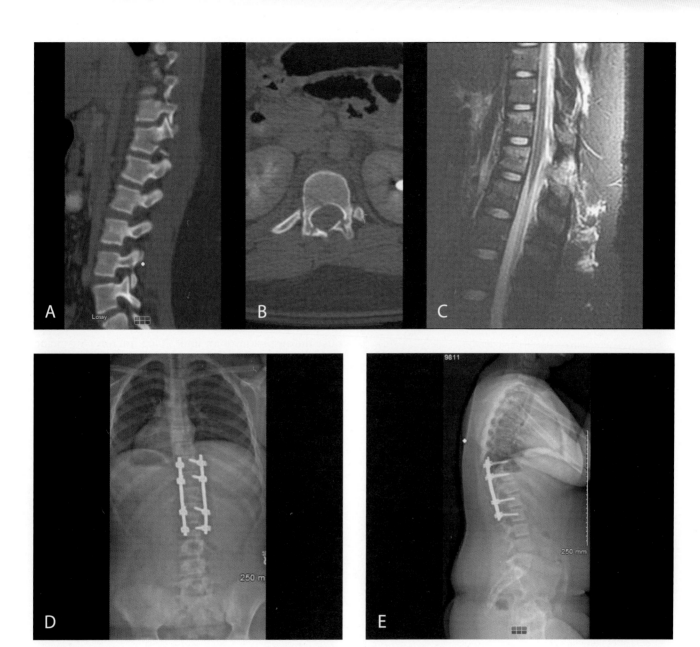

FIGURE 22-3 Chance fracture. A 13-year-old girl presented with a Chance fracture after a motor vehicle accident. Preoperative sagittal (**A**) and axial (**B**) CT images. Sagittal (**C**) MRI and postoperative anteroposterior (**D**) and lateral (**E**) radiographs after T10 to L2 posterior segmental stabilization

associated with ventricular arrhythmia and high rates of mortality.[24,25] This condition has been reported in a number of sports, including baseball, martial arts, and other sports with potential blunt force chest trauma. After commotion cordis, rapid cardiac defibrillation is advisable and can improve survival chances. Penetrating trauma or some blunt injuries (e.g., some rib fractures) can result in cardiac tamponade or pneumothorax, which may require lifesaving procedures (e.g., cardiocentesis or thoracostomy).

Athletes who demonstrate acute spinal cord dysfunction (e.g., partial or complete paralysis, sensory level, or bowel and bladder dysfunction) require emergent diagnostic imaging to evaluate for potential spinal compression or instability that could mandate emergency surgery for decompression or stabilization. Athletes with acute cardiopulmonary or neurologic dysfunction generally require rapid transportation to a hospital for diagnostic evaluation and definitive management. After initial evaluation and stabilization, the diagnostic workup for thoracic injuries depends on the nature and intensity of symptoms. Depending on the situation, the diagnostic workup

TABLE 22-1 Evaluation and initial management of thoracic injuries in athletes

Acute Thoracic Injuries

On Field

ABCs (airway, breathing, circulation)

Initial assessment and screening for systemic trauma and spine trauma

Spine precautions

General and neurologic examination assessment

History: timing, mechanism, symptoms, modifying factors

Bring player-patient to setting to be assessed and treated—sideline vs. stadium medical station vs. ED

Goals: resuscitate, stabilize patient, begin assessment of injuries, get player expeditiously and safely to setting best equipped to manage

In ED or Hospital

ABCs, systemic trauma evaluation, and spine precautions generally have already been addressed, but be careful not to assume

History: timing, mechanism, symptoms, modifying factors

Goals: direct workup to best evaluate thoracic symptoms to determine source(s) of symptoms (spine vs. paraspinal vs. other)

Outpatient Evaluation of Acute Thoracic Symptoms

ABCs, trauma evaluation, spine precautions generally already addressed

Neurologic Deficits: Rule Out Thoracic Spinal Cord Injury

Thoracic spinal MRI (consider CT or myelogram if MRI not possible)

CT of the thoracic spine

Goal: evaluate for compression and instability that could require intervention

Acute or Chronic Thoracic Pain without Neurologic Deficits

Consider nonspinal medical cause (PE, MI) with workup as appropriate

Consider paraspinal musculoskeletal causes (rib fx, muscle strain, soft tissue contusion)

Assess for thoracic spinal causes as appropriate

If fracture suspected: radiography, CT, and MRI if appropriate

ED = emergency department, MI = myocardial infarction, PE = pulmonary embolism.

may include plain radiographs and CT and MRI scans when indicated.

Approach to Chronic Thoracic Injuries

The evaluation of chronic thoracic injuries and symptoms is generally less time sensitive than for acute injuries. However, the clinician should remember that thoracic symptoms in athletes may reflect underlying serious medical conditions not related to injury. Pulmonary embolism, angina or coronary artery disease, myocarditis, and pneumothorax have been reported in athletes who present with thoracic pain or symptoms that could be mistakenly attributed to minor or occult injury. Although gross spinal instability is uncommon with chronic injuries, compromised stability may occur and require management. As with acute injuries, the diagnostic workup for thoracic injuries depends on the nature and intensity of symptoms but frequently includes MRI scanning. Plain radiographs and CT scans are used less frequently for chronic symptoms, and the value must be balanced with the risks of ionizing radiation.

Diagnostic Considerations

The thoracic spinal evaluation is primarily focused on assessing for structural compromise and neurologic compression. Intense acute focal pain or local tenderness to spinal palpation in a conscious and awake patient should raise the suspicion of an underlying fracture. Suspicion of a thoracic fracture based on the mechanism or severity of injury, neurologic deficit(s), or focal tenderness should prompt further evaluation with either plain film radiography or CT imaging. A patient with sternal or rib fractures or other spinal fractures should be considered at elevated risk for associated thoracic spinal injuries. Neurologic compression typically manifests as a deficit pattern associated with nerve root or spinal cord dysfunction and can occur without significant fracture. Thoracic radiculopathy can result in pain or numbness that radiates along a thoracic dermatome, which typically follows the associated rib level wrapping around to the lateral then anterior chest wall. As a result, thoracic radiculopathy can mimic symptoms from cardiac or other visceral pathology. Large thoracic disk herniations and epidural hematomas may develop without associated spinal fractures. Furthermore, aggravation of a preexisting, and often undiagnosed, condition such as dysraphism or severe spinal canal stenosis is also possible.

Neurologic assessment is required with any suspected or documented neurologic deficit. When the neurologic examination is limited by impaired consciousness, sedation, severe pain, hemodynamic instability, or associated injuries, one should maintain a healthy suspicion that a neurologic injury may have occurred. These patients may deteriorate rapidly and irreversibly, and MRI imaging should be considered to exclude the possibility of a time-sensitive condition.

Diagnostic Testing

When a spinal fracture is suspected (e.g., acute focal midline pain symptoms, point tenderness, or step-off or deformity), plain film radiographs should be strongly considered. Plain radiographic imaging is rapid and inexpensive, can demonstrate most significant thoracic fractures, and uses minimal radiation compared with CT scanning. However, some thoracic fractures are not well visualized on plain radiographs, for example, in the cervicothoracic and upper thoracic spinal regions, where the anatomy can provide radiographic interference.[44]

When a spinal fracture is suspected and plain radiographs are not available, conclusive, or adequate, CT imaging should be considered. CT scans with sagittal and coronal reformatting sequences represents the gold standard to diagnose and characterize most fractures.

Magnetic resonance imaging is useful in evaluating disks, nerve root and cord compression, and soft tissue abnormalities. Neurologic deficits from thoracic spinal cord injuries (SCIs) typically involve numbness and weakness in various patterns below the level of injury based on the nature of SCI. Bowel and bladder dysfunction (urinary or fecal incontinence or retention) as well as development of a thoracic sensory level are serious developments that also mandate advanced imaging with an MRI (or CT myelogram when MRI is unavailable, impractical, or contraindicated).

⬤ MANAGEMENT
General Principles

Acute thoracic injuries can result in structurally compromising fractures or neurologic deficits from spinal cord or nerve root compromise. Failure to rapidly identify and treat these injuries (sometimes with surgery) may result in permanent disability. However, most thoracic injuries are minor and can be conservatively managed. Management of extraspinal thoracic injuries (e.g., pulmonary, cardiac) should follow standard trauma care; the details are beyond the scope of this chapter. We will review the management considerations of the more common thoracic spinal injuries that can affect athletes. The primary goals are to minimize further injury and offer the patient the best chance at optimal recovery in the fastest way possible.

After injury, return to participation in athletic activities is an important yet often challenging and sometimes controversial topic.[45–49] After serious injury, return to play (RTP) may not be possible or advisable. Thankfully, after most injuries, RTP is possible, usually with gradual return to practice then play after symptoms have resolved. Although there have been a few articles discussing RTP after spine surgery in general, there has been little formal study of RTP after thoracic spine surgery. For all RTP decisions, a balanced approach with individualized risk-to-benefit analysis is warranted, including not only the ability to return to sport but also the ability to withstand reinjury. For obvious reasons, professional athletes whose livelihood is sports must assume some of the risk burden, and the physician's role is to adequately educate and guide them.

Superficial and Paraspinal Soft Tissue Injuries

Superficial soft tissue and paraspinal musculoskeletal injuries without underlying spinal column injury (e.g., contusions and muscle strains) are fairly common. The diagnosis is generally made clinically with diagnostic studies typically reserved to rule out occult deeper injuries when suspected. The clinician should consider some unique injury patterns, including rib stress fractures and the "slipping rib" syndrome.[50,51] Almost universally, these injuries are treated nonoperatively with symptomatic management (e.g., reduced activity, ice and heat medications, physical therapy, thoracic stabilization exercises, interventional pain procedures). After symptomatic improvement, RTP is a process involving progressive increase in activity under medical supervision in the absence of neurologic deficits or persistent structural concerns. Persistence of symptoms or setbacks in the recovery process should prompt clinical reevaluation and workup (e.g., imaging). Long-term considerations for these injuries are generally rare. Athletes with muscular injuries may be susceptible to reinjury and can benefit from enhanced muscular conditioning to help prevent recurrent or progressive injuries.

Thoracic Disk Herniations

Because of the increased stability from overall thoracic anatomy, thoracic disk herniations are relatively rare compared with herniations of other parts of the spine.[36] When they do occur, the main concerns are neurologic deficits from spinal cord impingement or radiculopathy from nerve root compression. Thoracic cord compression may present as varying combinations of pain, numbness, and weakness. Classic patterns include Brown-Séquard syndrome (spinal cord hemidysfunction) and varying degrees of spinal cord dysfunction below the level of injury, which may include bowel and bladder dysfunction. Thoracic root compression generally causes radicular pain without significant neurologic or functional deficits because the thoracic nerve roots (aside from T1) are not typically involved in major extremity function. The T1 root can be affected from a T1 to T2 disk herniation.[52] Also, there has been a report of a T2 to T3 distribution causing extremity weakness into the hand caused by a postfixed brachial plexus.[53] Midthoracic disk herniations are relatively rare and are typically associated with major trauma (acute) or degenerative spondylosis (chronic). Lower thoracic disk herniations, typically in the last T10 to T12 regions, can present with a picture resembling cauda equina syndrome.

As with other parts of the spine, thoracic disk herniations can often be managed nonoperatively with various modalities such as physical therapy and pain management. With time, many disk herniations can recede and become or remain asymptomatic.[54] When pain persists, there is level 3 evidence supporting the use of epidural injections.[55,56] Surgical decompression also may prove needed for refractory symptoms from a thoracic disk herniation. Similarly, at any point, surgical intervention is appropriate to consider when there is neurologic concerns. Acute or chronic (e.g., myelopathy) SCI from thoracic disk herniation frequently requires surgical intervention to promote recovery and prevent further injury. Similarly, sizable herniations with significant radiographic cord compression (sometimes with cord signal changes) also warrant consideration of surgery. When surgery is needed, the primary goal is safe and adequate decompression of the spinal cord or nerve roots (or both). A wide variety of surgical approach options can be broadly grouped into anterior or posterolateral approaches.

Although some surgeons advocate one approach for most or all cases, most surgeons tailor the choice of surgical approach based on injury characteristics. Anterior approaches are well-suited for disks that are large, midline, or calcified. Smaller, softer lateral disk herniations may be amenable to a posterior approach, which can avoid some of the additional morbidity associated with anterior thoracic approaches. Instability, either from the injury or surgical approach, may require concomitant stabilization as a secondary goal.

Return to play is based upon symptom improvement with gradual return to activity and competition as tolerated. Persistence of symptoms or setbacks in the recovery process should prompt additional workup (e.g., imaging). Although thoracic disk herniations are less common than herniations in other spinal regions, a study of disk herniations in NFL players found that they are associated with the longest time before RTP.[36]

Athletes with thoracic disk herniations may be susceptible to increased delayed degeneration from either latent instability or accelerated degenerative process. In addition, some athletes could have unrecognized thoracic disk herniations that prove significant later in life.

Thoracic Spinal Fractures

History (e.g., pain, injury mechanism) and physical examination findings (e.g., point tenderness, palpable step-off) can suggest that a thoracic fracture has occurred. Radiographic studies are needed for proper diagnosis and characterization for management. Traditionally radiographs have been used for the initial diagnosis of thoracic fractures, and they still have a role when rapid assessment of spinal alignment and potential fracture is needed. However, CT represents the gold standard to diagnose and characterize spinal fractures with far better sensitivity and specificity. MRI studies are less commonly used to diagnose spinal fractures, but they can be very helpful to assess important characteristics of thoracic fractures. Differentiating acute from chronic thoracic vertebral fractures is limited on plain film radiographs. MRI is currently the most commonly used technique to identify acuity of fractures, with hyperintense signal of marrow edema on short tau inversion recovery (STIR) sequences a sign of acuity. MRI can also evaluate ligamentous and cord injury, as well as canal and neural foraminal compromise.

Thoracic spinal fracture management is primarily based on instability and neurologic issues. Most transverse process, spinous process, laminar, facet fractures, and vertebral avulsion fracture are stable and able to be managed nonoperatively with symptomatic treatment. Vertebral body compression fractures generally do not demonstrate acute instability but should be monitored (clinically, radiographically, or both) for possible progression. Depending on the nature of the fracture and expected forces to be experienced in the athlete's sport, CT imaging may be advisable before RTP. Vertebral burst fractures must be differentiated from and managed differently than compression fractures. For many years, management of vertebral body burst fractures was primarily based on the three-column model of Denis[57] and the AO classification,[58] which both have limitations. In 2005, the Thoracolumbar Injury Classification and Severity Scale (TLICS) system was published by Vaccaro et al and has become a widely accepted grading system for thoracolumbar fractures (**Table 22-2**).[59] The TLICS score is calculated by first assigning three subgroup scores incorporating an assessment of the integrity of the posterior ligamentous complex (often through MRI). The TLICS has proven useful in deciding whether surgery is indicated without advocating which surgical approach is to be used, which

TABLE 22-2 Thoracolumbar Injury Classification and Severity (TLICS) grading system[52]

Points	Injury
Fracture Morphology	
1	Compression fracture
2	Burst fracture
3	Rotational injury
4	Distraction injury
Neurologic Deficits	
1	Neurologically intact
2	Nerve root injury or complete SCI
3	Cauda equina injury or incomplete SCI
Posterior Ligamentous Complex Injury	
0	No posterior ligamentous injury
2	Suspected posterior ligamentous injury
3	Posterior ligamentous injury

The subscores are totaled, and the resulting score is between 1 and 10. Treatment guidelines suggest:

   1–3: Surgery not required and can be treated nonoperatively (e.g., brace)
   4: Treated at the discretion of the surgeon (no clear treatment recommendation)
   5–10: Surgery for decompression and stabilization as injury dictates
SCI = spinal cord injury.

is left to surgeon choice. Regardless of which classification system is used, the main treatment principles depend on the degree of stability and neurologic deficits.[60] Unstable fractures typically require fusion surgery for stabilization, typically with spinal instrumentation. The goals of surgery include neurologic decompression, restoration of alignment, and stabilization. Depending on the type of injury and surgeon experience, anterior, posterior, or combined approaches may be selected.

Return to play for stable nonoperative fractures is based on fracture healing (generally documented on imaging) and symptom improvement with gradual return to activity and competition as tolerated depending on the nature of sport. For hairline fractures or nonstructural injuries such as transverse or spinous process fractures, 6 weeks of healing, possibly using a brace, should allow a healthy individual to recover to return to all but the most vigorous of activities. Athletes with stable fractures that heal completely may likely return to full activity and participation in their sports with the proper monitoring and progression through RTP protocols. Athletes with unstable fractures, which typically require surgical intervention, should have individualized RTP considerations and typically require longer periods of healing before they can safely return to competition. Persistence of symptoms

or setbacks in the recovery process should prompt additional workup (e.g., reimaging). However, the risks of ionizing radiation (particularly CT scans) must be balanced with the clinical utility and benefit. For athletes in contact sports with a higher likelihood of re-injury, follow-up imaging studies after RTP should routinely be considered to assess that the injury has remained healed (e.g., edema resolved).

Long-term considerations after thoracic fractures can include nonunion, refractures, and junctional fractures or spondylosis after a fusion at the injury site. Sometimes athletes can require secondary procedures to address these developments to achieve stabilization, improve alignment, or control pain (**Figure 22-4**).

Thoracic Spinal Cord Injuries

Acute thoracic SCIs are generally self-evident with significant motor (lower extremity paraparesis) or sensory deficits (often with a partial or complete level). Bowel and bladder function may be compromised and must be assessed. Initially, lower extremity reflexes are typically absent. The American Spinal Injury Association (ASIA) rating scale is frequently used to characterize the injury and has shown utility in predicting long-term outcome (**Table 22-3**). Chronic SCI (e.g., myelopathy) can be harder to diagnose and may be related to congenital or degenerative factors (e.g., herniated disk or spondylosis). With chronic spinal cord dysfunction, patients can exhibit similar deficits as acute injuries generally with less severe deficits and with development of hyperreflexia. For all these injuries, it is important to assess for possible ongoing sources of spinal injury related to fractures, cord compression, instability, and/or hematoma. Neurapraxic cord injuries (involving stretching of the spinal cord) are part of the spectrum of SCI and are generally transient and often without associated fractures or compression.

When acute neurologic compression exists, prompt surgical decompression remains the overriding treating principle with attention to correcting alignment or deformity where needed. Adjuncts such as high-dose methylprednisolone treatment and hypothermia (local or systemic) may be considered in conjunction with surgery in an attempt to improve outcomes. As with all treatments, the risk-to-benefit ratio must be carefully considered. Newer medications and transplant of stem cells and Schwann cells are under active investigation but are not established treatments. For all of these adjunct treatments, there is a lack of high level-of-evidence supportive studies, and not surprisingly, usage is variable and often controversial.

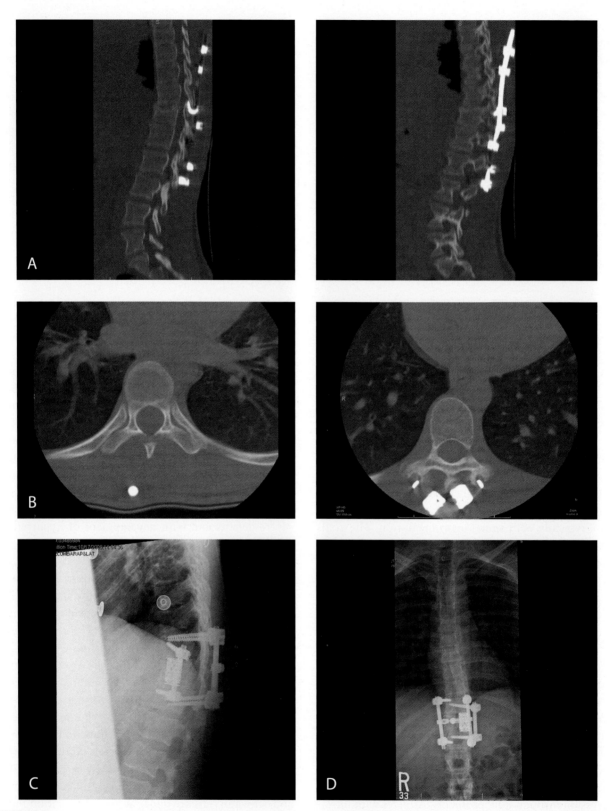

FIGURE 22-4 Burst fracture requiring revision surgery. A 19-year-old female elite sprinter developed a T12 burst fracture after a severe backward fall during plyometric workout. She was treated at an outside hospital with a T8 to L3 posterior rod and hook construct. She subsequently presented with increasing severe mechanical pain associated with progressive kyphosis, instability, and superior construct failure. She was treated with T12 corpectomy and T11 to L1 anteroposterior (AP) fusion–instrumentation construct. **A,** Preoperative sagittal CT. **B,** Preoperative axial CT image. **C,** Postoperative lateral radiograph. **D,** Postoperative AP radiograph.

TABLE 22-3	American Spinal Injury Association (ASIA) Rating Scale
Grade	Description
A	Complete lack of motor and sensory function below the level of injury (including the anal area)
B	Some sensation below the level of the injury (including anal sensation)
C	Some muscle movement is spared below the level of injury, but 50% of the muscles below the level of injury cannot move against gravity
D	Most (>50%) of the muscles that are spared below the level of injury are strong enough to move against gravity
E	All neurologic function has returned

Return to play is based on functional improvement with gradual return to activity and competition depending on not only return of function but also the ability to tolerate the risks of the sport with acceptably low risks of reinjury.

Long-term considerations after thoracic SCI depend on the specific injury deficits. Although some delayed neurologic improvement is possible, the magnitude is frequently limited because of the inherent central nervous system biologic properties. The potential long-term consequences of repeated neurapraxic injuries (sometimes described as spinal concussions) requires further study.

CONCLUSIONS

Evaluation and management of thoracic spinal and paraspinal injuries in athletes requires an understanding of the unique regional anatomy and injury patterns. Although rare, potentially life-threatening cardiovascular and pulmonary conditions need to be considered. Paraspinal injuries are generally able to be managed nonoperatively with full return to sport. Thoracic disk herniations can have acute and chronic presentations and sometimes require surgery for neurologic consequences or refractory symptoms. Degenerative thoracic spondylosis can be caused or accelerated by repetitive trauma, more commonly in high-intensity sports. Stable thoracic fractures require a period of recovery to heal but usually allow full return to sport without need for surgery. Unstable fractures typically require stabilization surgery with instrumentation and a more extensive recovery process with full return to sport possible but not guaranteed. With proper diagnosis and management, for most athletes, absent neurologic injury, a full return to sports participation is possible after most thoracic injuries.

ACKNOWLEDGMENTS

The authors would like to thank Asim Choudhri, MD, for review of manuscript, discussion of radiologic issues, and history and imaging related to Figures 22-2B and 22-3.

REFERENCES

1. Watkins R, Watkins R, Williams L, et al: Stability provided by the sternum and rib cage in thoracic spine. *Spine* 2005;30(11):1283–1286.

2. Oda I, Abumi K, Cunningham BW, et al: An in vitro Human cadaveric study investigating the biomechanical properties of the thoracic spine. *Spine* 2002;27: E64–E70.

3. Oda I, Abumi K, Lu D, et al: Biomechanical role of the posterior elements, costovertebral joints, and rib cage in stability of the thoracic spine. *Spine* 1996;21: 1423–1429.

4. Panjabi MM, Brand RA, White AA: Mechanical properties of the human thoracic spine: As shown by three-dimensional load-displacement curves. *J Bone Joint Surg* 1976;58(suppl A):642–652.

5. Panjabi MM, Hausfeld JN, White AA: A Biomechanical study of the ligamentous stability of the thoracic spine in man. *Acta Orthop Scand* 1981;52:315–326.

6. Fon GT, Pitt MJ, Thies AC: Thoracic kyphosis: Range in normal subjects. *AJR Am J Roentgenol* 1980;134:979–983.

7. Damborg F, Engell V, Andersen M, Kyvik KO, Thomsen K: Prevalence, concordance, and heritability of scheuermann kyphosis based on a study of twins. *J Bone Joint Surg Am* 2006;88:2133–2136.

8. Tall RL, DeVault W: Spinal injury in sport: Epidemiologic considerations. *Clin Sports Med* 1993;12:441–448.

9. Jonasson P, Halldin K, Karlsson J, Thoreson O, Hvannberg J, Sward L, Baranto A: Prevalence of joint-related pain in the extremities and spine in five groups of top athletes. *Knee Surg Sports Traumatol Arthrosc* 2011;19:1540–1546.

10. Fukuta S, Miyamoto K, Iwata A, Hosoe H, Iwata H, Shirahashi K, Shimizu K: Unusual Back pain caused by intervertebral disc degeneration associated with Schmorl node at Th11/12 in a young athlete, successfully treated by anterior interbody fusion: A case report. *Spine* 2009;34(5): E195–E198.

11. Videman T, Battie MC, Gibbons LE, Manninen H, Gill K, Fisher LD, Koskenvuo M: Lifetime exercise and disk degeneration: An MRI study of monozygotic twins. *Med Sci Sports Exerc* 1997;29(10):1350–1356.

12. Healy JF, Healy BB, Wong WH, Olson EM: Cervical and lumbar MRI in asymptomatic older male lifelong athletes: Frequency of degenerative findings. *J Comput Assist Tomogr* 1996;20:107–112.

13. Rachbauer F, Sterzinger W, Eibl GP: Radiographic abnormalities in the thoracolumbar spine of young elite skiers. *Am J Sports Med* 2001;29(4):446–449.

14. Daniels DJ, Luo TD, Puffer R, McIntosh AL, Larson AN, Wetjen NM, Clarke MJ: Degenerative changes in adolescent spines: A comparison of motocross racers and age-matched controls. *J Neurosurg Pediatrics* 2015;15:266–271.

15. Baranto A, Hellstrom M, Cederlund CG, Nyman R, Sward L: Back pain and MRI changes in the thoraco-lumbar spine of top athletes in four different sports: A 15 year follow-up study. *Knee Surg Sports Traumatol Arthrosc* 2009;17:1125–1134.

16. Baranto A, Hellstrom M, Nyman R, Lundin O, Sward L: Back pain and degenerative abnormalities in the spine of young elite divers. *Knee Surg Sports Traumatol Arthrosc* 2006;14(9):907–914.

17. Khan N, Husain S, Haak M: Thoracolumbar injuries in the athlete. *Sports Med Arthrosc* 2008;16(1):16–25.

18. Lundin O, Hellstrom M, Nilsson I, Sward L: Back pain and radiological changes in the thoraco-lumbar spine of athletes. A long-term follow-up. *Scand J Med Sci Sports* 2001;11:103–109.

19. McDonagh D, Zideman D: Thoracic injuries. In: *IOC Manual for Emergency Sports Medicine*. Hoboken, NJ: Wiley-Blackwell, 2015, pp 142–156.

20. Boden BP, Pasquina P, Johnson J, Mueller FO: Catastrophic injuries in pole-vaulters. *Am J Sports Med* 2001;29(1):50–54.

21. Boden BP, Boden MG, Peter RG, Mueller FO, Johnson JE: Catastrophic Injuries in pole vaulters: A prospective 9-year follow-up study. *Am J Sports Med* 2012;40(7):1488–1494.

22. Wasfy MM, Baggish A: Chest pain in athletes from personal history section (medical causes). *Curr Sports Med Rep* 2015;14(3):248–252.

23. Lolay GA, Abdel-Latif AK: Trauma induced myocardial infarction. *Int J Cardiol* 2016;203:19–21.

24. Maron BJ, Gohman T, Kyle SB, Estes NAM, Link MS: Clinical profile and spectrum of commotio cordis. *JAMA* 2002;287(9):1142–1146.

25. Lucena JS, Rico A, Salguero M, Blanco M, Vazquez R: Commotio cordis as a result of a fight: Report of a case considered to be imprudent homicide. *Forens Sci Int* 2008; 177(1):1–4.

26. Ahmadi H, Shirani S, Yazdanifard P: Aortic dissection type 1 in a weightlifter with hypertension: A case report. *Cases J* 2008;1(1):99.

27. Kahanov L, Daly T: Bilateral pulmonary emboli in a collegiate gymnast: A case report. *J Athl Train* 2009;44(6): 666–671.

28. Landesberg WH: Pulmonary embolism in a female collegiate cross-country running presenting as nonspecific back pain. *J Chiropr Med* 2012;11:215–220.

29. Hsing DD, Madikians A: True-true, unrelated: A case report. *Pediatr Emerg Care* 2005;21(11):755–759.

30. Soundappan SVS, Holland AJA, Browne G: Sports-related pneumothorax in children. *Pediatr Emerg Care* 2005; 21(4):259–260.

31. Keene JS, Albert MJ, Springer SL, Drummond DS, Clancy WG Jr: Back injuries in college athletes. *J Spinal Disorders* 1989;2(3):190–195.

32. Khadavi MJ, Fredericson M: Chest pain in athletes from personal history section (musculoskeletal causes). *Curr Sports Med Rep* 2015;14(3):252–254.

33. Mirkovic S, Cybulski GR: Thoracic disc herniations, in Garfin SR, Vaccaro AR, eds: *Orthopaedic Knowledge Update V*. Rosemont, IL, American Academy of Orthopaedic Surgeons, 1996.

34. Awwad EE, Martin DS, Smith KR Jr, Baker BK: Asymptomatic versus symptomatic herniated thoracic discs: Their frequency and characteristics as detected by computed tomography after myelography. *Neurosurgery* 1991;28(2):180–186.

35. Wood KB, Garvey TA, Gundry C, Heithoff KB: Magnetic resonance imaging of the thoracic spine. Evaluation of asymptomatic individuals. *J Bone Joint Surg Am* 1995; 77(11):1631–1638.

36. Gray BL, Buchowski JM, Bumpass DB, Lehman RA, Mall NA, Matava MJ: Disc herniations in the National Football League. *Spine* 2013;38(22):1934–1938.

37. Bartlett GR, Robertson PA: Acute thoracic disc prolapse with paraparesis following a rugby tackle: A case report. *N Z Med J* 1994;107(973):86–88.

38. Baranto A, Borjesson M, Danielsson, Hellstrom M, Sward L: Acute chest pain in a top soccer player due to thoracic disc herniation. *Spine* 2009;34(10):E359–E362.

39. Davies PR, Kaar G: High thoracic disc prolapse in a rugby player: The first reported case. *Br J Sports Med* 1993; 27(2):177–178.

40. Jamieson DR, Ballantyne JP: Unique presentation of a prolapsed thoracic disk: Lhermitte's symptom in a golf player. *Neurology* 1995;45(6):1219–1221.

41. Olivier EC, Muller E, Janse van Rensburg DC: Clay-shoveler fracture in a paddler: A case report. *Clin J Sport Med* 2016; 26(3):e69–e70.

42. Menzer H, Gill GK, Paterson A: Thoracic spine sports-related injuries. *Curr Sports Med Rep* 2015;14(1):34–40.

43. Boham M, O'Connell K: Unusual mechanism of injury resulting in a thoracic chance fracture in a rodeo athlete: A case report. *J Athl Train* 2014;49(2):274–279.

44. De Jonge MC, Kramer J: Spine and sport. *Semin Musculoskelet Radiol* 2014;18(3):246–264.

45. Abla AA, Maroon JC, Lochhead R, Sonntag VKH, Maroon A, Field M: Return to golf after spine surgery. *J Neurosurg Spine* 2011;14:23–30.

46. Burnett MG, Sonntag VKH: Return to contact sports after spinal surgery. *Neurosurg Focus* 2006;21(4):1–3.

47. Eck JC, Riley LH: Return to play after lumbar spine conditions and surgeries. *Clin Sports Med* 2004;23:367–370.

48. Eddy D, Congeni J, Loud K: A review of spine injuries and return to play. *Clin J Sport Med* 2005;15:453–458.

49. Huang P, Anissipour A, McGee W, Lemak L: Return-to-play recommendations after cervical, thoracic, and lumbar spine injuries: A comprehensive review. *Sports Health* 2016;8(1):19–25.

50. Gerrie BJ, Harris JD, Lintner DM, McCulloch PC: Lower thoracic rib stress fractures in baseball pitchers. *Physician Sportsmed* 2015;26:1–4.

51. Kingsley RA: A little-known cause of chest pain in a 14-year-old athlete. *J Pediatric Health Care* 2014;28(6):555–558.

52. Foss-Skiftesvik J, Hougaard MG, Larsen VA, Hansen K: Clinical reasoning: Partial Horner syndrome and upper right limb symptoms following chiropractic manipulation. *Neurology* 2015;84(21):e175–e180.

53. Kuzma SA, Doberstein ST, Rushlow DR: Postfixed brachial plexus radiculopathy due to a thoracic disc herniation in a collegiate wrestler: A case report. *J Athl Train* 2013;48(5):710–715.

54. Wood KB, Blair JM, Aepple DM, Schendel MJ, Garvey TA, Gundry CR, Heithoff KB: Natural history of asymptomatic thoracic disc herniations. *Spine* 1997;22(5):525–529.

55. Kaye AD, Machikanti L, Abdi S, et al: Efficacy of epidural injections in managing chronic spinal pain: A best evidence synthesis. *Pain Physician* 2015;18:E939–E1004.

56. Manchikanti L, Cash KA, McManus CD, Pampati V, Benyamin RM: Thoracic interlaminar epidural injections in managing chronic thoracic pain: A randomized, double-blind, controlled trial with a 2-year follow-up. *Pain Physician* 2014;17:E327–E338.

57. Denis F: The three column spine and its significance in the classification of acute thoracolumbar spinal injuries. *Spine* 1983;8(8):817–831.

58. Reinhold M, Audige L, Schnake KJ, Bellabarba C, Dai LY, Oner FC: AO Spine injury classification system: A revision proposal for the thoracic and lumbar spine. *Eur Spine J* 2013;22(10):2184–2201.

59. Vaccaro AR, Lehman RA, Hurlbert RJ, et al: A new classification of thoracolumbar injuries: The importance of injury morphology, the integrity of the posterior ligamentous complex, and neurologic status. *Spine* 2005;30(20):2325–2333.

60. Hitchon PW, Abode-Iyamah K, Dahdaleh NS, Shaffrey C, Noeller J, He W, Moritani T: Non-operative management in neurologically intact thoracolumbar burst fractures: Clinical and radiographic outcomes. *Spine* 2016;41(6):483–489.

SECTION 4

Concussion

23 Concussion: Introduction—The Controversy

Vin Shen Ban, MA, MB, BChir, MRCS, MSc AFHEA • Richard G. Ellenbogen, MD • H. Hunt Batjer, MD, FACS

According to the 1991 National Health Interview Survey, about 300,000 Americans sustain sports-related concussions each year.[1] This figure was then extrapolated to 1.6 to 3.8 million based on several other factors that were not taken into account previously.[2] The Centers for Disease Control and Prevention (CDC) estimated that, between 2001 and 2009, an annual average of 173,285 traumatic brain injury (TBI)–related emergency department (ED) visits were reported in those 19 years of age or younger.[3] This number grew from 153,375 in 2001 to 248,418 in 2009. The true incidence of concussion is difficult to ascertain, partly because of the lack of objective diagnostic criteria[4] and thus inconsistencies in reporting.[5] Furthermore, the majority of patients with a presumed concussion likely do not seek evaluation in the ED but instead are self-diagnosed or treated in their primary care physician's offices. The increasing trend in the reported ED visits is hypothesized to be the result of clearer, more publicized criteria for diagnosing concussions, and the media attention focused on concussions and their potential long- term effects on the athlete's health.[6–10] Outreach and educational events, especially those in the Internet and printed media, have also played a part in raising the public's awareness on the signs and symptoms of concussion.[11–13]

There has been an exponential increase in the number of peer reviewed articles published with the keyword "concussion" in the past 5 years (**Figure 23-1**), reflecting the growing interest in the subject, both from the scientific community and from the public at large.[8] Research in concussion and TBI in general has spanned the entire spectrum from the bench to the bedside, with an increasing number of large-scale initiatives attempting to bridge

---

None of the following authors or any immediate family member has received anything of value from or has stock or stock options held in a commercial company or institution related directly or indirectly to the subject of this article: Dr. Ban, Dr. Batjer, and Dr. Ellenbogen.

the extremes.[14,15] On the molecular level, scientists have provided us with a comprehensive review of the neurometabolic cascade of concussion.[16] In line with the overall objectives of this book, our focus in this section is on the practical aspects of the diagnosis and management of concussion, as relevant to clinicians caring for student and elite athletes.

The terms "concussion" and "mild TBI" (mTBI) are often used interchangeably.[4] Concussion is a form of TBI on the milder range of the spectrum of brain injury. The "mTBI" designation can be misleading because a minority of these can sustain significant sequelae of their injury.

DISTINGUISHING BETWEEN CERVICAL AND VESTIBULAR INJURY AND CONCUSSION

It is common for sports-related blows to the head to have a concomitant transfer of force to the cervical spine.[17,18] As it has been discussed in the section on cervical spine injuries, athletes may experience a range of symptoms from neck pain, dizziness, and cognitive disturbances to headaches. These whiplash-associated disorders (WADs) have common features with concussion,[19–21] and their mechanisms of injuries are often identical,[17,18] suggesting that concussions may not be purely a brain phenomenon.[22] If this is indeed true, that is, if concussion is a constellation of symptoms attributable, at least in part, to the type of cervical spinal injury seen in WAD, then there will be significant implications for the management of these patients. WAD has been treated with active mobilization, injections (steroids, botulinum toxin), manipulation techniques, and radiofrequency neurotomy,[23,24] while concussions are currently being treated with rest or active rehabilitation.[4]

Distinguishing between a head injury and a cervical spine injury by symptoms alone can be challenging.[19] Often, the mechanism of trauma is witnessed, and the patient can articulate his or her symptoms, making the diagnosis and treatment more straightforward. When there is any doubt, it is best to remain suspicious of both

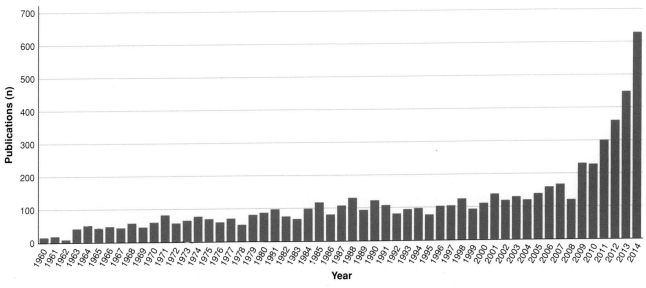

FIGURE 23-1 Number of publications by year through a MEDLINE search of "concussion" up until the end of 2014.

a spine and a head injury. Therefore, standard precautions should be taken to immobilize the cervical spine while removing the athlete from the field for further assessment. After clearing the primary survey, the sports clinician may then proceed to obtain a history and assess the cervical spine (as described in Chapters 9–15).

● THE CONTROVERSIES

Despite the growing literature, every aspect of concussion remains a controversial subject to include definition, diagnosis, treatment, and prognosis. Many groups have published their own guidelines and recommendations for sports-related concussions; these groups include the American Academy of Neurology,[25] the American Medical Society for Sports Medicine,[26] the International Conference on Concussion in Sport,[4] and the Brain Trauma Foundation.[27] A detailed comparison of the guidelines has been undertaken by West and Marion.[28]

In this section of the book, encompassing Chapters 23 through 28, we review the current state of knowledge and practice and highlight areas of controversy. For ease of reference, the chapters in this section are arranged according to the chronological order of events after a (suspected) concussion in an athlete. All of the authors here are leading experts in their fields, and they have provided authoritative overviews of their respective chapters. You will also recognize them as part of the writing committees developing the concussion guidelines mentioned earlier. It is important to emphasize that although much

remains to be uncovered in the world of concussions, it would simply be impossible to include everything that we do know in the space of these few chapters. The main purpose, therefore, is to highlight areas pertinent to the clinical practice of a healthcare expert caring for patients with sports related concussions.

Definition, Diagnosis, and On-Field Evaluation

The diagnosis is the first step in the concussion management pathway. In Chapter 24, Dr. Stan Herring and colleagues review the elements of the currently accepted diagnostic criteria, including the symptoms that are commonly reported and the physical signs to look out for. The role of commonly used assessment tools is also discussed, along with plans for preseason, on-the-field, and sideline assessments. This is then followed by a video by Leigh Weiss and Ronnie Barnes demonstrating the on-field assessment of an athlete with a suspected concussion. In the video, several key elements and tools are reviewed, including the Maddock's questionnaire, Sport Concussion Assessment Tool 3 (SCAT3), and National Football League (NFL) Sideline Assessment (Go v. No-Go, symptom inventory, Standardized Assessment of Concussion [SAC], memory recall), cervical spine and neurologic examinations, balance testing, and upper limb coordination testing.

Objective means of diagnosing concussions are currently being studied. There has been increasing interest in developing a biomarker that could either predict susceptibility to concussions or be used as part of the diagnostic criteria.[29] S100β,[30–41] glial fibrillary acidic protein

(GFAP),[34,37,39–42] neuron-specific enolase,[35–38] apolipoprotein E4,[43–45] neurofilament light protein,[40–42] amyloid beta,[39,41,42] tau protein,[39–42] brain-derived neurotrophic factor (BDNF),[37,39] creatinine kinase,[34,38] heart-type fatty acid binding protein (h-FABP),[37,41] prolactin,[31] cortisol,[38] and albumin[40] are among the biomarkers that have been studied. The number of references associated with each biomarker provides a relative indication on the frequency with which they have been studied, but they are by no means exhaustive. Most of these studies were small pilot studies with some conflicting evidence and are certainly of insufficient strength to support their use in clinical practice so far.

Imaging techniques represent another subset of interest in the field of concussions. Because concussion is considered to be a functional injury rather than a structural injury, structural imaging techniques such as conventional CT, MRI, and diffusion tensor imaging (DTI) have been used mainly to rule out any structural lesions[46] (e.g., subdural or epidural hematomas, contusions, colloid cysts). Functional imaging techniques have shown promising results with functional MRI (fMRI) leading the way.[47] Some studies have demonstrated some correlation between fMRI signal abnormalities, concussion symptom severity[48] and recovery time.[49] Other functional imaging techniques such as positron emission tomography (PET) and single-photon emission CT (SPECT) require intravenous injections of radioactive tracers, and therefore the risks outweigh any potential benefit. For concussions, all functional imaging techniques are currently only for experimental use in research settings.

Short-Term Prognosis and Return to Play

In Chapter 25, Dr. Margot Putukian takes us through the chronology of care after a diagnosis of concussion has been made. She discusses the initial treatment strategies and gives us a glimpse of the assessments that she routinely performs in her office setting. This is followed by the concepts of the return-to-play (RTP) protocol, including what she would do in anomalous cases with worrisome features that might delay RTP. Occasionally, athletes who undergo imaging as part of their concussion workup may have incidental findings. Dr. Putukian considers the factors that lead her to image a patient and make any subsequent referrals. She concludes the chapter by highlighting the effects of gender on concussion.

Neuropsychological Testing

Neuropsychological testing has evolved to become an integral part of concussion evaluation.[50] In Chapter 26, Dr. Michael McCrea and colleagues describe the role of the neuropsychologist in sports concussion. They also consider the evolution of neuropsychological testing with the advent of cheaper and more portable computers. With the ever-growing list of neuropsychological tests available on the market today,[51] understanding the strengths and limitations of these tests helps guide the selection of a test in a specific situation.

Baseline neuropsychological testing has been controversial.[4,51] McCrea et al review the arguments for and against baseline testing, as well as the alternative means of comparison using population-based normative data. They also highlight the issues surrounding the interpretation of neuropsychological testing data and finish off the chapter by discussing the use and interpretation of neuropsychological testing in the pediatric population.

Postconcussion Syndrome

Although most concussions in adults resolve symptomatically within 7 to 10 days,[4] a small cohort of patients have prolonged symptoms, leading to what is known as the postconcussion syndrome.[52] This topic is discussed by Dr. Javier Cárdenas in Chapter 27. He clarifies the differences between postconcussion *symptoms* versus postconcussion *syndrome* and discusses the various symptoms associated with postconcussion syndrome, including physical (including sleep disturbance), behavioral, and cognitive symptoms. Risk factors for postconcussion syndrome, especially postconcussion syndrome in children, and the challenges in their management, including the use of medication, are also discussed.

It is important to note that young collegiate athletes take longer (in the order of 2–3 weeks) to fully recover from a concussion compared with adults.[53] Similarly, younger athletes such as those younger than 15 years of age can take 3 or more weeks to fully recover.[54] This is probably attributable to the incomplete myelination of neurons in the growing brain.[55]

Long-Term Sequelae

Finally, in Chapter 28, Drs. Mitch Berger and Rajiv Saigal finish off this section with a review seeking to answer what is currently known and unknown about long-term sequelae of repeated mild TBI in sports. In their review, the authors examine leading questions such as what risk factors cause some to develop long-term sequelae and others not? How much risk does repeated head trauma entail? When is it safe for a concussed athlete to RTP? These remain important, unanswered questions that at the same time identify future directions for research and inform recommendations for treatment.

RELATIONSHIP WITH CHRONIC TRAUMATIC ENCEPHALOPATHY

The spectrum of long-term effects of TBI has garnered significant scientific and media attention. The entity called chronic traumatic encephalopathy (CTE) is a subject of intense study and discussion. The term CTE was historically used synonymously with *dementia pugilistica*[56,57] or the *punch drunk syndrome*,[58] a condition limited to boxers who had sustained repetitive blows to the head and were later found to have dysarthria and pyramidal dysfunction with or without cognitive decline.[59,60] The cognitive decline, when present, was detected 10 to 20 years after retirement and was associated with an overall clinical syndrome that was considered nonprogressive.[60] Recently, several groups have published histopathologic case series[61–63] in what has become known as "modern CTE," differentiating itself from the "classic" version previously described.[59] "Modern CTE," as reported by the groups of McKee et al,[61] Omalu et al,[62] and Hazrati et al,[63] demonstrates more neuropsychiatric (depression, paranoia, agitation, social withdrawal, aggression) and behavioral symptoms, with progressive cognitive decline and dementia.[59,64]

A comprehensive review and comparison of the "classic" and "modern" CTE was performed by Gardner et al.[59] The main criticisms against the conclusions drawn by the groups attempting to define "modern CTE" include case selection bias and the availability cascade,[65,66] the presence of other neurodegenerative disease processes confounding their findings (e.g., Alzheimer disease, frontotemporal dementia, Lewy body dementia, Parkinson disease, normal aging), inclusion of psychiatric symptoms that were too broad and therefore could be attributed to other neurodegenerative diseases, and the multifactorial nature of neurodegenerative disorders (e.g., alcohol or drug abuse). Because there appears to be a degree of discordance between the neuropathologic and clinical findings of several aging studies, we agree with Gardner and colleagues that correlating clinical presentation with previous neuropathologic findings in making the assumption (not diagnosis) of modern CTE should proceed with considerable caution. In any case, a true diagnosis of CTE will still have to come from the autopsy room.[59]

FUTURE DIRECTIONS FOR TRAUMATIC BRAIN INJURY RESEARCH

Although our knowledge in brain injury and concussion in particular has come a long way, there is clearly still a lot of work to be done. As we touched on briefly in the subsection on diagnosis and definition of concussion, the lack of clear and objective ways of classifying brain injury and concussions has led to the comparison of multiple heterogeneous endophenotypes as a single homogenous entity. The conflicting evidence on the best treatment for concussion[67,68] and the multivariable prognostication models[69] often found in the literature could at least partially be explained by this issue.

The other major stumbling block in current concussion research is the lack of a single outcome measure that is reliable and reflects recovery from concussion.[69] As a functional rather than a structural disorder, deficits can be subtle and difficult to assess objectively. The National Institute of Neurological Disorders and Stroke (NINDS) published a list of common data elements (CDEs) for TBIs with a subgroup specifically aimed at concussions.[70,71] This list contains about 185 outcome measure tools grouped into 24 subdomains (**Table 23-1**). Some of these measures, such as the Glasgow Outcome Scale and the Disability Rating Scale, are rather crude. Others, such as the Traumatic Brain

TABLE 23-1	List of outcome measure subdomains in the national institute of neurological disorders and stroke's common data elements for concussion research		
Activities of daily living	Deafness and communication disorders	Language and communication	Postconcussive-related symptoms
Global outcome	Effort or symptom validity	Military studies	Psychiatric and psychological status
Academics	End points	Neuropsychological impairment	Recovery of consciousness or memory recovery
Adaptive and daily living skills	Family and environment	Patient-reported outcomes	Social cognition
Behavioral function	Health-economic measures	Perceived generic and disease-specific health-related quality of life	Social role participation and social competence
Cognitive activity limitations	Infant and toddler measures	Physical function	Sports-related studies

Injury Multidimensional Quality of Life (TBI-QOL) and the Neurobehavioral Symptom Inventory, rely on patient self-reporting, which can be subjective, especially among patients. It would also be impossible to obtain data from all subdomains from a single patient. However, focusing on only a few would introduce bias in the results. Concussion research could substantially benefit from a form of outcome measure that is objective, reliable, and quick to administer.

For the time being, concussion research should focus on better defining the endophenotypes of concussion and their outcome measures. Rather than another randomized controlled trial (RCT), we need to have sufficient pilot data from prospective longitudinal studies to support the patient selection and treatment arm design of future RCTs. The Texas Institute of Brain Injury and Repair (TIBIR) has initiated a large-scale, multicenter, prospective concussion registry with this aim in mind.[72] The registry will be rolled out in phases and will evolve as new information from the data gathered becomes available.

● PREVENTION

Perhaps it goes without saying that preventing a concussion is more effective than trying to treat one. Football was almost banned in the beginning of the 20th century after a series of college on-field–related deaths. To reform the game to become safer, several meetings led by President Theodore Roosevelt were held, culminating in rule changes and the formation of the Intercollegiate Athletic Association of the United States, which was later renamed the National Collegiate Athletic Association (NCAA). Since then, multiple other rule changes have been implemented to prevent injuries and open up the passing game.[73] In more recent times, the moving of the restraining line up 5 yards during kickoff in the NFL has resulted in a 40% drop in concussion rate for that play. Establishing helmet standards and rules against head-down tackling (spearing) are among the other changes in football that have reduced the incidence of concussion and neck injuries.[74]

Outside of football, rule and guideline changes have helped to reduce the number of head injuries sustained by athletes. Helmet use has been found to reduce the number of head injuries in recreational skiers and snowboarders.[75] In soccer, the practice of elbowing the opponent while attempting to head the ball was expressly forbidden just before the 2006 FIFA World Cup. This used to account for up to 40% of head incidents in elite soccer.[76] After the rule change, fewer head injuries and concussions were observed in the 2006 (13 head injuries,

1 concussion) compared with the 2002 FIFA World Cup (25 head injuries, 4 concussions).[77] Although the 2014 FIFA World Cup saw 5 concussions, none were caused by the elbow.

Despite being primarily a noncollision sport, basketball has had its fair share of high-profile concussions. Only recently, in the National Basketball Association (NBA) Western Conference Finals' game 4 against the Houston Rockets, Golden State Warriors' Stephen Curry was involved in an awkward fall, which sparked some debate on the issue of concussion in the NBA.[78–81] The 2014 to 2015 Most Valuable Player attempted to block a field goal attempt by Trevor Ariza but ended up tumbling over Ariza, who ducked in anticipation of Curry's block attempt. Curry appeared to have landed on the top of his shoulder blades, with a follow-through impact to his occiput, and remained lying on the ground for several minutes. When he was finally able to get up and walk back to the locker room, it was reported that he appeared dazed. The Warriors labeled this event a "contusion," and Curry sat out the rest of the second quarter. Curry was then put through the SCAT, and was cleared to return in the third quarter. Deviating from his usual form, he made only 4 of 11 field goals (36.3%) for the rest of the game after his return. Before this, his season average was 48.7%.[82]

With that match being a best-of-seven playoff series for a spot in the NBA Finals and the Warriors being up 3 to 0 heading into it, losing their star player became a concern for the Warriors. A concussion diagnosis would have put Curry out for at least 5 to 7 days, possibly even missing game 1 of the Finals. The current NBA Concussion Protocol does not require an independent physician to clear an athlete with a suspected concussion to RTP.[83] This approach could create potential conflicts between the team's best interests versus the player's best interests. On a side note, the NFL has mandated clearance by an independent neurologic consultant for several years with the aim of eliminating this potential conflict.[84]

The Rockets survived a clean sweep, and 2 nights later in the fourth quarter of game 5, Curry's other half of the "Splash Brothers," Klay Thompson, was accidentally kneed in the ear, coincidentally by Trevor Ariza.[85] Thompson was taken to the locker room and cleared from a concussion, and he returned to the bench. As he was about to check back in to the game, he started bleeding profusely from his injured ear, leading to a trip back to the locker room for stitches. The Warriors went on to win the game and book themselves a trip to the NBA

Finals. Thompson returned for the team celebrations but started vomiting and could not drive home. The following day, he was reevaluated and was officially diagnosed with a concussion. Six days later, he was cleared to play in game 1 of the NBA Finals. This series of incidents led the NBA Players' Association to review its concussion protocol.[86]

● ADVOCACY

The Lystedt Law was passed in the State of Washington in May 2009 and was a provocative and innovative way of advocating and achieving youth sports safety. The law had three major tenets to benefit student athletes:

1. Education: All youth participants in athletics on state-sanctioned athletic arenas required education on the diagnosis and risks of concussion.
2. Advocacy: All youth athletes with a suspected concussion were to be removed from play immediately, without same-day RTP.
3. RTP: Clearance for return of a youth athlete after a concussion would be performed by a healthcare expert versed in the treatment of concussion.[87-89] Zackery Lystedt sustained an intracranial bleed (bilateral subdural hematoma) after being prematurely returned to play after sustaining a concussion.

Although legislation preventing premature RTP will go a long way toward minimizing preventable concussions, it is by no means sufficient.[12] Fundamentally, a change in mindset and attitude among athletes, parents, and coaches will be the driving force in tackling concussion.[11,90] Education of coaches, parents, and athletes on concussions also formed a component of this law, which has since been passed in all 50 states and the District of Columbia with the help of Mr. Jeff Miller and the NFL.[91] Educational efforts by the CDC, among other organizations, have played a huge role in raising awareness about concussions among athletes, parents, and coaches.[92] Ensuring familiarity with the current diagnostic criteria for concussion and the local RTP protocols will enable parents and teammates to help identify athletes who should be flagged for professional evaluation, especially in the high school and collegiate setting, where resources such as team physicians and video replays may not be available. As part of the culture change, it is important for everyone to understand that unlike a shoulder or a leg injury, you cannot just "play through" a head or spine injury. Medical health and safety issues always trump competitive issues in sporting events. Managing the concussion issue safely and effectively requires a team effort from all concerned—athletes, family members, coaches, school leadership, athletic associations, clinicians, and legislators.

REFERENCES

1. Sosin DM, Sniezek JE, Thurman DJ: Incidence of mild and moderate brain injury in the United States, 1991. *Brain Inj* 1996;10(1):47–54.

2. Langlois JA, Rutland-Brown W, Wald MM: The epidemiology and impact of traumatic brain injury: A brief overview. *J Head Trauma Rehabil* 2006;21(5):375–378.

3. Centers for Disease Control and Prevention: Nonfatal traumatic brain injuries related to sports and recreation activities among persons aged </=19 years—United States, 2001-2009. *MMWR Morbid Mortal Wkly Rep* 2011;60(39):1337–1342.

4. McCrory P, Meeuwisse WH, Aubry M, et al: Consensus statement on concussion in sport: The 4th International Conference on Concussion in Sport held in Zurich, November 2012. *J Am Coll Surg* 2013;216(5): e55–e71.

5. McCrea M, Hammeke T, Olsen G, Leo P, Guskiewicz K: Unreported concussion in high school football players: Implications for prevention. *Clin J Sports Med* 2004; 14(1):13–17.

6. Borland CL: Retirement: Is 24 too late to stop football brain damage? *NBC News*. Available at: http://www.nbcnews.com/health/health-news/borland-retirement-brain-damage-tk-n325866. Accessed June 9, 2015.

7. Belson K: Brain trauma to affect one in three players, N.F.L. agrees. *The New York Times*. Available at: http://www.nytimes.com/2014/09/13/sports/football/actuarial-reports-in-nfl-concussion-deal-are-released.html?_r=0. Accessed June 9, 2015.

8. NFL Brain Injuries. *Huffington Post*. Available at: http://www.huffingtonpost.com/news/nfl-brain-injuries. Accessed June 9, 2015.

9. Guskiewicz KM, Marshall SW, Bailes J, et al: Association between recurrent concussion and late-life cognitive impairment in retired professional football players. *Neurosurgery* 2005;57(4):719–726; discussion 719–726.

10. Guskiewicz KM, Marshall SW, Bailes J, et al: Recurrent concussion and risk of depression in retired professional football players. *Med Sci Sports Exerc* 2007;39(6): 903–909.

11. Chrisman SP, Schiff MA, Chung SK, Herring SA, Rivara FP: Implementation of concussion legislation and extent of concussion education for athletes, parents, and coaches in Washington State. *Am J Sports Med* 2014;42(5):1190–1196.

12. Rivara FP, Schiff MA, Chrisman SP, Chung SK, Ellenbogen RG, Herring SA: The effect of coach education on reporting of concussions among high school athletes after passage of a concussion law. *Am J Sports Med* 2014;42(5):1197–1203.

13. Sullivan SJ, Schneiders AG, Cheang CW, et al: "What's happening?" A content analysis of concussion-related traffic on Twitter. *Br J Sports Med* 2012;46(4):258–263.

14. TRACK-TBI. Available at: http://tracktbi.ucsf.edu. Accessed June 23, 2015.

15. CENTER-TBI. Available at: https://www.center-tbi.eu. Accessed June 23, 2015.

16. Giza CC, Hovda DA: The new neurometabolic cascade of concussion. *Neurosurgery* 2014;75(suppl 4):S24–S33.

17. Cooper MT, McGee KM, Anderson DG: Epidemiology of athletic head and neck injuries. *Clin Sports Med* 2003;22(3):427–443, vii.

18. Torg JS, Vegso JJ, O'Neill MJ, Sennett B: The epidemiologic, pathologic, biomechanical, and cinematographic analysis of football-induced cervical spine trauma. *Am J Sports Med* 1990;18(1):50–57.

19. Leddy JJ, Baker JG, Merchant A, et al: Brain or strain? Symptoms alone do not distinguish physiologic concussion from cervical/vestibular injury. *Clin J Sports Med* 2015;25(3):237–242.

20. McCrea M, Guskiewicz KM, Marshall SW, et al: Acute effects and recovery time following concussion in collegiate football players: The NCAA Concussion Study. *JAMA* 2003;290(19):2556–2563.

21. Spitzer WO, Skovron ML, Salmi LR, et al: Scientific monograph of the Quebec Task Force on Whiplash-Associated Disorders: Redefining "whiplash" and its management. *Spine* 1995;20(8 suppl):1S–73S.

22. Leslie O, Craton N: Concussion: Purely a brain injury? *Clin J Sports Med* 2013;23(5):331–332.

23. Verhagen AP, Scholten-Peeters GG, van Wijngaarden S, de Bie RA, Bierma-Zeinstra SM: Conservative treatments for whiplash. *Cochrane Database Syst Rev* 2007(2): CD003338.

24. van Suijlekom H, Mekhail N, Patel N, Van Zundert J, van Kleef M, Patijn J. 7. Whiplash-associated disorders. *Pain Pract* 2010;10(2):131–136.

25. Giza CC, Kutcher JS, Ashwal S, et al: Summary of evidence-based guideline update: Evaluation and management of concussion in sports: Report of the Guideline Development Subcommittee of the American Academy of Neurology. *Neurology* 2013;80(24):2250–2257.

26. Harmon KG, Drezner J, Gammons M, et al: American Medical Society for Sports Medicine position statement: Concussion in sport. *Clin J Sports Med* 2013;23(1):1–18.

27. Carney N, Ghajar J, Jagoda A, et al: Concussion guidelines step 1: Systematic review of prevalent indicators. *Neurosurgery* 2014;75(suppl 1):S3–15.

28. West TA, Marion DW: Current recommendations for the diagnosis and treatment of concussion in sport: A comparison of three new guidelines. *J Neurotrauma* 2014; 31(2):159–168.

29. Papa L, Ramia MM, Edwards D, Johnson BD, Slobounov SM: Systematic review of clinical studies examining biomarkers of brain injury in athletes after sports-related concussion. *J Neurotrauma* 2015;32(10):661–673.

30. Otto M, Holthusen S, Bahn E, et al: Boxing and running lead to a rise in serum levels of S-100B protein. *Int J Sports Med* 2000;21(8):551–555.

31. Dietrich MO, Tort AB, Schaf DV, et al: Increase in serum S100B protein level after a swimming race. *Can J Appl Physiol* 2003;28(5):710–716.

32. Mussack T, Dvorak J, Graf-Baumann T, Jochum M: Serum S-100B protein levels in young amateur soccer players after controlled heading and normal exercise. *Eur J Med Res* 2003;8(10):457–464.

33. Stalnacke BM, Tegner Y, Sojka P: Playing ice hockey and basketball increases serum levels of S-100B in elite players: A pilot study. *Clin J Sports Med* 2003;13(5):292–302.

34. Hasselblatt M, Mooren FC, von Ahsen N, et al: Serum S100beta increases in marathon runners reflect extracranial release rather than glial damage. *Neurology* 2004;62(9):1634–1636.

35. Stalnacke BM, Tegner Y, Sojka P: Playing soccer increases serum concentrations of the biochemical markers of brain damage S-100B and neuron-specific enolase in elite players: A pilot study. *Brain Inj* 2004;18(9):899–909.

36. Stalnacke BM, Ohlsson A, Tegner Y, Sojka P: Serum concentrations of two biochemical markers of brain tissue damage S-100B and neurone specific enolase are increased in elite female soccer players after a competitive game. *Br J Sports Med* 2006;40(4):313–316.

37. Zetterberg H, Tanriverdi F, Unluhizarci K, Selcuklu A, Kelestimur F, Blennow K: Sustained release of neuron-specific enolase to serum in amateur boxers. *Brain Inj* 2009;23(9):723–726.

38. Graham MR, Myers T, Evans P, et al: Direct hits to the head during amateur boxing is associated with a rise in serum biomarkers for brain injury. *Int J Immunopathol Pharmacol* 2011;24(1):119–125.

39. Neselius S, Zetterberg H, Blennow K, et al: Olympic boxing is associated with elevated levels of the neuronal protein tau in plasma. *Brain Inj* 2013;27(4):425–433.

40. Zetterberg H, Jonsson M, Rasulzada A, et al: No neurochemical evidence for brain injury caused by heading in soccer. *Br J Sports Med* 2007;41(9):574–577.

41. Neselius S, Brisby H, Theodorsson A, Blennow K, Zetterberg H, Marcusson J: CSF-biomarkers in Olympic boxing: Diagnosis and effects of repetitive head trauma. *PloS One* 2012;7(4):e33606.

42. Zetterberg H, Hietala MA, Jonsson M, et al: Neurochemical aftermath of amateur boxing. *Arch Neurol* 2006;63(9):1277–1280.

43. Kristman VL, Tator CH, Kreiger N, et al: Does the apolipoprotein epsilon 4 allele predispose varsity athletes to concussion? A prospective cohort study. *Clin J Sports Med* 2008;18(4):322–328.

44. Tierney RT, Mansell JL, Higgins M, et al: Apolipoprotein E genotype and concussion in college athletes. *Clin J Sports Med* 2010;20(6):464–468.

45. Terrell TR, Bostick RM, Abramson R, et al: APOE, APOE promoter, and Tau genotypes and risk for concussion in college athletes. *Clin J Sports Med* 2008;18(1):10–17.

46. Davis GA, Iverson GL, Guskiewicz KM, Ptito A, Johnston KM: Contributions of neuroimaging, balance testing, electrophysiology and blood markers to the assessment of sport-related concussion. *Br J Sports Med* 2009;43(suppl 1): i36–i45.

47. Chen JK, Johnston KM, Frey S, Petrides M, Worsley K, Ptito A: Functional abnormalities in symptomatic concussed athletes: an fMRI study. *NeuroImage* 2004; 22(1):68–82.

48. Chen JK, Johnston KM, Collie A, McCrory P, Ptito A: A validation of the post concussion symptom scale in the assessment of complex concussion using cognitive testing and functional MRI. *J Neurol Neurosurg Psychiatry* 2007;78(11):1231–1238.

49. Lovell MR, Pardini JE, Welling J, et al: Functional brain abnormalities are related to clinical recovery and time to return-to-play in athletes. *Neurosurgery* 2007;61(2):352–359; discussion 359–360.

50. Echemendia RJ, Iverson GL, McCrea M, et al: Role of neuropsychologists in the evaluation and management of sport-related concussion: An inter-organization position statement. *Clin Neuropsychol* 2011;25(8):1289–1294.

51. Echemendia RJ, Iverson GL, McCrea M, et al: Advances in neuropsychological assessment of sport-related concussion. *Br J Sports Med* 2013;47(5):294–298.

52. Morgan CD, Zuckerman SL, Lee YM, et al: Predictors of postconcussion syndrome after sports-related concussion in young athletes: A matched case-control study. *J Neurosurg Pediatr* 2015;15(6):589–598.

53. Cancelliere C, Hincapie CA, Keightley M, et al: Systematic review of prognosis and return to play after sport concussion: Results of the International Collaboration on Mild Traumatic Brain Injury Prognosis. *Arch Phys Med Rehabil* 2014;95(3 suppl):S210–S229.

54. Babcock L, Byczkowski T, Wade SL, Ho M, Mookerjee S, Bazarian JJ: Predicting postconcussion syndrome after mild traumatic brain injury in children and adolescents who present to the emergency department. *JAMA Pediatr* 2013;167(2):156–161.

55. Mayer AR, Ling JM, Yang Z, Pena A, Yeo RA, Klimaj S: Diffusion abnormalities in pediatric mild traumatic brain injury. *J Neurosci* 2012;32(50):17961–17969.

56. Corsellis JA, Bruton CJ, Freeman-Browne D: The aftermath of boxing. *Psychol Med* 1973;3(3):270–303.

57. Roberts GW, Allsop D, Bruton C: The occult aftermath of boxing. *J Neurol Neurosurg Psychiatry* 1990;53(5): 373–378.

58. Martland HS. Punch drunk. *JAMA* 1928;91(15): 1103–1107.

59. Gardner A, Iverson GL, McCrory P: Chronic traumatic encephalopathy in sport: A systematic review. *Br J Sports Med* 2014;48(2):84–90.

60. McCrory P: Sports concussion and the risk of chronic neurological impairment. *Clin J Sports Med* 2011;21(1):6–12.

61. McKee AC, Stern RA, Nowinski CJ, et al: The spectrum of disease in chronic traumatic encephalopathy. *Brain* 2013;136(Pt 1):43–64.

62. Omalu B, Bailes J, Hamilton RL, et al: Emerging histomorphologic phenotypes of chronic traumatic encephalopathy in American athletes. *Neurosurgery* 2011;69(1):173–183; discussion 183.

63. Hazrati LN, Tartaglia MC, Diamandis P, et al: Absence of chronic traumatic encephalopathy in retired football players with multiple concussions and neurological symptomatology. *Front Hum Neurosci* 2013;7:222.

64. Davis GA, Castellani RJ, McCrory P: Neurodegeneration and sport. *Neurosurgery* 2015;76(6):643–656.

65. Solomon GS, Sills A: Chronic traumatic encephalopathy and the availability cascade. *Physician Sportsmed* 2014; 42(3):26–31.

66. Barr WB: An evidence based approach to sports concussion: Confronting the availability cascade. *Neuropsychol Rev* 2013;23(4):271–272.

67. Comper P, Bisschop SM, Carnide N, Tricco A: A systematic review of treatments for mild traumatic brain injury. *Brain Inj* 2005;19(11):863–880.

68. Snell DL, Surgenor LJ, Hay-Smith EJ, Siegert RJ: A systematic review of psychological treatments for mild traumatic brain injury: An update on the evidence. *J Clin Exp Neuropsychol* 2009;31(1):20–38.

69. Silverberg ND, Gardner AJ, Brubacher JR, Panenka WJ, Li JJ, Iverson GL: Systematic review of multivariable prognostic models for mild traumatic brain injury. *J Neurotrauma* 2015;32(8):517–526.

70. Hicks R, Giacino J, Harrison-Felix C, Manley G, Valadka A, Wilde EA: Progress in developing common data elements for traumatic brain injury research: Version two—the end of the beginning. *J Neurotrauma* 2013; 30(22):1852–1861.

71. NINDS: NINDS Common Data Elements 2012; 2.0: Available at: http://www.commondataelements.ninds.nih.gov/tbi.aspx#tab=Data_Standards. Accessed June 17, 2015.

72. North Texas Sports Concussion Registry: Available at: http://www.utsouthwestern.edu/research/brain-injury/research/con-tex.html. Accessed June 23, 2015.

73. National Football Leauge: Evolution of the rules: from hashmarks to crackback blocks. Available at: http://www.nfl.com/news/story/0ap1000000224872/article/evolution-of-the-rules-from-hashmarksto-crackback-blocks. Accessed June 18, 2015.

74. Levy ML, Ozgur BM, Berry C, Aryan HE, Apuzzo ML: Birth and evolution of the football helmet. *Neurosurgery* 2004;55(3):656–661; discussion 661–652.

75. Haider AH, Saleem T, Bilaniuk JW, Barraco RD; Eastern Association for the Surgery of Trauma Injury ControlViolence Prevention C: An evidence-based review: efficacy of safety helmets in the reduction of head injuries in recreational skiers and snowboarders. *J Trauma Acute Care Surg* 2012;73(5):1340–1347.

76. Andersen TE, Arnason A, Engebretsen L, Bahr R: Mechanisms of head injuries in elite football. *Br J Sports Med* 2004;38(6):690–696.

77. Junge A, Dvorak J: Football injuries during the 2014 FIFA World Cup. *Br J Sports Med* 2015;49(9):599–602.

78. Davison A: How did Stephen Curry not get a concussion? Medical expert explains. Available at: http://www.sportingnews.com/nba/story/2015-05-26/stephen-curry-head-injury-contusion-concussion-protocol-warriors-rockets-game-4. Accessed June 2, 2015.

79. Press A: Why Stephen Curry is so sure he doesn't have a concussion. *New York Post.* Available at: http://nypost.com/2015/05/26/why-stephen-curry-is-so-sure-he-doesnt-have-a-concussion. Accessed June 2, 2015.

80. Boren C: Stephen Curry's scary fall raises concussion questions in NBA. *The Washington Post.* Available at: http://www.washingtonpost.com/blogs/early-lead/wp/2015/05/26/stephen-currys-scary-fall-raises-concussion-questions-in-nba. Accessed June 2, 2015.

81. Amick S: Klay Thompson's uncertain status highlights lack of understanding on concussions. *USA Today.* Available at: http://www.usatoday.com/story/sports/nba/playoffs/2015/06/02/klay-thompson-jeffrey-kutcher-concussion-nba-finals-warriors/28314221/. Accessed June 23, 2015.

82. NBA.com: Stats. Available at: http://stats.nba.com/game/#!/0041400314/?ID=3&StartRange=14400&EndRange=28800&RangeType=2. Accessed June 23, 2015.

83. National Basketball League: NBA Concussion Protocol. Available at: http://www.nba.com/official/concussion_policy_summary.html. Accessed June 23, 2015.

84. Bradley B: Independent concussion specialists ready to work NFL sidelines. Available at: http://www.nfl.com/news/story/0ap1000000237739/article/independent-concussion-specialists-ready-to-work-nfl-sidelines. Accessed June 24, 2015.

85. Cacciola S: Warriors' Klay Thompson Has a Concussion and Is Indefinitely Sidelined. *The New York Times.* Available at: http://www.nytimes.com/2015/05/30/sports/basketball/klay-thompson-does-have-a-concussion-the-warriors-say.html?_r=0. Accessed June 2, 2015.

86. Dubow J: NBPA set to investigate league's concussion protocol. Available at: http://www.nba.com/2015/news/06/02/nbpa-to-investigate-leagues-concussion-protocol.ap/index.html?cid=nba.2013. Accessed 06/03/2015.

87. Zackery Lystedt law. In: State W, ed. RCW 28A.600.190. Available at: http://apps.leg.wa.gov/rcw/default.aspx?cite=28A.600.1902009.

88. Ellenbogen RG: Concussion advocacy and legislation: a neurological surgeon's view from the epicenter. *Neurosurgery* 2014;75(suppl 4):S122–S130.

89. Ellenbogen RG, Berger MS, Batjer HH: The National Football League and concussion: leading a culture change in contact sports. *World Neurosurgery* 2010;74(6):560–565.

90. McKinlay A, Bishop A, McLellan T: Public knowledge of "concussion" and the different terminology used to communicate about mild traumatic brain injury (MTBI). *Brain Inj* 2011;25(7–8):761–766.

91. National Conference of State Legislatures: Traumatic brain injury legislation. Available at: http://www.ncsl.org/research/health/traumatic-brain-injury-legislation.aspx. Accessed June 25, 2015.

92. Centers for Disease Control and Prevention: CfDCaP. Heads Up. Available at: http://www.cdc.gov/headsup. Accessed June 18, 2015.

24 Definitions of Sports Concussion, Initial Diagnosis, and On-Field Evaluation

Leah G. Concannon, MD • Brian C. Liem, MD • Stanley A. Herring, MD
Video Authors: Ronnie Barnes, ATC • Leigh J. Weiss, ATC

Sports concussions account for 5% to 18% of all sports-related injuries in high school and collegiate athletes,[1-3] with an estimated 1.6 to 3.8 million sports-related concussions per year,[4] which is probably low. The annual incidence of sports concussions is apparently rising, but some attribute this trend to an increased awareness and reporting by athletes and healthcare professionals.[5] The greatest number of concussions occur in high school and collegiate football, with a rate of 0.60 per 1000 athletic exposures.[2,5,6,7] In one study of high school and collegiate football players, 14.7% of concussed players sustained a second injury during the same season.[6] Among high school female athletes, soccer players have the highest incidence of concussion.[2,5] Although the absolute number of concussions is highest in football, the rate of concussions is higher in women's collegiate soccer than in collegiate football (0.63 vs. 0.61 per 1000 athlete exposures).[2]

DEFINITIONS

The definition of a sports concussion continues to evolve. The Fourth International Conference on Concussion in Sport, held in Zurich in 2012, described a concussion as a subset of traumatic brain injury defined as a complex pathophysiological process affecting the brain induced,

by biochemical forces.[8] Four key features help to further clarify this definition:

1. May result from a direct blow to the head, face, neck, or body with "impulsive" force transmitted to the head
2. Rapid onset of short-lived impairment of neurologic function that resolves spontaneously but may progress over minutes to hours
3. Injury is largely functional rather than structural, which generally results in normal standard neuroimaging studies
4. Concussion results in a graded set of clinical and cognitive symptoms. These symptoms typically resolve in a sequential course, but some individuals may have a more prolonged course.[8]

DIAGNOSIS

Concussion remains a clinical diagnosis. Assessment includes recognition of mechanism of injury, assessment of symptoms, evaluation of cognitive function, and balance testing. Screening neurologic and physical examination are also performed to rule out other injuries, including more severe brain injury. Because concussion is largely a functional deficit, standard imaging, including CT and MRI, is routinely normal and does not rule out concussion.[9] However, CT may be used in the acute setting to evaluate for intracranial hemorrhage or skull fracture.[10] MRI may be better in the subacute setting to identify evidence of diffuse axonal injury. Magnetic resonance spectroscopy, diffusion tensor imaging, and functional MRI are promising imaging modalities that may be capable of detecting acute subtle neuropathologic changes, but further research is needed to determine their application in the clinical setting.[11]

An athlete suspected of concussion may report or display one or more elements from five clinical areas:

(1) symptoms, (2) physical signs, (3) behavioral changes, (4) sleep disturbance, and (5) cognitive impairment.[8]

Symptoms

Symptoms experienced in a concussion can be divided into three main categories: somatic, cognitive, and affective. The most common somatic symptom is headache, reported in up to 80% to 90% of concussed athletes.[6,12] Other somatic symptoms include nausea, dizziness, blurred vision, fatigue, and neck pain. Cognitive complaints can present as difficulty concentrating and remembering, confusion, feeling "foggy," and slowed down. Athletes may also have affective changes such as emotional lability, irritability, and anxiety.

Physical Signs

Physical signs may include loss of consciousness (LOC) and amnesia, but it is important to note that LOC is not necessary for the diagnosis of concussion. Studies have shown that only 4–8% of athletes diagnosed with concussion suffer LOC.[6,12] There is conflicting evidence on whether or not the presence of LOC is associated with prolonged symptom duration.[13,14]

Behavior Changes

Changes in behavior such as increased irritability or depressed mood may be evident in a concussed athlete. A study by Kontos et al found that concussed high school and college athletes had a statistically significant increase from baseline in reported depression symptoms 2, 7, and even 14 days after injury.[15]

Sleep Disturbance

Sleep disturbance in concussed athletes is common and may be caused by a neurophysiologic injury. In a study comparing concussed patients versus those with only orthopedic injuries, there was a statistically significant greater number of concussed individuals who reported difficulties with sleep initiation, frequent awakenings, increased sleep duration, and daytime sleepiness.[16]

Cognitive Impairment

Cognitive impairment is a frequent finding in concussed athletes. The areas of neurocognitive functioning most affected include attention and concentration, short-term memory, processing speed, and problem solving.[17] Studies suggest that recovery of cognitive deficits generally occurs within 3 to 7 days.[18] However, in 18% of athletes, recovery can last beyond 7 days.[19] It is important to note that in some cases, cognitive recovery may not

occur until up to 2 to 3 days after symptom resolution.[19] Therefore, it is important to not rely only on the athlete's symptom reporting when determining timing of return to play (RTP). The Standardized Assessment of Concussion (SAC) is a well-validated sideline tool used to evaluate an athlete's cognitive function immediately after a suspected concussion.[20] It includes assessments of orientation, immediate memory, concentration, and delayed recall.

Assessment Tools

A standardized instrument used to help assess all of the above is the Sports Concussion Assessment Tool version 3 SCAT3 published in 2013, an update to the SCAT2 published in 2009 (**Figure 24-1**).[21] A separate SCAT3 for children 12 years and younger has also been published to address differences in symptom reporting by children compared with adults (**Figure 24-2**).[22] The SCAT3 combines several concussion assessment measures and includes seven measures: Glasgow Coma Scale score, modified Maddock's questions for orientation, concussion symptom checklist, standardized assessment of concussion (SAC) to assess cognition, neck examination, modified Balance Error Scoring System (mBESS), and coordination testing. It takes approximately 8 to 10 minutes to administer the SCAT3 which is usually performed on the sideline or in the locker room. By combining the various concussion assessments into one tool, the goal is to improve the sensitivity and specificity of concussion diagnosis. The SCAT2 was found to have high sensitivity (83%) and specificity (91%) for concussion when using a cutoff score of 74.5.[23] However, there have been no similar studies yet published on the SCAT3 nor the Child-SCAT3. Comparison of sideline SCAT3 should be made to a baseline (preseason) assessment if available.

The National Football League (NFL) sideline concussion tool is similar to the SCAT3 with the additional component of six "No Go" criteria (**Figure 24-3**).[24] These criteria are not specific to football and can be used in any sport. If an athlete exhibits any one of the six "No Go" criteria outlined in **Table 24-1**, he or she is presumed to have sustained a concussion and prohibited from RTP in the same game or practice.

TABLE 24-1 NFL "No Go" criteria[24]
Loss of consciousness
Confusion
Amnesia
New symptoms on symptom checklist
Abnormal neurologic examination results
Progressive or worsening symptoms

Balance Impairment

Balance impairments have also been well documented after sport concussion.[25-27] Balance testing results typically return to normal after 3 days.[28] Assessment tools include the Sensory Organization Test (SOT), the BESS, and the mBESS. The SOT uses force-plate technology to assess overall balance and performance using six different conditions performed three times each.[29,30] Although this is a valid and reliable tool, it is not practical for sideline use. The BESS in an easy, rapid, 5- to 7-minute test that measures balance on two different surfaces (firm and soft foam) and in three different stances on the nondominant foot while the athlete's eyes are closed and hands are resting on the hips. Athletes are instructed to hold each stance for 20 seconds. Performance is assessed by assigning a point for each error (i.e., lifting hand off iliac crest, step, stumble, fall, open eyes, moving hip into >30° of abduction, lifting the forefoot or heel, remaining out of test position >5 seconds) for a maximum of 10 errors per stance. In a large study of football players, the BESS had a high specificity during the first 7 days after concussion (0.91–0.96), with the highest sensitivity (0.34) at the time of injury.[31] In this same study, researchers found that 36% of concussed athletes demonstrated balance impairments on BESS immediately after concussion. An alternative to the BESS is the mBESS, which only uses a firm surface. Currently, there is a lack of studies assessing intra- or interrater reliability of the mBESS.

PRESEASON MANAGEMENT

Proper management of concussions begins even before the season starts. The preparticipation examination (PPE) should include a discussion of any prior concussions, including the nature of injury and duration of symptoms. In population-based studies, the risk of future concussion is increased in a dose-dependent manner, although individual vulnerability may vary. Athletes with a history of three prior concussions have a threefold risk of sustaining a concussion over athletes without a prior history of concussion in population-based studies.[32] Additionally, the presence of learning disabilities, mood disorders, migraine headaches, attention deficit disorder (ADD), and attention deficit hyperactivity disorder (ADHD) in the athlete or family members should be recorded.[8,10,33] Screening for baseline headache is important as 18% of patients with headache after brain injury have reported preexisting headache.[34]

Part of the PPE may include baseline assessment, including symptom score (e.g., using concussion symptom checklist), balance testing (i.e., BESS or mBESS), and cognitive tests (either on paper or with computerized testing). Baseline assessment is an important step because many nonconcussed athletes report two or three symptoms at baseline and may have difficulty with balance and concentration testing at baseline.[35] It is still not clear if baseline testing should be performed in all athletes or only those in high-risk sports or with prior history of concussion.[10] Chapter 26 discusses baseline testing in further detail. The PPE also offers an opportunity for education of the athlete about signs and symptoms of a concussion and the importance of properly recognizing and treating any future concussions.

ON-THE-FIELD ASSESSMENT

An emergency action plan (EAP) should be in place before the start of the season. The EAP provides instructions for care of any medical emergency, but a dedicated concussion protocol should also be in place. The roles and responsibilities of each team member should be clearly outlined, including who evaluates the athlete on the field and on the sidelines, who may remove an athlete from play, and who may return an athlete to play. A plan for emergency transport of the athlete with more severe brain injury should also be in place and rehearsed by the team medical personnel.[36] The EAP should be reviewed on at least a yearly basis to ensure that it continues to reflect the most current recommendations.

The assessment of the collapsed or unconscious athlete on the field begins with evaluation of circulation, airway, breathing, and cervical spine status (Video 24-1). The unconscious athlete must always be treated as if he or she has sustained a cervical spine injury, with inline stabilization and transfer onto a backboard. Even in the collapsed but conscious athlete, care should be taken to protect the cervical spine while assessing cardiopulmonary function. Indications for emergency transport are highlighted in **Table 24-2**.

TABLE 24-2	Indications for emergency transport[19,37,38]
Cervical spine injury	
Focal neurologic deficit (pupillary abnormality, extraocular movement, motor-sensory screening examination)	
Persistent vomiting	
Declining mental status	
Severe, worsening headache	
Slurred speech	
Persistent gait unsteadiness	
Development of seizures or prolonged impact seizure	

● CLINICAL VIGNETTE

A collegiate basketball player is hit in the head while driving to the basket during the third quarter of a game. He falls to the ground holding his head and is slow to get up before being helped up by his teammates. As he comes off the court, he tells the athletic trainer that his head was hurting at the point of impact and felt like he "got the wind knocked out of me" but that he is fine now and wants to go back into the game.

What should the medical staff do next?

Sideline Assessment

After the primary survey above has been completed, the athlete may be moved to the sideline or training room for the secondary survey, with a more detailed history and physical examination focused on concussion. This should include a discussion of the mechanism of injury, particularly if it was unwitnessed. The athlete should be asked about any LOC and assessed for amnesia. The athlete should be asked about accompanying symptoms, including their severity. This is often accomplished with the use of a symptom checklist, such as that embedded in the SCAT3 or the NFL sideline concussion tool.[28,31] A complete neurologic exam, including cranial nerves (with an emphasis on pupillary reactions and extraocular movement) and upper and lower extremity strength and sensation, should also be performed.

Serial assessments evaluating cranial nerves, symptom checklist, cognitive function, and balance testing should be performed.[37] This is most often accomplished with the SCAT3 or other sideline assessment tool as discussed earlier. The athlete must not be left alone during this period, so as not to miss any signs of progressive neurologic compromise that would require emergency transport, as it can take some time for these symptoms to appear.

If any of the NFL "No Go" criteria (outlined in Table 24-1) are present, the athlete is presumed to have sustained a concussion and is immediately removed from play.[31] This is true even if the athlete has not shown any abnormalities on cognitive or balance testing. It is important to recognize that even in the absence of "No Go" criteria, a concussion may still be suspected based on mechanism of injury or performance on cognitive and balance testing. Indeed, the SCAT3 or other sideline tool may be at or even above baseline, and the athlete may still be concussed. Clinical judgment remains the ultimate method in diagnosing a suspected concussion rather than a reliance on sideline tools that are not sensitive enough to diagnose every concussion.[37]

Signs and symptoms of a concussion often develop over minutes to hours, and the athlete may have increasing symptoms several hours after the initial insult.[8] This is one reason that immediate removal from practice or play is essential when a concussion is suspected. There is no same-day return to practice or play at any level of sports participation with a suspected or confirmed concussion. There may be rare circumstances when a trained medical professional evaluates an athlete on the sideline or in the locker room and determines that a concussion has not occurred. Only in that situation should the player be allowed to return to practice or play the same day. Medical professionals must exercise extreme caution in these situations, however, recalling that symptom onset may be delayed.

Initial disposition of the injured athlete must be determined, either transfer to hospital or home with observation by a responsible adult.[33] In youth athletes, this is often the parents or guardians. In older athletes, this may be a friend, teammate, or spouse. If the athlete is discharged home, the adult must be educated on warning signs and indications for evaluation in the emergency department. The person should also be given instructions including topics such as initial physical rest, medication and alcohol use, and driving. There should be a plan in place for follow-up with a medical professional. It is also desirable to discuss relative cognitive rest and how it may pertain to the particular athlete and his or her school or work schedule. It must be understood that there is no RTP until the athlete is cleared by a medical professional trained in the management of concussion. This includes not just the sport of injury but also other recreational sports, as well as recess and gym class for student-athletes.

Sideline Assessment without a Healthcare Provider

Many youth sports do not have a healthcare provider at games and practices. Therefore, coach, parent, and athlete education is essential for recognition of when a concussion may have occurred. Athletes should be encouraged to report symptoms and to speak up if a teammate has sustained a concussion and has not reported it. This remains a challenge. In a study of high school football and girls soccer players in Washington State after passage of the Lystedt law, 69% of athletes continued playing with symptoms consistent with a concussion, and 40% did not report symptoms to their coach.[39] In general, athletes fail to report symptoms for multiple reasons, including not believing symptoms are serious, a desire to continue playing, and worry about letting down teammates.[40,41]

It is not the coach's job to diagnose a concussion but rather to recognize when a concussion may have occurred so that the athlete is removed from play at that time. Any athlete with new symptoms (e.g., headache, dizziness, confusion) after a blow to the head or body must be suspected of having sustained a concussion and removed from play. The athlete should not be left alone and should be monitored for the development of any worrisome signs that would require emergency transport (Table 24-2). The athlete must not be allowed to return to practice or play until evaluated and cleared by a healthcare professional trained in the management of concussions.[8] There is no same-day return to practice or play with a suspected or confirmed concussion.

The athlete denies any current symptoms and "passes" the sideline assessment, meaning that he is essentially at his baseline. He wants to go back into the game to help his team. What should the medical staff do at this point?

Return to Play

As previously noted, it is now recognized that any athlete who is suspected of having sustained a concussion is not to return to practice or play the same day, even if symptoms resolve quickly.[8] The National Collegiate Athletic Association (NCAA) and many professional sport organizations have policies to this effect.[37] All 50 states and the District of Columbia now also have legislation in place mandating removal from practice or play for athletes 18 years of age and younger who are suspected of having sustained a concussion.

It is well known that some signs and symptoms of concussion may become apparent only minutes to hours after the initial injury.[8] For this reason, it is always prudent to err on the side of caution if the diagnosis is in question. The mantra "When in doubt, sit them out" is especially important in youth athletes, who may be susceptible to second-impact syndrome. This is a rare but life-threatening injury thought to occur when an athlete sustains a second head injury while still symptomatic from a previous head injury. A loss of cerebral autoregulation leads to vascular congestion, increased intracranial pressure, and brain herniation, ultimately resulting in death or severe morbidity.[42]

If an athlete has had a concussion, RTP should only begin after the athlete has returned to baseline on symptom checklist as well as cognitive and balance testing. Student-athletes should be at baseline for all school, homework, and after-school activities before returning to play. Athletes must successfully progress through a graded return to exercise protocol (**Table 24-3**) under the direction of a healthcare provider before full RTP can resume.[8] There must be at least 24 hours between each step, and any return of symptoms must result in a reevaluation by a healthcare provider. RTP always requires medical clearance. A more detailed description of RTP is presented in Chapter 25.

After a thorough evaluation of the athlete, there are no concerning signs on examination that would require transfer to the hospital. Any sideline assessment tool is not 100% sensitive for diagnosing a concussion, and in this case, the mechanism of injury and the athlete's behavior immediately after the hit are suspicious for a concussion. Therefore, the athlete should be removed from play and should not return to the game. It is likely that his symptoms will increase over the next few hours. He can begin the RTP protocol when all symptoms are back to baseline.

● PITFALLS

A failure to identify any of the following situations may prolong recovery and can even lead to tragic consequences such as permanent disability or, rarely, death.

- Failure to suspect a concussion in the appropriate situation
- Failure to suspect a concussion because the athlete did not lose consciousness
- Failure to remove an athlete from play when a concussion is suspected or diagnosed
- Failure to recognize a possible cervical spine injury
- Failure to recognize a moderate or severe brain injury
- Failure of proper communication to the athlete or caregiver about postinjury expectations and restrictions

● **TABLE 24-3**	Return-to-play protocol[8]	
Stage	**Exercise Allowed at Each Step**	**Goal of Stage**
No activity	Physical and relative cognitive rest	Recovery
Light aerobic exercise	Walking, swimming, or stationary cycling; no resistance training	Increase heart rate
Sport-specific exercise	Running or skating drills	Introduce movement
Noncontact drills	More complex training drills; acceptable to introduce progressive resistance training	Coordination and cognitive load
Full-contact practice	Normal training activities *after* medical clearance	Exercise, coordination, and cognitive load
Return to play	Competition-level play	

SCAT3™

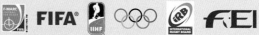

Sport Concussion Assessment Tool – 3rd Edition

For use by medical professionals only

Name	Date / Time of Injury:	Examiner:
	Date of Assessment:	

What is the SCAT3?[1]

The SCAT3 is a standardized tool for evaluating injured athletes for concussion and can be used in athletes aged from 13 years and older. It supersedes the original SCAT and the SCAT2 published in 2005 and 2009, respectively[2]. For younger persons, ages 12 and under, please use the Child SCAT3. The SCAT3 is designed for use by medical professionals. If you are not qualified, please use the Sport Concussion Recognition Tool[1]. Preseason baseline testing with the SCAT3 can be helpful for interpreting post-injury test scores.

Specific instructions for use of the SCAT3 are provided on page3. If you are not familiar with the SCAT3, please read through these instructions carefully. This tool may be freely copied in its current form for distribution to individuals, teams, groups and organizations. Any revision or any reproduction in a digital form requires approval by the Concussion in Sport Group.

NOTE: The diagnosis of a concussion is a clinical judgment, ideally made by a medical professional. The SCAT3 should not be used solely to make, or exclude, the diagnosis of concussion in the absence of clinical judgement. An athlete may have a concussion even if their SCAT3 is "normal".

What is a concussion?

A concussion is a disturbance in brain function caused by a direct or indirect force to the head. It results in a variety of non-specific signs and/or symptoms (some examples listed below) and most often does not involve loss of consciousness. Concussion should be suspected in the presence of **any one or more** of the following:

- Symptoms (e.g., headache), or
- Physical signs (e.g., unsteadiness), or
- Impaired brain function (e.g. confusion) or
- Abnormal behaviour (e.g., change in personality).

SIDELINE ASSESSMENT

Indications for Emergency Management

NOTE: A hit to the head can sometimes be associated with a more serious brain injury. Any of the following warrants consideration of activating emergency procedures and urgent transportation to the nearest hospital:

- Glasgow Coma score less than 15
- Deteriorating mental status
- Potential spinal injury
- Progressive, worsening symptoms or new neurologic signs

Potential signs of concussion?

If any of the following signs are observed after a direct or indirect blow to the head, the athlete should stop participation, be evaluated by a medical professional and **should not be permitted to return to sport the same day** if a concussion is suspected.

Any loss of consciousness?	Y	N
"If so, how long?" _____		
Balance or motor incoordination (stumbles, slow/laboured movements, etc.)?	Y	N
Disorientation or confusion (inability to respond appropriately to questions)?	Y	N
Loss of memory:	Y	N
"If so, how long?" _____		
"Before or after the injury?" _____		
Blank or vacant look:	Y	N
Visible facial injury in combination with any of the above:	Y	N

1 Glasgow coma scale (GCS)

Best eye response (E)	
No eye opening	1
Eye opening in response to pain	2
Eye opening to speech	3
Eyes opening spontaneously	4

Best verbal response (V)	
No verbal response	1
Incomprehensible sounds	2
Inappropriate words	3
Confused	4
Oriented	5

Best motor response (M)	
No motor response	1
Extension to pain	2
Abnormal flexion to pain	3
Flexion / Withdrawal to pain	4
Localizes to pain	5
Obeys commands	6

Glasgow Coma score (E + V + M)	of 15

GCS should be recorded for all athletes in case of subsequent deterioration.

2 Maddocks Score[3]

"I am going to ask you a few questions, please listen carefully and give your best effort."

Modified Maddocks questions (1 point for each correct answer)

What venue are we at today?	0	1
Which half is it now?	0	1
Who scored last in this match?	0	1
What team did you play last week / game?	0	1
Did your team win the last game?	0	1
Maddocks score		of 5

Maddocks score is validated for sideline diagnosis of concussion only and is not used for serial testing.

Notes: Mechanism of Injury ("tell me what happened"?):

_____

_____

_____

_____

Any athlete with a suspected concussion should be REMOVED FROM PLAY, medically assessed, monitored for deterioration (i.e., should not be left alone) and should not drive a motor vehicle until cleared to do so by a medical professional. No athlete diagnosed with concussion should be returned to sports participation on the day of Injury.

FIGURE 24-1 *(continued)*

© 2017 American Academy of Orthopaedic Surgeons

BACKGROUND

Name: ______ Date: ______
Examiner: ______
Sport / team / school: ______ Date / time of injury: ______
Age: ______ Gender: M F
Years of education completed: ______
Dominant hand: right left neither
How many concussions do you think you have had in the past? ______
When was the most recent concussion? ______
How long was your recovery from the most recent concussion? ______
Have you ever been hospitalized or had medical imaging done for a head injury? Y N
Have you ever been diagnosed with headaches or migraines? Y N
Do you have a learning disability, dyslexia, ADD / ADHD? Y N
Have you ever been diagnosed with depression, anxiety or other psychiatric disorder? Y N
Has anyone in your family ever been diagnosed with any of these problems? Y N
Are you on any medications? If yes, please list: Y N

SCAT3 to be done in resting state. Best done 10 or more minutes post excercise.

SYMPTOM EVALUATION

3 How do you feel?

"You should score yourself on the following symptoms, based on how you feel now".

	none	mild		moderate		severe	
Headache	0	1	2	3	4	5	6
"Pressure in head"	0	1	2	3	4	5	6
Neck Pain	0	1	2	3	4	5	6
Nausea or vomiting	0	1	2	3	4	5	6
Dizziness	0	1	2	3	4	5	6
Blurred vision	0	1	2	3	4	5	6
Balance problems	0	1	2	3	4	5	6
Sensitivity to light	0	1	2	3	4	5	6
Sensitivity to noise	0	1	2	3	4	5	6
Feeling slowed down	0	1	2	3	4	5	6
Feeling like "in a fog"	0	1	2	3	4	5	6
"Don't feel right"	0	1	2	3	4	5	6
Difficulty concentrating	0	1	2	3	4	5	6
Difficulty remembering	0	1	2	3	4	5	6
Fatigue or low energy	0	1	2	3	4	5	6
Confusion	0	1	2	3	4	5	6
Drowsiness	0	1	2	3	4	5	6
Trouble falling asleep	0	1	2	3	4	5	6
More emotional	0	1	2	3	4	5	6
Irritability	0	1	2	3	4	5	6
Sadness	0	1	2	3	4	5	6
Nervous or Anxious	0	1	2	3	4	5	6

Total number of symptoms (Maximum possible 22)
Symptom severity score (Maximum possible 132)

Do the symptoms get worse with physical activity? Y N
Do the symptoms get worse with mental activity? Y N

self rated — self rated and clinician monitored
clinician interview — self rated with parent input

Overall rating: If you know the athlete well prior to the injury, how different is the athlete acting compared to his / her usual self?
Please circle one response:

no different | very different | unsure | N/A

Scoring on the SCAT3 should not be used as a stand-alone method to diagnose concussion, measure recovery or make decisions about an athlete's readiness to return to competition after concussion. Since signs and symptoms may evolve over time, it is important to consider repeat evaluation in the acute assessment of concussion.

COGNITIVE & PHYSICAL EVALUATION

4 Cognitive assessment

Standardized Assessment of Concussion (SAC)[4]

Orientation (1 point for each correct answer)

What month is it?	0	1
What is the date today?	0	1
What is the day of the week?	0	1
What year is it?	0	1
What time is it right now? (within 1 hour)	0	1
Orientation score		of 5

Immediate memory

List	Trial 1		Trial 2		Trial 3		Alternative word list		
elbow	0	1	0	1	0	1	candle	baby	finger
apple	0	1	0	1	0	1	paper	monkey	penny
carpet	0	1	0	1	0	1	sugar	perfume	blanket
saddle	0	1	0	1	0	1	sandwich	sunset	lemon
bubble	0	1	0	1	0	1	wagon	iron	insect
Total									

Immediate memory score total of 15

Concentration: Digits Backward

List	Trial 1		Alternative digit list		
4-9-3	0	1	6-2-9	5-2-6	4-1-5
3-8-1-4	0	1	3-2-7-9	1-7-9-5	4-9-6-8
6-2-9-7-1	0	1	1-5-2-8-6	3-8-5-2-7	6-1-8-4-3
7-1-8-4-6-2	0	1	5-3-9-1-4-8	8-3-1-9-6-4	7-2-4-8-5-6
Total of 4					

Concentration: Month in Reverse Order (1 pt. for entire sequence correct)

Dec-Nov-Oct-Sept-Aug-Jul-Jun-May-Apr-Mar-Feb-Jan 0 1

Concentration score of 5

5 Neck Examination:

Range of motion Tenderness Upper and lower limb sensation & strength
Findings: ______

6 Balance examination

Do one or both of the following tests.
Footwear (shoes, barefoot, braces, tape, etc.) ______

Modified Balance Error Scoring System (BESS) testing[5]
Which foot was tested (i.e. which is the **non-dominant** foot) Left Right
Testing surface (hard floor, field, etc.) ______

Condition
Double leg stance: Errors
Single leg stance (non-dominant foot): Errors
Tandem stance (non-dominant foot at back): Errors

And / Or

Tandem gait[6,7]
Time (best of 4 trials): ______ seconds

7 Coordination examination

Upper limb coordination
Which arm was tested: Left Right
Coordination score of 1

8 SAC Delayed Recall[4]

Delayed recall score of 5

SCAT3 SPORT CONCUSSION ASSESSMENT TOOL 3 | **PAGE 2**

260

FIGURE 24-1 *(Continued)*

INSTRUCTIONS

Words in *Italics* throughout the SCAT3 are the instructions given to the athlete by the tester.

Symptom Scale

"You should score yourself on the following symptoms, based on how you feel now".

To be completed by the athlete. In situations where the symptom scale is being completed after exercise, it should still be done in a resting state, at least 10 minutes post exercise.

For total number of symptoms, maximum possible is 22.

For Symptom severity score, add all scores in table, maximum possible is 22 x 6 = 132.

SAC[4]

Immediate Memory

"I am going to test your memory. I will read you a list of words and when I am done, repeat back as many words as you can remember, in any order."

Trials 2 & 3:

"I am going to repeat the same list again. Repeat back as many words as you can remember in any order, even if you said the word before."

Complete all 3 trials regardless of score on trial 1 & 2. Read the words at a rate of one per second. **Score 1 pt. for each correct response.** Total score equals sum across all 3 trials. Do not inform the athlete that delayed recall will be tested.

Concentration
Digits backward

"I am going to read you a string of numbers and when I am done, you repeat them back to me backwards, in reverse order of how I read them to you. For example, if I say 7-1-9, you would say 9-1-7."

If correct, go to next string length. If incorrect, read trial 2. **One point possible for each string length**. Stop after incorrect on both trials. The digits should be read at the rate of one per second.

Months in reverse order

"Now tell me the months of the year in reverse order. Start with the last month and go backward. So you'll say December, November … Go ahead"

1 pt. for entire sequence correct

Delayed Recall

The delayed recall should be performed after completion of the Balance and Coordination Examination.

"Do you remember that list of words I read a few times earlier? Tell me as many words from the list as you can remember in any order."

Score 1 pt. for each correct response

Balance Examination

Modified Balance Error Scoring System (BESS) testing[5]

This balance testing is based on a modified version of the Balance Error Scoring System (BESS)[5]. A stopwatch or watch with a second hand is required for this testing.

"I am now going to test your balance. Please take your shoes off, roll up your pant legs above ankle (if applicable), and remove any ankle taping (if applicable). This test will consist of three twenty second tests with different stances."

(a) Double leg stance:

"The first stance is standing with your feet together with your hands on your hips and with your eyes closed. You should try to maintain stability in that position for 20 seconds. I will be counting the number of times you move out of this position. I will start timing when you are set and have closed your eyes."

(b) Single leg stance:

"If you were to kick a ball, which foot would you use? [This will be the dominant foot] Now stand on your non-dominant foot. The dominant leg should be held in approximately 30 degrees of hip flexion and 45 degrees of knee flexion. Again, you should try to maintain stability for 20 seconds with your hands on your hips and your eyes closed. I will be counting the number of times you move out of this position. If you stumble out of this position, open your eyes and return to the start position and continue balancing. I will start timing when you are set and have closed your eyes."

(c) Tandem stance:

"Now stand heel-to-toe with your non-dominant foot in back. Your weight should be evenly distributed across both feet. Again, you should try to maintain stability for 20 seconds with your hands on your hips and your eyes closed. I will be counting the number of times you move out of this position. If you stumble out of this position, open your eyes and return to the start position and continue balancing. I will start timing when you are set and have closed your eyes."

Balance testing – types of errors

1. Hands lifted off iliac crest
2. Opening eyes
3. Step, stumble, or fall
4. Moving hip into > 30 degrees abduction
5. Lifting forefoot or heel
6. Remaining out of test position > 5 sec

Each of the 20-second trials is scored by counting the errors, or deviations from the proper stance, accumulated by the athlete. The examiner will begin counting errors only after the individual has assumed the proper start position. **The modified BESS is calculated by adding one error point for each error during the three 20-second tests. The maximum total number of errors for any single condition is 10.** If an athlete commits multiple errors simultaneously, only one error is recorded but the athlete should quickly return to the testing position, and counting should resume once subject is set. Subjects that are unable to maintain the testing procedure for a minimum of **five seconds** at the start are assigned the highest possible score, ten, for that testing condition.

OPTION: For further assessment, the same 3 stances can be performed on a surface of medium density foam (e.g., approximately 50 cm x 40 cm x 6 cm).

Tandem Gait[6,7]

Participants are instructed to stand with their feet together behind a starting line (the test is best done with footwear removed). Then, they walk in a forward direction as quickly and as accurately as possible along a 38mm wide (sports tape), 3 meter line with an alternate foot heel-to-toe gait ensuring that they approximate their heel and toe on each step. Once they cross the end of the 3m line, they turn 180 degrees and return to the starting point using the same gait. A total of 4 trials are done and the best time is retained. Athletes should complete the test in 14 seconds. Athletes fail the test if they step off the line, have a separation between their heel and toe, or if they touch or grab the examiner or an object. In this case, the time is not recorded and the trial repeated, if appropriate.

Coordination Examination

Upper limb coordination
Finger-to-nose (FTN) task:

"I am going to test your coordination now. Please sit comfortably on the chair with your eyes open and your arm (either right or left) outstretched (shoulder flexed to 90 degrees and elbow and fingers extended), pointing in front of you. When I give a start signal, I would like you to perform five successive finger to nose repetitions using your index finger to touch the tip of the nose, and then return to the starting position, as quickly and as accurately as possible."

Scoring: 5 correct repetitions in < 4 seconds = 1
Note for testers: Athletes fail the test if they do not touch their nose, do not fully extend their elbow or do not perform five repetitions. **Failure should be scored as 0.**

References & Footnotes

1. This tool has been developed by a group of international experts at the 4th International Consensus meeting on Concussion in Sport held in Zurich, Switzerland in November 2012. The full details of the conference outcomes and the authors of the tool are published in The BJSM Injury Prevention and Health Protection, 2013, Volume 47, Issue 5. The outcome paper will also be simultaneously co-published in other leading biomedical journals with the copyright held by the Concussion in Sport Group, to allow unrestricted distribution, providing no alterations are made.

2. McCrory P et al., Consensus Statement on Concussion in Sport – the 3rd International Conference on Concussion in Sport held in Zurich, November 2008. British Journal of Sports Medicine 2009; 43: i76-89.

3. Maddocks, DL; Dicker, GD; Saling, MM. The assessment of orientation following concussion in athletes. Clinical Journal of Sport Medicine. 1995; 5(1): 32 – 3.

4. McCrea M. Standardized mental status testing of acute concussion. Clinical Journal of Sport Medicine. 2001; 11: 176 – 181.

5. Guskiewicz KM. Assessment of postural stability following sport-related concussion. Current Sports Medicine Reports. 2003; 2: 24 – 30.

6. Schneiders, A.G., Sullivan, S.J., Gray, A., Hammond-Tooke, G. & McCrory, P. Normative values for 16-37 year old subjects for three clinical measures of motor performance used in the assessment of sports concussions. Journal of Science and Medicine in Sport. 2010; 13(2): 196 – 201.

7. Schneiders, A.G., Sullivan, S.J., Kvarnstrom. J.K., Olsson, M., Yden. T. & Marshall, S.W. The effect of footwear and sports-surface on dynamic neurological screening in sport-related concussion. Journal of Science and Medicine in Sport. 2010; 13(4): 382 – 386

© 2013 Concussion in Sport Group
261

FIGURE 24-1 *(Continued)*

ATHLETE INFORMATION

Any athlete suspected of having a concussion should be removed from play, and then seek medical evaluation.

Signs to watch for

Problems could arise over the first 24–48 hours. The athlete should not be left alone and must go to a hospital at once if they:

- Have a headache that gets worse
- Are very drowsy or can't be awakened
- Can't recognize people or places
- Have repeated vomiting
- Behave unusually or seem confused; are very irritable
- Have seizures (arms and legs jerk uncontrollably)
- Have weak or numb arms or legs
- Are unsteady on their feet; have slurred speech

Remember, it is better to be safe.
Consult your doctor after a suspected concussion.

Return to play

Athletes should not be returned to play the same day of injury.
When returning athletes to play, they should be **medically cleared and then follow a stepwise supervised program,** with stages of progression.

For example:

Rehabilitation stage	Functional exercise at each stage of rehabilitation	Objective of each stage
No activity	Physical and cognitive rest	Recovery
Light aerobic exercise	Walking, swimming or stationary cycling keeping intensity, 70 % maximum predicted heart rate. No resistance training	Increase heart rate
Sport-specific exercise	Skating drills in ice hockey, running drills in soccer. No head impact activities	Add movement
Non-contact training drills	Progression to more complex training drills, eg passing drills in football and ice hockey. May start progressive resistance training	Exercise, coordination, and cognitive load
Full contact practice	Following medical clearance participate in normal training activities	Restore confidence and assess functional skills by coaching staff
Return to play	Normal game play	

There should be at least 24 hours (or longer) for each stage and if symptoms recur the athlete should rest until they resolve once again and then resume the program at the previous asymptomatic stage. Resistance training should only be added in the later stages.

If the athlete is symptomatic for more than 10 days, then consultation by a medical practitioner who is expert in the management of concussion, is recommended.

Medical clearance should be given before return to play.

Scoring Summary:

Test Domain	Score		
	Date: _____	Date: _____	Date: _____
Number of Symptoms of 22			
Symptom Severity Score of 132			
Orientation of 5			
Immediate Memory of 15			
Concentration of 5			
Delayed Recall of 5			
SAC Total			
BESS (total errors)			
Tandem Gait (seconds)			
Coordination of 1			

Notes:

_____
_____
_____
_____
_____
_____
_____
_____
_____
_____
_____
_____
_____
_____
_____
_____

✂ ---

CONCUSSION INJURY ADVICE

(To be given to the **person monitoring** the concussed athlete)

This patient has received an injury to the head. A careful medical examination has been carried out and no sign of any serious complications has been found. Recovery time is variable across individuals and the patient will need monitoring for a further period by a responsible adult. Your treating physician will provide guidance as to this timeframe.

If you notice any change in behaviour, vomiting, dizziness, worsening headache, double vision or excessive drowsiness, please contact your doctor or the nearest hospital emergency department immediately.

Other important points:

- Rest (physically and mentally), including training or playing sports until symptoms resolve and you are medically cleared
- No alcohol
- No prescription or non-prescription drugs without medical supervision. Specifically:
  · No sleeping tablets
  · Do not use aspirin, anti-inflammatory medication or sedating pain killers
- Do not drive until medically cleared
- Do not train or play sport until medically cleared

Clinic phone number _____

Patient's name _____

Date/time of injury _____

Date/time of medical review _____

Treating physician _____

Contact details or stamp

SCAT3 SPORT CONCUSSION ASSESSMENT TOOL 3 | **PAGE 4**   © 2013 Concussion in Sport Group

FIGURE 24-1 (Continued)

Child-SCAT3™

Sport Concussion Assessment Tool for children ages 5 to12 years

For use by medical professionals only

What is ChildSCAT3?[1]

The ChildSCAT3 is a standardized tool for evaluating injured children for concussion and can be used in children aged from 5 to 12 years. It supersedes the original SCAT and the SCAT2 published in 2005 and 2009, respectively [2]. For older persons, ages 13 years and over, please use the SCAT3. The ChildSCAT3 is designed for use by medical professionals. If you are not qualified, please use the Sport Concussion Recognition Tool[1]. Preseason baseline testing with the ChildSCAT3 can be helpful for interpreting post-injury test scores.

Specific instructions for use of the ChildSCAT3 are provided on page 3. If you are not familiar with the ChildSCAT3, please read through these instructions carefully. This tool may be freely copied in its current form for distribution to individuals, teams, groups and organizations. Any revision and any reproduction in a digital form require approval by the Concussion in Sport Group.
NOTE: The diagnosis of a concussion is a clinical judgment, ideally made by a medical professional. The ChildSCAT3 should not be used solely to make, or exclude, the diagnosis of concussion in the absence of clinical judgement. An athlete may have a concussion even if their ChildSCAT3 is "normal".

What is a concussion?

A concussion is a disturbance in brain function caused by a direct or indirect force to the head. It results in a variety of non-specific signs and/or symptoms (like those listed below) and most often does not involve loss of consciousness. Concussion should be suspected in the presence of any one or more of the following:

- Symptoms (e.g., headache), or
- Physical signs (e.g., unsteadiness), or
- Impaired brain function (e.g. confusion) or
- Abnormal behaviour (e.g., change in personality).

SIDELINE ASSESSMENT

Indications for Emergency Management

NOTE: A hit to the head can sometimes be associated with a more severe brain injury. If the concussed child displays any of the following, then do not proceed with the ChildSCAT3; instead activate emergency procedures and urgent transportation to the nearest hospital:

- Glasgow Coma score less than 15
- Deteriorating mental status
- Potential spinal injury
- Progressive, worsening symptoms or new neurologic signs
- Persistent vomiting
- Evidence of skull fracture
- Post traumatic seizures
- Coagulopathy
- History of Neurosurgery (eg Shunt)
- Multiple injuries

1 | Glasgow coma scale (GCS)

Best eye response (E)

No eye opening	1
Eye opening in response to pain	2
Eye opening to speech	3
Eyes opening spontaneously	4

Best verbal response (V)

No verbal response	1
Incomprehensible sounds	2
Inappropriate words	3
Confused	4
Oriented	5

Best motor response (M)

No motor response	1
Extension to pain	2
Abnormal flexion to pain	3
Flexion/Withdrawal to pain	4
Localizes to pain	5
Obeys commands	6
Glasgow Coma score (E + V + M)	**of 15**

GCS should be recorded for all athletes in case of subsequent deterioration.

Potential signs of concussion?

If any of the following signs are observed after a direct or indirect blow to the head, the child should stop participation, be evaluated by a medical professional and **should not be permitted to return to sport the same day** if a concussion is suspected.

Any loss of consciousness?	Y	N
"If so, how long?" _____		
Balance or motor incoordination (stumbles, slow/laboured movements, etc.)?	Y	N
Disorientation or confusion (inability to respond appropriately to questions)?	Y	N
Loss of memory:	Y	N
"If so, how long?" _____		
"Before or after the injury?" _____		
Blank or vacant look:	Y	N
Visible facial injury in combination with any of the above:	Y	N

2 | Sideline Assessment – child-Maddocks Score[3]

"I am going to ask you a few questions, please listen carefully and give your best effort."
Modified Maddocks questions (1 point for each correct answer)

Where are we at now?	0	1
Is it before or after lunch?	0	1
What did you have last lesson/class?	0	1
What is your teacher's name?	0	1
child-Maddocks score		**of 4**

Child-Maddocks score is for sideline diagnosis of concussion only and is not used for serial testing.

Any child with a suspected concussion should be REMOVED FROM PLAY, medically assessed and monitored for deterioration (i.e., should not be left alone). No child diagnosed with concussion should be returned to sports participation on the day of Injury.

BACKGROUND

Name: _____	Date/Time of Injury: _____
Examiner: _____	Date of Assessment: _____
Sport/team/school: _____	
Age: _____	Gender: M F
Current school year/grade: _____	
Dominant hand:	right left neither

Mechanism of Injury ("tell me what happened"?): _____

For Parent/carer to complete:

How many concussions has the child had in the past? _____
When was the most recent concussion? _____
How long was the recovery from the most recent concussion? _____

Has the child ever been hospitalized or had medical imaging done (CT or MRI) for a head injury?	Y	N
Has the child ever been diagnosed with headaches or migraines?	Y	N
Does the child have a learning disability, dyslexia, ADD/ADHD, seizure disorder?	Y	N
Has the child ever been diagnosed with depression, anxiety or other psychiatric disorder?	Y	N
Has anyone in the family ever been diagnosed with any of these problems?	Y	N
Is the child on any medications? If yes, please list:	Y	N

_____

© 2013 Concussion in Sport Group
263

FIGURE 24-2 *(continued)*

© 2017 American Academy of Orthopaedic Surgeons

SYMPTOM EVALUATION

3 Child report

Name:	never	rarely	sometimes	often
I have trouble paying attention	0	1	2	3
I get distracted easily	0	1	2	3
I have a hard time concentrating	0	1	2	3
I have problems remembering what people tell me	0	1	2	3
I have problems following directions	0	1	2	3
I daydream too much	0	1	2	3
I get confused	0	1	2	3
I forget things	0	1	2	3
I have problems finishing things	0	1	2	3
I have trouble figuring things out	0	1	2	3
It's hard for me to learn new things	0	1	2	3
I have headaches	0	1	2	3
I feel dizzy	0	1	2	3
I feel like the room is spinning	0	1	2	3
I feel like I'm going to faint	0	1	2	3
Things are blurry when I look at them	0	1	2	3
I see double	0	1	2	3
I feel sick to my stomach	0	1	2	3
I get tired a lot	0	1	2	3
I get tired easily	0	1	2	3
Total number of symptoms (Maximum possible 20)				
Symptom severity score (Maximum possible 20 x 3 = 60)				

self rated ⬜ clinician interview ⬜ self rated and clinician monitored

4 Parent report

The child	never	rarely	sometimes	often
has trouble sustaining attention	0	1	2	3
Is easily distracted	0	1	2	3
has difficulty concentrating	0	1	2	3
has problems remembering what he/she is told	0	1	2	3
has difficulty following directions	0	1	2	3
tends to daydream	0	1	2	3
gets confused	0	1	2	3
is forgetful	0	1	2	3
has difficulty completing tasks	0	1	2	3
has poor problem solving skills	0	1	2	3
has problems learning	0	1	2	3
has headaches	0	1	2	3
feels dizzy	0	1	2	3
has a feeling that the room is spinning	0	1	2	3
feels faint	0	1	2	3
has blurred vision	0	1	2	3
has double vision	0	1	2	3
experiences nausea	0	1	2	3
gets tired a lot	0	1	2	3
gets tired easily	0	1	2	3
Total number of symptoms (Maximum possible 20)				
Symptom severity score (Maximum possible 20 x 3 = 60)				

Do the symptoms get worse with physical activity? ⬜ Y ⬜ N
Do the symptoms get worse with mental activity? ⬜ Y ⬜ N

parent self rated ⬜ clinician interview ⬜ parent self rated and clinician monitored

Overall rating for parent/teacher/coach/carer to answer.
How different is the child acting compared to his/her usual self?
Please circle one response:

no different	very different	unsure	N/A

Name of person completing Parent-report: _____

Relationship to child of person completing Parent-report: _____

Scoring on the ChildSCAT3 should not be used as a stand-alone method to diagnose concussion, measure recovery or make decisions about an athlete's readiness to return to competition after concussion.

COGNITIVE & PHYSICAL EVALUATION

5 Cognitive assessment
Standardized Assessment of Concussion – Child Version (SAC-C)[4]

Orientation (1 point for each correct answer)

What month is it?	0	1
What is the date today?	0	1
What is the day of the week?	0	1
What year is it?	0	1
Orientation score		of 4

Immediate memory

List	Trial 1		Trial 2		Trial 3		Alternative word list		
elbow	0	1	0	1	0	1	candle	baby	finger
apple	0	1	0	1	0	1	paper	monkey	penny
carpet	0	1	0	1	0	1	sugar	perfume	blanket
saddle	0	1	0	1	0	1	sandwich	sunset	lemon
bubble	0	1	0	1	0	1	wagon	iron	insect
Total									

Immediate memory score total — of 15

Concentration: Digits Backward

List	Trial 1		Alternative digit list		
6-2	0	1	5-2	4-1	4-9
4-9-3	0	1	6-2-9	5-2-6	4-1-5
3-8-1-4	0	1	3-2-7-9	1-7-9-5	4-9-6-8
6-2-9-7-1	0	1	1-5-2-8-6	3-8-5-2-7	6-1-8-4-3
7-1-8-4-6-2	0	1	5-3-9-1-4-8	8-3-1-9-6-4	7-2-4-8-5-6
Total of 5					

Concentration: Days in Reverse Order (1 pt. for entire sequence correct)

Sunday-Saturday-Friday-Thursday-Wednesday-Tuesday-Monday	0	1
Concentration score		of 6

6 Neck Examination:

Range of motion   Tenderness   Upper and lower limb sensation & strength
Findings: _____

7 Balance examination
Do one or both of the following tests.
Footwear (shoes, barefoot, braces, tape, etc.) _____

Modified Balance Error Scoring System (BESS) testing[5]
Which foot was tested (i.e. which is the **non-dominant** foot) ⬜ Left ⬜ Right
Testing surface (hard floor, field, etc.) _____
Condition

Double leg stance:	Errors
Tandem stance (non-dominant foot at back):	Errors

Tandem gait[6,7]
Time taken to complete (best of 4 trials): _____ seconds
If child attempted, but unable to complete tandem gait, mark here ⬜

8 Coordination examination
Upper limb coordination

Which arm was tested: ⬜ Left ⬜ Right
Coordination score — of 1

9 SAC Delayed Recall[4]

Delayed recall score — of 5

Since signs and symptoms may evolve over time, it is important to consider repeat evaluation in the acute assessment of concussion.

264

CHILD-SCAT3 SPORT CONCUSSION ASSESSMENT TOOL 3 | PAGE 2

© 2013 Concussion in Sport Group

FIGURE 24-2 (Continued)

INSTRUCTIONS

Words in *Italics* throughout the ChildSCAT3 are the instructions given to the child by the tester.

Sideline Assessment – child-Maddocks Score

To be completed on the sideline/in the playground, immediately following concussion. There is no requirement to repeat these questions at follow-up.

Symptom Scale[8]

In situations where the symptom scale is being completed after exercise, it should still be done in a resting state, at least 10 minutes post exercise.

On the day of injury
- the child is to complete the Child Report, according to how he/she feels now.

On all subsequent days
- the child is to complete the Child Report, according to how he/she feels today, **and**
- the parent/carer is to complete the Parent Report according to how the child has been over the previous 24 hours.

Standardized Assessment of Concussion – Child Version (SAC-C)[4]

Orientation
Ask each question on the score sheet. A correct answer for **each question scores 1 point.** If the child does not understand the question, gives an incorrect answer, or no answer, then the score for that question is 0 points.

Immediate memory
"I am going to test your memory. I will read you a list of words and when I am done, repeat back as many words as you can remember, in any order."

Trials 2 & 3:
"I am going to repeat the same list again. Repeat back as many words as you can remember in any order, even if you said the word before."

Complete all 3 trials regardless of score on trial 1 & 2. Read the words at a rate of one per second. **Score 1 pt. for each correct response.** Total score equals sum across all 3 trials. Do not inform the child that delayed recall will be tested.

Concentration
Digits Backward:

"I am going to read you a string of numbers and when I am done, you repeat them back to me backwards, in reverse order of how I read them to you. For example, if I say 7-1, you would say 1-7."

If correct, go to next string length. If incorrect, read trial 2. **One point possible for each string length.** Stop after incorrect on both trials. The digits should be read at the rate of one per second.

Days in Reverse Order:

"Now tell me the days of the week in reverse order. Start with Sunday and go backward. So you'll say Sunday, Saturday ... Go ahead"

1 pt. for entire sequence correct

Delayed recall

The delayed recall should be performed after completion of the Balance and Coordination Examination.
"Do you remember that list of words I read a few times earlier? Tell me as many words from the list as you can remember in any order."

Circle each word correctly recalled. **Total score equals number of words recalled.**

Balance examination

These instructions are to be read by the person administering the ChildSCAT3, and each balance task **should be demonstrated to the child.** The child should then be asked to copy what the examiner demonstrated.

Modified Balance Error Scoring System (BESS) testing[5]

This balance testing is based on a modified version of the Balance Error Scoring System (BESS)[5]. A stopwatch or watch with a second hand is required for this testing.

"I am now going to test your balance. Please take your shoes off, roll up your pant legs above ankle (if applicable), and remove any ankle taping (if applicable). This test will consist of two different parts."

(a) Double leg stance:
The first stance is standing with the feet together with hands on hips and with eyes closed. The child should try to maintain stability in that position for 20 seconds. You should inform the child that you will be counting the number of times the child moves out of this position. You should start timing when the child is set and the eyes are closed.

(b) Tandem stance:
Instruct the child to stand heel-to-toe with the non-dominant foot in the back. Weight should be evenly distributed across both feet. Again, the child should try to maintain stability for 20 seconds with hands on hips and eyes closed. You should inform the child that you will be counting the number of times the child moves out of this position. If the child stumbles out of this position, instruct him/her to open the eyes and return to the start position and continue balancing. You should start timing when the child is set and the eyes are closed.

Balance testing – types of errors - Parts (a) and (b)

1. Hands lifted off iliac crest
2. Opening eyes
3. Step, stumble, or fall
4. Moving hip into > 30 degrees abduction
5. Lifting forefoot or heel
6. Remaining out of test position > 5 sec

Each of the 20-second trials is scored by counting the errors, or deviations from the proper stance, accumulated by the child. The examiner will begin counting errors only after the child has assumed the proper start position. **The modified BESS is calculated by adding one error point for each error during the two 20-second tests. The maximum total number of errors for any single condition is 10.** If a child commits multiple errors simultaneously, only one error is recorded but the child should quickly return to the testing position, and counting should resume once subject is set. Children who are unable to maintain the testing procedure for a minimum of **five seconds** at the start are assigned the highest possible score, ten, for that testing condition.

OPTION: For further assessment, the same 2 stances can be performed on a surface of medium density foam (e.g., approximately 50 cm x 40 cm x 6 cm).

Tandem Gait[6,7]

Use a clock (with a second hand) or stopwatch to measure the time taken to complete this task. Instruction for the examiner – **Demonstrate the following to the child:**

The child is instructed to stand with their feet together behind a starting line (the test is best done with footwear removed). Then, they walk in a forward direction as quickly and as accurately as possible along a 38mm wide (sports tape), 3 meter line with an alternate foot heel-to-toe gait ensuring that they approximate their heel and toe on each step. Once they cross the end of the 3m line, they turn 180 degrees and return to the starting point using the same gait. A total of 4 trials are done and the best time is retained. Children fail the test if they step off the line, have a separation between their heel and toe, or if they touch or grab the examiner or an object. In this case, the time is not recorded and the trial repeated, if appropriate.

Explain to the child that you will time how long it takes them to walk to the end of the line and back.

Coordination examination

Upper limb coordination
Finger-to-nose (FTN) task:

The tester should **demonstrate it to the child.**

"I am going to test your coordination now. Please sit comfortably on the chair with your eyes open and your arm (either right or left) outstretched (shoulder flexed to 90 degrees and elbow and fingers extended). When I give a start signal, I would like you to perform five successive finger to nose repetitions using your index finger to touch the tip of the nose as quickly and as accurately as possible."

Scoring: 5 correct repetitions in < 4 seconds = 1
Note for testers: Children fail the test if they do not touch their nose, do not fully extend their elbow or do not perform five repetitions. **Failure should be scored as 0.**

References & Footnotes

1. This tool has been developed by a group of international experts at the 4th International Consensus meeting on Concussion in Sport held in Zurich, Switzerland in November 2012. The full details of the conference outcomes and the authors of the tool are published in The BJSM Injury Prevention and Health Protection, 2013, Volume 47, Issue 5. The outcome paper will also be simultaneously co-published in other leading biomedical journals with the copyright held by the Concussion in Sport Group, to allow unrestricted distribution, providing no alterations are made.

2. McCrory P et al., Consensus Statement on Concussion in Sport – the 3rd International Conference on Concussion in Sport held in Zurich, November 2008. British Journal of Sports Medicine 2009; 43: i76-89.

3. Maddocks, DL; Dicker, GD; Saling, MM. The assessment of orientation following concussion in athletes. Clinical Journal of Sport Medicine. 1995; 5(1): 32–3.

4. McCrea M. Standardized mental status testing of acute concussion. Clinical Journal of Sport Medicine. 2001; 11: 176–181.

5. Guskiewicz KM. Assessment of postural stability following sport-related concussion. Current Sports Medicine Reports. 2003; 2: 24–30.

6. Schneiders, A.G., Sullivan, S.J., Gray, A., Hammond-Tooke, G. & McCrory, P. Normative values for 16-37 year old subjects for three clinical measures of motor performance used in the assessment of sports concussions. Journal of Science and Medicine in Sport. 2010; 13(2): 196–201.

7. Schneiders, A.G., Sullivan, S.J., Kvarnstrom. J.K., Olsson, M., Yden. T. & Marshall, S.W. The effect of footwear and sports-surface on dynamic neurological screening in sport-related concussion. Journal of Science and Medicine in Sport. 2010; 13(4): 382–386

8. Ayr, L.K., Yeates, K.O., Taylor, H.G., & Brown, M. Dimensions of post-concussive symptoms in children with mild traumatic brain injuries. Journal of the International Neuropsychological Society. 2009; 15:19–30.

CHILD-SCAT3 SPORT CONCUSSION ASSESSMENT TOOL 3 | **PAGE 3**

© 2013 Concussion in Sport Group
265

FIGURE 24-2 *(Continued)*

CHILD ATHLETE INFORMATION

Any child suspected of having a concussion should be removed from play, and then seek medical evaluation. The child must NOT return to play or sport on the same day as the suspected concussion.

Signs to watch for

Problems could arise over the first 24–48 hours. The child should not be left alone and must go to a hospital at once if they develop any of the following:

- New Headache, or Headache gets worse
- Persistent or increasing neck pain
- Becomes drowsy or can't be woken up
- Can not recognise people or places
- Has Nausea or Vomiting
- Behaves unusually, seems confused, or is irritable
- Has any seizures (arms and/or legs jerk uncontrollably)
- Has weakness, numbness or tingling (arms, legs or face)
- Is unsteady walking or standing
- Has slurred speech
- Has difficulty understanding speech or directions

Remember, it is better to be safe.
Always consult your doctor after a suspected concussion.

Return to school

Concussion may impact on the child's cognitive ability to learn at school. This must be considered, and medical clearance is required before the child may return to school. **It is reasonable for a child to miss a day or two of school after concussion, but extended absence is uncommon.** In some children, a graduated return to school program will need to be developed for the child. The child will progress through the return to school program provided that there is no worsening of symptoms. If any particular activity worsens symptoms, the child will abstain from that activity until it no longer causes symptom worsening. Use of computers and internet should follow a similar graduated program, provided that it does not worsen symptoms. This program should include communication between the parents, teachers, and health professionals and will vary from child to child. The return to school program should consider:

- Extra time to complete assignments/tests
- Quiet room to complete assignments/tests
- Avoidance of noisy areas such as cafeterias, assembly halls, sporting events, music class, shop class, etc
- Frequent breaks during class, homework, tests
- No more than one exam/day
- Shorter assignments
- Repetition/memory cues
- Use of peer helper/tutor
- Reassurance from teachers that student will be supported through recovery through accommodations, workload reduction, alternate forms of testing
- Later start times, half days, only certain classes

The child is not to return to play or sport until he/she has successfully returned to school/learning, without worsening of symptoms. Medical clearance should be given before return to play.

If there are any doubts, management should be referred to a qualified health practitioner, expert in the management of concussion in children.

Return to sport

There should be no return to play until the child has successfully returned to school/learning, without worsening of symptoms.
Children must not be returned to play the same day of injury.
When returning children to play, they should **medically cleared and then follow a stepwise supervised program,** with stages of progression.

For example:

Rehabilitation stage	Functional exercise at each stage of rehabilitation	Objective of each stage
No activity	Physical and cognitive rest	Recovery
Light aerobic exercise	Walking, swimming or stationary cycling keeping intensity, 70 % maximum predicted heart rate. No resistance training	Increase heart rate
Sport-specific exercise	Skating drills in ice hockey, running drills in soccer. No head impact activities	Add movement
Non-contact training drills	Progression to more complex training drills, eg passing drills in football and ice hockey. May start progressive resistance training	Exercise, coordination, and cognitive load
Full contact practice	Following medical clearance participate in normal training activities	Restore confidence and assess functional skills by coaching staff
Return to play	Normal game play	

There should be approximately 24 hours (or longer) for each stage and the child should drop back to the previous asymptomatic level if any post-concussive symptoms recur. Resistance training should only be added in the later stages.
If the child is symptomatic for more than 10 days, then review by a health practitioner, expert in the management of concussion, is recommended.
Medical clearance should be given before return to play.

Notes:

_____
_____
_____
_____
_____

CONCUSSION INJURY ADVICE FOR THE CHILD AND PARENTS / CARERS
(To be given to the **person monitoring** the concussed child)

This child has received an injury to the head. A careful medical examination has been carried out and no sign of any serious complications has been found. It is expected that recovery will be rapid, but the child will need monitoring for the next 24 hours by a responsible adult.

If you notice any change in behavior, vomiting, dizziness, worsening headache, double vision or excessive drowsiness, please call an ambulance to transport the child to hospital immediately.

Other important points:

- Following concussion, the child should rest for at least 24 hours.
- The child should avoid any computer, internet or electronic gaming activity if these activities make symptoms worse.
- The child should not be given any medications, including pain killers, unless prescribed by a medical practitioner.
- The child must not return to school until medically cleared.
- The child must not return to sport or play until medically cleared.

Patient's name _____

Date/time of injury _____

Date/time of medical review _____

Treating physician _____

```
                                          Contact details or stamp
```

Clinic phone number _____

CHILD-SCAT3 SPORT CONCUSSION ASSESSMENT TOOL 3 | **PAGE 4**   © 2013 Concussion in Sport Group

FIGURE 24-2 (Continued)

This tool does not constitute, and is not intended to constitute, a standard of medical care. It is a guide derived from the Standardized Concussion Assessment Tool 2 (SCAT2) (McCrory, et al, BJSM '09) and represents a standardized method of evaluating NFL players for concussion consistent with the reasonable, objective practice of the healthcare profession. This guide is not intended to be a substitute for the clinical judgment of the treating healthcare professional and should be interpreted based on the individual needs of the patient and the specific facts and circumstances presented.

NFL Sideline Concussion Assessment Tool: Completed by healthcare professional. Athlete completes symptoms at bottom.

Athlete _____ Position _____ Team _____ Evaluator _____ ATC / MD / DO

Evaluation date____ time ____ am / pm **Injury date** ____ time ____ am / pm **during** ☐ Game ☐ Practice ☐ Other _____

Mechanism of injury ☐ head to head ☐ elbow to head ☐ knee to head ☐ ground to head ☐ blow to body

☐ other mechanism _____ ☐ unknown mechanism

Penalty called ☐ Yes ☐ No   Other circumstances _____

This concussion assessment tool contains an assessment of orientation, memory, concentration, balance & symptoms. This tool is intended to be used in conjunction with your clinical judgment. If <u>ANY</u> significant abnormality is found, a conservative, "safety first" approach should be adopted. An athlete suspected of sustaining a concussion is a "No Go" and does not return to play in the same game or practice.

ANY OF THE FOLLOWING ARE OBVIOUS SIGNS OF DISQUALIFICATION (i.e. "No Go"):

1) **LOC or unresponsiveness?** (for any period of time) If so, how long? _____   ☐   Y   N
2) **Confusion?** (any disorientation or inability to respond appropriately to questions)   ☐   Y   N
3) **Amnesia (retrograde / anterograde)?** If so, how long? _____   ☐   Y   N
4) **New and/or persistent symptoms: see checklist?** (e.g. headache, nausea, dizziness)   ☐   Y   N
5) **Abnormal neurological finding?** (any motor, sensory, cranial nerve, balance issues, seizures) **or**   ☐   Y   N
6) **Progressive, persistent or worsening symptoms? If so, consider cervical spine and/or**
     a more serious brain injury (See box below)   ☐   Y   N

Other _____   Total Physical Signs Score: (total above ☐ Yes scores) of 6 = _____

Neurological Screen for Cervical Spine and/or More Serious Brain Trauma

Deteriorating mental status?	Y	N
Any reported neck pain, cervical spine tenderness or decreased range of motion?	Y	N
Pupil reaction abnormal or pupils unequal?	Y	N
Extra-ocular movements abnormal and/or cause double vision? (difficulty tracking and/or reading)	Y	N
Asymmetry or abnormalities on screening motor or sensory exam?	Y	N

ORIENTATION / SAC	of 5 = ____		**ORIENTATION / Maddock's Questions**	of 5 = ____
What month is it?	0 1		Where are we?	0 1
What is the date today?	0 1		What quarter is it right now?	0 1
What is the day of the week?	0 1		Who scored last in the practice / game?	0 1
What year is it?	0 1		Who did we play last game?	0 1
What time is it right now? (within an hour)	0 1		Did we win the last game?	0 1

SAC / Word Recall: Read list of 5 words 1 per second, ask athlete to repeat list, in any order. (Use of specific lists below optional). For Trial 2 & 3, read the same list of words again and have athlete repeat them back, in any order. One point for each word remembered. You must conduct all 3 trials regardless of their success on trial 1. **Do not tell athlete that delayed recall will be tested**

List 1	Immediate Recall Trials			Alternative Lists		Delayed recall (perform at end of all sideline testing, at least > 5 minutes)
	#1	#2	#3			
elbow	____	____	____	candle	baby	____
apple	____	____	____	paper	monkey	____
carpet	____	____	____	sugar	perfume	____
saddle	____	____	____	sandwich	sunset	____
bubble	____	____	____	wagon	iron	____
Total of all three immediate word recalls: out of 15 = ____						Total delayed recall: out of 5 = ____

FIGURE 24-3 (continued)

NFL Sideline Concussion Assessment Tool (continued)

Overall Rating; If you know the athlete well p/t the injury, how different is the athlete acting compared to his usual self?

Check one; ☐ No different ☐ Very different ☐ Unsure

SAC / Concentration: Read string of numbers, ask athlete to repeat backwards. (Use of specific numbers below optional). If correct go to the next string length. If incorrect, read second string (same length) 1 point for each string length correct. Stop after incorrect on both trials. Read digits at rate of 1 digit /sec

Digits Backward:		Alternative digit lists	
4-9-3	0 1	6-2-9	5-2-6
3-8-1-4	0 1	3-2-7-9	1-7-9-5
6-2-9-7-1	0 1	1-5-2-8-6	3-8-5-2-7
7-1-8-4-6-2	0 1	5-3-9-1-4-8	8-3-1-9-6-4

1 point for each sequence correct of 4 = _____

SAC / Concentration cont. Months in reverse order
Dec - Nov - Oct - Sept - Aug - Jul - Jun - May - Apr - Mar - Feb - Jan

1 point for months in reverse correctly (<30 sec) = _____

Total of SAC Concentration of 5 = _____

Modified BESS: This is calculated by adding 1 error point for each error during the three 20-sec tests. The maximum total # of errors for any single condition is 10. The higher the score, the worse is the player's balance.

Balance testing – types of errors
1. Hands lifted off iliac crest
2. Opening eyes
3. Step, stumble, or fall
4. Moving hip into > 30 degrees abduction
5. Lifting forefoot or heel
6. Remaining out of test position > 5 sec

Which foot tested (non-dominant foot) ☐ L ☐ R
Double leg stance (feet together) # errors ___
Single leg stance (non dominant foot) # errors ___
Tandem stance (non dominant foot at back) # errors ___
BALANCE SCORE: (summed # of errors) = _____

Signs and symptoms of concussion may be delayed, and therefore it may be prudent to remove an athlete from play, not leave them alone, and serially monitor them over a period of time. WHEN IN DOUBT, TAKE A "TIME OUT"

SCORING
All Physical Signs Score: (total # ☐ Yes) = ___ of 6
Maddock's score: = ___ of 5
All SAC scores: (summed orange boxes) = ___ of 30
Balance Score: (summed BESS Errors) = ___
Symptom Score: (# symptoms reported) = ___ of 24
ALL SCORES SHOULD BE COMPARED WITH BASELINE VALUES FOR THE INDIVIDUAL ATHLETE

The following symptom checklist should be completed by the athlete

How do you feel? The athlete should score themselves on the following symptoms, as applicable, based on how they feel at the time. (i.e. 0 = not present, 1 = mild, 3 = moderate, 6 = severe)

Symptom	Score	Symptom	Score
Headache / head pressure	0 1 2 3 4 5 6	Feeling slowed down	0 1 2 3 4 5 6
Nausea / vomiting	0 1 2 3 4 5 6	Sensitivity to noise	0 1 2 3 4 5 6
Neck pain	0 1 2 3 4 5 6	Sensitivity to light	0 1 2 3 4 5 6
Drowsiness	0 1 2 3 4 5 6	Visual problems/ blurred vision	0 1 2 3 4 5 6
Balance problems	0 1 2 3 4 5 6	Sleeping more than usual	0 1 2 3 4 5 6
Dizziness	0 1 2 3 4 5 6	Sleeping less than usual	0 1 2 3 4 5 6
Fatigue / low energy	0 1 2 3 4 5 6	Trouble falling asleep	0 1 2 3 4 5 6
Confusion	0 1 2 3 4 5 6	Sadness	0 1 2 3 4 5 6
"Don't feel right"	0 1 2 3 4 5 6	Nervous or anxious	0 1 2 3 4 5 6
Feeling "in a fog"	0 1 2 3 4 5 6	Feeling more emotional	0 1 2 3 4 5 6
Difficulty remembering	0 1 2 3 4 5 6	Irritability	0 1 2 3 4 5 6
Difficulty concentrating	0 1 2 3 4 5 6	Numbness or tingling	0 1 2 3 4 5 6

Do symptoms worsen with physical activity? Y N | Total # symptoms = _____ of 24
Do symptoms worsen with mental activity? Y N | Symptom Severity (max 24 X max 6) = _____ of 144

FIGURE 24-3 *(Continued)*

REFERENCES

1. Powell JW, Barber-Foss KD: Traumatic brain injury in high school athletes. *JAMA* 1999 Sep 8;282(10):958–963.

2. Gessel LM, Fields SK, Collins CL, et al: Concussions among United States high school and collegiate athletes. *J Athl Train* 2007;42(4):495–503.

3. Bompadre V, Jinguji TM, Yanez ND, et al: Washington State's Lystedt law in concussion documentation in Seattle public high schools. *J Athl Train* 2014;49(4):486–492.

4. Langlois JA, Rutland-Brown W, Wald MM: The epidemiology and impact of traumatic brain injury: a brief overview. *J Head Trauma Rehabil* 2006;21(5):375–378.

5. Lincoln AE, Caswell SV, Almquist JL, et al: Trends in concussion incidence in high school sports: a prospective 11-year study. *Am J Sports Med* 2011;39(5):958–963.

6. Guskiewicz KM, Waver NL, Padua DA, et al: Epidemiology of concussion in collegiate and high school football players. *Am J Sports Med* 2000;28(5):643–650.

7. Gilchrist J, Thomas KE, Wald M, Langlois J: Nonfatal traumatic brain injuries from sports and recreation activities: United States, 2001-2005. *MMWR Morbid Mortal Wkly Rep* 2007;56(29):733–737.

8. McCrory P, Meeuwise WH, Aubry M, et al: Consensus statement on concussion in sport: The 4th International Conference on Concussion in Sport, held in Zurich, November 2012. *Br J Sports Med* 2013;47(5):250–258.

9. Gonzales, P, Walker M: Imaging modalities in mild traumatic brain injury and sports concussion. *PM R* 2011;3(10 suppl 2):S413–S424.

10. Harmon KG, Drezner JA, Gammons M, et al: American Medical Society for Sports Medicine position statement: Concussion in sport. *Br J Sports Med* 2013;47(1):15–26.

11. Bigler E: Neuroimaging in sports concussion, in: The Oxford Handbook of Sports-Related Concussion. *Oxford Handbooks Online* 2014;Sep;1–17.

12. Meehan WP, d'Hemecourt P, Comstock D, et al: High school concussions in the 2008-2009 academic year: mechanism, symptoms, and management. *Am J Sports Med* 2010;38(12):2405–2409.

13. Meehan, WP, Mannix RC, Stracciolini A, et al: Symptom severity predicts prolonged recovery after sport-related concussion, but age and amnesia do not. *J Pediatr* 2013;163(3):721–725.

14. McCrea M, Guskiewicz K, Randolph C, et al: Incidence, clinical course, and predictors of prolonged recovery time following sport-related concussion in high school and college athletes. *J Int Neuropsychol Soc* 2013;19(1):22–33.

15. Kontos A, Covassin T, Elbin RJ, et al: Depression and neurocognitive performance after concussion among male and female high school and collegiate athletes. *Arch Phys Med Rehabil* 2012;93(10):1751–1756.

16. Perlis, M, Artiola, L, Giles D: Sleep complaints in chronic postconcussion syndrome. *Percept Mot Skills* 1997;84(2):595–599.

17. Coppel D: Use of neuropsychological evaluations. *Phys Med Rehabil Clin North Am* 2011;22(4):653–664, viii.

18. Bleiberg J, Cernich AN, Cameron K, et al: Duration of cognitive impairment after sports concussion. *Neurosurgery* 2004;54(5):1073–1078.

19. Makdissi, M, Darby D, Maruff, P, et al: Natural history of concussion in sport: Markers of severity and implications for management. *Am J Sports Med* 2010;38(3):464–471.

20. McCrea M: Standardized mental status testing of acute concussion. *Clin J Sport Med* 2001;11(3):176–181.

21. SCAT 3. *Br J Sports Med* 2013;47(5):259.

22. Child SCAT3. *Br J Sports Med* 2013;47(5):263.

23. Putukian M, Echemendia R, Dettwiler-Danspeckgruber A, et al: Prospective clinical assessment using Sideline Concussion Assessment Tool-2 testing in the evaluation of sport-related concussion in college athletes. *Clin J Sport Med* 2015;25(1):36–42.

24. National Football League: NFL Sideline Concussion Assessment Tool. Available at: http://nflps.org/wp-content/uploads/2012/08/NFL_SIDELINE_TOOL-POST_INJURY_Final.pdf. Accessed January 19, 2016.

25. Peterson CL, Ferrara MS, Mrazik M, et al: Evaluation of neuropsychological domain scores and postural stability following cerebral concussion in sports. *Clin J Sport Med* 2003;13(4):230–237.

26. Guskiewicz KM, Perrin DH, Gansneder BM: Effect of mild head injury on postural stability in athletes. *J Athl Train* 1996;31(4):300–306.

27. Register-Mihalik JK, Mihalik JP, Guskiewicz KM: Balance deficits after sports-related concussion in individuals reporting posttraumatic headache. *Neurosurgery* 2008;63(1):76–80.

28. McCrea M, Guskiewicz KM, Marshall SW, et al: Acute effects and recovery time following concussion in collegiate football players: The NCAA concussion study. *JAMA* 2003;290(19):2556–2563.

29. Guskiewicz KM, Riemann BL, Perrin DH, et al: Alternative approaches to the assessment of mild head injury in athletes. *Med Sci Sports Exerc* 1997;29(suppl 7):S213–S221.

30. Guskiewicz KM, Register-Mihalik JK: Postconcussive impairment differences across a multifaceted concussion assessment protocol. *PM R* 2011;3(10 suppl 2):S445–S451.

31. McCrea M, Barr W, Guskiewicz K: Standard regression-based methods for measuring recovery after sport-related concussion. *J Int Neuropsychol Soc* 2005;11(1):58–69.

32. Guskiewicz, K, McCrea, M, Marshall SW, et al: Cumulative effects associated with recurrent concussion in collegiate football players: The NCAA Concussion study. *JAMA* 2003;290(19):2549–2555.

33. Herring SA, Cantu RC, Guskiewicz KM, et al: Concussion (mild traumatic brain injury) and the team physician: A consensus statement—2011 update. *Med Sci Sports Exerc* 2011;43(12):2412–2422.

34. Hoffman J, Lucas S, Dikemen S, et al: Natural history of headache after traumatic brain injury. *J Neurotrauma* 2011;28(9):1719–1725.

35. Jinguji T, Bompardre V, Harmon K, et al: Sports concussion assessment Tool-2: Baseline values for high school athletes. *Br J Sports Med* 2012;46(5):365–370.

36. Herring SA, Kibler W, Putukian M, et al: Sideline preparedness for the team physician: A consensus statement—2012 update. *Med Sci Sports Exerc* 2012;44(12):2442–2445.

37. Putukian M, Raftery M, Guskiewicz K, et al: Onfield assessment of concussion in the adult athlete. *Br J Sports Med* 2013;47(5):285–288.

38. Makdissi M, Davis G, Jordan B, et al: Revisiting the modifiers: how should the evaluation and management of acute concussions differ in specific groups? *Br J Sports Med* 2013;47(5):314–320.

39. Rivara FP, Schiff MA, Chrisman SP, et al: The effect of coach education on reporting of concussions among high school athletes after passage of a concussion law. *Am J Sports Med* 2014;42(5):1197–203.

40. Chrisman SP, Quitiquit C, Rivara FP: Qualitative study of barriers to concussive symptom reporting in high school athletics. *J Adolesc Health* 2013;52(3):330–335.e3.

41. McCrea M, Hammeke T, Olsen G, et al: Unreported concussion in high school football players: implications for prevention. *Clin J Sport Med* 2004;14(1):13–17.

42. Cantu RC: Recurrent athletic head injury: risks and when to retire. *Clin Sports Med* 2003;22(3):593–603, x.

25 Determining Short-Term Prognosis and Return to Play

Margot Putukian, MD, MSPH • Siatta B. Dunbar, DO, CAQSM

INTRODUCTION

Concussion has been characterized by the 4th International Conference on Concussion in Sport (CIS) as a "subset of traumatic brain injury" and is defined as "a complex pathophysiological process affecting the brain, induced by biomechanics forces."[1] The Centers for Disease Control and Prevention, through the National Electronic Injury Surveillance System—All Injury Program (NEISS-AIP), during the period of 2001 to 2009, estimated that 173,285 persons younger than 19 years old were treated for nonfatal traumatic brain injury (TBI).[2] Overall there has been an increase in TBI-related emergency department (ED) visits from 153,375 in 2001 to 248,418 in 2009.[2] Concussion and TBI represent a significant injury for athletes at all levels, including youth, high school, college, and professional. The diagnosis of a concussion can be challenging and remains a clinical diagnosis based on a constellation of subjective and objective data. After a concussion, there are typically alterations in function that cover several domains, including athlete-reported symptoms; physical signs; and behavioral, postural, and cognitive changes. Risk factors for concussion as well as risk factors that may prolong recovery, often termed "modifiers," have been reviewed,[3–8] and return to play (RTP) protocols after concussion have been published,[1,8–12] though much is still unknown regarding the natural history of concussion. This chapter focuses on the current understanding of RTP decision making and short-term prognosis after concussion.

Dr. Putukian or an immediate family member serves as a board member, owner, officer, or committee member of the Journal of Athletic Training. *Neither Dr. Dunbar nor any immediate family member has received anything of value from or has stock or stock options held in a commercial company or institution related directly or indirectly to the subject of this article.*

CHRONOLOGY OF CARE

The diagnosis of *concussion* and *sideline management* are discussed in the chapter by Herring et al. After the diagnosis of a concussion is made, there is clear consensus that an athlete should not return to activity or play the same day, and this holds true at all levels of competition, including youth, college, and professional sports.[1,8,13,14] Each concussion should be treated individually, taking into account the characteristics of the athlete (e.g., age, sport, position, gender, specific modifying variables), as well as his or her injury and prior history.[1,6,8] There is likely a spectrum of concussive injury that exists, from mild to more severe, and at this point, it remains unclear as to what factors definitively predict recovery.

ROLE OF IMAGING

The role of imaging initially and in the first several weeks after concussion is frequently considered. Current research and guidelines do not support obtaining imaging when an athlete is diagnosed with concussion without any other indication of potential serious brain injury.[1,6,8,10] However, if at initial presentation the history or clinical examination findings are concerning for cervical spine, intracranial bleeding, or skull fracture, then advanced imaging—in most cases, a CT scan—should be obtained emergently given the ability to demonstrate both bony injury as well as bleeding.[1]

Several studies have compared MRI with CT findings after minor head injury.[15–18] Abdul Rahman and coworkers evaluated 152 patients with blunt head trauma and Glasgow Coma Scale (GCS) scores of 13 to 15 and found that the most common symptoms were headache (61%) followed by loss of consciousness (LOC) (45%), vomiting (39%), amnesia (29%), and convulsions (4%).[18] Although this patient setting may include more severe brain injury, convulsions were the most predictive of positive CT finding (80%), and history of

LOC was least predictive (29%). The presence of two or more clinical findings increased the likelihood of abnormality.[18] In another study, abnormal MRI findings were noted in 10% of patients with mild head injury who had normal CT results, and abnormalities on imaging were most common in patients with LOC, symptoms longer than 2 weeks, those with skull fracture, and those with multiple associated injuries.[17]

Lyttle et al[19] evaluated three pediatric clinical decision rules—CATCH (Canadian Assessment of Tomography for Childhood Head Injury), CHALICE (Children's Head Injury Algorithm for the Prediction of Important Clinical Events Rule), and PECARN (Pediatric Emergency Care Applied Research Network)—to determine what clinical findings warrant imaging in the setting of head trauma. They concluded that a GCS score less than 15 two hours after the injury, worsening headache, irritability on examination, LOC for more than 5 minutes, vomiting more than three times, and seizure activity were the findings in which imaging should be obtained. When an athlete with suspected cervical spine or more serious brain injury is transported for more advanced care, it is important to consider a facility with both emergent imaging as well as specialty physician (e.g., onsite spine surgeons and neurosurgeons) capabilities.

In less acute settings (e.g., after 2–3 weeks), with persistent or worsening symptoms, an MRI should be considered, given this modality's predilection for demonstrating subtle abnormalities and the avoidance of radiation exposure.[20] The decision making regarding when MRI is indicated should be individualized. If there are abnormal findings on MRI, depending on if they are causative versus incidental, referral to additional members of the healthcare team, such as neurologists or neurosurgeons, should be considered.

● INITIAL ASSESSMENT OF CONCUSSION

The assessment often includes documenting symptoms, cognitive function, and balance. It also involves using several standardized tools, such as the Sideline Concussion Assessment Tool 3 (SCAT 3),[21] which has been shown to be both sensitive and specific to concussion.[22] When baseline assessments are available and compared with postinjury assessments, a drop in score of 3.5 points on the SCAT 2 demonstrated a sensitivity and specificity of the SCAT 2 of 96% and 81%, respectively. When a baseline assessment is not available, sensitivity and specificity were 91% and 83%, respectively, when a cutoff value is used.[22] The utility of a sideline assessment in

predicting severity is unknown at this time. As important as the sideline assessment, the in-office evaluation should include a thorough history of the concussion, including the mechanism of injury, immediate treatment, the athlete's sport and position, and any symptoms immediately thereafter and progression or regression since onset. The presence of amnesia or LOC should be explored and documented.

Additionally, a complete personal and family medical, social, and academic history should be obtained. The clinician should also have a clear understanding of all current and upcoming academic demands. An evaluation for the presence of any concussion risk factors or modifiers[3] should occur, and a standardized symptom checklist should be completed. A complete neurologic examination, including ocular motor screening, cognitive assessment, and balance and postural examination, should be performed. A symptom checklist (either Post Concussion Symptom Scale [PCSS] or SCAT 3) that can be compared with the sideline assessment, and ideally with a baseline, preinjury assessment, is useful to evaluate for improving or worsening symptoms across domains: cognitive-sensory (sensitivity to light, difficulty concentration), sleep arousal (drowsiness, sleeping more than usual), vestibular-somatic (headache, dizziness), and affective (sadness, nervousness).[23] The role of symptoms in diagnosis of concussion is reviewed elsewhere.[24,25]

The cognitive assessment is important, and the SAC,[26] which is a component of the SCAT 3, can be used in the office. Consideration should be given for more sophisticated postinjury computerized or paper-pencil neuropsychological (NP) testing. These tests are more comprehensive measures of brain behavior relationship that assess cognitive function, and they can provide an additional value to the brief cognitive tests performed on the sideline or at baseline. In addition, compared with similar tests performed at baseline, they can provide additional information that can be used to assess the severity of injury as well as recovery from injury.[27,28] The evidence for or against NP testing and the timing is being addressed by Melissa et al in Chapter 26.

During the initial in-office visit after the diagnosis of a concussion, a balance and postural examination should be conducted. This may vary from the on-field assessment, as demonstrated by Herring et al in Chapter 24. The in-office postural assessment may be completed in a variety of manners, including using the Balance Error Scoring System (BESS) or Biosway.[29,30] The BESS includes postural testing, with eyes closed, for 20 seconds on a hard surface and foam, in three different stance positions.

A trained observer records errors, inclusive but not limited to, opening eyes, removing hands from hips, and stumbling or swaying from midline. BESS testing has been shown to have varying inter- and intrarater reliability (0.57–0.85 and 0.60–0.92, respectively),[30] and having the same individual administer serial and repeated testing is useful. Additionally, there is a "learning effect"[31] with multiple administrations of BESS testing. An alternative is to assess postural sway using a Clinical Test for Sensory Interaction and Balance (CTSIB) combined with a force platform as integrated in the Biosway system. Additional research is needed to determine if the CTSIB combined with the BESS protocol is a reliable way to assess postural sway and if it addresses the learning effect of BESS testing alone. The utility of using a multimodal approach of symptoms, cognitive function, and balance testing in assessing and tracking recovery in concussion has been demonstrated using meta-analysis.[32,33]

The final examination that should be considered in the in-office evaluation is a vestibular-ocular motor screen (VOMS) as detailed by Mucha et al.[34] Concussion may lead to impairment in postural control as well as ocular impairments, with up to 30% of concussed individuals reporting visual problems, including "blurry vision, diplopia, difficulty reading, dizziness, headache, ocular pain and poor visual concentration, all within the first week following a concussion."[34] Screening includes five domains, with near-point convergence of 5 cm or greater increasing the diagnosis of concussion by 34%.[34] Beyond the initial screening and diagnosis, Heitger et al[35] explored the presence of impaired ocular function in postconcussion syndrome (PCS). Comparing 36 individuals with postconcussion syndrome at 140 days postinjury with matched control participants showed that the postconcussion syndrome group scored worse on saccades and smooth pursuits. This research is very encouraging and begins to explore the role of serial ocular screening in tracking recovery from concussion. At the present time, it is yet unknown how important ocular screening is in the RTP decision; therefore, in the interim, reliance on more validated modalities is recommended.

The diagnosis of a concussion is a multifaceted clinical decision requiring evaluation of mechanism, presence of symptoms and severity, presence of risk factors or modifiers and any resultant cognitive, and postural impairment. The same in-depth clinical thinking should occur during follow-up examinations, which should occur serially and at weekly intervals or time frames that are flexible, including when the athlete is back to his or her baseline level of symptoms; when the athlete is able to tolerate cardiovascular activities without difficulties; and when the athlete has tolerated noncontact, sport-specific activities and is ready to participate in contact play. In general, when an athlete reports being back to her or his baseline level of symptoms; when results of neurologic examination, including NP testing and postural examinations, have returned to baseline; and when the athlete is functioning at her or his baseline with academics, then she or he can be cleared to begin their RTP protocol. An exception to this, as discussed later, cardiovascular exercise may be considered a component of treatment, prior to resolution of symptoms and separate from the RTP protocol.

● RETURN TO PLAY

The RTP decision after concussion is ideally a gradual, stepwise progression that includes an incremental increase in both the level of exertion and the risk for contact. Each step typically occurs over 24 hours, while a PCSS is documented before and after activity.[9] Although several position statements have supported this concept,[1,6–8,10–12] it is worth noting that there is little evidence-based data to support this approach. Nonetheless, all of the RTP guidelines agree with the CIS group statements[1,9] that recommends a graduated RTP protocol beginning with light aerobic activity of sufficient intensity to maintain a heart rate below 70% of maximum. If the athlete tolerates this activity, the following day he or she is progressed to sport-specific exercises and then noncontact drills. If at any point the athlete develops symptoms of any severity level, she or he is returned to the previous level of exertion that caused no symptoms. Before returning to full contact sport, the athlete should fell like they are back to feeling normal, and they should be considered back to their baseline level of function in terms of their cognitive and balance function. If baseline tests of cognitive or postural function are performed, the postinjury tests should be compared with the baseline tests. Overall, the RTP progression is individualized to take into account the severity of injury (e.g., the nature, burden, and duration of symptoms) as well as other "modifiers" such as the concussion history or a history of attention deficit hyperactivity disorder (ADHD) or other learning disabilities, history of depression or anxiety, or history of migraine headaches.[1,8] As detailed later, risk factors and modifiers can affect an athlete's baseline scores, progression, and recovery from a concussion. Therefore, a comprehensive treatment plan, sometimes in concert with an athlete's parents, will need to be developed, including focused rehabilitation if necessary. For example, if the athlete has evidence of persistent ocular findings or irregularities as determined by the VOMS,[34] he or she may benefit from specialized vestibulo-ocular rehabilitation. Generally, concussive symptoms resolve within 7 to 10 days[5,29,36–38]; however, in some cases, symptoms can persist for weeks or months, known as postconcussion syndrome. Predictors for the development of postconcussion syndrome in young athletes include a prior history of concussion, premorbid mood disorder, and other psychiatric illness or significant life stressors, along with a family history of mood disorders, other psychiatric illness, and migraine.[39] For the management of postconcussion syndrome, it is helpful and recommended to institute a multidisciplinary treatment program, including neuropsychology, rehabilitation, psychology and psychiatry, and academic support. Chapter 27 provides a very detailed description and management strategy for athletes with postconcussion syndrome.

RISK FACTORS AND MODIFIERS: INCIDENCE OF CONCUSSION

There may be certain risk factors that increase the likelihood or incidence of concussion, including the sport played, prior history of concussion, and gender. According to the Institute of Medicine Brief,[40] at the high school and collegiate levels, male athletes have the highest incidence of concussion when participating in football, ice hockey, lacrosse, wrestling, and soccer. For female athletes, the sports with the highest incidence are soccer, lacrosse, basketball, and ice hockey. Additionally, data suggest that a history of concussion increases the risk for future concussions compared with individuals who have not had a prior concussion.[4,5] Guskiewicz et al[5] showed that those with a history of at least three concussions had a threefold greater chance of sustaining another concussion. In the National Collegiate Athletic Association (NCAA) study, 90% of athletes who sustained a second concussion did so within 10 days of a prior concussion diagnosis, suggesting that many RTP decisions might have been premature.[5]

Finally, on preliminary analysis, gender appears to increase the risk for reported incidence of concussion in sports with the same rules (e.g., soccer and basketball).[41,42] Speculated explanations for the increased incidence of concussion in female athletes include the possibility of selection bias, with women more likely to report concussion symptoms; effects of sex hormones, most notably progesterone[43,44]; and the biomechanical differences that exist between the genders.[45–49]

RISK FACTORS AND MODIFIERS: RATE OF RECOVERY

The "modifiers" that may prolong recovery include number of symptoms reported after concussion; history of prior concussion(s); female gender; known history of depression; attention deficit disorder, ADHD, or migraines; or an athlete younger than 18 years old.[3,50,51] Makdissi et al[51] showed a correlation between the number of symptoms after sustaining a concussion and the rate of recovery. Guskiewicz et al[5] showed in their cohort of college football players that those with three or more concussions had a prolonged recovery (>7 days) compared with athletes with one previous concussion. Discerning other modifiers, especially gender, mental health issues, headache disorder, and ADHD, is more challenging, especially when taking into account differences in baseline measures, which are not always available.

According to the World Health Organization,[52] "major depression carries the heaviest burden of disability" that "affects 350 million people . . . and is 50% higher in females than males." Given this prevalence, it is important to know if an athlete has premorbid symptoms of depression. This can be determined during the athlete's baseline preseason physical examination and evaluation. Covassin et al researched how depression may affect baseline NP testing and PCSS. Immediate post concussion assessment and cognitive testing (ImPACT), PCSS, and the Beck Depression Inventory were completed by a total of 1616 collegiate and high school athletes.[53] Those with severe depression "scored worse on visual memory" and endorsed symptoms in the "somatic (headache, dizziness), cognitive (memory problems, fogginess), emotional (anxiety, depression) and sleep (more/less sleep, trouble sleeping) domains of the PCSS." Female athletes overall had more symptoms in the "cognitive, emotional and sleep clusters," but there was no correlation to the presence of depression. A study completed by Putukian et al[22] showed a statistically significant correlation between the presence of more symptoms and of greater severity on SCAT 2 and higher patient health questionnaire-9 (PHQ-9) and generalized anxiety disorder-7 (GAD-7) scores.

Similarly, a prospective study completed by Yang et al[54] evaluated baseline and postconcussion data from male and female college athletes. Results showed that preexisting depression, as defined by the Center of Epidemiological Studies Depression (CESD) scale, was the "strongest predictor of postconcussion depression," and these athletes were almost five times more likely to develop symptoms postinjury. Interestingly, these same athletes were almost 3.5 times more likely to develop postanxiety symptoms, as defined by the State-Trait Anxiety Inventory. The same did not hold true for preexisting anxiety, which conferred no increased risk for developing either depression or anxiety symptoms after concussion.

The importance of baseline measures is also demonstrated when evaluating for the presence of symptoms overall, especially given the nonspecific nature of several symptoms included in the PCSS. Covassin et al[55] evaluated 1209 collegiate athletes with baseline computerized NP testing and PCSS. A total of 68% of male participants and 76% of female participants endorsed at least one symptom. Additionally, 30–50% of the 1209 athletes reported mild symptoms (rated 1 or 2 on a symptom score) of fatigue, sleep difficulty, drowsiness, and difficulty concentrating. In terms of NP tests, female participants performed better on verbal memory and male participants better on visual memory. There were no significant differences in reaction time and processing speed. These data demonstrate the importance of an individualized approach to concussion management and the need to compare results of postconcussion NP testing and PCSS with baseline values.

There have also been reported gender differences in the both NP tests and PCSS after concussion.[55-58] Broshek et al[56] showed that male and female athletes had a similar number of reported symptoms, 5.07 and 6.66, respectively, but female athletes self-reported "concentration problems, fatigue, lightheadedness and seeing flyspecks" compared with male athletes. The most reported symptom postinjury was headache at 82% for male athletes and 86% for female athletes. Covassin et al[57] studied 79 concussed collegiate athletes and showed that male athletes reported vomiting and sadness more than female athletes, both in frequency and intensity. When evaluating gender differences in similar sports, as was done by Colvin et al,[42] female athletes endorsed more symptoms. The study evaluated 234 soccer players (93 male and 141 female) ranging from 8 to 24 years old and found that female athletes endorsed significantly higher total PCSS, 25.6 compared with 14.0 reported by male athletes.

As related to postconcussion NP testing, Broshek et al found that female athletes had cognitive decline 1.7 times more frequently than male athletes and had more decline in reaction time compared with baseline.[56] In an attempt to quantify the degree and domains of greatest cognitive impairment, Covassin et al[57] demonstrated that female athletes had a lower score in only visual memory. Therefore, in relation to sport-related concussion and when comparing gender across similar sports, there does appear to be a difference with baseline and postconcussion PCSS and NP testing. However, there does not appear to be a predilection for certain postconcussion symptom at baseline and postinjury, based purely on gender. These data again underscore the importance of an individualized approach to managing concussive injury and including baseline measures when possible.

Lange et al[59] evaluated a cohort of patients who had sustained mTBI, not limited to sport-related concussion, to assess depression and the development of postconcussion symptoms. Four distinct groups were established: mTBI depressed, mTBI no depression, depressed outpatient, and healthy. A statistically significant percentage of the mTBI patients with depression, as determined by the British Columbia Major Depression Inventory, were found to be more symptomatic and could be diagnosed with "postconcussion disorder" per ICD-10 (International Classification of Diseases 10) symptom criteria. Results were that 87% of the mTBI with depression group reported 10 or more symptoms as compared with 24.3% of the patients who sustained mTBI without a diagnosis of depression. Additionally, the depressed mTBI group met diagnostic criteria at 95.7% compared with 48.6% for the nondepressed mTBI patients.

Given that depression is common in the general population, a baseline screen should be included for all athletes, inclusive of family history of mood or other psychiatric disorders.[39] Additionally, the overlap between depressive symptoms (trouble sleeping, difficulty concentrating, fatigue or low energy, more emotional, sadness) and concussion makes management of concussed athletes with preexisting mental health issues more challenging. Although we believe that Lange et al's[59] research can be extrapolated to sports-related concussion, it is not conclusive. To that end, more research about preexisting depression and the associated recovery pattern after sports-related concussion is warranted.

In regards to ADD and ADHD, when the diagnosis is present before sustaining a concussion, Zuckerman et al[60] have demonstrated that NP testing is adversely impacted. A total of 6636 youth athletes, ages 14 to 19 years, completed ImPACT testing at baseline, of which 262 athletes had a self-reported diagnosis of ADHD. A control group was established, which was matched by age, years of education, and number of prior concussions, and the results demonstrated that the ADHD group's NP scores across all six domains were significant lower. Similarly, Elbin et al[61] evaluated 2377 athletes, high school and college age, who had completed ImPACT over a 2-year period. The total was divided into four groups based on their self-reported diagnosis of learning disability (LD), ADHD, LD and ADHD, and control. The results show that athletes with a self-reported diagnosis scored significantly lower on all domains of ImPACT and that the ADHD group had the highest mean symptom score of 4.5. These data support the concept of baseline testing for athletes so their individual postinjury evaluations can be compared with their preinjury baseline tests instead of using group-based norms, which has been presented as an alternative.[62]

Although preexisting ADHD has been shown to effect baseline NP testing, it is unclear whether it leads to prolonged recovery after sustaining a concussion. Mautner et al[63] investigated this by conducting a retrospective study that included 70 high school athletes who sustained a concussion and had a self-reported diagnosis of ADHD. The results demonstrated a longer recovery, although not statistically significant in the ADHD group at 16.5 days versus 13.5 days. Given the limited power, additional research is needed before concluding that a history of ADHD is a modifier that leads to prolonged recovery. However, at minimum, one can clearly see how a diagnosis of ADHD may complicate the management of a concussed athlete because of the overlap of symptoms such as difficulty concentrating, difficulty remembering, and trouble falling asleep. Knowing baseline symptom scores can help to extrapolate if postinjury scores are the same or worsening and if specialized or focused rehabilitation would be of benefit.

Although headaches are one of the most reported symptoms after concussion,[51] migraine headaches represent a different entity and carry different risks and possible treatment and management strategy. A retrospective study completed by Morgan et al[39] sought to evaluate risk factors for developing postconcussive syndrome, which was described as symptoms being present longer than 3 months postinjury. The study included 40 patients, ages 9 to 18 years old, and demonstrated a statistically significant correlation between family, not personal history, of migraines and development of postconcussive symptoms. This study highlights the importance of not only an athlete's personal history but also her or his family history, especially for youth athletes. Studies on postconcussive symptoms completed in the adult population are generally done after a nonsport injury, with data derived from emergency department charts after an individual sustains an mTBI. By limiting the results to those with postconcussive symptoms lasting longer than 3 months,[64-66] there is no statistically significant correlation with migraines and development of postconcussive symptoms. There were correlations with early positive VOMS, individuals having a negative perception about their injury, female sex, and

LOC. Therefore, it appears that preexisting migraines in families may pose a risk for youth athletes, but they may be less important or nonexistent as a risk factor for adults.

There has been recent speculation that the development of prolonged symptoms after concussion is more common in female athletes.[58,67,68] A statistically significant correlation exists between postconcussion syndrome, defined as the presence of symptoms for 12 to 18 months postinjury, and female gender with a mean age of 35.9 years.[67] This gender difference also exists in the adolescent population, age 11 to 18 years, where 41.2% of girls and young women took more than 2 months to return to baseline.[68] Although the research supports a correlation between female gender and concussion incidence, severity, and later development of postconcussion syndrome, there is not a clear consensus of why this relationship exists. As stated earlier, one possibility is the protective effect of sex hormones; the other possibility is biomechanical differences.

There has been speculation that the difference in gender for incidence as well as recovery from concussion may be explained by differences in the strength or mass of the head–neck segment in female athletes compared with their male counterparts.[45-47,49] Eckner et al[47] showed when the force is known, a higher head–neck mass with subsequent muscle activation led to decreased linear and angular velocity. Schmidt et al[49] demonstrated that neck stiffness rather than neck strength and size was more protective. Collins et al[48] showed that across both genders and specifically with soccer, the neck strength between athletes with a history of concussion versus those without was not statistically significant. More research is needed to determine how to mitigate concussion risk along with any avenues for possible interventions to protect athletes in their sports participation.

Youth athletes may take longer to recover from concussion than older athletes.[1-3,10] In a prospective study of 670 children who presented to the ED with mTBI, 13.7% still had symptoms longer than 3 months after their injury with an overall prevalence of postconcussion syndrome at 14% to 29%.[69,70] Babcock et al[71] also concluded that adolescent age (11–18 years old), female gender, and the presence of a headache at presentation to the ED was significant for later postconcussion syndrome. A recent meta-analysis demonstrated that although cognitive recovery in high school compared with college athletes was similar at 5 versus 7 days postinjury and that the high school athletes had self-reported symptoms for 15 days compared with 6 days for college athletes.[33] Given that youth athletes may take longer to recover and may be more vulnerable to developing postconcussion syndrome, it is recommended that youth athletes should be treated with caution.

Last, the presence of certain symptoms on the PCSS has been shown to lead to a risk of prolonged recovery. According to Makdissi et al,[3] if the athlete has four or more symptoms at the time of diagnosis, they are more likely to have a prolonged recovery. Other specific symptoms that will lead to a longer recovery time, according to Makdissi et al,[51] include having a headache for longer than 60 hours or having symptoms in the cognitive domain of the PCSS, such as fatigue or fogginess.

As discussed earlier, the RTP progression typically starts with a low-intensity cardiovascular challenge. More recent data suggest that this can be initiated after the acute period after injury has passed and before complete resolution of symptoms.[1] There has not been any advantage to having a "symptom-free interval,"[72] and additional studies have emphasized the importance of exercise in recovery. Another recent study demonstrated no benefit

for "strict rest" after a concussion, which was defined as no activity for 5 days, compared with rest for 1 to 2 days before beginning a gradual return to activity.[73] Return to exercise can be extremely supportive for any injured athlete and potentially prevent psychological distress.[74] In addition, the resumption of normal academics can occur after the first few days, and the recommendation of the American Academy of Pediatrics is that priority should be given to normal return of academics before RTP to sports.[75] They recommend a multidisciplinary team to facilitate "return to learn" and distinguish making academic adjustments and academic accommodations.[75] The NCAA has similarly encouraged a return to academics as a component of the return to sports activity after concussion.[11]

For each individual concussion, the RTP progression should be modified based on the severity of injury,

TABLE 25-1   Return to play algorithm

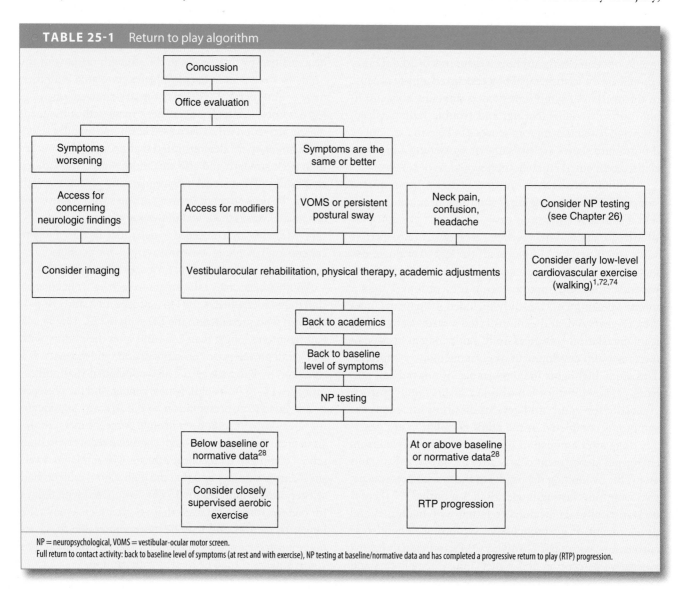

NP = neuropsychological, VOMS = vestibular-ocular motor screen.
Full return to contact activity: back to baseline level of symptoms (at rest and with exercise), NP testing at baseline/normative data and has completed a progressive return to play (RTP) progression.

which is determined by the nature, burden, and duration of symptoms, as well as by other risk factors or modifiers. After the acute injury, athletes may be allowed back into academic and low-level exercise within a few days as long as this does not make them significantly worse. If there is a significant burden or severity of symptoms, it may be prudent to wait for a longer period. Using additional objective measures of cognitive function, postural stability, and vestibular-ocular function, the athlete can be followed and allowed back into more sport-specific and finally contact activities. There may be variations in terms of the rate of progression depending on individual factors; an athlete with very minimal symptom burden and duration without any prior history of injury or other modifiers can likely be returned much more quickly than an athlete

with several weeks of symptoms and prior concussion, especially if recent. These are the issues that must be considered in the "art" of RTP decision making.

The risk factors for concussion that may prolong recovery are previous history of concussion, female gender, youth athletes, preexisting depression in the athlete, migraines, and history of mental health and migraines in family members. It is inconclusive as to whether a history of ADHD will lead to a prolonged recovery. There are few criteria that predictably determine a prolonged recovery. Ongoing research is needed to validate and confirm risk factors and modifiers before using any to make significant changes in management. Each athlete is unique, each concussion for an individual is also unique, and their treatment and return to academics and sports should be individualized (**Table 25-1**).

REFERENCES

1. McCrory P, Meeuwisse WH, Aubry M, et al: Consensus statement on concussion in sport: The 4th International Conference on Concussion in Sport held in Zurich, November 2012. *Br J Sports Med* 2013;47(5):250–258.

2. Centers for Disease Control and Prevention: Nonfatal traumatic brain injuries related to sports and recreation activities among persons aged <19 years—United States, 2001–2009. *MMWR Morb Mortal Wkly Rep* 2011;60(39):1337–1342.

3. Makdissi M, Davis G, Jordan B, Patricios J, Purcell L, Putukian M: Revisiting the modifiers: How should the evaluation and management of acute concussions differ in specific groups? *Br J Sports Med* 2013;47:314–320.

4. Gerberich SG, Priest JD, Boen JR, et al: Concussion incidences and severity in secondary school varsity football players. *Am J Public Health* 1983;73:1370–1375.

5. Guskiewicz KM, McCrea M, Marshall S, et al: Cumulative effects associated with recurrent concussion in collegiate football players: The NCAA Concussion Study. *JAMA* 2003;290:2549–2555.

6. Harmon KG, Drezner JA, Gammons M, et al: American Medical Society for Sports Medicine position statement: Concussion in sport. *Br J Sports Med* 2013;47:15–26.

7. Giza CC, Kutcher JS, Ashwal S, et al: Summary of evidence-based guideline update: Evaluation and management of concussion in sports. *Neurology* 2013;80:2250–2257.

8. Herring SA, Cantu RC, Guskiewicz KM, et al: Concussion (mild traumatic brain injury) and the team physician: a consensus statement—2011 update. *Med Sci Sports Exerc* 2011;43(12):2412–2422.

9. Aubry M, Cantu R, Dvorak J, et al: Summary and agreement statement of the first International Conference on Concussion in Sport, Vienna 2001. *Br J Sports Med* 2002;36(6–7):6–10.

10. Broglio SP, Cantu RC, Gioia GA, et al; National Athletic Trainer's Association: National Athletic Trainer's Association position statement: Management of sport concussion. *J Athl Train* 2014;49(2):245–265.

11. National Collegiate Athletics Association: *Concussion Guidelines; Diagnosis & Management of Sport-Related Concussion.* Available at: http://www.ncaa.org/health-and-safety/concussion-guidelines. Accessed June 5, 2015.

12. National Football League: *Head Neck & Spine Committee; Return to Play Policy after Concussion.* Available at: http://www.nflhealthplaybook.com/article/2014-nfl-return-to-play-protocol?ref=0ap3000000381612. Accessed August 20, 2015.

13. NFL.com: *League Announces Stricter Concussion Guidelines.* Available at: http://blogs.nfl.com/2009/12/02/league-announces-stricter-concussion-guidelines. Accessed August 20, 2015.

14. Baugh CM, Kroshus E, Daneshvar DH, Filali NA, Hiscox MJ, Glantz LH: Concussion management in united states college sports. *Am J Sports Med* 2015;43(1):47–56.

15. Smits M, Dippel DW, de Haan GG, et al: External validation of the Canadian CT Head Rule and the New Orleans Criteria for CT scanning in patients with minor head injury. *JAMA* 2005;294:1519–1525.

16. Smits M, Dippel DW, Steyerberg EW, et al: Predicting intracranial traumatic findings on computed tomography in patients with minor head injury: The CHIP prediction rule. *Ann Intern Med* 2007;146:397–405.

17. Kim DS, Kong MH, Jang SY, et al: The usefulness of brain magnetic resonance imaging with mild head injury and the negative findings of brain computed tomography. *J Korean Neurosurg Soc* 2013;54(2):100–106.

18. Abdul Rahman YS, Al Den AS, Mauli KI: Prospective study of validity of neurologic signs in predicting positive cranial computed tomography following minor head trauma. *Prehosp Disaster Med* 2010;25(1):59–62.

19. Lyttle MD, Crowe L, Oakley E, Dunning J, Babl FE: Comparing CATCH, CHALICE and PECARN clinical decision rules for pediatric head injuries. *Emerg Med J* 2012;29:785–794.

20. Foerster BR, Petrou M, Lin D, et al: Neuroimaging evaluation of non-accidental head trauma with correlation to clinical outcomes: A review of 57 cases. *J Pediatr* 2009; 154(4):573–577.

21. SCAT-3. *Br J Sports Med* 2013;47:259.

22. Putukian M, Echemendia R, Dettwiler-Danspeckgruber A, et al: Prospective clinical assessment using Sideline Concussion Assessment Tool-2 (SCAT-2) Testing in the evaluation of sport related concussion in college athletes. *Clin J Sports Med* 2015;25(1):36–42.

23. Kontos AP, Covassin T, Elbin RJ, Parker T: Depression and neurocognitive performance after concussion among male and female high school and collegiate athletes. *Arch Phys Med Rehabil* 2012;93:1751–1756.

24. Putukian M: The acute symptoms of sport-related concussion: Diagnosis and the on-field management. *Clin Sports Med* 2011;30:49–61.

25. Putukian M, Raftery M, Guskiewicz K, et al: On field assessment of concussion in the adult athlete. *Br J Sports Med* 2013;47:285–288.

26. McCrea M: Standardized mental status testing on the sideline after sport-related concussion. *J Athl Train* 2001; 36(3):274–279.

27. Putukian M: Neuropsychological testing as it relates to recovery from sports-related concussion. *PM R* 2011;3: S425–432.

28. Echemendia RJ, Iverson GL, McCrea M, et al: Advances in neuropsychological assessment of sport-related concussion. *Br J Sports Med* 2013;47:294–298.

29. Guskiewicz KM, Ross SE, Marshall SW: Postural stability and neuropsychological deficits after concussion in collegiate athletes. *J Athl Train* 2001;36:263–273.

30. Bell DR, Guskiewicz KM, Clark MA, Padua DA: Systematic review of the balance error scoring system. *Sports Health* 2011;3(3):287–295.

31. Ruhe A, Fejer R, Gänsslen A, Klein W: Assessing postural stability in the concussed athlete: What to do, what to expect, and when. *Sports Health* 2014;6(6):427–433.

32. Broglio SP, Puetz TW: The effect of sport concussion on neurocognitive function, self report symptoms and postural control: A meta-analysis. *Sports Med* 2008;38(1): 53–67.

33. Williams RM, Puetz TW, Giza C, Broglio SP: Concussion recovery time among high school and collegiate athletes: A systematic review and meta-analysis. *Sports Med* 2015;45(6):893–903.

34. Mucha, A, Collins MW, Elbin RJ, et al: A Brief Vestibular/Ocular Motor Screening (VOMS) assessment to evaluate concussions: Preliminary findings. *Am J Sports Med* 2014;42(20):2479–2486.

35. Heitger MH, Jones RD, Macleod AD, Snell DL, Frampton CM, Anderson TJ: Impaired eye movements in post-concussion syndrome indicate suboptimal brain function beyond the influence of depression, malingering or intellectual ability. *Brain* 2009;132:2850–2870.

36. McCrory P, Johnston K, Meeuwisse W, et al: Summary and agreement statement of the 2nd International Conference on Concussion in Sport, Prague 2004. *Br J Sports Med* 2005;39:196–204.

37. McCrea M, Guskiewicz KM, Marshall SW, et al: Acute effects and recovery time following concussion in collegiate football players; the NCAA Concussion Study. *JAMA* 2003;290:2556–2563.

38. Iverson GL, Brooks BL, Collins MW, et al: Tracking neuropsychological recovery following concussion in sport. *Brain Inj* 2006;20:245–252.

39. Morgan CD, Zuckerman SL, Lee YM, King L, Beaird S, Sills AK, Solomon GS: Predictors of postconcussion syndrome after sports-related concussion in young athletes: A matched case-control study. *J Neurosurg Pediatric* 2015;15:589–598.

40. The Institute of Medicine of the National Academies: Sports-Related Concussion in Youth. In Graham R, Rivara F, Ford M, Spicer C (eds). *Improving the Science, Changing the Culture* 2013.

41. Dick RW: Is there a gender difference in concussion incidence and outcomes? *Br J Sports Med* 2009;43(suppl I):i460–i50.

42. Colvin AC, Mullen J, Lovell MR, West RV, Collins MW, Groh M, et al: The role of concussion history and gender in recovery from soccer-related concussion. *Am J Sports Med* 2009;37(9):1699–1704.

43. Djebailia M, Guo Q, Pettus EH, Hoffman SW, Stein DG: The neurosteroids progesterone and allopregnanolone reduce cell death, gliosis, and functional deficits after traumatic brain injury in rats. *J Neurotrauma* 2005;22(1):106–118.

44. Wunderle K, Hoeger KM, Wasserman E, Bazarian JJ: Menstrual phase as predictor of outcome after mild traumatic brain injury in women. *J Head Trauma Rehabil* 2014;29(5):E1–E8.

45. Tierney RT, Sitler MR, Swanik CB, Swanik KA, Higgins M, Torg J: Gender differences in head-neck segment dynamic stabilization during head acceleration. *Med Sci Sports Exerc* 2005:272–279.

46. Mansell J, Tierney RT, Sitler MR, Swanik KA, Stearne D: Resistance training and head-neck segment dynamic stabilization in male and female collegiate soccer players. *J Athl Train* 2005;40(4):310–319.

47. Eckner JT, Oh YK, Joshi MS, Richardson JK, Ashton-Miller JA: Effect of neck muscle strength and anticipatory cervical muscle activation on the kinematic response of the head to impulsive loads. *Am J Sports Med* 2014;42(3):566–576.

48. Collins MW, Kontos AP, Reynolds E, Murawski CD, Fu FH: A comprehensive, targeted approach to the clinical care of athletes following sport-related concussion. *Knee Surg Sports Traumatol Arthrosc* 2014;22:235–246.

49. Schmidt JD, Guskiewicz KM, Blackburn JT, Mihalik JP, Siegmund GP, Marshall SW: The influence of cervical muscle characteristics on head impact biomechanics in football. *Am J Sports Med* 2014;42(9):2056–2066.

50. McCrory P, Meeuwisse W, Johnston K, et al: Consensus statement on concussion in sport: The 3rd International Conference on Concussion in Sport. Zurich, Switzerland, November 2008. *Br J Sports Med* 2009;43:i76–i84.

51. Makdissi M, Darby D, Maruff P, Ugoni A, Brukner P, McCrory PR: Natural history of concussion in sport: Markers of severity and implications for management. *Am J Sports Med* 2010;38(3):464–471.

52. World Federation for Mental Health: *Depression: A Global Crisis*. Available at: http://www.who.int/mental health/management/depression/wfmh paper depression wmhd 201 2.pdf?ua=1. Accessed August 20, 2015.

53. Covassin T, Elbin R, Larson E, et al: Sex and age differences in depression and baseline sport-related concussion neurocognitive performance and symptoms. *Clin J Sport Med* 2012;22:98–104.

54. Yang J, Peek-Asa C, Covassin T, Torner JC: Post-concussion symptoms of depression and anxiety in division I collegiate athletes. *Dev Neuropsychol* 2015;40(1):18–23.

55. Covassin T, Swanik CB, Sachs M, Kendrick Z, Schatz P, Zillmer E, Kaminaris C: Sex differences in baseline neuropsychological function and concussion symptoms of collegiate athletes. *Br J Sports Med* 2006;40:923–927.

56. Broshek DK, Kaushik T, Freeman JR, Erlanger D, Webbe F, Barth JT: Sex differences in outcome following sports-related concussion. *J Neurosurg* 2005;102:856–863.

57. Covassin T, Schatz P, Swanik CB: Sex differences in neuropsychological function and post-concussion symptoms of concussed collegiate athletes. *Neurosurgery* 2007;61:345–351.

58. Bazarian JJ, Blyth B, Mookerjee S, He H, McDermott MP: Sex differences in outcome after mild traumatic brain injury. *J Neurotrauma* 2010;27:527–539.

59. Lange RT, Iverson GL, Rose A: Depression strongly influences postconcussion symptom reporting following mild traumatic brain injury. *J Head Trauma Rehabil* 2011;26(2):127–137.

60. Zuckerman SL, Lee YM, Odom MJ, Solomon GS, Sills AK: Baseline neurocognitive scores in athletes with attention deficit-spectrum disorders and/or learning disability. *J Neurosurg* 2013;12:103–109.

61. Elbin RJ, Kontos AP, Kegel N, Johnson E, Burkhart S, Schatz P: Individual and combined effects of LD and ADHD on computerized neurocognitive concussion test performance: Evidence for separate norms. *Arch Clin Neuropsychol* 2013;28:476–484.

62. Echemendia RJ, Bruce JM, Bailey CM, Sanders JF, Arnett P, Vargas G: The utility of post-concussion neuropsychological data in identifying cognitive change following sports-related MTBI in the absence of baseline data. *Clin Neuropsychol* 2012;26:1077–1091.

63. Mautner K, Sussman WI, Axtman M, Al-Farsi Y, Al-Adawi S: Relationship of attention deficit hyperactivity disorder and postconcussion recovery in youth athletes. *Clin J Sports Med* 2015;25:355–360.

64. Heitger MH, Jones RD, Anderson TJ: A new approach to predicting postconcussion syndrome after mild traumatic brain injury based upon eye movement function. Presented at the 30th Annual International IEEE EMBS Conference. Vancouver; BC, Canada, 2008, pp 3570–3573.

65. Hou R, Moss-Morris R, Peveler R, Mogg K, Bradley BP, Belli A: When a minor head injury results in enduring symptoms: A prospective investigation of risk factors for postconcussional syndrome after mild traumatic brain injury. *J Neurosurg Psychiatry* 2012;83:217–223.

66. Preiss-Farzanegan S, Chapman B, Wong TM, Wu J, Bazarian JJ: The relationship between gender and post concussion symptoms after sport-related mild traumatic brain injury. *PM R* 2009;1:245–253.

67. King NS: A systematic review of age and gender factors in prolonged post-concussion symptoms after mild head injury. *Brain Inj* 2014;28(13–14):1639–1645.

68. Kostyun RO, Hafeez I: Protracted recovery from a concussion: A focus on gender and treatment interventions in an adolescent population. *Sports Health* 2015;7(1):52–57.

69. Barlow K, Crawford S, Stevenson A, Sandhu SS, Belanger F, Dewey D: Epidemiology of post concussion syndrome in pediatric mild traumatic brain injury. *Pediatrics* 2010;126(2):e374–381.

70. Barlow KM: Postconcussion syndrome: A review. *J Child Neurol* 2014;1–11.

71. Babcock L, Byczkowski T, Wade SL, Ho M, Mookerjee S, Bazarian JJ: Predicting postconcussion syndrome after mild traumatic brain injury in children and adolescents who present to the emergency department. *JAMA Pediatr* 2013;167(2):156–161.

72. McCrea M, Guskiewicz K, Randolph C, et al: Effects of a symptom-free waiting period on clinical outcome and risk of re-injury after sport related concussion. *Neurosurgery* 2009;65(5):876–882.

73. Thomas DG, Apps JN, Hoffmann RG, McCrea M, Hammeke T: Benefits of strict rest after acute concussion: a randomized controlled trail. *Pediatrics* 2015;135(2):213–223.

74. Herring SA, Boyajian-O'Neill, Coppel D, et al: Psychological issues related to injury in athletes and the team physician: A consensus statement. *Med Sci Sports Exer* 2006;38(11):2030–2034.

75. Halstead ME, McAvoy K, Devore CD, et al: Returning to learning following a concussion. *Pediatrics* 2013;132:948–957.

26 Neuropsychological Testing in the Treatment and Management of Sport-Related Concussion

Melissa A. Lancaster, PhD • Lindsay D. Nelson, PhD • Michael A. McCrea, PhD

INTRODUCTION

After sustaining a sport-related concussion (SRC), the nervous system begins a complex sequence of neurochemical and metabolic processes that result in adverse physical, cognitive, and emotional sequelae.[1] As a result, a multidimensional assessment approach is needed that takes into account an athlete's past history in addition to current report of symptoms, neurologic status, postural stability, and cognitive functioning in order to make an accurate diagnosis and proper treatment recommendations (**Figure 26-1**). Regarding cognitive functioning, common symptoms include memory disturbance, impaired vigilance, heightened distractibility, difficulty forming cohesive thoughts, slowed processing speed, and inability to carry out sequences of goal-directed movements.[2,3] Although self-report measures are a simple and convenient way to screen for cognitive symptoms, their reliability and sensitivity may be diminished because athletes sometimes fail to recognize these symptoms or may be motivated to underreport symptoms in order to return to play (RTP).[4] As a result, objective, standardized measurement of cognitive symptoms by a trained neuropsychologist can be valuable for evaluating concussed athletes and informing RTP because repeat injuries appear most likely while athletes are early in their recovery.[5]

The purpose of this chapter is to describe how the field of neuropsychology contributes to the diagnosis

and treatment of SRC. Within the sections below, the following will be discussed: the role of the neuropsychologist and neuropsychological (NP) testing in treatment of SRC, points of NP intervention, issues surrounding interpretation of NP data, and factors to consider when assessing pediatric populations.

ROLE OF THE NEUROPSYCHOLOGIST IN THE ASSESSMENT OF SPORT-RELATED CONCUSSION

Neuropsychologists are the healthcare professionals best trained to assess cognitive and emotional functioning in individuals who have sustained SRCs.[6] Beginning with the work of Barth and colleagues, who first used NP tests to monitor the acute effects of SRC and recovery in collegiate athletes in the 1980s,[7] neuropsychologists have been essential to the study of assessment and treatment of SRC.[8] Neuropsychologists receive doctoral-level training in the field of clinical psychology in addition to

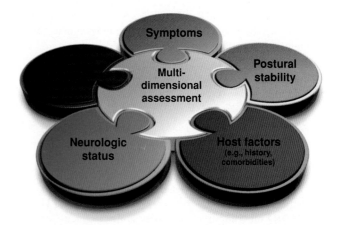

FIGURE 26-1 Multidimensional approach to the assessment of sport-related concussion.

specialized training in brain–behavior relationships and the science of assessment. As described by Barth et al[9]:

> Clinical neuropsychologists use this knowledge in the assessment, diagnosis, treatment, and/or rehabilitation of patients across the lifespan with neurological, medical, neurodevelopmental and psychiatric conditions, as well as other cognitive and learning disorders. The clinical neuropsychologist uses psychological, neurological, cognitive, behavioral, and physiological principles, techniques, and tests to evaluate patients' neurocognitive, behavioral, and emotional strengths and weaknesses and their relationship to normal and abnormal nervous system functioning (p. 16).

Neuropsychologists are also well-qualified to assess for preexisting factors, such as attention deficit hyperactivity disorder (ADHD), learning disability, and other developmental conditions, which may complicate interpretation of cognitive test data.

In addition to cognitive disturbance, individuals with SRC can present with emotional symptoms such as depression, fear, and anxiety.[10] Also, athletes have been documented to respond differently to their injury than would nonathletes and have difficulty coping with restriction in activity after SRC and other lifestyle changes during recovery.[11] Furthermore, a positive relationship has been established between the presence of mood symptoms and length of recovery.[12–14] Neuropsychologists, who are trained in the fundamentals of clinical psychology, are highly competent in the assessment of emotional factors that may be impacting cognitive functioning and injury recovery, and they are able to make appropriate recommendations for treatment of mood symptoms if deemed necessary.

As the consequences of improper treatment of SRC gain more attention, several states have enacted legislation mandating that student athletes with SRC be removed from play until cleared by a healthcare provider. It is the official position of the main governing bodies in neuropsychology, the American Academy of Clinical Neuropsychology (AACN), the American Board of Neuropsychology (ABN), the Society for Clinical Neuropsychology (SCN) of the American Psychological Association (APA), and the National Academy of Neuropsychology (NAN), that neuropsychologists be included among the healthcare professionals authorized to participate in SRC evaluation and management.[6]

The American Academy of Neurology (AAN) also cites that NP testing is likely useful in identifying the presence of concussion,[15] and the American Medical Society for Sports Medicine (AMSSM)[16] has concluded

that NP testing may be especially helpful in informing RTP decisions in high-risk athletes with prior concussion. In line with these views, professional organizations such as the National Football League (NFL), Major League Baseball, National Hockey League, and Major League Soccer all include NP assessment in their concussion management protocols. As evidenced by these endorsements, neuropsychologists have played an important role in the development of current guidelines for assessment of SRC.[17]

APPROACHES TO NEUROPSYCHOLOGICAL ASSESSMENT OF SPORT-RELATED CONCUSSION

Neuropsychologists assess cognitive functioning with standardized measures of a range of abilities (e.g., memory, attention, reasoning, visuospatial ability). Patients' abilities are examined compared with demographically adjusted normative data or patients' individual premorbid baselines (frequently available in the context of SRC). Taken with other relevant information such as patient history, neuroimaging, and laboratory findings, neuropsychologists make inferences about the presence of dysfunction in certain cognitive domains and sometimes specific neuroanatomical regions and brain circuits. Depending on a patient's presenting condition, clinical profile, and goals for assessment, NP testing may facilitate differential diagnosis, inform prognosis, and guide appropriate treatment planning.

Traditional Pencil-and-Paper Neuropsychological Testing

Traditionally, the field of neuropsychology has used pencil-and-paper testing methods that have since been borrowed or adapted for assessment of athletes with SRC, especially instruments that measure functions affected by acute head injury (e.g., new learning and memory, attention, processing speed, and executive functioning). Most of these measures have demonstrated acceptable psychometric properties and are at least moderately sensitive to SRC early after injury (see Randolph et al[18] for an overview of these measures). Although several athletic organizations have used fixed batteries composed of such tests,[19] neuropsychologists may modify fixed batteries depending on each patient's individual cognitive symptoms and other relevant factors (e.g., learning disability, physical limitations). This testing format has a number of advantages over computerized testing in that the one-on-one testing format may maximize participant performance (e.g., clinicians can respond to participants' needs for breaks between subtests), allows for clinicians to obtain valuable behavioral observations, allows more flexibility for examiners to test cognitive domains relevant to each patient, and tends to allow for the assessment of a wider range of neurocognitive domains. A negative attribute of traditional NP testing, however, is the amount of time and expertise needed to test athletes.[16,20]

Computerized Neurocognitive Testing

Because traditional NP assessment is not feasible to perform on large groups of athletes or by sports medicine practitioners, several companies have devised computerized neurocognitive tests (CNTs) for SRC assessment. Currently, the most widely used CNTs in the United States include ANAM (Automated Neuropsychological Assessment Metrics), Axon Sports, and ImPACT (Immediate Postconcussion and Cognitive Testing Test Battery), with ImPACT the most widely used.[21,22] Since their appearance in the 1990s, CNTs have become considerably more popular with sports medicine professionals (e.g., athletic trainers) because of their ease of administration (especially to large groups of athletes preseason), transportability (with easy access through the internet or computer hard drive), and availability of alternate forms to reduce practice effects. Although strongly discouraged, CNTs can be interpreted more readily than paper-and-pencil measures by non-neuropsychologists, making them more accessible in many sports medicine settings.[22]

However, several disadvantages to cognitive assessment via CNT have been noted. For example, environmental distractions (especially when testing several athletes at once in a room), difficulty understanding test instructions, and computer issues may introduce errors into the measurement of cognitive functioning and result in a higher number of invalid test results.[23] Another criticism of CNTs is the fact that studies of reliability and validity of these measures have been highly variable, with all CNTs containing some subtest and summary scores that do not meet acceptable levels of psychometric quality.[22] However, it should be noted that some traditional NP measures also have psychometric limitations, especially in the context of SRC assessment.[18,20] Other limitations of CNTs include a lack of norms corresponding to specific age groups and poor indices of inadequate effort. Finally, there has been concern about non-neuropsychologists such as athletic trainers, who are not trained in psychometrics and test interpretation, interpreting CNT test data.[16]

NEUROCOGNITIVE RECOVERY FROM SPORT-RELATED CONCUSSION

As prior work has demonstrated in high school and collegiate samples, most athletes demonstrate a return to baseline in reported symptoms, cognition, and postural stability within 7 to 14 days of injury.[24,25] In support of this finding, a meta-analysis by Broglio and Puetz[26] found that the cognitive effects of SRC are large (Hedge's g = −0.81) immediately postinjury but minimal after 7 days (Hedge's g = −0.22), with effects of such small proportion that differences between injured and noninjured athletes would be difficult to detect at the individual case level. Furthermore, after 1 month, the cognitive effects of SRC are nearly nonexistent at a group level (Hedge's g = −0.12). That said, it is recognized that a minority of athletes experience more prolonged recovery that is obscured in such group-level analyses.[27] For those that do not recover within the typical 1-week to 1-month window, several factors may contribute to prolonged recovery, with initial concussive symptom burden most consistently predictive of prolonged symptoms. Other markers of injury severity (e.g., posttraumatic amnesia, loss of consciousness) have been predictive in some studies.[28] Furthermore, as mentioned earlier, preexisting or postinjury emotional factors may also contribute significantly to recovery time.

As acknowledged in the AMSSM guidelines, comprehensive NP evaluation is valuable when managing athletes with more prolonged or complicated recoveries.[16] In these cases, neuropsychologists may provide insight into the nature and severity of residual cognitive and emotional symptoms and make recommendations about what other treatment options (e.g., psychotherapy in the case of mood disturbance) may be most beneficial to such athletes. These comprehensive evaluations are typically performed in medical or private-practice settings and should involve well-validated, traditional NP measures.

NEUROPSYCHOLOGICAL TESTING PROTOCOL CONSIDERATIONS

Because recovery from SRC is complex and depends on several individual and injury-specific factors, there are multiple time points in which a neuropsychologist may intervene after injury. However, given the fact that each individual and injury differs, there is no "one size fits all" method for assessing cognitive recovery, and practical considerations must also be made. Points when a neuropsychologist may intervene include at baseline (before

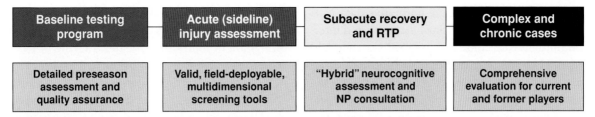

FIGURE 26-2 Multitiered approach to neuropsychological assessment of sport-related concussion. NP = neuropsychological; RTP = return to play.

the commencement of activity), immediately after injury, in the subacute recovery phase, and several months after injury in the case of prolonged recovery (**Figure 26-2**). These assessment points are discussed in detail next.

Baseline Testing

Since the introduction of the Sport as Laboratory Assessment Model (SLAM) in the 1980s,[7] preseason baseline testing teams of athletes has become increasingly common. In this model, an athlete is tested before the season and retested after injury to determine if he or she has experienced a decline. Such testing may be administered using paper-and-pencil, computerized, or mixed formats. Because an individual is being compared to his or her own performance, this method theoretically has a greater ability to detect true cognitive impairment, as factors such as preexisting cognitive limitations (e.g., ADHD or learning disability) can be controlled.

Despite the potential benefits of the use of baseline testing, a number of potential issues may limit its added value over traditional approaches. For example, several factors complicate the interpretation of repeated testing, including practice effects that may be present even if alternate forms are used.[29] In addition, measures with poor reliability have greater measurement error, which translates to (1) larger changes in cognition needed for postinjury scores to be statistically different from baseline scores and (2) increased regression to the mean, a phenomenon in which extreme test scores at one test period revert toward the mean of the normative group at repeat testing.[30] When multiple athletes are baseline tested together using CNTs, environmental distractors and computer problems may also lead to invalid data; furthermore, because athletes are often tested alone after injury, many of these factors are not present during post-testing, creating difficulty in comparing scores. Finally, athletes' motivation to avoid being removed from play or even losing their positions has led to the phenomenon of "sandbagging," or purposefully giving poor effort on preseason testing to decrease the chances of looking

impaired after SRC, further complicating interpretation of change from baseline performance. Along this line, approximately half of athletic trainers using ImPACT report not screening baseline assessments for validity.[31]

Given some of the complicating factors in interpreting change from baseline performance, methods have been proposed to reduce some individual and measurement error. For example, two baseline assessments can be collected with the latter serving as a "true" baseline to reduce the influence of practice effects.[30] Furthermore, methods exist for calculating change that statistically account for measurement error and regression to the mean,[32,33] and multiple regression formulas predicting postinjury performance may also be helpful in accounting for individual variables such as age, education, socioeconomic status, and history of prior head injury.[34]

In contrast to baseline testing, another method of determining cognitive impairment after SRC is the use of normative data, as is common practice in the field of neuropsychology at large. Using this approach, measurements of premorbid functioning are obtained, and scores on testing that fall statistically below one's expected functioning (usually measured as 1 to 2 standard deviations) are examined in more detail. A neuropsychologist will consider a person's history, including medical, psychological, psychosocial, and educational factors, to determine if a decline from the person's premorbid function has occurred. A well-trained neuropsychologist looks for patterns in test data indicative of dysfunction in distinct neural circuits and does not overinterpret individual impaired scores in isolation because most individuals who complete a comprehensive NP examination will obtain at least one low score, with the likelihood of this occurring increasing with the number of tests given.[35] One criticism of using norm-based methods is illustrated in the work of Schatz and Robertshaw,[36] who demonstrated that this method may lead to false-positive errors in individuals whose normal baseline cognitive functioning is below average and to greater false-negative errors in above-average athletes.

It has been argued that if using normative data is as effective as baseline testing, the time, financial, and interpretation burdens that come with baseline testing could be avoided. However, few studies have been conducted to compare the ability of these two methods to actively detect the cognitive effects of SRC, and findings have been mixed, with some studies finding that applying normative cut scores to postinjury scores produces comparable sensitivity over baseline-adjusted methods[37,38] and others suggesting a small gain for some individuals when baseline information is available.[39] This information, in addition to the findings of Schatz and Robertshaw, indicate that baseline testing may not be necessary for identifying impairment unless there is reason to believe the individual falls atypically above or below the normative sample at baseline for a number of reasons (e.g., intellectual giftedness, ADHD, a learning or developmental disorder, emotional disturbance).

● POSTINJURY SIDELINE COGNITIVE SCREENING

Per widely accepted guidelines from organizations such as the AAN and AMSSM, any athlete suspected of concussion during play should be removed from the game and assessed by a licensed healthcare provider. Athletic trainers, team physicians, and other sports medicine professionals are often the first available providers to assess concussed athletes immediately after injury. A number of screening tools have been developed for such professionals that are intended for rapid sideline assessment of athletes' symptoms, cognition, and postural stability. The most widely used and studied sideline neurocognitive measure is the Standardized Assessment of Concussion (SAC), which takes approximately 6 minutes to administer and assesses four neurocognitive domains: orientation, immediate memory, concentration, and delayed recall.[40] The SAC is designed to be administered by practitioners not heavily trained in psychometric assessment. The SAC has shown excellent sensitivity and specificity immediately after SRC.[3,41,42] A critical review of the literature on the effectiveness of sideline measures[43] illustrated that clinical sequelae of concussion vary across individuals and therefore are best assessed using a multifactorial approach (i.e., considerations of physical symptoms, balance, and cognitive symptoms). As a result, measures such as the Sport Concussion Assessment Tool, 3rd edition (SCAT 3[17]) and the NFL Sideline Concussion Assessment Tool include the SAC with measures of other signs and symptoms of concussion to yield a multidimensional screen of numerous common sequelae of concussion.

Postinjury Neurocognitive Testing

Although sideline measures are very useful for early estimation of injury severity and tracking of changes in symptoms, cognition, and balance, their brevity results in more psychometric limitations than longer tests (e.g., restricted range of scores on the SAC, which will limit its maximal reliability and validity). Consequently, more comprehensive NP testing is sometimes warranted to more conclusively establish when athletes have returned to normal levels of cognitive functioning and to better understand their strengths and weaknesses across a broad array of neurocognitive abilities. After sideline cognitive assessment, some differences in opinion exist as to when to retest symptomatic athletes. We believe that it is unnecessary to routinely administer neurocognitive tests to injured athletes who remain symptomatic because repeat testing early postinjury may create unnecessary stress on recovering athletes, introduces unnecessary practice effects, and is irrelevant in informing RTP decisions because of current guidelines that preclude athletes from returning to play while symptoms persist. In most cases of SRC, when an athlete reports that he or she is symptom free, NP testing can be used to determine if the athlete continues to show objective cognitive impairment. However, testing symptomatic athletes may be helpful to determine classroom accommodations for student athletes, if the athlete's organization requires status updates, or in cases of prolonged recovery.[44]

● NEUROPSYCHOLOGICAL ASSESSMENT OF PEDIATRIC SPORT-RELATED CONCUSSION

The majority of research studies investigating SRC in athletes have used high school, collegiate, and professional athletes, and findings are often generalized and used to inform treatment recommendations for athletes of all ages. However, there is growing evidence that younger brains have a differential propensity to concussive injury and may not recover in the same fashion as that of adults. In smaller brains, for example, more force is necessary to cause a concussion, yet when holding the force of the impact constant, young brains show more damage than those of adults.[45] Other factors that may lead younger children to be more vulnerable to concussion include larger head-to-body ratio, weaker neck muscles, and thinner skulls.[15] Furthermore, incomplete myelination of neurons in younger athletes may contribute not only to an increased risk of SRC but also affect cognitive recovery. Although some studies have found slightly slower recovery in high school athletes versus collegiate athletes (in the order of a few days), they do not appear to differ in risk for prolonged recovery (>4 weeks), and this effect has not been studied adequately in younger children.[46]

There are several developmental factors to consider when assessing symptoms of younger athletes with SRC. One consideration is that children may not be reliable historians who can accurately describe what they are experiencing, or they may not fully understand the concept of concussion and its related symptoms.[47] Another factor to consider is the inclination of some children and young adults to minimize symptoms for fear of being pulled from a game. As such, obtaining collateral reports of perceived symptoms by parents, coaches, or teachers may facilitate the assessment in children.[48]

Regarding formalized NP testing, it is important to consider developmental factors when assessing children and adolescents. For example, younger individuals have shorter attention spans, may be more tired or unmotivated later in the day, may have difficulty understanding task instructions, and may be more prone to responding in a way to please the examiner.[15] Furthermore, assessment measures must take into account reading, language, and physical development.[49] Because of differences in the assessment of children and adults, cognitive evaluation of children should be completed by a trained pediatric neuropsychologist who is able to properly consider all developmental factors when interpreting test results. Given their training in the impact of head injury on neurodevelopment, pediatric neuropsychologists have vital roles in the acute, postacute, and long-term management of children with SRC.[50]

A major challenge in performing neurocognitive assessment of concussed children and adolescents is that there is a paucity of research on concussion response and recovery in young athletes, and there are few well-validated measures for children with SRC. Although the SCAT 3 has recently been modified for use in children aged 5 to 13 years (Child-SCAT 3[17]), the measure was developed by expert consensus (rather than empirically) and remains to be validated. Normative data for other existing computerized testing programs is being collected and validated; one caveat is that younger children show higher rates of invalid results on computerized testing designed for adults.[51] Fortunately, many traditional pediatric NP measures with appropriate normative data exist and have been validated in pediatric concussion, but their administration and interpretation requires a pediatric neuropsychologist.[52]

SUMMARY

Neuropsychologists are a valuable part of sports medicine teams for the evaluation and management of SRC across many stages of injury, including baseline assessment of at-risk athletes, immediate sideline injury assessment, tracking recovery to inform RTP decisions, and treatment of individuals who experience prolonged recovery. As clinicians who are well-trained in assessment methods and their application to psychiatric and neurologic cases, they are best able to interpret NP measures in the context of each test's limitations and complicating factors unique to each injured athlete (e.g., neurodevelopmental disorders, motivational and emotional factors). Furthermore, neuropsychologists have the proper background in psychometric considerations important when making determinations about cognitive change, regardless of whether baseline or normative data are used. As the importance of proper assessment and treatment of SRC continues to be of widespread concern, the field of neuropsychology will be called upon to deliver evidence-based approaches toward improving assessment measures and further studying cognitive and emotional factors important to optimal recovery after SRC.

REFERENCES

1. Giza CC, Hovda DA: The new neurometabolic cascade of concussion. *Neurosurgery* 2014;75(suppl 4):S24–S33.

2. Kelly JP, Rosenberg JH: Diagnosis and management of concussion in sports. *Neurology* 1997;48(3):575–580.

3. McCrea M, Kelly JP, Randolph C, Cisler R, Berger L: Immediate neurocognitive effects of concussion. *Neurosurgery* 2002;50(5):1032–1040; discussion 1040–1032.

4. McCrea M, Hammeke T, Olsen G, Leo P, Guskiewicz K: Unreported concussion in high school football players: implications for prevention. *Clin J Sport Med* 2004;14(1):13–17.

5. Guskiewicz KM, McCrea M, Marshall SW, et al: Cumulative effects associated with recurrent concussion in collegiate football players: The NCAA Concussion Study. *JAMA* 2003;290(19):2549–2555.

6. Echemendia RJ, Iverson GL, McCrea M, et al: Role of neuropsychologists in the evaluation and management of sport-related concussion: An inter-organization position statement. *Clin Neuropsychol* 2011;25(8):1289–1294.

7. Barth JT, Alves WM, Macciocchi SN, Rimel RW, Jane JA, Nelson WE: Mild head injury in sports: Neuropsychological sequelae and recovery of function, in: Levin H, Eisenberg J, Benton A (eds): *Mild Head Injury*. New York, Oxford University Press, 1989, pp 257–275.

8. Webbe FM, Zimmer A: History of neuropsychological study of sport-related concussion. *Brain Inj* 2015;29(2): 129–138.

9. Barth JT, Pliskin N, Axelrod B, et al: Introduction to the NAN 2001 Definition of a clinical neuropsychologist. NAN Policy and Planning Committee. *Arch Clin Neuropsychol* 2003;18(5):551–555.

10. Putukian M, Echemendia RJ: Psychological aspects of serious head injury in the competitive athlete. *Clin Sports Med* 2003;22(3):617–630, xi.

11. Smith AM, Scott SG, Wiese DM: The psychological effects of sports injuries. Coping. *Sports Med* 1990;9(6): 352–369.

12. Mooney G, Speed J, Sheppard S:Factors related to recovery after mild traumatic brain injury. *Brain Inj* 2005; 19(12):975–987.

13. Ponsford J, Cameron P, Fitzgerald M, Grant M, Mikocka-Walus A, Schonberger M: Predictors of postconcussive symptoms 3 months after mild traumatic brain injury. *Neuropsychology* 2012;26(3):304–313.

14. Satz P, Forney DL, Zaucha K, et al: Depression, cognition, and functional correlates of recovery outcome after traumatic brain injury. *Brain Inj* 1998;12(7):537–553.

15. Giza CC, Kutcher JS, Ashwal S, et al: Summary of evidence-based guideline update: Evaluation and management of concussion in sports: report of the Guideline Development Subcommittee of the American Academy of Neurology. *Neurology* 2013;80(24):2250–2257.

16. Harmon KG, Drezner J, Gammons M, et al: American Medical Society for Sports Medicine position statement: Concussion in sport. *Clin J Sport Med* 2013;23(1):1–18.

17. McCrory P, Meeuwisse WH, Aubry M, et al: Consensus statement on concussion in sport: The 4th International Conference on Concussion in Sport held in Zurich, November 2012. *Br J Sports Med* 2013;47(5): 250–258.

18. Randolph C, McCrea M, Barr WB: Is neuropsychological testing useful in the management of sport-related concussion? *J Athl Train* 2005;40(3):139–152.

19. Lovell MR, Collins MW: Neuropsychological assessment of the college football player. *J Head Trauma Rehabil* 1998; 13(2):9–26.

20. Iverson GL, Schatz P: Advanced topics in neuropsychological assessment following sport-related concussion. *Brain Inj* 2015;29(2):263–275.

21. Meehan WP 3rd, d'Hemecourt P, Collins CL, Taylor AM, Comstock RD: Computerized neurocognitive testing for the management of sport-related concussions. *Pediatrics* 2012;129(1):38–44.

22. Resch JE, McCrea MA, Cullum CM: Computerized neurocognitive testing in the management of sport-related concussion: An update. *Neuropsychol Rev* 2013; 23(4):335–349.

23. Schatz P, Neidzwski K, Moser RS, Karpf R: Relationship between subjective test feedback provided by high-school athletes during computer-based assessment of baseline cognitive functioning and self-reported symptoms. *Arch Clin Neuropsychol* 2010;25(4):285–292.

24. Macciocchi SN, Barth JT, Alves W, Rimel RW, Jane JA: Neuropsychological functioning and recovery after mild head injury in collegiate athletes. *Neurosurgery* 1996; 39(3):510–514.

25. McCrea M, Guskiewicz KM, Marshall SW, et al: Acute effects and recovery time following concussion in collegiate football players: The NCAA Concussion Study. *JAMA* 2003;290(19):2556–2563.

26. Broglio SP, Puetz TW: The effect of sport concussion on neurocognitive function, self-report symptoms and postural control: A meta-analysis. *Sports Med* 2008;38(1): 53–67.

27. Iverson GL, Brooks BL, Collins MW, Lovell MR: Tracking neuropsychological recovery following concussion in sport. *Brain Inj* 2006;20(3):245–252.

28. Nelson LD, Janecek JK, McCrea MA: Acute clinical recovery from sport-related concussion. *Neuropsychol Rev* 2013;23(4):285–299.

29. Benedict RH, Zgaljardic DJ: Practice effects during repeated administrations of memory tests with and without alternate forms. *J Clin Exp Neuropsychol* 1998;20(3): 339–352.

30. Collie A, Maruff P, Makdissi M, McStephen M, Darby DG, McCrory P: Statistical procedures for determining the extent of cognitive change following concussion. *Br J Sports Med* 2004;38(3):273–278.

31. Covassin T, Elbin RJ 3rd, Stiller-Ostrowski JL, Kontos AP: Immediate post-concussion assessment and cognitive testing (ImPACT) practices of sports medicine professionals. *J Athl Train* 2009;44(6):639–644.

32. Chelune GJ, Naugle RI, Luders H, Sedlak J, Awad IA: Individual change after epilepsy surgery: Practice effects and base-rate information. *Neuropsychology* 1993;7(1): 41–52.

33. Jacobson NS, Truax P: Clinical significance: A statistical approach to defining meaningful change in psychotherapy research. *J Consult Clin Psychol* 1991;59(1):12–19.

34. Temkin NR, Heaton RK, Grant I, Dikmen SS: Detecting significant change in neuropsychological test performance: A comparison of four models. *J Int Neuropsychol Soc* 1999; 5(4):357–369.

35. Schretlen DJ, Testa SM, Winicki JM, Pearlson GD, Gordon B: Frequency and bases of abnormal performance by healthy adults on neuropsychological testing. *J Int Neuropsychol Soc* 2008;14(3):436–445.

36. Schatz P, Robertshaw S: Comparing post-concussive neurocognitive test data to normative data presents risks for under-classifying "above average" athletes. *Arch Clin Neuropsychol* 2014;29(7):625–632.

37. Echemendia RJ, Bruce JM, Bailey CM, Sanders JF, Arnett P, Vargas G: The utility of post-concussion neuropsychological data in identifying cognitive change following sports-related MTBI in the absence of baseline data. *Clin Neuropsychol* 2012;26(7):1077–1091.

38. Schmidt JD, Register-Mihalik JK, Mihalik JP, Kerr ZY, Guskiewicz KM: Identifying Impairments after concussion: Normative data versus individualized baselines. *Med Sci Sports Exerc* 2012;44(9):1621–1628.

39. Roebuck-Spencer TM, Vincent AS, Schlegel RE, Gilliland K: Evidence for added value of baseline testing in computer-based cognitive assessment. *J Athl Train* 2013;48(4):499–505.

40. McCrea M, Kelly JP, Randolph C, Kluge J, Bartolic E, Finn G, Baxter B: Standardized assessment of concussion (SAC): On-site mental status evaluation of the athlete. *J Head Trauma Rehabil* 1998;13(2):27–35.

41. Barr WB, McCrea M: Sensitivity and specificity of standardized neurocognitive testing immediately following sports concussion. *J Int Neuropsychol Soc* 2001;7(6):693–702.

42. McCrea M: Standardized mental status testing on the sideline after sport-related concussion. *J Athl Train* 2001;36(3):274–279.

43. McCrea M, Iverson GL, Echemendia RJ, Makdissi M, Raftery M: Day of injury assessment of sport-related concussion. *Br J Sports Med* 2013;47(5):272–284.

44. Pardini JE, Johnson EW, Lovell MR: Concussion management programs in college and professional sport, in: Webbe FM (ed): *The Handbook of Sport Neuropsychology*. New York, Springer Publishing, 2011.

45. Ommaya AK, Goldsmith W, Thibault L: Biomechanics and neuropathology of adult and paediatric head injury. *Br J Neurosurg* 2002;16(3):220–242.

46. Foley C, Gregory A, Solomon G: Young age as a modifying factor in sports concussion management: What is the evidence? *Curr Sports Med Rep* 2014;13(6):390–394.

47. Moser RS, Fryer AC, Berardinelli S: Youth sport concussion: A heads up on the growing public health concern, in: Webbe FM (ed): *The Handbook of Sport Neuropsychology*. New York, Springer Publishing, 2011.

48. Gioia GA, Vaughan CG, Sady MDS: Developmental considerations in pediatric concussion evaluation and management, in: Niskala J, Walter KD (eds): *Pediatric and Adolescent Concussion: Diagnosis, Management, and Outcomes*. New York, Springer Science+Business Media, 2011.

49. Davis GA, Purcell LK: The evaluation and management of acute concussion differs in young children. *Br J Sports Med* 2014;48(2):98–101.

50. Kirkwood MW, Yeates KO, Taylor HG, Randolph C, McCrea M, Anderson VA: Management of pediatric mild traumatic brain injury: A neuropsychological review from injury through recovery. *Clin Neuropsychol* 2008;22(5):769–800.

51. Lichtenstein JD, Moser RS, Schatz P: Age and test setting affect the prevalence of invalid baseline scores on neurocognitive tests. *Am J Sports Med* 2014;42(2):479–484.

52. Kegel NE, Lovell MR: Methods of formal neurocognitive assessment of concussion, in: Apps JN, Walter KD (eds): *Pediatric and Adolescent Concussion: Diagnosis, Management, and Outcomes*. New York, Springer, 2011.

27 Postconcussion Syndrome

Javier Cárdenas, MD

CASE VIGNETTE

A 19-year-old female soccer player for a division 1 National Collegiate Athletic Association university was referred to the clinic by the team athletic trainer 1 month after sustaining a concussion for persistent headaches. The student-athlete's initial complaints were headache, insomnia, anxiety, and a decline in academic performance. Headaches were described as a pressure sensation with photophobia but no nausea or vomiting. Frequency was daily with an intolerance to physical and cognitive activity. Headaches were partially relieved with daily ibuprofen. Her cognitive complaints were notable for word-finding and short-term memory problems. Academic adaptations were provided by the institution for note taking and additional time for assignments and tests. She described her insomnia as difficulty falling asleep but not staying asleep. Appropriate sleep hygiene was practiced, but she reported that she could not "shut off my brain." Her history was notable for premorbid migraine headaches with a frequency of one per month and anxiety. Her examination was normal with the exception of photosensitivity on ophthalmologic examination and imbalance.

The student athlete's evaluation and treatment plan included noncontrast MRI of the brain with susceptibility imaging, low-dose nortriptyline, physical and vestibular therapy, sports psychology consultation, and neuropsychological (NP) evaluation. MRI results were normal, and NP testing revealed inattention, but otherwise intact cognitive function. Within 1 week of treatment, she reported a decrease in headache frequency and intensity, as well as an improvement in sleep. She was able to tolerate physical and cognitive exertion, and her balance improved with therapy. When symptom free with heavy noncontact physical activity and no

longer requiring academic adaptations, she successfully returned to competition. Her anxiety resolved when she returned to physical activity, but she continued sports psychology for treatment of her premorbid anxiety.

DEFINITION

The challenges in defining postconcussion syndrome (PCS) are similar to the challenges in defining concussion. The timeline in which the symptoms of a concussion begin are typically within minutes of the injury but can sometimes take hours and (less commonly) days to develop. The symptoms that patients report in the days and weeks after a concussion are typically referred to as *postconcussive symptoms*. This is distinguished from *postconcussion syndrome*, which is defined by the *Diagnostic and Statistical Manual IV* as physical, behavioral, and cognitive symptoms that "last at least three months."[1] Although clinicians and researchers fret and debate the definition, patients are equally, if not more confused, often asking, "Do I *have* a concussion?" when referring to their existing symptomatology regardless of timeframe. For the sake of argument, this chapter refers to postconcussive syndrome and persistent postconcussive symptoms as the physical, behavioral, and cognitive symptoms that persist (or worsen) beyond the typical recovery as defined earlier in the book (**Table 27-1**). This is particularly relevant when treating student athletes because the timing of intervention is critical to the academic success of the patient.

Generally, symptoms associated with concussion fall into three broad categories: physical, behavioral, and cognitive. Physical symptoms include headaches, dizziness, visual disturbance, and sleep disturbance. Seizures and endocrine disturbances are uncommonly a result of concussion but are addressed later in the chapter because they can be a consequence of moderate and severe traumatic brain injury (TBI). Behavioral symptoms typically include irritability, depression, and anxiety. Less frequently, psychosis can occur after concussion but should be addressed when present. Last, the cognitive symptoms after concussion include problems with focus, short-term

Neither Dr. Cárdenas nor any immediate family member has received anything of value from or has stock or stock options held in a commercial company or institution related directly or indirectly to the subject of this article.

TABLE 27-1	Clinical approach to postconcussion syndrome		
Domain	Physical	Behavioral	Cognitive
Symptoms	Headache, dizziness, sleep disturbance, vision change, seizures, endocrine abnormalities	Irritability, anxiety, depression, psychosis	Inattention, memory deficit, word-finding difficulty, slow processing speed
Evaluation	Examination, imaging, laboratory testing, electrophysiology	Psychiatric consultation, psychological evaluation	Neuropsychological testing
Treatment	Medications, physical and vestibular therapy, occupational therapy	Medications, behavioral psychology, counseling	Speech and cognitive therapy, medication

memory, and word finding, although more specific disturbances in cognition have been described in the literature and are elicited by NP evaluation.

While evaluating a patient with PCS (or any TBI, for that matter), it is important to recognize that the symptoms have overlapping influence like that of a Venn diagram. As such, headaches and migraines can negatively affect mood as well as impair cognitive performance.[2] Additionally, depression and anxiety can influence focus and academic performance and result in a lower threshold for pain.[3] The overlap in symptomatology underscores the importance of taking a holistic approach to evaluation and management of patients with persistent postconcussive symptoms. Finally, the most relevant risk factors for developing PCS are the presence of conditions *before* the concussion. For example, patients with a history of migraine typically have worsening of their headaches after a concussion, and those with attention and learning problems have worsening academic and cognitive performance.[4] The most at risk for developing long-term symptoms are those with a history of anxiety or depression because psychological disturbance is the most common cause of PCS.[5]

● PHYSICAL SYMPTOMS
Headache

Postconcussive headache is the most common symptom reported by individuals who sustain a concussion. Interestingly, this is a less common feature of those with moderate or severe TBIs.[6] Postconcussive headaches affect 30% to 90% of athletes after a head injury.[7] The description of the headaches is most like that of migraine. Specifically, photophobia, phonophobia, nausea, and vomiting are commonly associated with the headache.[8] In contrast, persistent headaches in PCS have features of chronic daily headache and medication overuse headache.[9]

The evaluation of an individual with persistent headache associated with a concussion includes a detailed history, particularly noting a personal and family history of migraine. Adolescence is the most common time for migraines to present,[10] and concussion can often be the inciting event for those with a strong family history. Worsening of migraine headaches in frequency, intensity, or both is common for those with a personal history of migraine. Modifying factors often include worsening with bright lights, loud noise, physical exertion, and cognitive exertion. Others may also report feeling car sick or bothered by rapid movements. Associated physical symptoms such as dizziness and visual disturbance may exacerbate symptoms. Improvement is commonly associated with sleep, analgesic medication, and avoiding exacerbating environments. Red flags in the history include disturbances in other neurologic function, such as altered mental status, seizures, worsening of vision, and weakness.

The physical examination of a patient with postconcussive headaches is key to determining further treatment and testing. General observation of distress or pain is common with postconcussive headaches, especially under the bright fluorescent lights typically found in a clinical setting. As such, pupillary evaluation and funduscopic examination tend to elicit a negative physical response. It is critically important to perform a complete cranial nerve evaluation because headache may represent an underlying intracranial abnormality. Red flags on neurologic examination in the presence of persistent headache include papilledema, hyperreflexia, and any cranial neuropathy.

Management of postconcussive headaches depends largely on the history and physical examination findings. Those with persistent or worsening headaches warrant neurologic imaging. Although CT scan of the head is valuable in the acute setting, the risks of radiation exposure, especially in a young population, far outweigh the benefit.[11] MRI of the brain can provide greater detail of intracranial structures while avoiding unnecessary radiation exposure. MRI studies for trauma do not require contrast enhancement but should include gradient echo sequences.

Gradient echo sequences are readily available sequences and can detect hemosiderin deposition such as those found in shear injury and diffuse axonal injury. A host of emerging techniques and sequences appear to confer greater sensitivity to concussion, but they are not widely commercially available. These include, but are not limited to, susceptibility-weighted imaging, diffusion tensor imaging, and diffusion kurtosis imaging.[12] Lumbar puncture is infrequently indicated but should be considered if headaches worsen or are not responsive to treatment or if funduscopic examination demonstrates papilledema.

Medication treatment of postconcussive headaches can often be a challenging effort of trial and error. Analgesic medications are typically helpful in the early course of injury recovery but can lead to rebound headaches if overused. "Headache prevention" medications are often indicated for those whose headaches fail to improve with time or have an exacerbation of their underlying migraines.[13] These medications are almost exclusively off label for headache prevention and have other primary indications. Starting doses tend to be fractions of what are used for their primary indications. They are taken on a daily basis to reduce the frequency and intensity of headaches. Common examples of "headache prevention" medications include topiramate, nortriptyline, amitriptyline, valproate, gabapentin, propranolol, and verapamil. Consideration of medication requires a thorough understanding of each medication's side effect profile and the other symptoms the patient is experiencing. For example, an athlete who is experiencing insomnia in addition to headaches may benefit from a tricyclic antidepressant (TCAs) such as nortriptyline because sleepiness is a common side effect of the medication. Conversely, nortriptyline may exacerbate symptoms in those are experiencing hypersomnia. Tricyclic medications should be avoided in those with a cardiac history because they can cause prolongation of the QT interval. Equally important is a time frame for discontinuation of the medication. There should be an established period of headache freedom before weaning and discontinuing the medication.

Dizziness

Dizziness after a concussion is an often ill-defined descriptor for patients. Therefore, it is imperative that a detailed history of the reported symptomatology be performed. Postural dizziness, or feeling "lightheaded" when changing from a seated (or lying) position to a standing position, is most common. It should be noted that the adolescent population has a high incidence of postural orthostatic tachycardia syndrome (POTS) and typically has low resting blood pressure even in the absence of injury.[14] Dizziness as a result of vestibular dysfunction is present in more than of 80% of athletes after concussion.[15] Athletes often complain of symptoms if trying to track objects or watching television with an excessive amount of movement displayed. Dizziness as a result of posttraumatic vertigo is less common in young athletes but can happen nonetheless. Patients tend to report dizziness with a change in head position, such as rolling over in bed, tilting their heads back (in the shower), and bending over. These descriptions are of dizziness that tends to be intense and episodic, often rendering the patient incapable of movement until the vertigo has resolved.[16] Finally, dizziness can be a component of other symptoms, such as postconcussive headaches. This can occur in the absence of movement and is often accompanied by nausea. These patients also report experiencing motion sickness when traveling in a car.

The physical examination of the patients with concussion experiencing dizziness should be done in a detailed fashion. Cranial nerve examination, specifically extraocular movements, are particularly helpful to evaluate for nystagmus. Smooth pursuits and saccades are often impaired in the patients with concussion who have vestibular symptoms. Vestibular ocular reflex testing is especially useful in eliciting symptoms in postconcussive dizzy patients.[17] The intent of these maneuvers is to suppress the natural tendency to keep one's eyes fixed on an object while moving the head. An extreme example of this is evaluating a comatose patient for brainstem injury using what is commonly termed the "doll's head" maneuver. Those with an intact vestibular ocular reflex demonstrate eye movement when the head is moved in horizontal and vertical planes. In a patient with an impaired reflex (injured brainstem), the eyes remain in a fixed position. Although the details of these pathways are not suited for this chapter, this reflex is best illustrated in the conscious patient by maintaining visual fixation on a stationary object while moving the head in a horizontal or vertical plane. Suppression of the vestibular ocular reflex involves maintaining visual fixation on a moving object while moving the head in same direction as the object. For those complaining of symptoms consistent with vertigo, the Dix-Halpike maneuver can be diagnostic and provide an opportunity for immediate treatment. This should not be performed in patients with cervical spine injuries.

Treatment for dizziness is primarily focused on physical therapy. This is performed by therapists who specialize in vestibular therapy. For patients with postconcussive vertigo and demonstrate nystagmus with the Dix-Halpike maneuver, canalith repositioning (Epley maneuver) can be immediately therapeutic.[18] Medications for dizziness should be used sparingly because the side effects of these medications often exacerbate the other symptoms of postconcussive syndrome, especially fatigue.

Visual Disturbance

Visual disturbance in postconcussion patients can present in many forms, including blurry vision, double vision, or visual disturbance associated with other symptoms such as headache or dizziness.[19] Accommodation is commonly affected immediately after concussion and may manifest as difficulty with reading independent of comprehension. A lack of visual focus, near or far, is most common and typically self-resolves. The history should focus on characterizing the visual disturbance. Red flags include double vision in primary gaze, vertical skew, visual field loss, or monocular visual disturbance. These should all be indications for urgent neuroimaging and subspecialty assessment with ophthalmology or neuro-ophthalmology.

Examination of the athlete with visual disturbance begins with standard measures of acuity. An extraocular movement examination evaluating for cranial neuropathy is necessary. The assessment should also include smooth pursuits, saccadic movements, visual field testing by confrontation, and funduscopic examination. Reference to vestibular-ocular reflex suppression is described earlier in the section addressing dizziness. Dynamic visual acuity measures may be especially useful in evaluating an athlete who reports visual disturbance in his or her sport.[20] This is done by combining a physical task of movement with visual acuity. An example of this is a horizontal head movement while reading a Snellen chart.

Treatment for visual disturbances begins with vision therapy, often performed by occupational therapists. Activities typically focus on integrating eye movement activities with a motor task, such as touching a moving light on a large, fixed board. Such exercises are designed to address deficits in scanning, tracking, and visual fixation. For more persistent or challenging vision deficits, specific vision therapy by a trained optometrist may be indicated.[21]

Sleep Disturbance

Sleep disturbance after concussion is a statistically significant consequence of concussion independent of other physical symptoms and is often cited as such. Typically, a period of hypersomnia precedes some degree of insomnia. For those whose recovery is prolonged, insomnia with daytime fatigue is most common.[22] The history of a patient with insomnia should focus on stages of sleep.

Although most report difficulty initiating sleep, many report trouble maintaining sleep or have restless sleep. A history of premorbid sleep disturbance is useful in determining risk factors for delayed recovery. Questions should also focus on the nighttime habits, including watching television at night or a lack of a routine before going to bed. An assessment of the total amount of sleep in a 24-hour period may reveal compensation during the day with naps. Additional modifying factors often include head or neck pain that prevents patients from falling asleep as well as anxiety that keeps them preoccupied at night.

Treatment and management of sleep disturbance can be challenging but may result in improvement of other associated symptoms, including headaches, fatigue, and cognitive impairment. "Sleep hygiene" is a nonpharmacologic approach to managing sleep. A behavioral approach to sleep management, sleep hygiene focuses on the environmental factors that promote sleep.[23] This includes establishing deliberate routine for sleep, such as going to bed at the same time, turning down the lights in the evening, avoiding caffeine after noon, and engaging in relaxing activities such as bathing. Pharmacologic management of sleep disturbance is less well defined. Medications that treat concussion comorbidities such as headache may be helpful in reducing multiple symptoms while limiting exposure to medication and side effects. The TCAs, often used for headache prevention in low doses, produce the side effect of fatigue, which may be mutually beneficial to the patient. Medications that are designed specifically for sleep may result in undesirable side effects. However, they may be helpful in rare postconcussion patients who complain of insomnia in isolation. Studies are underway to evaluate the efficacy of melatonin on insomnia in postconcussive patients.[24]

Endocrine Disturbance

Hormonal deficits are among the most overlooked and undiagnosed consequences of TBI.[25] This is particularly relevant for patients whose symptoms persist for months to years. Given the location of the pituitary gland within the sella turcica and thin connection to the hypothalamus via the pituitary stalk, the neuroendocrine system is susceptible to traumatic injury and dysfunction. Such dysfunction may present as fatigue and changes in weight, menses, and libido. Physical examination tends to be unrevealing in these cases, but evaluation for neuroendocrine dysfunction includes serum hormonal analysis, specifically thyroid hormones (thyroid-stimulating hormone), follicle stimulating hormone, luteinizing hormone, and growth hormone.[26] When hypopituitarism is detected, referral to an endocrinologist for hormone replacement is indicated.

Seizures

In contrast to moderate and severe TBI, seizures and posttraumatic epilepsy are an uncommon consequence of mild TBI. The incidence ranges from 2% to 4% of those who have a history of concussion.[27] A seizure occurring immediately after a concussion is considered part of the injury and does not confer an increased risk for epilepsy.[28] When evaluating patients for posttraumatic seizures, a history of staring spells, lip smacking, and nocturnal enuresis may represent more subtle indications of seizure activity. Generalized tonic-clonic movements of the extremities are more obvious signs of seizure. When concerned for seizure, electroencephalography and neuroimaging (preferably with MRI) are indicated.

Treatment for seizures with anticonvulsant medication should be initiated and managed by a neurologist. Posttraumatic seizures are typically localized in nature, so the choice of antiepileptic medication should cover localization related seizures.

● BEHAVIORAL SYMPTOMS

Behavioral changes after a concussion are among the most common and most disturbing to a family. They also represent the most common reason for PCS.[5] Although irritability is the most common symptom immediately after an injury, anxiety and depression represent the most common long-term problems.[29]

Irritability

Patients and their family members often describe irritability as having a "short fuse," moody, and impulsive. Modifying factors include the physical factors that influence mood, including insomnia, headaches, and musculoskeletal pain. History should include input from loved ones, but if they are not available, patients should be asked how family members perceive their mood. Efforts to manage irritability include treating the primary medical condition and directly addressing the behavioral health needs of the patient with psychology and psychiatry.

Depression

Depression can occur as a direct or indirect consequence of TBI. In patients with PCS, a sense of feeling depressed may not always be expressed.[30] However, patients may report feeling sad and constantly fatigued. Many report hypersomnia but often have restless sleep. Although they may have not been clinically diagnosed with depression, attention should be paid to a history of depressive symptoms as well as a family history of depression. Red flags include suicidal or homicidal ideation, as well as a sense of hopelessness. Examination findings include a flat affect and emotional lability. Treatment for depression may be initiated with antidepressants, though psychiatrists are best suited to manage medication. Similarly, psychotherapy should be used early to address depressive symptomatology.

Anxiety

Patients with anxiety after a concussion report a sense of feeling "overwhelmed." This is especially true of high-performing athletes who also excel academically. These student athletes become consumed with the physical and cognitive consequences of injury and fall behind in their studies. This often leads to increased stress manifesting as insomnia, panic attacks, and heightened emotions. Addressing the modifying factors can significantly impact outcomes. This includes treating the physical symptoms, addressing the cognitive symptoms, and providing academic accommodations to alleviate external pressures. Additionally, introducing noncontact physical activity can often serve as an outlet for physical and emotional stress. Emphasis should be placed on avoiding contact while monitoring for exacerbation of symptoms. Although short-term anxiolytics should be used with caution in young populations, pharmacologic management may be useful in addressing acutely stressful situations, such as panic attacks.[31] As with depression, psychiatry and behavioral psychology are valuable resources for continued treatment.

Psychosis

Psychosis as an element of postconcussive syndrome is a rare, often acute event that requires inpatient psychiatric management. Red flags include bizarre affect, visual, and auditory hallucinations.[32] Excluding structural lesions is recommended in this setting, though they are rarely found.

● COGNITIVE SYMPTOMS

The cognitive deficits associated with postconcussive syndrome are among the most common and pertinent to student athletes.[33] Lack of focus, short-term memory deficits, and slowed processing speed are the most common cognitive deficits after a concussion. When they persist,

NP testing, academic accommodations, and speech therapy are the gold standards for evaluation, management, and treatment respectively.[34–36]

Focus and Attention

Trouble with focus and inattention are the most common reported cognitive symptoms postconcussion. Attentional deficits are often misdiagnosed as memory deficits because the lack of focus keeps one from efficiently creating new memories. Many student athletes report a limited ability to stay focused when reading book passages or paying attention in class. They often feel that they lose their train of thought when speaking or have an inability to follow conversations. Parents typically report that their children miss details and repeat questions.

Academic accommodations at any point in the recovery process are helpful to struggling student athletes. Specifically, preferential seating (front of the class) and additional time for assignments and tests help to minimize distractions and allow for adequate time to complete work.[37] Rarely, stimulants can be helpful with inattention. However, because most are controlled substances, they should be reserved for those who have a preexisting comorbid diagnosis of attention deficit hyperactivity disorder.[38] Use of such medications can also impact eligibility to participate in collegiate and professional sports. Therefore, one should become familiar with specific guidelines before prescribing these medications.

Memory

Although impaired memory for the injury is a hallmark of concussion, persistent memory deficits are often reported in PCS.[39] As previously mentioned, deficits in attention are often confused for memory deficits. However, short-term memory deficits often coexist with attentional ones. One should be wary of long-term memory deficits because they are highly atypical for concussion and are likely to represent psychological disturbance or, rarely, a structural lesion. NP testing should be used to distinguish verbal memory deficits from visual memory deficits.[40] Such details are useful in prescribing specific academic accommodations. Examples of accommodations for visual memory deficits include recording lectures and using note takers. For those with verbal memory deficits, written distribution of materials can be beneficial. Speech therapists with special training and certification in cognition are crucial in the neurologic rehabilitation of patients with memory deficits.

Word-Finding and Processing Speed

Word-finding processing speed deficits are an often frustrating experience for those recovering from concussion. Many patients with PCS report greater trouble finding words when under pressure and in stressful situations. They also report feeling "stupid" as their working vocabulary decreases temporarily. Processing speed deficits manifest as accurate but slow completion of tasks.[41] Student athletes tend to have trouble completing in-class assignments and tests, though the questions answered are often correct. As with other aspects of cognition, NP evaluation and speech therapy are particularly useful for assessment and treatment, respectively. Academic accommodations for such deficits include increased time to complete assignments and tests.

● CONCLUSION

Postconcussion syndrome and persistent postconcussive symptoms require an understanding of the physical, behavioral, and cognitive symptoms associated with the injury. History and examination are keys to determining the most pressing and relevant symptoms to assess, manage, and treat. Comprehensive evaluations include detailed neurologic examination, neuroimaging, NP evaluation, and psychiatric consultation. As such, the multidisciplinary setting provides the most comprehensive approach to this disorder. When not available in a single setting, access to the disciplines of neurology, neuropsychology, psychiatry, and psychology are necessary to assess and manage the complex medical needs of the patient. Equally important are therapists who specialize in concussion (physical, occupational, and speech). Although the long-term consequences of prolonged recovery from concussion are not entirely understood, it is important to address them presently with the best available resources and treatments.

REFERENCES

1. American Psychiatric Association: *Diagnosis and Statistical Manual of Mental Disorders (DSM-IV-TR),* ed 4. Washington, DC, American Psychiatric Association, 2000.

2. Gil-Gouveia R, Oliveira AG, Martins IP: Assessment of cognitive dysfunction during migraine attacks: a systematic review. *J Neurol* 2015;262(3):654–665.

3. Lange RT, Brickell TA, Kennedy JE, et al: Factors influencing postconcussion and posttraumatic stress symptom reporting following military-related concurrent polytrauma and traumatic brain injury. *Arch Clin Neuropsychol* 2014;29(4):329–347.

4. Morgan CD, Zuckerman SL, Lee YM, King L, Beaird S, Sills AK, Solomon GS: Predictors of postconcussion syndrome after sports-related concussion in young athletes: A matched case-control study. *J Neurosurg Pediatr* 2015;15(6):589–598.

5. Prigatano GP, Gale SD: The current status of postconcussion syndrome. *Curr Opin Psychiatry* 2011;24(3):243–250.

6. Riechers RG 2nd, Walker MF, Ruff RL: Post-traumatic headaches. *Handb Clin Neurol* 2015;128:567–578.

7. Solomon S: Posttraumatic headache. *Med Clin North Am* 2001;85:987–996, vii–viii.

8. Anderson K, Tinawi S, Lamoureux J, Feyz M, de Guise E: Detecting migraine in patients with mild traumatic brain injury using three different headache measures. *Behav Neurol* 2015:1–7.

9. Kjeldgaard D, Forchhammer H, Teasdale T, Rigmor H, Jensen R: Chronic post-traumatic headache after mild head injury: A descriptive study. *Cephalalgia* 2014;34(3):191–200.

10. Sangermani R and Boncimino A: Adolescent migraine: Diagnostic and therapeutic approaches. *Neurol Sci* 2015;36:S89–S92.

11. Pearce M, Salotti J A, Little M P, et al: Radiation exposure from CT scans in childhood and subsequent risk of leukaemia and brain tumours: A retrospective cohort study. *Lancet* 2012;380:499–505.

12. Delouche A, Attyé A, Heck O, et al: Pitfalls, literature review and future directions of research in mild traumatic brain injury. *Eur J Radiol* 2016;85(1):25–30.

13. Lew HL, Lin P-H, Fuh J-L, Wang S-J, Clark DJ, Walker WC: Characteristics and treatment of headache after traumatic brain injury: A focused review. *Am J Phys Med Rehabil* 2006;85:619–627.

14. Kizilbash S J, Ahrens SP, Bruce BK: Adolescent fatigue, POTS, and recovery: A guide for clinicians. *Curr Probl Pediatr Adolesc Health Care* 2014;44:108–133.

15. Corwin DJ, Wiebe DJ, Zonfrillo MR, Grady MF, Robinson RL, Goodman AM, Master CL: Vestibular deficits following youth concussion. *J Pediatr* 2015;166(5):1221–1225.

16. Pisani V, Mazzone S, Di Mauro R, Giacomini PG, Di Girolamo S: A survey of the nature of trauma of posttraumatic benign paroxysmal positional vertigo. *Int J Audiol* 2015;54(5):329–333.

17. Mucha A, Collins MW, Elbin RJ, et al: A brief vestibular/ocular motor screening (VOMS) assessment to evaluate concussions: Preliminary findings. *Am J Sports Med* 2014;42(10):2479–2486.

18. Teixeira LJ, Machado JN: Maneuvers for the treatment of benign positional paroxysmal vertigo: A systematic review. *Braz J Otorhinolaryngol* 2006;72(1):130–139.

19. Master CL, Scheiman M, Gallaway M, Goodman A, Robinson RL, Master SR, Grady MF: Vision diagnoses are common after concussion in adolescents. *Clin Pediatr (Phila)* 2016;55(3)260–267.

20. Kaufman DR, Puckett MJ, Smith MJ, Wilson KS, Cheema R, Landers MR: Test-retest reliability and responsiveness of gaze stability and dynamic visual acuity in high school and college football players. *Phys Ther Sport* 2014;15(3):181–188.

21. Barnett BP, Singman EL: Vision concerns after mild traumatic brain injury. *Curr Treat Options Neurol* 2015;17(2):329.

22. Theadom A, Cropley M, Parmar P, Barker-Collo S, Starkey N, Jones K, Feigin VL: Sleep difficulties one year following mild traumatic brain injury in a population-based study. *Sleep Med* 2015;15:926–932.

23. Trauer JM, Qian MY, Doyle JS, W Rajaratnam SM, Cunnington D: Cognitive behavioral therapy for chronic insomnia: A systematic review and meta-analysis. *Ann Intern Med* 2015;163(3):191–204.

24. Barlow KM, Brooks BL, McMaster FP, et al: A double-blind, placebo-controlled intervention trial of 3 and 10 mg sublingual melatonin for post-concussion syndrome in youths (PLAYGAME): Study protocol for a randomized controlled trial. *Trials* 2014;15:271.

25. Gaddam SS, Buell T, Robertson CS: Systemic manifestations of traumatic brain injury. *Handb Clin Neurol* 2015;127:205–218.

26. Fernandez-Rodriguez E, Bernabeu I, Castro AI, Casanueva FF: Hypopituitarism after traumatic brain injury. *Endocrinol Metab Clin North Am* 2015;44(1):151–159.

27. Lowenstein DH: Epilepsy after head injury: An overview. *Epilepsia* 2009;50(suppl 2):4–9.

28. Treiman DM: Current treatment strategies in selected situations in epilepsy. *Epilepsia* 1993;34(suppl 5):S17–S23.

29. Chrisman SP, Richardson LP: Prevalence of diagnosed depression in adolescents with history of concussion. *J Adolesc Health* 2014;54(5):582–586.

30. Lange RT, Brickell TA, Kennedy JE, et al: Factors influencing postconcussion and posttraumatic stress symptom reporting following military-related concurrent polytrauma and traumatic brain injury. *Arch Clin Neuropsychol* 2014;29(4):329–347.

31. Mott TF, McConnon ML, Rieger BP: Subacute to chronic mild traumatic brain injury. *Am Fam Physician* 2012;86(11):1045–1051.

32. Sherer M, Yablon SA, Nick TG: Psychotic symptoms as manifestations of the posttraumatic confusional state: Prevalence, risk factors, and association with outcome. *J Head Trauma Rehabil* 2014;29(2):E11–E18.

33. Macciocchi SN, Barth JT, Alves W, Rimel RW, Jane JA: Neuropsychological functioning and recovery after mild head injury in collegiate athletes. *Neurosurgery* 1996;39(3):510–514.

34. Echemendia RJ, Iverson GL, McCrea M, Macciocchi SN, Gioia GA, Putukian M, Comper P: Advances in neuropsychological assessment of sport-related concussion. *Br J Sports Med* 2013;47(5):294–298.

35. Bennett TD, Niedzwecki CM, Korgenski EK, Bratton SL: Initiation of physical, occupational, and speech therapy in children with traumatic brain injury. *Arch Phys Med Rehabil* 2013;94(7):1268–1276.

36. Hall EE, Ketcham CJ, Crenshaw CR, Baker MH, McConnell JM, Patel K: Concussion management in collegiate student-athletes: Return-to-academics recommendations. *Clin J Sport Med* 2015;25(3):291–296.

37. Popoli DM, Burns TG, Meehan WP 3rd, Reisner A; Children's Health of Atlanta (CHOA) Concussion Consensus: Establishing a uniform policy for academic accommodations. *Clin Pediatr (Phila)* 2014;53(3):217–224.

38. Brooks BL, Iverson GL, Atkins JE, Zafonte R, Berkner PD: Sex differences and self-reported attention problems during baseline concussion testing. *Appl Neuropsychol Child* 2016;5(2):119–126.

39. Sherer M, Davis LC, Sander AM, Nick TG, Luo C, Pastorek N, Hanks R: Factors associated with word memory test performance in persons with medically documented traumatic brain Injury. *Clin Neuropsychol* 2015;29(4):522–541.

40. McCauley SR, Wilde EA, Barnes A, Hanten G, Hunter JV, Levin HS, Smith DH: Patterns of early emotional and neuropsychological sequelae after mild traumatic brain injury. *J Neurotrauma* 2014;31(10):914–925.

41. Carlozzi NE, Kirsch NL, Kisala PA, Tulsky DS: An examination of the Wechsler Adult Intelligence Scales, Fourth Edition (WAIS-IV) in individuals with complicated mild, moderate and severe traumatic brain injury (TBI). *Clin Neuropsychol* 2015;29(1):21–37.

28 Concussion: Long Term Sequelae—The Controversy

Rajiv Saigal, MD, PhD • Mitchel Berger, MD

INTRODUCTION

The possibility of long-term neurologic deficits from repetitive head trauma first appeared in medical literature in the 1920s, but it has gained considerable public attention in recent years. First described as "punch-drunk syndrome" in boxers by Martland in 1928,[1] chronic traumatic encephalopathy (CTE) is the modern term for this neurodegenerative disorder. Yet this clinical entity that is nearly a century old remains controversial. Although there are increasing neuropathological data from deceased, former athletes, there remains a paucity of systemic or prospective studies to understand who is at risk or why some develop the condition and some do not. Many athletes who sustain repeated head impacts do not go on to develop CTE. Although most recent media attention has focused on CTE, other possible long-term sequelae exist across a spectrum from mild cognitive impairment (MCI) to Alzheimer disease to CTE. What risk factors cause some to develop long-term sequelae and others not? How much risk does repeated head trauma entail? When is it safe for a concussed athlete to return to play (RTP)? These remain important, unanswered questions. This review seeks to answer what is currently known and unknown about the long-term sequelae of repeated mild traumatic brain injury (mTBI) in sports.

CONCUSSION

Contact sports are highly popular, and approximately 300,000 to 3.8 million sports-related concussions occur annually in the United States.[2-5] In the subset of American high school athletes, approximately 63,000 sports-related concussions occur annually and require removal from play; 63% of these are in football.[6] Female athletes have higher concussion rates than male athletes in common sports: 0.85 concussions per 1000 games in female versus 0.45 per 1000 in male basketball players and 1.8 per 1000 in female versus 1.38 per 1000 in male soccer players.[7]

Concussion is closed mTBI with posttraumatic amnesia or confusion.[8] Common clinical symptoms in the postconcussive syndrome include impaired attention and concentration, headache, impaired memory, cognitive dysfunction, nausea, vomiting, mood changes, irritability, light and sound sensitivity, sleep disturbance, and fatigue.[8] *Concussion* and *mTBI* are most often used interchangeably, although some groups define subtle distinctions between the two.[9] The Fourth International Conference on Concussion in Sport defined concussion broadly as a "complex pathophysiological process affecting the brain, induced by biomechanical forces."[9] Rapid symptom onset, loss of consciousness (LOC), direct impact to the head, and relatively quick recovery (often <10 days) may occur but are not required to meet the formal definition.[9] Postconcussive symptoms affect up to 50% of patients 1 year after injury.[10]

The exact force and acceleration required to cause a concussion remains a topic of study. Accelerometers placed in football helmets have yielded quantitative information regarding forces and acceleration required for concussion. **Table 28-1** shows these values. National Football League (NFL) studies showed concussive impacts average 98 times gravitational acceleration (98 × 9.8 m/sec^2, or 98 g), and nonconcussive impacts average 60 g.[11] Additional study is needed to gather similar information from other levels of competition and other sports.

CONTROVERSIES

Several controversial subtopics are related to potential long-term sequelae from repetitive head trauma in sports.

Neither of the following authors nor any immediate family member has received anything of value from or has stock or stock options held in a commercial company or institution related directly or indirectly to the subject of this article: Dr. Berger and Dr. Saigal.

TABLE 28-1	Impact characteristics predictive of concussion in football
Rotational acceleration	5582.3 rad/sec^2
Linear acceleration	96.1 g
Location	Top, front, and back of helmet

Data from Bailes JE, Petraglia AL, Omalu BI, Nauman E, Talavage T: Role of subconcussion in repetitive mild traumatic brain injury. *J Neurosurg* 2013;119(5):1235–1245 and Broglio SP, Schnebel B, Sosnoff JJ, Shin S, Fend X, He X, Zimmerman J: Biomechanical properties of concussions in high school football. *Med Sci Sports Exerc* 2010;42(11):2064–2071.

These include subconcussion, MCI, CTE, apolipoprotein E4 (ApoE4), dementia, and RTP guidelines. Each is discussed separately in this chapter.

SUBCONCUSSION

Subconcussion is a milder form of TBI not meeting the formal diagnostic criteria for concussion. The characteristic concussion symptoms of headache, visual disturbance, amnesia, confusion, gait or postural instability, and dizziness do not occur in subconcussion.[12] Regardless, there is now some evidence that subconcussive blows may also lead to long-term sequelae.[13–15]

Boxers were the first group of athletes noted to have potential long-term neurodegeneration from repeated head trauma, and research has continued to corroborate this early finding. The degree to which this risk is due to concussive or subconcussive trauma is unknown. In one report, neuropsychological (NP) tests, CT, and electroencephalography (EEG)-based evidence showed more bouts correlated with higher cognitive impairment even in young fighters.[16] The authors speculated that this could be due to repeated subconcussion.[16] In the absence of quantitative data on subconcussions and concussions sustained during training and competition, there are insufficient data to support this claim.

Helmet accelerometer data showed that football players experience between 100 head impacts per season in youth and 1000 in college.[12] Even in the absence of concussion, these impacts can cause lasting sequelae. Nonconcussed college athletes scored lower in NP tests and memory than control participants.[12,17] Even at the high school level, there is a subset of football players who have no history of diagnosed concussion yet demonstrate altered activation of the prefrontal cortex and impaired visual memory on neurocognitive testing.[18] This same group of athletes had higher numbers of accelerometer-recorded impacts to the front and top of the head.[18] Follow-up studies using magnetic resonance spectroscopy showed metabolic abnormalities in high school football players after subconcussive trauma.[19] Short-term abnormalities in connectivity were seen on functional MRI (fMRI).[20] If validated through further study, this presents an opportunity for rules changes to improve player safety, such as decreasing the number of full contact practices in order to decrease the total number of head impacts.

MILD COGNITIVE IMPAIRMENT

Mild cognitive impairment is a memory deficit beyond age-related norms, corroborated by either neurocognitive testing or family but with insufficient symptoms to meet diagnostic criteria for dementia; impairment is mild enough that the patient can still complete activities of daily living.[21] A 2005 survey-based study assessed whether MCI was associated with repeated concussion in retired professional football players.[22] A total of 24% sustained at least three concussions during their professional careers, and this group had a fivefold increased prevalence of MCI.[22] Only 17.6% of players with history of concussion believed that it had an enduring effect on cognition. For a survey-based study, there was a relatively high participation rate of 69% (2552 of 3683) in the concussion questionnaire. However, less than 30% (758 of 2552) of the entire cohort completed the MCI-based questionnaire, limiting the interpretation of these data.[22]

Amateur athletes are also subject to risks of repeated mild TBI. High school athletes with at least three prior concussions showed increased concussion severity, including anterograde amnesia, confusion, and LOC, compared with those without concussion.[23] These data support the argument that RTP should be disallowed after three concussions in a season.[8,24] According to data recorded from helmet accelerometers in high school football players, there does not appear to be a correlation between number of prior hits to the head and impact threshold for a new concussion.[25] In other words, the same magnitude of head impact is required to cause a concussion, whether or not the player has sustained prior concussions. In a comparison of amateur boxers with matched soccer and track athletes, boxers had inferior finger-tapping scores and slight EEG abnormalities but no other difference in neurologic examination findings.[26]

CHRONIC TRAUMATIC ENCEPHALOPATHY

Chronic traumatic encephalopathy is a progressive neurodegenerative disorder caused by perivascular tau-positive neurofibrillary tangles, with an absence of the amyloid beta deposits seen in Alzheimer disease.[27,28] Gross brain disturbances may include atrophy of frontal and temporal lobes, cavum septum pellucidum, ventriculomegaly, corpus callosum thinning, and white matter loss.[27] Clinically, patients with CTE may exhibit components of cognition, mood, behavior, and motor dysfunction.[27] Case reports from the Center for the Study of Traumatic Encephalopathy (CSTE) at Boston University have shown evidence of CTE pathology in a subset of retired athletes.[5,14,28-37] These former athletes with CTE had a mean exposure to repetitive head trauma of 15.4 years with symptom onset 14.5 years after initial exposure.[27] A total of 92% (33 or 36) of cases displayed clinical symptoms before death.[30] **Table 28-2** shows clinical findings in one case series on CTE.[30] Nonetheless, data on CTE correlation to repetitive concussion remain mixed and controversial. Although 84% of diagnosed cases had history of concussion, the remaining ones did not, raising the possibility that subconcussive trauma or other factors may also cause risk.[27]

A 2013 CSTE study compared 85 deceased cases with history of TBI (94% former athletes) against 18 deceased control cases (matched for age and gender) without history of TBI.[28] Although 61% (11 of 18) of control participants had evidence of Alzheimer pathology, none met diagnostic criteria for CTE. A total of 80% (68 of 85) of TBI participants had pathologic evidence of CTE, including phosphorylated tau neurofibrillary tangles and astrocytic tangles.[22] Of these, CTE cases carried an additional diagnosis, including Lewy body disease ($n = 11$), Alzheimer disease ($n = 7$), and frontotemporal lobar dementia ($n = 4$). Comparison of CTE prevalence in the two groups by the Fisher exact test leads to a significant difference with P less than 0.0001, but the result is misleading. The main criticism of these case series is the high risk of selection bias.[38] Former athletes who sustained neurocognitive impairment during their lives may be more likely to donate their brains for postmortem study. Although there is no doubt CTE exists in some former athletes, we are unable to assess the exact prevalence or how number of prior concussion correlates with risk of CTE development. An unbiased, broad sample of former athletes would be necessary to better address these questions.

Reports from other centers have shown confounding data. One recent small case series ($n = 6$) assessed former Canadian Football League players who all had history of repetitive head trauma and cognitive decline. Half of the former CFL players had CTE pathology on postmortem

TABLE 28-2	Clinical symptoms and signs during life in postmortem-confirmed diagnosis of chronic traumatic encephalopathy, displayed in order of decreasing prevalence

Sign or Symptom	Prevalence (%)
Execution and memory impairment	100
Language deficits	70
Gait difficulty	40
Physically violent	40
History of falls	30
Visuospatial deficits	20
Verbally violent	20
Tremor	10

Data from Stern RA, Daneshvar DH, Baugh CM, et al: Clinical presentation of chronic traumatic encephalopathy. *Neurology* 2013;81(13):1122–1129.

neuropathologic examination; the other half did not, despite similar exposure.[39]

From 1954 to 2013, there were 153 published, neuropathologically confirmed CTE cases, 86% of whom played football or boxed.[38] A total of 70% of deaths were from natural causes, 17% were accidental, and 12.6% were suicides. A total of 19.6% abused a substance, including alcohol, painkillers, and marijuana. A total of 61% were homozygous for ApoE3, and all had at least either one allele of ApoE3 or one allele of ApoE4.

There are 63 former football players with pathology-confirmed CTE, two thirds of whom played in the NFL. Nearly 80% of cases since 2002 have been in former football players. It is unclear if this high number reflects a changing incidence rate or rather a selection bias toward autopsy, as mentioned earlier. About one third of cases are in former athletes younger than 50 years of age.[38] The 2012 international consensus statement on concussion in sports stated that the cause-and-effect relationship between repeated athletic head trauma and subsequent development of CTE is not yet established.[9]

At present, the diagnosis of CTE may only be confirmed postmortem. Novel imaging modalities may eventually offer diagnostic options during life. fMRI is one modality to assess for abnormal brain connectivity. An fMRI study of former NFL players showed hypoconnectivity of the dorsolateral frontal and frontopolar cortices compared with control participants.[20] As mentioned earlier, connectivity abnormalities have been documented in high school athletes after subconcussive blows,[20] so diagnostic imaging techniques to separate those with mild connective impairment versus more advanced neurodegeneration or CTE require further study.

Other imaging modalities may better delineate neuropathology after repeated mTBI. Diffusion tensor imaging (DTI) was used to show subcortical grey matter and white matter abnormalities in boxers. A history of more knockouts, but not higher fight numbers, correlated with these changes.[40] The posterior cingulate gyrus showed abnormal transversal diffusivity in mixed martial artists.[40] Follow-up studies showed abnormal putaminal and callosal transverse diffusivity, associated with number of bouts, and reduced putamenal resting state connectivity.[41] White matter integrity was associated with depressive symptoms in a small case series of NFL retirees.[42] DTI fractional anisotropy (DTI FA) assessment of forceps major white matter disruption was 95% specific and 100% sensitive in identifying depression in NFL retirees.[42] Prospective, randomized studies are needed to further examine white matter and other changes seen in this group of former athletes.

DOES ApoE4 CARRY ADDED RISK?

Cholesterol-carrier proteins called apolipoproteins (Apo) have been associated with certain neurodegenerative disorders. In particular, ApoE4 allele is associated with a twofold increase in the risk of Alzheimer disease. In patients with ApoE4 and history of TBI, this jumps to a 10-fold risk. Boxers with at least 12 professional bouts and an ApoE ε4 allele score worse (higher) on chronic brain injury scores (0–9 scale) than those without the allele (3.9 vs. 1.8, respectively; $P = 0.04$).[43] The score difference is comparable to the 2.3 score improvement in those with fewer bouts (2.6 vs. 0.3, respectively; $P < 0.001$).[43] In a study of 53 active NFL players, those with the ApoE ε4 allele and age older than 27.1 years (the mean age for the study group) had poorer memory and attention scores but not spatial ability or reasoning.[44] Age was used as a proxy for contact exposure, but it is a crude proxy and likely not true in all cases, even within the same sport.

The exact mechanism by which ApoE4 affects long-term outcomes from repeated head injury is unknown. It may be due to ε4 allele-specific inhibition of neurite outgrowth,[45,46] astrocyte dysfunction or endoplasmic reticulum stress,[47] impaired dendritic arborization,[48] or other mechanisms. Although the ApoE4 allele has been associated with these changes, it does not show added risk for development of CTE ($P = 0.26$).[38] McKee et al

also found no evidence of increased ApoE4 in CTE cases compared with control participants ($P = 0.33$).[28]

DEMENTIA

A 2008 questionnaire-based study of 1063 former NFL players found a 6.1% rate of dementia in retirees older than 50 years of age compared with 1.2% in the general U.S. male population.[49] Although it is tempting to assign causation to repetitive head trauma, available data were insufficient to do so. First, the study relied on self-reporting from players or proxy family members rather than objective data. Second, it is unclear if head trauma, training regimen, performance enhancing supplements, genetic predisposition, or other factors led to this increased prevalence. The same study showed similar rates of current depression (3.9% for NFL players aged 30–49 years vs. 3.0% of control participants; 3.6% for NFL players aged ≥50 years vs. 3.6% of control participants) between the two groups, although former NFL players had higher rates on depression screening questions (75.3% for NFL players aged 30–49 years vs. 61.2% of control participants; 63.3% for NFL players aged ≥50 years vs. 58.1% of control participants).[49] NFL players had lower rates of intermittent explosive disorder (uncontrollable, unprovoked anger) based on screening questions (31% for NFL players aged 30 to 49 years vs. 55% of control participants; 29% for NFL players older than 50 years versus 29.3% of control participants).[49]

A statistically insignificant trend between recurrent concussion and subsequent development of Alzheimer disease in retired professional football players was seen compared with an age-matched general population (prevalence ratio, 1.37; confidence interval [CI], 0.98–1.56). There was no association between number of prior concussions and development of Alzheimer disease.[22]

RETURN-TO-PLAY GUIDELINES

Given the potential risk for long term sequelae without sufficient cognitive rest, the consensus guidelines state that players who sustain a concussion should not be allowed to RTP on the same day.[9] Consensus statements recommend a six-step, graduated protocol for RTP in which players progress from no activity to light exercise (aerobic and then sport specific) to noncontact drills to full contact and finally RTP.[9] The recommended time period between steps is at least 1 day, and a player should progress to the next level only if asymptomatic. However, this recommendation is only at the level of expert opinion, with a lack of evidence to support specific time frames for rest or types of activity. Further study is needed to see if the recommended protocol is superior to other options for gradual RTP. Please see Chapter 25 for a detailed discussion on this topic.

FUTURE DIRECTIONS FOR RESEARCH

Although published reports show examples of CTE and other neurodegenerative disorders in some retired athletes, the exact risk remains controversial. Retired NFL players have received great attention recently because of publicity regarding CTE. Nonetheless, published case series must be interpreted with caution in light of possible selection bias. Some studies suggest increased risk because the overall standardized mortality ratio (SMR) from neurodegenerative disorders is higher for NFL players 2.83 (CI, 1.36–5.21) as are mortality ratios for specific diseases, such as Alzheimer disease (SMR, 3.86; CI, 1.55–7.95) and amyotrophic lateral sclerosis (SMR, 4.31; CI, 1.73–8.87).[50] Conversely, NFL players carry a lower SMR than the general public (SMR, 0.53; CI, 0.48–059).[50]

Concussion, or mTBI, consists of at least two phases that offer opportunities for research and possible intervention. Primary injury occurs as a result of mechanical stress and strain on the brain from rapid rotational forces or linear acceleration-deceleration.[15,51] The potential targets for intervention here are preventative ones: neck strengthening and novel helmet designs to help absorb the blow, altered techniques to limit head contact (e.g., starting lineman in a standing rather than three point stance at the line of scrimmage), and rules changes to decrease number and velocity of head impacts (e.g., moving the kickoff from the 30- to 35-yard line).[12,52] Concussion rates were lowered from 7.6% to 5.4% in high school football players by using helmets with thicker internal padding and greater offset.[53] In collegiate football players, the concussion rate was reduced from 8.4 to 3.9 concussions per 100,000 head impacts with a new, more padded helmet design.[52]

The secondary injury phase involves neuronal and axonal injury, disruption to the blood–brain barrier, and excitotoxicity. Neuroinflammation is a prominent component of either this or a chronic, tertiary phase, depending on semantic definitions. Each of these pathophysiological mechanisms offers potential for pharmaceutical development to lessen deleterious impacts on the brain. Additionally, the treating clinician can help protect the brain by diagnosing concussion and limiting RTP while the brain is in a vulnerable state.

RECOMMENDATIONS

- Any athlete with suspected concussion should be evaluated by a medical professional.
- After a diagnosed concussion, an athlete should be removed from play for the remainder of the game.
- Strong consideration should be given to removing an athlete from the remainder of the season after three concussions, with the understanding that even fewer numbers may carry cumulative risks.
- Although athletes should be aware of potential risks from repetitive traumatic head injury, this should not be taken as a societal call to ban contact sports. Besides risks, there are also health benefits to athletic competition, as seen in the net overall decrease in mortality in NFL retirees.
- Knowledge of potential long-term neurologic sequelae presents an opportunity to improve player safety through education, rule adjustments, and safety equipment, as needed.

REFERENCES

1. Martland HS: Punch drunk. *JAMA* 1928;91(15):1103–1107.

2. Langlois JA, Rutland-Brown W, Wald MM: The epidemiology and impact of traumatic brain injury: A brief overview. *J Head Trauma Rehabil* 2006;21(5):375–378.

3. Gessel LM, Fields SK, Collins CL, Dick RW, Comstock RD: Concussions among United States high school and collegiate athletes. *J Athl Train* 2007;42(4):495–503.

4. Sosin DM, Sniezek JE, Thurman DJ: Incidence of mild and moderate brain injury in the United States, 1991. *Brain Inj* 1996;10(1):47–54.

5. Daneshvar DH, Nowinski CJ, McKee AC, Cantu RC: The epidemiology of sport-related concussion. *Clin Sports Med* 2011;30(1):1–17, vii.

6. Powell JW, Barber-Foss KD: Traumatic brain injury in high school athletes. *JAMA* 1999;282(10):958–963.

7. Giza CC, Kutcher JS, Ashwal S, et al: Summary of evidence-based guideline update: evaluation and management of concussion in sports: Report of the Guideline Development Subcommittee of the American Academy of Neurology. *Neurology* 2013;80(24):2250–2257.

8. Practice parameter: The management of concussion in sports (summary statement). Report of the Quality Standards Subcommittee. *Neurology* 1997;48(3):581–585.

9. McCrory P, Meeuwisse WH, Aubry M, et al: Consensus statement on concussion in sport: The 4th International Conference on Concussion in Sport held in Zurich, November 2012. *Br J Sports Med* 2013;47(5):250–258.

10. Middleboe T, Andersen HS, Birket-Smith M, Friis ML: Minor head injury: Impact on general health after 1 year. A prospective follow-up study. *Acta Neurol Scand* 1992; 85(1):5–9.

11. Pellman EJ, Viano DC, Tucker AM, Casson IR, Waeckerle JF: Concussion in professional football: Reconstruction of game impacts and injuries. *Neurosurgery* 2003;53(4):799–812; discussion 812–814.

12. Bailes JE, Petraglia AL, Omalu BI, Nauman E, Talavage T: Role of subconcussion in repetitive mild traumatic brain injury. *J Neurosurg* 2013;119(5):1235–1245.

13. Broglio SP, Schnebel B, Sosnoff JJ, Shin S, Fend X, He X, Zimmerman J: Biomechanical properties of concussions in high school football. *Med Sci Sports Exerc* 2010;42(11):2064–2071.

14. Baugh CM, Stamm JM, Riley DO, et al: Chronic traumatic encephalopathy: Neurodegeneration following repetitive concussive and subconcussive brain trauma. *Brain Imaging Behav* 2012;6(2):244–254.

15. Gavett BE, Stern RA, McKee AC: Chronic traumatic encephalopathy: A potential late effect of sport-related concussive and subconcussive head trauma. *Clin Sports Med* 2011;30(1):179–188, xi.

16. Casson IR, Siegel O, Sham R, Campbell EA, Tarlau M, DiDomenico A: Brain damage in modern boxers. *JAMA* 1984;251(20):2663–2667.

17. Killam C, Cautin RL, Santucci AC: Assessing the enduring residual neuropsychological effects of head trauma in college athletes who participate in contact sports. *Arch Clin Neuropsychol* 2005;20(5):599–611.

18. Talavage TM, Nauman EA, Breedlove EL, et al: Functionally-detected cognitive impairment in high school football players without clinically-diagnosed concussion. *J Neurotrauma* 2014;31(4):327–338.

19. Poole VN, Breedlove EL, Shenk TE, et al: Sub-concussive hit characteristics predict deviant brain metabolism in football athletes. *Dev Neuropsychol* 2015;40(1):12–17.

20. Abbas K, Shenk TE, Poole VN, Robinson ME, Leverenz LJ, Nauman EA, Talavage TM: Effects of repetitive sub-concussive brain injury on the functional connectivity of Default Mode Network in high school football athletes. *Dev Neuropsychol* 2015;40(1):51–56.

21. Petersen RC, Stevens JC, Ganguli M, Tangalos EG, Cummings JL, DeKosky ST: Practice parameter: Early detection of dementia: Mild cognitive impairment (an evidence-based review). Report of the Quality Standards Subcommittee of the American Academy of Neurology. *Neurology* 2001;56(9):1133–1142.

22. Guskiewicz KM, Marshall SW, Bailes J, McCrea M, Cantu RC, Randolph C, Jordan BD: Association between recurrent concussion and late-life cognitive impairment in retired professional football players. *Neurosurgery* 2005;57(4):719–726; discussion 719–726.

23. Collins MW, Lovell MR, Iverson GL, Cantu RC, Maroon JC, Field M: Cumulative effects of concussion in high school athletes. *Neurosurgery* 2002;51(5):1175–1179; discussion 1180–1181.

24. Schneider RC: *Head and Neck Injuries in Football: Mechanisms, Treatment, and Prevention.* Baltimore, Williams & Wilkins, 1973.

25. Eckner JT, Sabin M, Kutcher JS, Broglio SP: No evidence for a cumulative impact effect on concussion injury threshold. *J Neurotrauma* 2011;28(10): 2079–2090.

26. Haglund Y, Eriksson E: Does amateur boxing lead to chronic brain damage? A review of some recent investigations. *Am J Sports Med* 1993;21(1):97–109.

27. Stein TD, Alvarez VE, McKee AC: Concussion in chronic traumatic encephalopathy. *Curr Pain Headache Rep* 2015; 19(10):522.

28. McKee AC, Stern RA, Nowinski CJ, et al: The spectrum of disease in chronic traumatic encephalopathy. *Brain* 2013;136(Pt 1):43–64.

29. McKee AC, Daneshvar DH, Alvarez VE, Stein TD: The neuropathology of sport. *Acta Neuropathol* 2014;127(1): 29–51.

30. Stern RA, Daneshvar DH, Baugh CM, et al: Clinical presentation of chronic traumatic encephalopathy. *Neurology* 2013;81(13):1122–1129.

31. Stein TD, Alvarez VE, McKee AC: Chronic traumatic encephalopathy: A spectrum of neuropathological changes following repetitive brain trauma in athletes and military personnel. *Alzheimers Res Ther* 2014;6(1):4.

32. Mez J, Stern RA, McKee AC: Chronic traumatic encephalopathy: Where are we and where are we going? *Curr Neurol Neurosci Rep* 2013;13(12):407.

33. Goldstein LE, Fisher AM, Tagge CA, et al: Chronic traumatic encephalopathy in blast-exposed military veterans and a blast neurotrauma mouse model. *Sci Transl Med* 2012;4(134):134ra60.

34. Stern RA, Riley DO, Daneshvar DH, Nowinski CJ, Cantu RC, McKee AC: Long-term consequences of repetitive brain trauma: chronic traumatic encephalopathy. *PM R* 2011;3(10 suppl 2):S460–S467.

35. Gavett BE, Cantu RC, Shenton M, Lin AP, Nowinski CJ, McKee AC, Stern RA: Clinical appraisal of chronic traumatic encephalopathy: Current perspectives and future directions. *Curr Opin Neurol* 2011;24(6): 525–531.

36. McKee AC, Gavett BE, Stern RA, et al: TDP-43 proteinopathy and motor neuron disease in chronic traumatic encephalopathy. *J Neuropathol Exp Neurol* 2010;69(9): 918–929.

37. McKee AC, Cantu RC, Nowinski CJ, et al: Chronic traumatic encephalopathy in athletes: progressive tauopathy after repetitive head injury. *J Neuropathol Exp Neurol* 2009;68(7):709–735.

38. Maroon JC, Winkelman R, Bost J, Amos A, Mathyssek C, Miele V: Chronic traumatic encephalopathy in contact sports: A systematic review of all reported pathological cases. *PLoS One* 2015;10(2):e0117338.

39. Hazrati LN, Tartaglia MC, Diamandis P, et al: Absence of chronic traumatic encephalopathy in retired football players with multiple concussions and neurological symptomatology. *Front Hum Neurosci* 2013;7:222.

40. Shin W, Mahmoud SY, Sakaie K, et al: Diffusion measures indicate fight exposure-related damage to cerebral white matter in boxers and mixed martial arts fighters. *AJNR Am J Neuroradiol* 2014;35(2):285–290.

41. Bernick C, Banks SJ, Shin W, et al: Structural and functional brain changes in boxers and mixed martial arts fighters are correlated with fight exposure. Presented at the American Academy of Neurology Annual Meeting, San Diego, CA, 2013.

42. Strain J, Didehbani N, Cullum CM, et al: Depressive symptoms and white matter dysfunction in retired NFL players with concussion history. *Neurology* 2013;81(1):25–32.

43. Jordan BD, Relkin NR, Ravdin LD, Jacobs AR, Bennett A, Gandy S: Apolipoprotein E epsilon4 associated with chronic traumatic brain injury in boxing. *JAMA* 1997;278(2):136–140.

44. Kutner KC, Erlanger DM, Tsai J, Jordan B, Relkin NR: Lower cognitive performance of older football players possessing apolipoprotein E epsilon4. *Neurosurgery* 2000;47(3):651–657; discussion 657–658.

45. Pitas RE, Ji ZS, Weisgraber KH, Mahley RW: Role of apolipoprotein E in modulating neurite outgrowth: Potential effect of intracellular apolipoprotein E. *Biochem Soc Trans* 1998;26(2):257–262.

46. Hussain A, Luong M, Pooley A, Nathan BP: Isoform-specific effects of apoE on neurite outgrowth in olfactory epithelium culture. *J Biomed Sci* 2013;20:49.

47. Zhong N, Ramaswamy G, Weisgraber KH: Apolipoprotein E4 domain interaction induces endoplasmic reticulum stress and impairs astrocyte function. *J Biol Chem* 2009;284(40):27273–27280.

48. Jain S, Yoon SY, Leung L, Knoferle J, Huang Y: Cellular source-specific effects of apolipoprotein (apo) E4 on dendrite arborization and dendritic spine development. *PLoS One* 2013;8(3):e59478.

49. Weir D, Jackson JS, Sonnega A: *Study of Retired NFL Players*. Michigan, MI: University of Michigan Institute for Social Research, 2009.

50. Lehman EJ, Hein MJ, Baron SL, Gersic CM: Neurodegenerative causes of death among retired National Football League players. *Neurology* 2012;79(19):1970–1974.

51. Dashnaw ML, Petraglia AL, Bailes J: An overview of the basic science of concussion and subconcussion: Where we are and where we are going. *Neurosurg Focus* 2012;33(6):E5:1–9.

52. Rowson S, Duma SM, Greenwald RM, et al: Can helmet design reduce the risk of concussion in football? *J Neurosurg* 2014;120(4):919–922.

53. Collins M, Lovell MR, Iverson GL, Ide T, Maroon: Examining concussion rates and return to play in high school football players wearing newer helmet technology: A three-year prospective cohort study. *Neurosurgery* 2006;58(2):275–286; discussion 275–286.

SECTION 5

Roundtable Discussion of the Experts

29 Spine and Sports: A Roundtable Discussion

Andrew C. Hecht, MD • Alexander R. Vaccaro, MD, PhD, MBA • Wellington Hsu, MD • Robert G. Watkins, MD • Andrew Dossett, MD

Spine injuries are, unfortunately, a common problem for athletes who participate in contact sports such as football, hockey, and rugby. One of the most challenging roles for the physician team that cares for elite athletes is the decision making regarding spine injuries and return to play considerations. In this chapter, a group of spine surgeons who care for elite and professional athletes discuss this issue. Moderating the discussion and presenting a series of case studies was **Andrew C. Hecht, MD,** chief of spine surgery, associate professor of orthopaedic and neurosurgery, and director of the spine center at Mount Sinai Hospital, New York City. Dr. Hecht is the spine surgeon for the NY Jets and NY Islanders professional teams and sits on the NFL Brain and Spine Committee. He is also spine surgical consultant for the USTA. Joining him were the following:

- **Alexander R. Vaccaro, MD, PhD, MBA** the Richard H. Rothman Professor and chairman, department of orthopaedic surgery and professor of neurosurgery at Thomas Jefferson University in Philadelphia.

Dr. Alexander Vaccarro is spine surgeon for the Philadelphia Eagles.

- **Wellington K. Hsu, MD,** the Clifford C. Raisbeck, distinguished professor of orthopaedic surgery at Northwestern Medicine in Chicago. Dr. Wellington Hsu is spine surgeon for Northwestern University.
- **Andrew Dossett, MD,** a spine surgeon at the W.B. Carrell Memorial Clinic, in Dallas. Dr. Drew Dossett is Spine surgeon for the Dallas Cowboys.
- **Robert G. Watkins III, MD,** co-director of the Marina Spine Clinic and a member of the Association of Professional Team Physicians, in Marina Del Rey, California. Dr. Robert Watkins is Spine Surgeon is member of the NFL Brain and Spine Committee, and spine surgical consultant for numerous professional and collegiate teams.

Dr. Hecht: Let's discuss some challenging management scenarios, beginning with a professional football player with a C4 to C5 posterolateral disk herniation with weakness in his deltoid who has exhausted all conservative care. What kind of surgery would you perform?

Dr. Vaccaro: I would perform an anterior cervical decompression and fusion (ACDF) using an allograft bone and a cervical plate. I would allow him to return to play 6 to 9 months after that procedure after he has completed rehabilitation and has full range of motion (ROM) and his strength back.

Dr. Watkins: My recommendation is a one-level anterior cervical fusion using allograft and a plate. I use a cortical allograft packed with autogenous cancellous bone from the iliac crest.

I would not recommend a total disk replacement. I think the unknown factors of artificial disk replacement preclude its use in high-performance athletes, and certainly not in those in sports that potentially involve head contact, including those playing in the National Basketball Association (NBA), National Hockey League (NHL), and Major League Baseball (MLB) players.

I would not perform a foraminotomy and posterior disk excision. The potential risk of instability and reherniation is too high in this athlete.

Dr. Dossett: I would also perform an ACDF with autologous iliac crest graft and a plate.

Dr. Hecht: I agree with the ACDF with allograft and instrumentation. I would not do a foraminotomy or disk replacement in a football player with a disk herniation. Would total disk replacement in this scenario be appropriate for a player in any other sport?

Dr. Vaccaro: If the player were involved in a noncontact sport, I would perform a disk replacement if the patient preferred it after I explained the risks and benefits. In athletes involved in sports that involve significant contact, I would avoid disk replacement.

Dr. Hsu: Although both foraminotomy and ACDF have been successful for National Football League players, they both have their challenges. ACDF can lead to adjacent segment degeneration and ultimately a two-level fusion that is currently incompatible with return to play.

Posterior foraminotomies also lead to problems because it's been shown that up to 50% of professional athletes may require surgery at that index level in their lifetimes. ACDF probably has better long-term results in football players, but total disk arthroplasty is not indicated at this time.

Dr. Hecht: Even though there is adjacent segment degeneration after ACDF (2.9%/year), there is also an overlooked rate of adjacent segment degeneration after foraminotomy (1.8%/year). I would not perform a cervical disk replacement in any athlete with a risk of contact or collision. The success rate after ACDF is so high that I do not see any good reason to introduce this yet unknown risk of device failure in contact sports.

Dr. Hecht: Do you think a CT scan that shows definitive fusion is needed before you would allow this athlete to return to contact sports even if he is asymptomatic?

Dr. Vaccaro: I would always get a CT scan in a professional athlete, primarily as documentation. If a CT scan taken at 10 months after surgery showed a nonhealed union and the athlete had good isometric strength and symmetric ROM, I would tell that athlete that significant contact may disrupt a stable, nonhealed fusion, and he may become symptomatic, which may affect his ability to play. If he agreed and understood that, I would allow him to return to play. But, I would document it thoroughly.

Dr. Watkins: I don't think it is imperative that a patient have a radiographic solid fusion before returning to play. An asymptomatic patient with full ROM and full strength and conditioning, after completing a rehabilitation program for his sport, could return to play.

Dr. Hsu: I would say that a CT scan is definitely indicated. I know a number of physicians don't necessarily agree with that. But certainly knowing that someone has a pseudarthrosis before returning to the field is important.

Dr. Hecht: I would document a healed fusion with CT in an athlete returning to contact sports. The gold standard today is not motion on flexion-extension radiographs but fusion on coronal and sagittal reconstructed CT scans. I would be less concerned with a tennis player than an athlete involving collision and contact.

Dr. Hecht: Let's expand on the situation. The player had an ACDF, and he has no motion on flexion-extension films, but his CT scan shows a nonunion, with haloing around the screws of the anterior cervical plate and radiolucent lines. However, he's completely asymptomatic. Would you let him return to contact sports?

Dr. Watkins: A patient with an obvious nonunion who is completely asymptomatic and passes all of his conditioning and sport-specific training may return to play. He is at risk of becoming symptomatic at the operated level, just as he is at risk at becoming symptomatic at the adjacent level. Part of the problem at times is trying to sort out whether symptoms are at an adjacent level or the prior operated level.

Dr. Vaccaro: In contact sports, the potential exists that the player may develop neck pain and experience a symptomatic pseudarthrosis that may limit ROM. At that point, the player has to make a decision, if he wants to go back or not. He's not at risk of a catastrophic neurologic deficit.

He may or may not be at risk for developing arm discomfort, which can be seen due to inflammation associated with pseudarthrosis. I would clearly document this, and the patient would have to sign off to return to play. If he became concerned, he could opt to not return to contact sports or to have additional surgery. I would supplement posteriorly to allow the anterior fusion to eventually heal over time. I would allow that patient to return to sports.

Dr. Dossett: I'd say this: If the player had a cervical procedure other than an anterior autograft and a symptomatic nonunion developed, I'd go back in anteriorly with an autograft.

Dr. Hecht: If I had a patient with a nonunion autograft or allograft, I would almost universally use a posterior approach unless there was an adjacent segment problem with radiculopathy. If it was just the index level, I would treat that posteriorly. The union rate has been shown to be nearly 99% with a posterior augmentation of an anterior fusion. Despite the posterior dissection, athletes can return to play without limitation. The union rate is statistically significantly lower with revision anterior approaches for anterior nonunions, but the outcomes are similar once fused. Both approaches would be acceptable.

Dr. Watkins: If the patient has an anterior nonunion, I would generally recommend a posterior fusion. If the complex becomes solidly fused, I would clear him to return to play.

Dr. Hecht: What about a player who has a two-level ACDF? Is this still a relative contraindication for returning to play collision contact sports?

Dr. Dossett: My personal belief is that an athlete with a two-level cervical fusion should not play collision sports because the next injury that requires surgery dramatically reduces cervical function.

Dr. Watkins: My opinion is that a two-level cervical fusion is a contraindication to return to a head contact sport. Even in a noncontact sport, such as professional baseball, the problem in letting an athlete return after a two-level fusion is the increased risk of adjacent level injury. Then you have a young guy with a three-level neck problem. That is not good for his health and future outside of his professional sport.

If it were possible to sort out which is the symptomatic level when an adjacent level has degenerative changes, we would recommend fusing only the symptomatic level. If the adjacent level becomes symptomatic, the patient should definitely retire.

Dr. Vaccaro: I'm not as afraid to let an athlete with a healed two-level ACDF return to football. I agree that ROM may be decreased, but I'm not sure how significant that decreased ROM is. I agree also that, if junction disease develops, a three-level fusion would not allow a return to play.

Dr. Hecht: I would let him go back to playing, even with a two-level ACDF, but counsel him that symptoms may develop and force him to stop playing. I would also state that he is at increased risk of becoming symptomatic. This was looked at in rugby players, and those with two levels had new symptoms whereas the single levels were able to return to play. What about a football player who has recurring stingers? You're sure they're stingers, but an MRI shows congenital cervical stenosis.

Dr. Dossett: Those are unrelated conditions, and the risk doesn't impact each other. When the player can demonstrate normal ROM, resistance with isometrics and all kinds of combinations thereof and has a normal neurologic examination, he can return to play.

Dr. Hsu: The physical examination and the history are important because many of the reported symptoms can be mixed up with a transient cord neurapraxia episode. These are separate entities. If everybody with that scenario was held out, I think half the league would probably be affected.

Dr. Vaccaro: When I see patients with multiple stingers, I tell them that many studies have shown that the more stingers you have, the greater the likelihood of future chronic neck pain and referred arm discomfort from symptomatic degenerate disease as they age.

Dr. Watkins: A football player with multiple stingers may have a positive MRI for congenital stenosis. However, that is not a contraindication for returning to play. However, most stingers in adults in my experience, are foraminal stenosis problems, and they occur with extension and rotation toward the arm with the stingers. It closes the foramen. They need a very thorough workup, CT scan and MRI measurements, and a careful history and physical examination.

Dr. Hecht: What about a patient who has a cervical cord neurapraxia (CCN)? Let's look at two possible scenarios—one in which the patient has no congenital stenosis or herniation of any kind and one in which he has stenosis. So, a player with congenital cervical stenosis has his first episode of a CCN. How many episodes would you allow?

Dr. Hsu: In my opinion, it is not safe for that player to return to a collision sport because that incident is a harbinger for a permanent neurologic injury from a spinal cord injury (SCI). I think that player should have the cord decompressed before returning to the field. If more than one level is affected, the athlete should not return to play, as we've already established.

Dr. Vaccaro: If a player has a transient cervical spinal cord neurapraxia in the setting of cervical stenosis, I would strongly argue to keep that patient from playing. It could predispose the individual to a future spinal cord neurapraxia.

If the patient has no evidence of congenital spinal stenosis, he would have to complete a thorough rehab program and demonstrate symmetrical motion and normal strength before I would allow him to return to sports. After a second episode, I would counsel against return.

Dr. Watkins: I think the equivocal factor is the severity of the episode. It varies from mild quadriparesthesia that goes away immediately to being transported off the field as a SCI and being paralyzed for 1 to 6 hours, hospitalized, and having burning upper extremity symptoms for months after the episode. This can become a chronic problem. I would take all the appropriate measurements and evaluate for a spinal column injury such as ligamentous

disruption, disk herniation, or lateral mass fracture. If the episode is mild and transitory and the cervical stenosis is not significant, I would allow the patient to return to professional football. A second episode would disqualify him from the sport.

Unfortunately, when the patient comes to you, the history is often somewhat confusing. The patient may attempt to deny having significant symptoms. The history from the team's healthcare providers is very important.

Under the scenario of congenital stenosis without degenerative change, transitory minor episode, I would let the player return. If he has a significant SCI, such as transported as a SCI with residual symptoms, I would not let him return.

Dr. Hecht: Even though Dr. Torg's famous studies from the mid-1990s of quadriplegia in athletes, none of these patients had a so-called heralding even or warning shot before their devastating injury. Also, none of the patients who had CCN event went on to a devastating quadriplegic injury. Common sense dictates otherwise, that patients with multiple CCN (i.e., >1) in setting of congenital stenosis should be advised not to return to play contact sports.

Dr. Hecht: Is there a role for laminoplasty in an athlete with congenital cervical stenosis who's had a cord neurapraxia?

Dr. Hsu: I know of one NBA player who returned to play after a laminoplasty. I think a laminoplasty is consistent with return to play, even in a collision sport, as long as a CT scan demonstrates complete healing on that hinge side.

Dr. Watkins: We performed a laminoplasty on a top-level National Collegiate Athletic Association basketball player after a history of seven or eight transitory episodes that the player was not sure were happening—until the last significant one. His healthcare providers were not sure what was happening. We returned him to play with full confidence. I think he is at greater risk for a fracture-dislocation, but in professional basketball, the incidence of that occurring is remote, to say the least.

Dr. Vaccaro: If I saw someone with a history of a cervical spinal cord neurapraxia who had a laminoplasty, and the hinged side healed, I would clear that athlete to play, as long as I didn't see any cord atrophy or edema.

However, if I saw the patient up front with a SCI, I would take a more pessimistic approach because there are too many "ifs." Would I be able to operate and be successful? Would there be a risk of a C5 palsy? Will I be sure that the CT scan confirms adequate healing of the hinge side or be deceived because of volume averaging? With all of these variables, I would say that it's probably not a good idea to return to sports.

Dr. Hecht: I would let him return to play after a laminoplasty with reconstruction but not to a high-contact sport such as football or rugby or hockey.

Dr. Hecht: What about a player who has cord neurapraxia and a disk herniation? After the disk herniation was addressed, we would let him return to play, but what if there was a small spot of myelomalacia in the cord? Would you let the athlete return to play, assuming he has painless ROM and is neurologically normal?

Dr. Watkins: If the patient has an area of myelomalacia and a disk herniation, we would treat him with an ACDF. If the patient has a residual area of myelomalacia and a solid fusion, I would not let him return to professional football.

Dr. Vaccaro: No, I know what myelomalacia represents, and I probably would not let him play.

Dr. Hsu: I would let him play, as long as the amount of space around that myelomalacia was significant and he had a normal canal. I don't see any reason why the myelomalacia would prevent him from playing if it were treated successfully.

Dr. Hecht: I would not let him return with myelomalacia because it represents an injury to the cord. I would let him return to noncontact sports.

Dr. Hecht: Let's consider an elite 18-year-old tennis player ranked number 2 in the United States who presents with low back and acute fracture of the pars interarticularis that is nondisplaced. The MRI reveals edema in both pars with new defects.

Dr. Hsu: I would also obtain a SPECT (single-photon emission computed tomography) bone scan or CT scan to see if there is increased activity, and if positive, I would treat the patient in a brace for 3 to 5 months and restrict his or her activity. I would reevaluate after the bracing period, and if the athlete has painless ROM, I would gradually increase her or his activity to get the athlete back to sport.

Dr. Dossett: I would also get radiographs and a SPECT to make sure the facture is acute and the only fracture. I then would shut the athlete down without a brace for 3 months unless it involves L5.

Dr. Watkins: I would recommend an MRI and SPECT CT scan. I want to show the acute lesion. Sometimes I see an old L5 to S1 spondylolysis and then an acute lesion

forming at another level. I do not use immobilization as a method of curing spondylolysis. We have not been able to show there is anything a physician can do to cure a spondylolysis. I also never use electrical stimulation. If a corset or brace is used, it is for the person to go to class and get in and out of car or perform activities of daily living if very symptomatic.

1. Stop the sport.
2. Put the patient in the hands of a skilled physical therapist that begins in neutral position, isometric control system of core strengthening. Then the return to activity depends on their ability to do the rehab program. I use a core strengthening endurance program that is based on five progressive levels of activity. If the athlete can get to a level 3 and is asymptomatic, we never restudy the patient. If the athlete can do level 3, he or she can normally return to play and do a lightweight program. Most collegiate and pro athletes can get to level 5 of this program. At level 3, they can start sport-specific training programs. The key is to get the athlete, the parents, and the coaches to buy into the need for this rehab program. As for the timing of the return to play, that is a critical factor. Parents are often anxious about the upcoming season, the evaluation by college scouts, the potential for a scholarship, or tryouts for the team. Spinal disorders do not fit into the timetable for your sport. I tell them that the problem will take a certain amount of time to heal and recover from. You are going to have to work harder and put more time in than any of your teammates or competitors. Do not worry about the start of the season or the evaluation by the scout because if you play with a painful back, you are not going to perform well, and you may get labeled as a "back patient." The key is the rehab program!

Dr. Vaccaro: I moved away from bone cans and use MRI exclusively, particularly 3-tesla scans. I also use the MRI to evaluate the status of the disk. If its acute, I shut him down and put him in brace to ensure compliance. I brace for 3 months and modify activities. I do not start therapy for 3 months.

Dr. Hecht: My approach is nearly identical to Dr. Watkins' approach. I use MRI with stir sequences and agree 3-tesla scans are ideal. I get SPECT if MRI is negative. In about 8% to 10% of cases, the SPECT lights up, and the MRI was nondiagnostic. I then put the athlete in a brace only for 1 month simply to cool down the athlete and restrict activity. It adds a certain gravitas to the patient and family. After 1 month, the athlete is usually asymptomatic. I then start the athlete on the same protocol

Dr. Watkins discussed (it is actually called the Watkins-Randall protocol). If the athlete is then asymptomatic at level 3, I start getting him or her ready to return to play. The brace does nothing other than provide a restriction of activity reminder. I remove it in 95% of patients after 4 weeks and start rehab. If the patient returns and is still symptomatic after being in the brace for 4 weeks, I will then continue for another 4 weeks. I cannot emphasize enough the need to get the athlete as well as the parents to buy into the rehab program. I do not think anything we do influences the actual healing of the fracture. We influence the symptoms, and they are not one in the same.

Dr. Hecht: When is surgery indicated to treat a pars fracture? How long would you give the athlete to get better?

Dr. Vaccaro: At least a year.

Dr. Dossett: In 20 years, I have never had to operate on one. I see more than 100 stress fractures a year. The natural history is on our side.

Dr. Hecht: These rarely ever need surgery. I have only had to fix a handful of these over the past 15 years at most. The pain has to be fairly severe and incapacitating with activities of life.

Dr. Watkins: I agree; these rarely need surgery, and it's extraordinarily rare to need to fix this problem with surgery.

Dr. Hecht: Now, you have a collegiate hockey player who has possible NHL career ahead of him, and he has an L5 to S1 lytic spondylolisthesis. He has low back pain and leg pain (radiculopathy). When is surgery an option for this person, and how would you counsel him in regards to his future with a spinal fusion?

Dr. Watkins: If the patient has bilateral spondylitic spondylolisthesis, we use exactly the same treatment, exactly the same rehabilitation program, exactly the same return to sport-specific training that we would with an acute unilateral spondylolysis. Bob Kerlan once told me that he never had an athlete whose professional career was shortened by spondylolisthesis. That was his opinion, and I never forgot it. We have operated on a very small number of professional athletes. I think the younger the fusion is performed, the better. A midcareer professional athlete who needs a spinal fusion is unlikely, to put it mildly, to return to perform. A professional athlete at the end of his career who wants to have a fusion so he can play a couple more years is a contraindication to doing a fusion.

Dr. Vaccaro: I would do a transforaminal lumbar interbody fusion on this patient only after exhausting all

conservative care. I would tell him to expect a decrease in performance of approximately 10% to 15% in the studies I have reviewed and professional athletes. After he is healed, I would let him return to play.

Dr. Watkins: Foraminal stenosis at the level of a spondylitic spondylolisthesis, in my opinion, is not amenable to a foraminal decompression. Obviously, I have attempted it and failed. Just the approach makes it unstable. Lots of injections, lots of core strengthening, and I have had some dramatic famous athletes who have returned to full performance and a couple who have retired midcareer. As far as an athlete who is in his professional career and a condition that would be amenable to a spinal fusion under other circumstances, the chance of getting a fusion and returning to prior performance is not good. It is hard to have time off for a surgery like that and to return anyway. Hopefully, the consideration of a very young athlete has time to get well and the skills to attempt to return to his sport. It is a pretty rare situation. The most important thing is you have got to have a patient who buys into core stabilization training and a team environment that allows an intensive rehabilitation program.

Dr. Hsu: I think fusion in hockey do mix, so I would.

Dr. Hecht: If I changed the scenario and elevated the level of contact to football, would that change any of your recommendations? A lot of professional athletes think that if they have a spinal fusion, it's a "game over" scenario and that they will never return to play, mostly because of performance-related issues.

Dr. Vaccaro: I would allow any contact athlete go back to play football with lumbar fusion as long as he can make the grade and he demonstrates a functional ability to play. I'm not worried about future injury. I'm worried about him not being able to perform his function on the field. But, if he demonstrates to me that he can perform his function, I'd let any position go back to play with a stable lumbar fusion.

Dr. Dossett: It's rare that people get out from a lumbar fusion and play contact sports. I only know of one, and I have a vast experience. And I had one MLB player get back to the major leagues after a lumbar fusion. It changes your skill set. And so, yes, you feel better, but, a lot of times, you just can't do what you used to be able to do.

Dr. Hecht: I have a Division 1 wrestler who had a microdiscectomy, developed a pars fracture on the other side, and started developing a little bit of a slip. We did it with an instrumentation and fusion and he went back to wrestling once he developed a solid fusion radiographically. He's probably young enough, and it healed, and he went back to Division 1 wrestling. It really depends on the athlete; the likelihood of returning may be low, but it's not…I would say it's not a contra-indication to returning, but I would emphasize that the odds are not in the athlete's favor, mostly from the time it takes to return (nearly 1 year) and the performance reduction that accompanies most fusions.

Dr. Hecht: Let's talk about some cervical trauma questions that are more common and subtle than the devastating fractures that are more direct to deal with. What about a football player who has a cervical facet fracture that has healed with incongruity and has neck pain? Can he return to play?

Dr. Vaccaro: The literature is poor with this entity, but it says that a patient with facet fracture that healed with incongruity with continued pain would not be an optimal candidate to return to play sports. If I thought the patient was stable on flexion-extension radiographs, that the neck discomfort did not impeded his ROM to perform his function, and he was adequately rehabilitated, then I would allow that athlete to return to play.

Dr. Dossett: I agree and would allow him to play if he was stable and could tolerate the mild neck pain.

Dr. Hecht: What about a C5 and C6 spinous process fracture nonunion with minimal pain, but when you obtain flexion and extension radiographs, there is wide splaying of the spinous processes? There are no other problems or issues with the canal.

Dr. Hsu: If there were no instability or spondylolisthe-sis I would allow the athlete to return if asymptomatic.

Dr. Vaccaro: I would let the patient play.

Dr. Hecht: I would allow him to play; I had a baseball player with a clay shoveler's facture at C7 that did not heal that remained symptomatic after 1 year. He had pain whenever he swung a bat. We excised the nonunited frag-ment, and he returned to play without symptoms. Again, I would allow this athlete to return to play.

Dr. Hecht: The final scenario involves a football player who sustains a devastating incomplete SCI on the field. What are your thoughts on the administration of steroids?

Dr. Hsu: This population does not have comorbidities or other multitrauma issues, and we are talking about an iso-lated cervical spine injury. I would give that patient steroids.

Dr. Dossett: I would also give that patient steroids.

Dr. Vaccaro: In a word, yes. In the surgical timing in acute spinal cord injury study (STASCIS) trial that was published in *PLoS One*, we found that steroids combined with early surgery had a more rapid neurologic improve-ment and a lower complication rate. We actually saw the very subtle beneficial effect of the steroids.

Dr. Hecht: The recent outcome of the Arbeits-gemeinschaft für Osteosynthesefragen, or AOSPINE guidelines were to give methylprednisolone only if within 8 hours using the National Acute Spinal Cord Injury Study-2 (NASCIS-2) protocol as well as early surgery as reaffirmed the STASCIS trial. I think the key thing to remember that is unique about athletic spine injuries is that care is usually provided nearly instantly in the professional and collegiate setting. We have phy-sicians, athletic trainers, and paramedics standing by to administer care within minutes. This is not a roll-over motor vehicle crash that takes hours to extricate or a polytrauma case with other medical issues. In the spinal cord trauma protocols established for the New York Jets and New York Islanders, we give steroids as indicated.

Dr. Hecht: What about thermal cooling? Is there any role for this novel approach at this time?

Dr. Hsu: I don't think there's any clinical evidence to support the use of cooling. So, I would not recommend that for this patient.

Dr. Vaccaro: I agree. At Jefferson, which is a regional SCI center, we do not use thermal cooling.

Dr. Dossett: I agree. The Dallas Cowboys do not use this technique either. It remains experimental at this time.

Dr. Hecht: Although some basic science work suggests a potential rationale for the use of local or systemic hypo-thermia in acute traumatic SCI, this literature is contro-versial and includes many negative studies. There is little published research that justifies the use of hypothermia for SCI in the clinical setting. There are potential com-plications associated with systemic hypothermia (e.g., cardiac arrhythmias, increased susceptibility to infection, impaired coagulation); therefore, the use of this modality in the setting of SCI should be viewed as experimental. I think a "wait and see" approach makes the most sense at this time.

Index

Note: Page number followed by f and t indicates figure and table only.

A

Abdominal bracing technique (ABT), 27
Abdominal muscles, 22
ABN. *See* American Board of
  Neuropsychology
ACDF. *See* Anterior cervical discectomy
  and fusion
Acetabular stress fracture, 185–186, 186f
ADHD. *See* Attention deficit hyperactivity
  disorder
Aerobic conditioning, 29
Aging athlete, 194–195. *See also* Athletes
American Academy of Clinical
  Neuropsychology (AACN), 255
American Academy of Neurology
  (AAN), 255
American Association of Neurological
  Surgeons (AANS), 42
American Board of Neuropsychology
  (ABN), 255
American football, 3, 16, 32, 33, 86, 123,
  135, 166, 173, 198
American Medical Society for Sports
  Medicine (AMSSM), 255
American Psychological Association
  (APA), 255
American Spinal Injury Association
  (ASIA), 43
  rating scale, 211, 213t
AMSSM. *See* American Medical Society
  for Sports Medicine
Anterior cervical discectomy and fusion
  (ACDF), 103–107, 279–280
Anxiety after concussion, 266
APA. *See* American Psychological
  Association
ApoE4 allele, 275
Arnold-Chiari syndrome, 113
Articular pillars, cervical spine, 13
ASIA. *See* American Spinal Injury
  Association
Athletes
  aging, 194–195
  cervical disk herniation in, 100, 102
    cervical disk replacement, 108–109
    nonoperative management, 102–103
    operative management, 103–107
    posterior cervical foraminotomy,
      107–108
  cervical spine injuries in
    burners, 86–91
    cervical stenosis, 123–132
    congenital cervical anomalies, 112–121

degenerative disorders, 123–132
disk herniation, 100–109
fractures, 134–142
neurapraxia, 92–98
special needs, 112–121
stingers, 86–91
upper extremity disorders (neck and
  arm pain), 74–84
fractures of cervical spine and spinal
  cord injuries, 134
  burst fractures, 137, 139f
  epidemiology of, 134–135
  hyperextension injuries, 137–139, 140f
  hyperflexion injuries, 136, 138, 138f
  mechanism of injuries, 135
  precautions in, 135
  return to play, 139–140, 141t
  upper cervical spine fractures,
    135–136, 136f
low back pain in (*See* Low back pain
  (LBP))
lumbar degenerative disk disease in
  diagnosis, 175–177, 176f, 176t
  disk pathology, 173–175, 173f–174f
  epidemiology, 172–173
  normal aging *vs.* disk degeneration,
    175t
  return to play, 178
  treatment, 177–178
lumbar disk herniation in, 163
  case presentations, 165–168,
    165f–166f, 168f–169f
  clinical presentation, 164, 165t
  pathoanatomy, 163–164, 164f
lumbar spine disorders in aging, 194–196
  bone mineral density and, 198,
    200–201
  low back pain, 196–197, 196t
  musculoskeletal manifestations, 194,
    195t
  radiographic abnormalities, 197–198,
    199f
  with spinal cord injury, 47t
spinal stenosis in
  diagnosis, 175–177, 176f, 176t
  disk pathology, 173–175, 173f–174f
  epidemiology, 172–173
  normal aging *vs.* disk degeneration,
    175t
  return to play, 178
  treatment, 177–178
spondylolisthesis in (*See*
  Spondylolisthesis)
spondylolysis in (*See* Spondylolysis)

thoracic injuries in (*See* Thoracic injuries
  in athletes)
  thoracic pain in, 203–204
  thoracic spinal degeneration in, 204
Atlantoaxial instability, 119–121, 121f
Atraumatic back pain, 54–55
Attention deficit hyperactivity disorder
  (ADHD), 241, 246–249
Axial neck pain, 124
Axonotmesis, 86

B

Back pain, low. *See* Low back pain (LBP)
Balance Error Scoring System (BESS),
  245–246
Basilar invagination, 113–114, 114f
BESS. *See* Balance Error Scoring System
Biomechanics, 11
  patient characteristics, 17–18
  regional, of spine, 14
    cervical, 14–15, 15f
    lumbar spine, 16
    lumbo-sacro-pelvic spine, 16
    thoracic spine, 15
    thoracolumbar junction, 16
  sport-specific, 16
    contact sports and gymnastics, 17
    cycling, 17
    golf and swimming, 17
    running and weight lifting, 16
Bone mineral density (BMD), 195
  in athletes, 198, 200–201
Bony injuries, spine, 13–14
Brachial plexus neurapraxia. *See* Stingers
Buckling, concept of, 14, 15f
Burners. *See* Stingers
Burst fractures, 137, 139f

C

Canadian Assessment of Tomography
  for Childhood Head Injury
  (CATCH), 245
Canadian C-spine rules criteria, 53
Canadian Ice Hockey Spinal Injuries
  Registry, 3
Cardiac shock, 35
Carpal tunnel syndrome, 81–82
CATCH. *See* Canadian Assessment of
  Tomography for Childhood
  Head Injury
CCN. *See* Cervical cord neurapraxia
CDR. *See* Cervical disk replacement
Cell-based therapies, 45, 46t–47t

Center of Epidemiological Studies Depression (CESD) scale, 247
Cervical burst fractures, 137
Cervical cord neurapraxia (CCN), 5, 51, 86, 92, 281
  expert-based recommendations, 96–98, 97t
    economic considerations, 98
    medicolegal considerations, 98
  mechanism of injury in, 92–93
  return to play, 95–96, 97t
  risk factors for, 93, 93f
    spinal stenosis, 94–95, 94f, 95f
  symptoms, 92
  treatment, 95
Cervical disk herniation in athletes, 3, 100, 102
  cervical disk replacement, 108
    evidence-based review, 109
    return to play, recommendations for, 109
  nonoperative management, 102
    case examples, 103, 103f
    evidence-based review, 102–103
    return to play, recommendations for, 101f, 103
  operative management, 103
    anterior cervical discectomy and fusion, 103–107
    case examples, 105–106, 105f, 106f
    evidence-based review, 104–105
    return to play, recommendations for, 106–107
  posterior cervical foraminotomy, 107
    anterior cervical discectomy and fusion, 108
    case examples, 107, 108f
    evidence-based review, 107
Cervical disk replacement (CDR), 108–109
Cervical hyperextension injuries, 60–61
Cervical nerve root neurapraxia. See Stingers
Cervical spinal stenosis, 94–95, 94f, 95f
Cervical spine, 14–15, 15f
  buckling, 14, 15f
  degenerative disorders of, 123–125
    case examples, 126–127, 127f–131f, 129
    diagnosis, 125–126
    return to play after, 126
    treatment, 125–126
  injuries, 3, 14–15, 15f, 32 (See also Spinal cord injuries (SCI))
    burners, 86–91
    catastrophic, 3, 5
    cervical stenosis, 123–132
    congenital cervical anomalies, 112–121
    degenerative disorders, 123–132
    disk herniation, 100–109
    football-specific, 3–5, 4t, 6f
    fractures, 134–142
    neurapraxia, 92–98
    pediatric, 60–61, 60f
    special needs, 112–121
    stingers, 86–91

upper extremity disorders (neck and arm pain), 74–84
  myelopathy test for, 77t
  rehabilitation, 29–31, 30f, 31f
    chest-out posture exercises, 29–30
    doorway stretch, 29–30, 30f
    foam roller stretch, 30, 30f
    postsurgical, 29
    strength exercises, 30
    y's and t's exercises, 30–31, 31f
Cervical spine trauma, 51–53, 52f, 51t, 53
  pediatric, 60–61, 60f
Cervical spondylotic myelopathy (CSM), 124–125
Cervical stenosis, 124
Cethrin, 44
CHALICE. See Children's Head Injury Algorithm for the Prediction of Important Clinical Events Rule
Chiari malformations, 113
Children's Head Injury Algorithm for the Prediction of Important Clinical Events Rule (CHALICE), 245
Chondroitinase ABC, 45
Chronic back pain, 55
Chronic traumatic encephalopathy (CTE), 221
Clay-shoveler fractures, 13
Clinical Test for Sensory Interaction and Balance (CTSIB), 246
CNS. See Congress of Neurological Surgeons
Commotio cordis, 35
Compression fractures, 13–14
Concussion, 218, 219f
  advocacy, 223
  chronic traumatic encephalopathy, relationship with, 221
  controversies, 219
  definition, 219
  diagnosis, 219–220
  incidence of, 247
  long term sequelae, 220, 272
    ApoE4 allele, 275
    chronic traumatic encephalopathy, 273–275, 274t
    controversies, 272–273
    dementia, 275
    mild cognitive impairment, 273
    subconcussion, 273
  neuropsychological testing, 220
  on-field evaluation, 219–220
  postconcussion syndrome, 220
  prevention, 222
  rate of recovery, 247–251, 250t
  return to play, 220, 246–247, 275–276
  short-term prognosis, 220, 244
    chronology of care, 244
    imaging, role of, 244–245
    initial assessment, 245–246
  sports (See Sports concussions)
  vs. cervical and vestibular injury, 218–219
Congenital cervical anomalies, 112
  atlantoaxial instability, 118–121

Basilar invagination, 113–114, 114f
  clinical evaluation, 112–113
  Down syndrome, 119–121, 120f, 121f, 121t
  Klippel-Feil syndrome, 117–118, 119t
  os odontoideum, 114–117, 115f
Congress of Neurological Surgeons (CNS), 42
Contact sports, 17
Cordless screwdrivers, 37
Corticosteroids, for spinal cord injuries, 37
CSM. See Cervical spondylotic myelopathy
CTE. See Chronic traumatic encephalopathy
CTSIB. See Clinical Test for Sensory Interaction and Balance
Cycling, 11, 17

D

Decompression of spinal cord, 42
Degenerative cervical disorders, 123–125
  case examples, 126–127, 127f–131f, 129
  diagnosis, 125–126
  return to play after, 126
  treatment, 125–126
Dementia pugilistica, 221, 275
Depression, 266
DIM. See Draw-in maneuver
Disk herniations, 8–9, 12–13
Dizziness, 264–265
Down syndrome, 118–121
  atlantoaxial instability on flexion, 121f
  radiographic guidelines for, 121t
  return-to-play algorithm for, 120f
Draw-in maneuver (DIM), 27

E

Emergency Action Plan (EAP), 33, 229
Emergency medical services (EMS), 32, 33
EMS. See Emergency medical services
Endocrine disturbance, 265–266
Erb's palsy (traumatic upper brachial plexus injury), 81
Exercycle, 29

F

FABER test, 187
Facet joint fracture, 13
Female athlete triad, 18
Femoroacetabular impingement
  case presentation, 186
  diagnosis and decision making, 187–188, 187f
  etiology, 186–187
  treatment, 188
Fibroblast growth factors (FGF), 45
FLAIR. See Flexion-adduction-internal rotation
Flexion-adduction-internal rotation (FLAIR), 187
Football, and cervical spine injuries, 3–5, 4t, 6f, 32
Fractures. See also specific types
  acetabular stress, 185–186
  cervical burst, 137, 139f
  cervical spine, 134–142

pelvic stress, 185–186
sacral stress, 13, 151–152
spinal cord, 134–142
thoracic spinal, 210–211
upper cervical spine, 135–136, 136f
vertebral body apophyseal avulsion, 62, 62f
Functional spinal unit (FSU), 12

G

G-CSF. *See* Granulocyte colony-stimulating factor
Glasgow Coma Scale (GCS), 244
Glutamate-related excitotoxicity, 44
Gluteal muscles, 22, 23
Granulocyte colony-stimulating factor (G-CSF), 44
Greater trochanteric pain syndrome (GTPS), 183
case presentation, 188
diagnosis and decision making, 188–189
etiology, 188, 189f
treatment for, 190
GTPS. *See* Greater trochanteric pain syndrome
Gymnastics, 17, 172

H

Hamstrings, 22, 23
stretching, 25, 25f
Head abduction injury, 87, 87f
Headache, 263–264
Heads-up block, 15
Helmet, removal of, 37
Hip flexors, 22
stretch, 25–26, 26f
Thomas test, 23
Hoping test, 152
Hyperesthesia, 176
Hyperextension injuries, 135, 137–139, 140f
Hyperflexion injuries, 135, 136, 137, 138f
Hypothermia, induced, 42

I

Ice hockey, 33
Induced hypothermia, 42
Inflammatory/degenerative arthritis, 76
Intervertebral disk, functions of, 12
Intrasubstance muscle rupture, 76
Irritability, 266
Isthmic spondylolisthesis, 17, 151, 154

J

Jaw thrust, 35
Joint injuries, 12–13

K

Key hole, 107
Klippel-Feil syndrome, 117–118
contraindications to return to athletic activity, 119t
return-to-play algorithm for, 118f
Klumpke's paralysis, 82

L

LBP. *See* Low back pain
Levitation technique, for shoulder pad removal, 37
Lift and slide technique, 36
Ligament sprains, 150
LOC. *See* Loss of consciousness
Log roll technique, 35, 36
Loss of consciousness (LOC), 228, 244–245
Low back pain (LBP), 6–7, 13, 18, 146
differential diagnosis of, 150, 150t
degenerative disk disease, 150–151
disk herniation, 151, 151f
ligament sprains, 150
muscle strains, 150
sacral stress fractures, 151–152
spondylolisthesis, 151
spondylolysis, 151
evaluation
history, 147–148
imaging, 148–150, 149f
physical examination, 148, 148f, 149f
in golfers, 17
incidence, 146–147
with associated leg pain, 147
influence of sports type, 147
lumbar strain and, 12
stress fractures and, 8
Lumbar degenerative disk disease in athletes
diagnosis
clinical presentation, 175, 176f
physical examination, 176
radiologic manifestations, 176–177, 176t
disk pathology
disk degeneration in aging athletes, 174–175, 175t
mechanism of disk degeneration, 173–174, 174f
epidemiology, 172–173
return to play
after surgery, 178
prevention, 178
rehabilitation, 178
treatment
nonoperative management, 177
operative management, 177–178
Lumbar disk herniation (LDH), 8, 163
case presentations, 165–168, 165f–166f, 168f–169f
clinical presentation, 164, 165t
pathoanatomy, 163–164, 164f
Lumbar facet joint injury, 13
Lumbar spine, 16
evaluation, 22
history, 22
physical examination, 22–23, 23f
straight-leg raise, 23
rehabilitation program, 23–29, 23f–29f, 24t
aerobic exercise, 29
ball exercises, 28
neutral pain-free position, 23–24, 23f, 25f

pelvic tilt maneuver, 26–27, 27f
postsurgical, 24–25
quadruped exercises, 29, 29f
return to play (RTP), 27
stretching exercises, 25–26, 25f, 26f
trunk stabilization program, 24t, 26, 26f, 27, 28f
wall slide exercises, 28
trauma, 54, 54t
Lumbar spine disorders in aging athletes, 194–196
bone mineral density and, 198, 200–201
low back pain
differential diagnosis of, 196t
epidemiology of, 196–197
musculoskeletal manifestations, 194, 195t
radiographic abnormalities, 197–198, 199f
Lumbar spondylolysis, 55, 62, 63f, 154–155
etiology, 62–63
evaluation
history, 63, 155
imaging, 63
physical examination, 63, 155, 156f
imaging studies
magnetic resonance imaging, 156–157, 157t
plain radiography, 156
single-photon emission computed tomography, 157, 158f
pathoanatomy, 62–63
treatment, 65–66, 66f, 158–159
acute lesions, 159, 159f
chronic lesions, 159–160, 160f
nonoperative, 63–64
operative, 64, 64f
surgical intervention, 160–161, 160f
Lumbar strain injuries, 17
Lystedt Law, 223

M

Magnesium (Mg), 44
Major League Baseball (MLB), 8
Manual muscle test, 23
Mean arterial pressure (MAP), 41–42
Methylprednisolone (MP), 37, 43
Mild cognitive impairment, 273
Minocycline, 43–44
Mononeuropathy, 76
MP. *See* Methylprednisolone
Muscle strains, 150
Musculoligamentous injuries, to spine, 12
Myopathy/myositis, 76

N

National Academy of Neuropsychology (NAN), 255
National Basketball Association (NBA), 222
National Collegiate Athletic Association (NCAA), 222
National Football League (NFL), 2, 3
National Institute of Neurological Disorders and Stroke (NINDS), 221, 221t

National Spinal Cord Injury Statistics
    Center (NSCISC), 2
NBA. *See* National Basketball Association
NCAA. *See* National Collegiate Athletic
    Association
Neck Disability Index (NDI) scores, 104
Neck injuries, 15
Neurapraxic injury, 86
Neuropathic pain, 74, 76
Neuroprotective pharmaceutical agents,
    42–43. *See also specific agents*
Neuropsychologists, 254–255
Neurotmesis, 86
Neutral cervical stabilization, 35
NINDS. *See* National Institute of
    Neurological Disorders and Stroke
N-methyl-D-aspartate receptor (NMDA), 44
Nogo-A inhibitors, 45
Non-neuropathic pain, 76

O

Obers test, 23
Os odontoideum, 114–117, 115f

P

Padding, on-field management of, 37
Paraspinal soft tissue injuries, 209
Pars interarticularis, 154, 155f, 282
    defects in, 13
PCS. *See* Postconcussion syndrome
PCSS. *See* Post Concussion Symptom Scale
PECARN (Pediatric Emergency Care
    Applied Research Network), 245
Pediatric spine
    anatomy, 59–60
    injuries
        cervical spine, 60–61, 60f
        return-to-play guidelines, 65
        spondylolysis, 62–64, 63f
        thoracolumbar spine, 61–62, 61f
        treatment, 65–66, 66f
        vertebral body apophyseal avulsion
            fracture, 62, 62f
Pedicle stress fractures, 8
PEG. *See* Polyethylene glycol
Pelvic stress fracture, 185–186, 186f
Pelvic tilt maneuver, 26–27, 27f
Persistent ossiculum terminale, 114, 115f
Piriformis syndrome
    case presentation, 181
    diagnosis and decision making, 183, 183f
    etiology, 181–183, 182f
    treatment, 183–184
PLL. *See* Posterior longitudinal ligament
Polyethylene glycol (PEG), 44
Polyneuropathy, 76
Pool walking, 29
Post Concussion Symptom Scale (PCSS),
    245
Postconcussion syndrome (PCS), 246
    approach, 263t
    behavioral symptoms
        anxiety, 266
        depression, 266

irritability, 266
    psychosis, 266
case vignette, 262
cognitive symptoms, 266–267
    focus and attention, 267
    memory, 267
    word-finding processing speed, 267
definition, 262–263, 263t
physical symptoms
    dizziness, 264–265
    endocrine disturbance, 265–266
    headache, 263–264
    seizures, 266
    sleep disturbance, 265
    visual disturbance, 265
Postconcussive headaches
    adolescence, 263
    evaluation of, 263
    management of, 263–264
    medication treatment of, 264
    physical examination, 263
    symptom, 263
Postconcussive symptoms, 262
Posterior cervical foraminotomy (PCF),
    107–108
Posterior interosseous nerve (PIN) palsy, 82
Posterior longitudinal ligament (PLL),
    12, 13
Pronator syndrome, 81
Prone log roll technique, 35
Psychosis, 266
Punch drunk syndrome, 221

Q

Quadriceps, stretching of, 26, 26f
Quadriplegic injuries, 3

R

Radiculopathy, 124
Range of motion (ROM), 60, 77
Red flag symptoms, 55
Return to play (RTP), 3, 8, 27, 70–71
    after cervical cord neurapraxia,
        95–96, 97t
    after cervical disk herniation in athletes,
        101f, 103, 106–107, 109
    after concussion, 220, 246–247, 275–276
    after degenerative cervical disorders, 126
    after fractures of spinal cord injuries in
        athletes, 139–140, 141t
    after lumbar degenerative disk disease,
        178
    after spondylolisthesis, 158–161
    after spondylolysis, 158–161
    after stingers, 89–90
    algorithm for Down syndrome, 120f
    guidelines, 64–65
    pitfalls, 231
Rhabdomyolysis, 76
Rho inhibitors, 44
Riluzole, 43
ROM. *See* Range of motion
Rotator cuff tears, 81
Rowing, 12

RTP. *See* Return to play
Running, 16

S

SAC. *See* Standardized Assessment
    of Concussion
Sacral stress fractures, 13, 151–152
    acetabular stress fracture, 185–186, 186f
    case presentation, 184
    diagnosis and decision making, 185
    etiology of, 184–185
    pelvic stress fracture, 185–186, 186f
    treatment of, 185
Sacroiliac (SI) joint dysfunction, 13
Safety Towards Other Players (STOP)
    Patch Program, 33
Scaffolds, 45, 47
Scapular set, 30
SCAT 3. *See* Sideline Concussion
    Assessment Tool 3
SCI. *See* Spinal cord injury
SCN. *See* Society for Clinical
    Neuropsychology
Scoliosis, 16
Scotty dog sign, 63
Seizures, 266
Sensory Organization Test (SOT), 241
Shoulder depression injury, 87, 87f
Shoulder pads, removal of, 37
Sideline Concussion Assessment Tool 3
    (SCAT 3), 245
Single-photon emission computed
    tomography (SPECT), 55, 157,
    158f, 282
Skipping rope, 29
SLAM. *See* Sport as Laboratory
    Assessment Model
Sleep disturbance, 265
Society for Clinical Neuropsychology
    (SCN), 255
Soft tissue injuries, to spine, 12
SOT. *See* Sensory Organization Test
Spearing, 33
Spear tackler's spine, 137
Spear tackling technique, 3, 5, 14, 51
SPECT. *See* Single-photon emission
    computed tomography
Spinal cord injury (SCI), 2–3, 14, 32,
    40. *See also* Spine
    athletes with, 47t
    cervical spine injuries, 3–5, 4t, 6f,
        32, 134
        burst fractures, 137, 139f
        common mechanism of, 135
        epidemiology of, 134–135
        hyperextension injuries, 137–139, 140f
        hyperflexion injuries, 136, 137, 138f
        precautions in, 135
        return to play, 139–140, 141t
        upper cervical spine fractures,
            135–136, 136f
    epidemiology of, 2–9
    neuroprotection, 40, 46t
        decompression of spinal cord, 42

glutamate-related excitotoxicity, 44
granulocyte colony-stimulating
    factor, 44
induced hypothermia, 42
methylprednisolone, 43
minocycline, 43–44
pharmaceutical agents for, 42–43
riluzole, 43
supportive measures, 40–42
on-field management of, 32–39
    initial assessment, 34, 34f
    pregame planning, 33–34
    prevention of injury, 33
    protective padding and, 37
    stabilization and transport of
      athlete, 35–37
pathophysiology of, 40, 41f
in pediatric athletes, 59–66
    cervical spine, 60–61, 60f
    return-to-play guidelines, 65
    spondylisthesis, 62–64, 63f
    spondylolysis, 62–64, 63f
    thoracolumbar spine, 61–62, 61f
    treatment, 65–66, 66f
    vertebral body apophyseal avulsion
      fracture, 62, 62f
primary, 40, 41f
regenerative therapies for, 44, 46t–47t
    cell-based therapies, 45, 46t–47t
    chondroitinase ABC, 45
    fibroblast growth factors, 45
    Nogo-A inhibitors, 45
    Rho inhibitors, 44
    scaffolds, implanted, 45, 47
secondary, 40, 41f
sports-related, 51
    atraumatic back pain, 54–55
    cervical spine trauma, 51–53, 52f,
      51t, 53
    chronic back pain, 55
    lumbar spine trauma, 54, 54t
    thoracic spine trauma, 54
thoracolumbar spine injuries, 6–9, 7t
Spinal ligamentous injuries, 12
Spinal stenosis in athletes
diagnosis
    clinical presentation, 175, 176f
    physical examination, 176
    radiologic manifestations, 176–177, 176t
disk pathology
    disk degeneration in aging athletes,
      174–175, 175t
    mechanism of disk degeneration,
      173–174, 174f
epidemiology, 172–173
return to play
    after surgery, 178
    prevention, 178
    rehabilitation, 178
treatment
    nonoperative management, 177
    operative management, 177–178
Spine
biomechanical functions, 12
functional spinal unit (FSU), 12

injuries to, 12
    bony injuries, 13–14
    joint injuries, 12–13
    soft tissue injuries, 12
    spinal cord injury, 14
protective function, 12
regional biomechanics of, 14
    cervical, 14–15, 15f
    lumbar spine, 16
    lumbo-sacro-pelvic spine, 16
    thoracic spine, 15
    thoracolumbar junction, 16
Spine surgeon, role of
communication with concerned
    people, 71
estimating players risk in return to
    sport, 71
players and, 69–70
postoperative rehabilitation, understand
    and control of, 70
relationship with players, 69
within structure of team, 70
surgery, 69–70
Spinous process avulsion fracture, 13
Spondylolisthesis, 8, 62–65, 151, 154–155,
    283
evaluation
    history, 155
    physical examination, 155, 156f
imaging studies
    magnetic resonance imaging,
      156–157, 157t
    plain radiography, 156
    single-photon emission computed
      tomography, 157, 158f
Meyerding classification, 65f
return to play, 158–161
treatment, 158–159
    acute lesions, 65–66, 66f, 159, 159f
    chronic lesions, 159–160, 160f
    surgical intervention, 160–161, 160f
Spondylolysis, 7–8, 13, 55, 62, 63f, 151,
    154–155
etiology, 62–63
evaluation
    history, 63, 155
    imaging, 63
    physical examination, 63, 155, 156f
imaging studies
    magnetic resonance imaging, 156–157,
      157t
    plain radiography, 156
    single-photon emission computed
      tomography, 157
pathoanatomy, 62–63
return to play, 158–161
treatment, 158–159
    acute lesions, 159, 159f
    chronic lesions, 159–160, 160f
    nonoperative, 63–64
    operative, 64, 64f
    surgical intervention, 160–161, 160f
Spondylosis, 123, 154
Sport as Laboratory Assessment Model
    (SLAM), 257

Sports concussions, 227
assessment of
    approaches to neuropsychological,
      255–256
    baseline testing, 257–258
    computerized neurocognitive tests, 256
    multidimensional approach to, 254f
    neuropsychologist role in, 254–255
    pencil-and-paper neuropsychological
      testing, 255–256
clinical vignette, 230–231
    return to play, 231, 231t
    sideline assessment, 230
    sideline assessment without healthcare
      provider, 230
definitions, 227
diagnosis, 227–228
    assessment tools, 229
    balance impairments, 229
    behavior changes, 228
    cognitive impairment, 228
    physical signs, 228
    sleep disturbance, 228
    symptoms, 228
neurocognitive recovery from, 256
neuropsychological testing protocol
    considerations, 256–258
on-the-field assessment, 229
pediatric, neuropsychological assessment
    of, 258–259
postinjury neurocognitive testing, 258
postinjury sideline cognitive screening,
    258
preseason management, 229
Sports-related spinal injury, 51, 279–285
atraumatic back pain, 54–55
cervical spine trauma, 51–53, 52f, 51t, 53
chronic back pain, 55
lumbar spine trauma, 54, 54t
thoracic spine trauma, 54
STACIS trial, 284
Standardized Assessment of Concussion
    (SAC), 258
Stem cells, 45
Stenosis
of cervical spine, 123–132, 124
spinal, 94–95, 94f, 95f
Stingers, 5, 6f, 86, 280–281
equipment modifications for, 89
evaluation, 87
    diagnosis, 89
    diagnostic testing, 88–89
    physical examination, 87–88, 88f
mechanisms of injury, 86–87, 87f
neural injury patterns, 86
prevention from, 89
return to play, 89–90
symptoms of, 86
treatment, 89
Straight-leg raise test, 23
Stress fractures, 8, 13
Stress reaction, 155
Subconcussion, 273
Superficial soft tissue injuries, 209
Swimming, 17

T

TAL. *See* Transverse atlantal ligament
TBIs. *See* Traumatic brain injuries
Teardrop fragment, 136
Tendinitis, 76
Tendinopathy, 76
Tenosynovitis, 76
Thomas test, 23
Thoracic disk herniations, 8–9, 209–210
Thoracic injuries in athletes, 203
  anatomy, 203
  evaluation, 206, 208t
    of acute thoracic injuries, 206–208
    of chronic thoracic injuries, 208
    diagnostic considerations, 208
    diagnostic testing, 208–209
  management
    of disk herniations, 209–210
    general principles, 209
    of paraspinal soft tissue injuries, 209
    of spinal cord injuries, 211, 213
    of spinal fractures, 210–211, 211t, 212f
    of superficial soft tissue injuries, 209
  patterns of, 204–206, 205f, 206f, 207f
  spinal degeneration, 204
  spinal pain, 203–204
Thoracic spinal degeneration in athletes, 204
Thoracic spinal fractures, 210–211
Thoracic spine, sports-related injuries to, 15
Thoracic spine trauma, 54
  pediatric, 61–62, 61f
Thoracolumbar junction, 15
Thoracolumbar spine injuries, 6–9, 7t

Thoracolumbosacral orthosis (TLSO), 61
TLICS grading system, 211t
TLSO. *See* Thoracolumbosacral orthosis
Torso-lift technique, for shoulder pad removal, 37
Transient quadriplegia. *See* Cervical cord neurapraxia (CCN)
Transverse atlantal ligament (TAL), 114
Traumatic brain injuries (TBIs), 42, 218
  research, 221–222, 221t

U

Ulnar nerve entrapment, 82–83
Upper cervical spine fractures, 135–136, 136f
Upper extremity disorders, differential diagnosis of, 74
  additional workup for, 83
  clinical case example, 83–84, 83f, 84f
  diagnostic dilemmas, 78–79, 81–83
    carpal tunnel syndrome, 81–82
    C5 radiculopathy, 79
    C6 radiculopathy, 81
    C7 radiculopathy, 81, 82
    C8 radiculopathy, 82
    Erb's palsy (traumatic upper brachial plexus injury), 81
    Klumpke's paralysis, 82
    posterior interosseous nerve (PIN) palsy, 82
    pronator syndrome, 81
    rotator cuff tears, 81
    suprascapular nerve entrapment, 79, 81
    ulnar nerve entrapment, 82–83

myelopathy test for cervical spinal cord, 77t
neck *vs.* arm *vs.* shoulder pain in athletes, 75t
patient history, 74, 75t
  neuropathic pain, 74, 76
  neuropathic weakness, 76
  non-neuropathic pain, 76
peripheral nerves
  compression neuropathies, 80t
  test for, 78t
physical examination, 76–78, 78f
skin lesions and implications, 77t

V

Vacuum phenomenon, 165
VersaClimber, 29
Vertebral body apophyseal avulsion fracture, 62, 62f
Vestibular-ocular motor screen (VOMS), 246
Visual disturbance in postconcussion, 265
VOMS. *See* Vestibular-ocular motor screen

W

WADs. *See* Whiplash-associated disorders
Water sports, 17
Weight lifting, 16
Whiplash-associated disorders (WADs), 218

Z

Zygapophyseal joints (facets), 12